Paediatric Forensic Medicine and Pathology

*This book is dedicated to
the memory of those invited
contributors who died during
its preparation
DOUGLAS BAIN,
paediatric pathologist
HUGH JOHNSON,
forensic pathologist
and
JØRGEN VOIGT,
forensic pathologist.*

Paediatric Forensic Medicine and Pathology

Edited by

J.K. Mason

Regius Professor (Emeritus) of Forensic Medicine
Faculty of Law, Old College
University of Edinburgh

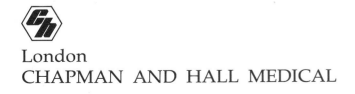

London
CHAPMAN AND HALL MEDICAL

First published in 1989 by Chapman and Hall Ltd
11 New Fetter Lane, London EC4P 4EE
Published in the USA by Van Nostrand Reinhold
115 Fifth Avenue, New York, NY 10003

© 1989 Chapman and Hall

Typeset in 10/12pt Palatino by
EJS Chemical Composition, Bath
Printed in Great Britain at the
University Press, Cambridge

ISBN   0 412 29160 6
0 442 31147 8 (USA)

British Library Cataloguing in Publication Data

Paediatric forensic medicine and pathology.
1. Forensic medicine
I. Mason, J.K. (John Kenyon), *1919–*
614'.1

ISBN 0-412-29160-6

Library of Congress Cataloging in
Publication Data available

Contents

PART FOUR ETHICAL CONSIDERATIONS

Contributors

Berry, C.L., MD, PhD, FRCPath. Professor of Morbid Anatomy, The London Hospital Medical College. Address: Department of Morbid Anatomy, The London Hospital, London, England E1 1BB

Bowen, D.A.Ll., MA, MB, FRCP, FRCP(E), FRCPath, DMJ. Professor of Forensic Medicine, Charing Cross and Westminster Medical School. Address: Department of Forensic Medicine and Toxicology, Charing Cross Hospital, Fulham Palace Road, London, England W6 8RF

Coe, John I., MD, FCAP. Professor of Pathology, University of Minnesota Medical School; formerly, Chief of Pathology and Medical Examiner, Hennepin County Medical Center, Minneapolis. Address: Medical Examiner's Office, 730 S. 7th Street, Minneapolis, Minnesota 55415, USA

Craft, Alan W., MD, FRCP. Consultant Paediatrician. Address: Department of Child Health, Royal Victoria Infirmary, Newcastle upon Tyne, England NE1 4LP

Dodd, Barbara E., MSc, PhD, DSc. Professor (Emeritus) of Blood Group Serology in the Department of Haematology and Honorary Adviser to the Department of Forensic Medicine. Address: The London Hospital Medical College, Turner Street, London, England E1 2AD

Downie, R.S., MA, BPhil, FRSE. Professor of Moral Philosophy and, currently, Stevenson Lecturer in Medical Ethics, University of Glasgow. Address: Department of Philosophy, University of Glasgow, Glasgow, Scotland G12 8QQ

Emery, John L., MD, FRCPath, DCH. Emeritus Professor of Paediatric Pathology, currently Honorary Lecturer in Paediatrics, University of Sheffield. Address: Wolfson Unit, Department of Paediatrics, University of Sheffield, 312 Fulwood Road, Sheffield, England S10 3BN

Evans, K.T., FRCP, FRCR. Professor of Diagnostic Radiology in the University of Wales College of Medicine. Address: Department of Diagnostic Radiology, University of Wales College of Medicine, Heath Park, Cardiff, Wales CF4 4XN

Froede, Richard C., MD. Armed Forces Medical Examiner, Armed Forces Institute of Pathology; lately, Chief of Forensic Sciences, Department of

Pathology, University of Arizona. Address: Armed Forces Institute of Pathology, Washington, DC 20306-6000, USA

Furrow, Barry R., JD. Professor of Law, Widener University School of Law. Address: PO Box 7474, Concord Pike, Wilmington, DE 19803, USA

Gath, Ann, DM, FRCPsych, DCH. Consultant in the Psychiatry of Mental Handicap in Childhood and Adolescence, The Maudsley and Bethlem Hospitals; formerly, Consultant Child Psychiatrist, West Suffolk Hospital. Address: Hilda Lewis House, Bethlem Royal Hospital, Beckenham, Kent, England

Golding, M. Jean, MA, PhD. Wellcome Senior Lecturer in the Department of Child Health at the University of Bristol; Editor-in-chief of the *Journal of Paediatric and Perinatal Epidemiology*. Address: Department of Child Health, Royal Hospital for Sick Children, Bristol, England BS2 8BJ

Henry, Thomas E., MD. Deputy Chief Medical Examiner, County of Pima; Assistant Clinical Professor of Pathology, University of Arizona. Address: University of Arizona College of Medicine, Tucson, Arizona 85724, USA

Hilton, J.M.N., MB, BCh, FRCPA. Chief Forensic Pathologist, State Health Laboratory Services, Western Australia. Address: Forensic Pathology Department, State Health Laboratory Services, Box F312, GPO Perth, Western Australia 6001

Hirsh, Harold, MD, JD, FCLM. Distinguished Visiting Professor, George Washington University; Diplomate, American Board of Internal Medicine; Diplomate, American Board of Legal Medicine; Editor-in-Chief, *TRAUMA*; President Elect, American College of Legal Medicine. Address: 2801 New Mexico Avenue NW, # 1009, Washington, DC 20007, USA

Knight, Bernard, MD, MRCP, FRCPath, DMJ, Barrister. Professor of Forensic Pathology, University of Wales College of Medicine. Address: Institute of Pathology, Royal Infirmary, Cardiff, Wales CF2 1SZ

Knoppers, Bartha M., Doctor en Droit (Paris), DLS (Cantab), DEA (Paris), BCL, LLB (McGill), MA (University of Alta), BA (McMaster University). Assistant Professor of Law, University of Montreal. Address: Faculté de Droit, 3101 Chemin de la Tour, Montreal, Quebec, Canada H3C 3J7

Laing, Ian A., MA, MB, BCh, MRCP. Consultant Neonatologist, Lothian Health Board. Address: Neonatal Intensive Care Unit, Simpson Memorial Maternity Pavilion, Lauriston Place, Edinburgh, Scotland EH3 9EF

Larkin, Glenn M., MD. Consultant in Forensic Pathology; formerly Chief Deputy Coroner, Allegheny County, Pennsylvania and Medical Examiner, Mecklenburg County, North Carolina. Address: 4000-E Providence Road, Charlotte, North Carolina 28111–4406, USA

Larson, Eunice J., MD. Associate Clinical Professor of Pediatrics and Pathology, University of California School of Medicine, Irvine. Address: Memorial Medical

Center of Long Beach, 2801 Atlantic Avenue, PO Box 1428, Long Beach, California 90801–1428, USA

McCall Smith, R.A., LLB, PhD. Senior Lecturer in Civil Law, University of Edinburgh. Address: Faculty of Law, Old College, South Bridge, Edinburgh, Scotland EH8 9YL

McLay, W.D.S., MB, ChB, LLB, FRCS. Chief Medical Officer, Strathclyde Police; Editor *The Police Surgeon*; Lecturer in Forensic Medicine, Strathclyde University; External examiner, Diploma in Forensic Medicine, University of Glasgow. Address: Police Headquarters, 173 Pitt Street, Glasgow, Scotland G2 4JS
FM/Prelims/7

Mancer, Kent, MD, BSc(Med), FRCPC. Associate Professor of Pathology, University of Toronto; Professor of Pathology, Unversiti Kebangsaan Malaysia; currently, Senior Staff Pathologist, The Hospital for Sick Children, Toronto. Address: Jabatan Patologi, Fakulti Perubatan, UKM, Jalan Raja Muda, 50300 Kuala Lumpur, Malaysia

Mason, J.K., CBE, MD, LLD, FRCPath, DMJ. Professor (Emeritus) of Forensic Medicine and, currently, Honorary Fellow, Faculty of Law in the University of Edinburgh. Address: Faculty of Law, Old College, South Bridge, Edinburgh, Scotland EH8 9YL

Meyers, David W., BA (Redlands), JD (U. Calif., Berkeley), LLM (Edinburgh). Active member, California Bar; Adjunct Lecturer, Department of Medical Ethics, University of California, San Francisco. Address: 809 Coombs Street, Napa, California 94559, USA

Patrick, W.J.A., MB, FRCS, FRCS(E), MRCPath. Consultant Perinatal and Paediatric Pathologist, Greater Glasgow Health Board; Honorary Clinical Lecturer, University of Glasgow. Address: Department of Pathology, Royal Hospital for Sick Children, Yorkhill, Glasgow, Scotland G3 8SJ

Pearn, John A.M., Professor and Head, Department of Child Health, Royal Children's Hospital, Brisbane. Address: Department of Child Health, Royal Children's Hospital, Brisbane, Queensland, Australia 4029

Proudfoot, A.T., BSc, FRCP. Consultant Physician, Regional Poisoning Treatment Centre; Director, The Scottish Poisons Information Bureau, Royal Infirmary of Edinburgh. Address: The Royal Infirmary, Edinburgh, Scotland EH3 9YW

Raeburn, J.A., MB, ChB, PhD, FRCPE. Senior Lecturer in Human Genetics, University of Edinburgh and Honorary Consultant, Clinical Genetics Service, Lothian Health Board. Address: Clinical Genetics Service, Western General Hospital, Crewe Road, Edinburgh, Scotland EH4 2XU

Roberts, G.M., FRCP, FRCR. Consultant Radiologist in the University Hospital of Wales. Address: Department of Radiology, University Hospital of Wales, Heath Park, Cardiff, Wales CF4 4XN

Sims, Bernard G., BDS, LDSRCS(Eng.), Dip F Od. Honorary Senior Lecturer in Forensic Odontology, London Hospital Medical College and Honorary Lecturer to the Combined Medical and Dental Schools of Guy's and St. Thomas' Hospitals; Honorary Consultant to the Home Office in Forensic Odontology. Address: Department of Forensic Medicine, London Hospital Medical College, Turner Street, London, England E1 2AD

Stephens, Boyd G., MD. Chief Medical Examiner, City and County of San Francisco; Fellow American Academy of Forensic Sciences; Member of the National Association of Medical Examiners; Assistant Clinical Professor of Pathology, University of California. Address: Chief Medical Examiner, 850 Bryant Street, San Francisco, California 94103, USA

Sutherland, Elaine E., LLB, LLM. Lecturer in Scots Law, Faculty of Law, University of Edinburgh. Address: Department of Scots Law, Old College, South Bridge, Edinburgh, Scotland EH8 9YL

Swinburne, Layinka M., BSc, MB, ChB, FRCP, FRCPath, DCH. Consultant Immuno-pathologist, Co-director of Haemophilia Unit, St James' University Hospital; Senior Clinical Lecturer, University of Leeds. Address: Department of Pathology, St James' University Hospital, Leeds, England LS9 7TF

Wecht, Cyril H., MD, JD, FCAP, FCLM. Clinical Adjunct Professor of Pathology, University of Pittsburgh Schools of Medicine and Dental Medicine; Adjunct Professor of Law, Duquesne University School of Law; former President, American Academy of Forensic Sciences and American College of Legal Medicine. Address: Department of Pathology, Central Medical Center and Hospital, 1200 Center Avenue, Pittsburgh, Pennsylvania 15219, USA

Whittaker, D.K., BDS, PhD, FDS, RCS, DFOdont. Reader in Oral Biology, University of Wales College of Medicine. Adviser in Forensic Dentistry to the Home Office. Address: Department of Basic Dental Science, Dental School, Heath Park, Cardiff, Wales CF4 4XY

Whittington, R.M., MA, BM, BCh, DObstRCOG, DCH, DMJ, MRCGP. HM Coroner, Birmingham and Solihull Districts. Address: Coroner's Court, Newton Street, Birmingham, England B4 6NE

Preface

I have felt for some time that there was a need for a book devoted to paediatric forensic medicine and pathology and I am grateful to the publishers for providing the opportunity. I also express my very deep appreciation of the efforts of contributors from three continents. Some have stepped into the breach at short notice; all have had to put up with, and have accepted with good heart, an unusual degree of editorial fancy. There has, however, been no editing of opinions. There are bound to be positional differences in a work of this type and it is emphasized that the views expressed are those of the individual authors – and not necessarily those of other contributors or of the editor.

The format of the book does, however, affirm my own strongly held concepts of the scope of forensic medicine. The modern forensic physician or pathologist is clearly not confined to problems of the criminal law and those involving the civil law cover a wide variety of interests. If there are those who would cavil at the inclusion of some of the titles, I can only restate my belief that forensic medicine should be looked on as a discipline which offers a wide-ranging service to the community rather than one which is confined within pathology and this is nowhere more evident than in the field of paediatrics. The forensic medical practitioner must also have a working knowledge of the law and I have tried to emphasize this by incorporating several chapters by legal authors. Finally, I believe that legal medicine – and the law itself – depends upon and reflects the ethics of society; the in-depth study of forensic medicine must include an interest in medical ethics and, for this reason, I am delighted that many contributors have not flinched from introducing and discussing moral issues that arise in paediatric practice.

One of the major disadvantages of 'status emeritus' is that one loses much of the administrative and secretarial support which one accepts as a natural accompaniment of working life. In this respect, I owe a debt of gratitude to Mrs Mary Schofield who, at a late stage, accepted the secretarial challenge with great spirit and without whose help this book would never have come to fruition. And, as always, I acknowledge with deep gratitude the continued and unstinting support of an elderly retainer which has been given by the Faculty of Law in the University of Edinburgh.

JKM
Edinburgh

PART 1

Introduction

CHAPTER 1

The role of the expert witness in paediatric forensic practice

Cyril H. Wecht and Glenn M. Larkin

The terms forensic medicine and forensic pathology imply an interface between medical practice and the application of the law. The training of the medical man impels him to seek the truth as to diagnosis and prognosis; the function of the lawyer, however, whether it be in the civil or the criminal courts, is to convince a tribunal that his argument, or interpretation of the facts, is to be preferred to that of his or her adversary. The doctor who is untrained in the law is often ill-prepared for this conflict of motives and may find himself both aggrieved and confused in the witness-box. The clinical and pathological aspects of forensic paediatrics are discussed in the second part of this book; the state of the law is considered in the third. The purpose of this introductory chapter is to indicate some of the difficulties which arise at this interface and to suggest how they may be overcome to the benefit of both disciplines.

1.1 TRAUMA AND THE CHILD

Trauma is the child's fifth Horseman of the Apocalypse; he roams the world with his squires – Accident, Neglect and Abuse. More deaths are caused by accident in the paediatric age-group – up to 14 years old – than by all other causes combined, including cancer, tuberculosis and pneumonia. Children in their curiosity find strange ways to cut, shoot, fracture, poison and otherwise maim themselves and other youngsters. A momentary lapse of supervision provides enough time for a toddler to stick his finger in the electric socket or meat grinder; his fifth Horseman is seldom far away.

In the United States, and elsewhere where firearms are easily accessible, children even kill each other occasionally; the files of every metropolitan medicolegal investigative office contain multiple instances of children shooting others both accidentally and homicidally, and each case is as, or more, tragic than the previous one:

Case 1.1
Three children from the same family came home when school was closed because of a snowstorm. Both parents were at work, leaving a 13-year-old girl and her two brothers, aged 12 and 10 years, unsupervised in a house full of both firearms and mischief. The girl was shot in the face by a shotgun [1].

The child can also enter the medicolegal arena through more conventional doors. He may be victim of an assault, of a product defect or be the central figure in one of the newly charted journeys through the legal system – wrongful life or wrongful conception. Each condition raises a host of medicolegal issues that defy classification before the fact. For example, he may claim damages from any of the following after a motor vehicular collision:

(i) the driver of the car in which he was a passenger;
(ii) the manufacturer of the seat-belt that failed to restrain him properly;
(iii) the paramedic who did not brace his neck properly;
(iv) the emergency-room physician who did not recognize his injury or who failed to treat it properly;
(v) anyone else even remotely connected with his traumatic quadriplegia.

The fact that the injured party was a child is fortuitous in this set of hypothetical circumstances but there are times when the entry to the legal arena is *because* the patient or victim is a child – small size and immature metabolic systems give rise to a limitless spectrum of lesions when associated with injury, ranging from cephalhaematoma to apodia. Dramatic advances in neonatal therapy have resulted in more and more children, who would previously have died at or near birth, surviving with some form of impairment. As the cost of caring for such children increases, trial lawyers look for innovative theories of liability through which to obtain large awards for alleged medical malpractice or negligence. Forensic physicians or pathologists are valuable witnesses in all such proceedings because of their knowledge of trauma. Their evaluation of injuries and assignment of 'causality' to the trauma or negligence should help the courts to determine the validity of whatever claims are asserted.

1.2 THE FORENSIC PHYSICIAN IN PAEDIATRICS

Paediatric forensic medicine represents the fusion of several overlapping disciplines: clinical paediatrics; anatomic, clinical and forensic pathology; gynaecology; psychiatry and psychology; internal medicine and surgery. This mixture involves a complex synthesis to which there may be clinical, pathological and legal approaches. At times, these approaches are in conflict with one another. Paediatrics is a challenging branch of medicine because of the endless variety of changes which are to be seen in the growing child. Each child changes by the moment and the different kaleidoscopes often defy rational evaluation. Changes take place with extreme suddenness; a healthy child in a closed car on a hot day can overheat to death in hours or minutes – yet the hot and dehydrated baby responds just as quickly to appropriate fluid and electrolyte therapy, often without serious sequelae [2]. The forensic physician or pathologist must rely on other professional investigators to help him arrive at his conclusions. The contribution of others involved in the investigation is recognized in most American jurisdictions as being inseparable from the pathologist's post-mortem protocol and is generally accepted as providing an exception to the hearsay rule of evidence.

Paediatric forensic medicine probably evolved as a separate entity from the need for a king to be certain that his new prince was, indeed, his child. Elaborate procedures developed during the Middle Ages by which to witness a royal birth and to retain an absolute chain of custody for the infant prince. The concept of *parens patriae* was not formalized in England until the reign of George II [3] but, even then, was restricted to protection of the children of the nobility. Fatal child abuse in the general population was treated as straight murder [4]; a hazy line separated legitimate punishment from abuse – in a society where whipping both children and adults was common, the courts took no notice of the former unless it was clearly offensive and lethal.

A very different climate exists today. The child's medical clock starts to tick before birth and even before conception [5]. The difficulties encountered and the consequent parchment of contradictory court decisions which have been reached in this area are considered in detail elsewhere in this book (see Chapters 25 and 26). For present purposes, two examples will suffice to illustrate the importance of witness evidence in the relevant court proceedings.

In *Commonwealth of Pennsylvania* v. *Laufe* [6], the defendant performed an abortion by a new hysterotomy technique and followed it by a hysterectomy. His surgical technique involved clamping the uterine and ovarian arteries early in the procedure so that the fetus, when it was removed, had been without oxygen for at least 10 minutes. Dr Laufe had a motion picture of his procedure made for teaching purposes and this figured prominently in the subsequent Coroner's inquest. A nurse in attendance asserted that the infant was born alive and her testimony was corroborated by a gynaecologist from a local medical school who commented on the motion picture. The defence countered with its own witnesses who used the same motion picture to assert that the fetus was dead. The Coroner's jury took a short time to rule that the infant was stillborn, thereby cutting off further adjudication.

A similar allegation was made against the treating physician in *Commonwealth of Pennsylvania* v. *Melnick* [7]. The major issue, again, was whether the fetus was 'alive' or 'stillborn' at the time of delivery. While this would seem to be a clear-cut legal 'either/or' situation, it may not be so clear to the doctor at the time of an elective abortion; philosophical theories and the physician's ability to

resuscitate ever younger newborns advance hand in hand and the differences between life and stillbirth progressively appear to be more semantic than real. Unfortunately, a great deal depends on the preconceived notions of the witness to pathology; consciously or subconsciously, these are usually the expression of his personal ethical and religious beliefs rather than an objective, scientifically determined, intellectual conclusion:

Case 1.2
A 13-year-old, unwed girl admitted to the hospital for an elective abortion. After removal of the 1545-g, approximately 32-week gestation fetus, allegations were made by the nurse, anaesthesiologist, intern and resident who were present that the fetus was alive and that the defendant obstetrician had 'let it die'. To complicate matters, someone in the delivery-room made out a certificate of stillbirth which was later torn up and birth and death certificates were substituted.

Pertinent original autopsy microscopic findings related to the lungs: '… Some areas in several slides show only congestion while other areas show patchy expansion of alveoli and compression of lining epithelial cells. Relatively mature lung. Some areas show patchy interstitial hemorrhage occasionally rather pronounced … These findings are consistent with spontaneous and/or mechanical expansion of the lungs in a somewhat immature infant with decreased availability of surfactant …'

The Medical Examiner's final comments were: 'This 32 week old gestation female infant was delivered of a 13 year old mother following prostaglandin-induced labor. After delivery, despite the fact that respirations and occasional heart beats were noted, no resuscitative efforts were undertaken. Further investigation is requested by the Homicide Squad …' [7]

Dr Melnick was charged with criminal homicide – a loose charge that could range from first-degree murder to involuntary manslaughter. Testimony to the effect that the infant had a 'heartbeat' for an hour and a half after delivery – and, therefore, was alive – was offered by several witnesses who were present at the abortion. It was noted that none of these witnesses had made any attempt to resuscitate an infant they swore was alive – the very same act of omission that formed the basis of the homicide charges against Dr Melnick.

The defence offered its own expert witness to refute the State's case:

DEFENCE ATTORNEY: From your examination, could you determine the cause of death?

EXPERT WITNESS: No.

DEFENCE: Why not?

EW: There were no markings of any sort on the body, no evidence of physical trauma, injury or external defects on the body.

In the opinion of the authors, the courts place too much emphasis on the 'presence of air' in the lungs. The literature cautions that the presence of air in the alveolar sacs has no absolute diagnostic value in the determination of 'live birth' [8–11]:

DEFENCE: What did the examination of the lungs show?

EW: The lungs were solid and collapsed; they showed no evidence of aeration. They had a rather dull, dark reddish brown to reddish purple colour …

DEFENCE: Now, when you say 'no evidence of aeration', what does that mean?

EW: When examining the lungs grossly, if there is air present, there will be signs such as crepitation on palpation. That is a tactile sensation that the trained pathologist obtains by feeling and gently squeezing different portions of the lungs to ascertain whether there is air present in the lung tissue.

DEFENCE: Does that have anything to do with whether or not there is evidence of ante-mortem breathing?

EW: Yes. The presence of air, of course, is a physiological process of respiration … but one has to examine the [lung] slides microscopically. Gross perceptions and impressions may be correct, and frequently are, but they may be modified or changed dramatically upon microscopic examination. You would want to do a microscopic study before you made a final determination.

The witness continued that he had found no evidence of definitive aeration in the lungs. Note that total expansion of the lungs would mean either that, the lungs had never mean either that the lungs had never expanded or that they were expanded and had collapsed subsequently. The intermediate state between these extremes – partial expansion – has no probative value in and of itself.

DEFENCE: Were you able to come to a conclusion as to the cause of death?

EW: … It was the abortion process … the use of a prostaglandin suppository, and pitocin, meperidine and prochlorperazine, both of which are central nervous system depressants – all of which, acting in concert, resulted in the fetus being a stillborn.

The prosecutor, who prefaced his cross-examination with a disclaimer that he was not interested in a technical debate regarding the definition of life, then proceeded to do just that:

DISTRICT ATTORNEY: Define life for me.

EW: Life is an ongoing process of respiration and cardiac activity with oxygen getting to the organs, including the heart itself, the lungs and, most importantly, the brain. You must have some pumping mechanism from the heart, and some respiratory movement, so that oxygenation and a blood–gas exchange take place and oxygenated blood keeps getting pumped round the body. There is no evidence of that in this case, with one respiration per minute. That's not life under the circumstances of this case.

DA: You said 'ongoing'. Are you telling me that if a newborn comes out, or anybody exhibits life for however short a time, that doesn't constitute life because it isn't ongoing?

EW: Oh, no. I don't want to get into a complex philosophical discussion. We're talking about a fetus that has been deliberately and knowingly removed in [an] abortion process that comes out with no evidence of life. I'm not talking about someone who has a heart attack in the courtroom.

DA: We're talking about signs of life now …

EW: Are you talking about this case specifically?

DA: I'm talking about this case. Was the positive APGAR score a sign of life?

EW: It depends on what you know as to what was being done clinically … what your entire mindset is.

DA: Why is the mindset important?

EW: The mindset is that you are there to perform an abortion. The fetus comes out and is apparently not alive. You have no reason to think that it is alive because there are no movements going on at the time. The fact that an APGAR score was obtained cannot be divorced from what is well-known and documented in this case, namely, that Dr Melnick had contracted with the patient and her parents to perform a therapeutic abortion, not deliver a viable premature infant.

DA: You never asked Dr Melnick if he saw the baby move or breathe. You got all the background information that attempts to establish that Dr Melnick was doing the right thing but you didn't ask him about whether he saw signs of life.

There was then the following exchange between the lawyers and the Court:

THE COURT: Is it that the State seeks to prove to me that, at the time of birth, this was an alive baby/human being as contained within the murder statutes; and/or does the State seek to prove to me that, according to documents supplied with somebody's signature [referring to a birth certificate that was made out by 'someone'], this was a live baby, a human being?

DA: Clearly, the former.

COURT: So that, when you're interrogating with respect to APGAR scores, you are attempting, by virtue of the fact that a number is affixed to the APGAR score, to prove that the baby is a human being, an alive baby? Is that correct?

DA: Yes. I have two purposes. One, I'm making a correlation of the APGAR and a birth certificate filled out by the defendant. As far as the State is concerned, when he filled out that APGAR [score], that was as good as coming to the police department and saying 'I observed this, and I observed that'. Two, I'm getting independent evidence from other witnesses who have testified as to the baby's colour and movement and heartbeats.

COURT: Would it not be true that, taking everything you have said into consideration, that would be a presumption which, legally, I could not give to the State … the presumption of life ? …

DA: I am having difficulty understanding the defence expert witness' opinion that there is absence of life here. He says there is death, yet there are signs of life. To me, these terms are mutually exclusive.

A lawyer is taught to obfuscate the issues when the facts go against him and the District Attorney has done this successfully.

The issue is not whether the abortus was 'alive' or not, but whether: (a) the abortion was a legal procedure and properly authorised – the answer is 'yes' – and (b) whether the doctor/defendant was acting under the belief that the abortion was successfully performed – yes, he was. The other issues – defining life and what the resident physician heard or thought he heard – are irrelevant. It is a further question of medical reality whether an immature heart can sustain a heartbeat of '20 beats per minute' without converting to ventricular fibrillation. In this case, factors other than medical reality were at issue, to the detriment of all concerned.

The road out of the uterus to independent existence is rough and unpredictable. Even in the best possible circumstances, the act of birth is a potentially hazardous process. In areas where prenatal visits are routine, fetal–pelvic disproportion, transverse lie, placenta praevia or any obstructive lesion can and should be diagnosed. Both uterine inertia and hypertonicity are potential problems to the mother and her fetus. Subdural haemorrhage due to dural laceration, traction lesions of the neck, Erb's paralysis and funicular strangulation should be avoidable by careful obstetric control of delivery. Forceps-associated lesions should be preventable now that the use of forceps is usually restricted to outlet procedures. The reader is directed to the important British case of *Whitehouse* v. *Jordan* [12] which indicates the difficulties the court faces in such adjudications.

Problems related to analgesia during vaginal delivery or during an elective or emergency caesarean delivery are more difficult to control and are an ever-present source of fetal and neonatal morbidity and mortality. An empty stomach is more important at the time of delivery than is an empty bowel or bladder, and aspiration caused by failure to ensure a patent airway in a woman who ate recently is a leading cause of morbidity in the mother – as well as in the child.

The 'why's and 'hows' are sought when the pathologist enters the picture after the fetus has died. A thorough examination, even when the cause of death is clinically obvious, will yield much helpful information in

exchange for the time and effort extended. The causes of perinatal death are legion, and often complex. This chapter merely mentions what other chapters discuss in greater detail. A simple classification divides these cases into the following categories:

(1) *Cause of death is obvious, expected and untreatable.* The clinician is aware of the anencephalus or other lethal condition and is powerless to prevent death; many congenital and genetic defects fall into this category. An autopsy may yield information regarding causality and may, perhaps, provide useful information both to the paediatrician and to the parents of the dead child. The obstetrician is not at risk in these situations, unless his failure to diagnose such a condition early enough to allow of an abortion becomes a relevant medicolegal question (see Chapter 2).

(2) *'Something' happens during pregnancy, labour, or delivery that compromises the fetus.* This 'something' is not diagnosed in time for appropriate treatment and the fetus is fatally injured during delivery. Such life-threatening problems may arise with amazing speed. Liability would attach if:

(i) The 'something' was diagnosable and treatable before it could cause damage.
(ii) The treatment of a properly diagnosed problem was too late or inappropriate through lack of the necessary equipment, diagnostic acumen or other error.

Examples include the definitive development of a prediagnosed marginal feto-pelvic disproportion if pregnancy is prolonged or the development of full-blown eclampsia during labour in a pre-eclamptic mother.

(3) *Previously undiagnosed and unanticipated problems during delivery.* These 'complications' are the source of considerable grief for the obstetrician. Even with much experience, he or she can confuse an undeliverable mento-

posterior presentation with a deliverable mento-anterior or full breech presentation.

The desire to intervene and to 'speed things up' is natural to most obstetricians, especially during a long or difficult labour, or one in which the fetus exhibits distress. He must remember that, once he applies forceps – or intervenes in any other manner – he is increasing the risk of complications and a greater likelihood of morbidity and mortality. Conversely, the reasons for intervention themselves may demand prompt and aggressive action. Faced with a dead neonate, the following questions arise:

(i) What is the cause of death ?
(ii) Are there any pre-existing anomalies, lesions or defects and, if so, how are they related to the cause of death, if at all?
(iii) Did any active injury which is seen occur before the onset of labour?
(iv) Is the discovered injury a proximate cause of death? The pathologist must be able to evaluate the degree of injury and its secondary consequences in the light of legal 'causality'.

The great majority of fetal injuries will manifest themselves through cerebral anoxia – haemorrhagic brain compression, shock and pulmonary insufficiency will all lead to an oxygen-deprived brain and the common pathway can be grafted on to maternal causes of anoxia-hypoxia. Prematurity makes the fetus more vulnerable to oxygen lack; what would be minimal damage in a full-term fetus may be lethal to one which is 2 months premature.

Infants who survive a partial lack of oxygen are host to a variety of neurological and psychological deficits, some with a poor prognosis. Children so injured have frequently brought obstetricians to court for damages and the flood of delivery-related cases has contributed significantly to the so-called medical malpractice crisis in the United States today. Full review and clear analysis of these cases will allow separation of the valid case from the frivolous one.

Some of the common causes of perinatal death are listed in Table 1.1.

The pathologist is often asked if the baby is stillborn. The question is of major practical importance since a stillbirth is *nullius bonis* whereas a live-born, even though alive for just a fleeting minute, can be murdered or inherit a kingdom. Unfortunately, there is no absolute test for a live birth, and the grey zone in the middle of the spectrum between absolute certainty of a live birth and a stillbirth continues to pose diagnostic uncertainty (see Chapters 4 and 5). The evidentiary question was addressed particularly in *Commonwealth of Pennsylvania* v. *Laufe* [6] and *Commonwealth of Pennsylvania* v. *Melnick* [7] (see above, p. 5).

The general pathologist, in a community hospital, will see much paediatric material, but may be uneasy dealing with an obscure tumour or a complex congenital heart malformation. He is further hampered by a general lack of agreement concerning 'normal values' in children, since no two textbooks even agree on basic facts such as average organ weights in children. Even the usual growth charts, compiled from measurements of 'healthy' children over the years, may be greatly misleading in the individual case.

To add to his problems, the general pathologist may be asked to perform forensic autopsies in suspected cases of child abuse or other traumatic deaths. He will be asked about the amount of force needed to cause a given result – but few such quantitative measurements are available because any prospective experiments involving children are clearly unethical. Information is, therefore, mostly anecdotal or is derived from bizarre experiments on baby cadavers which, apart from being misleading, are not to be encouraged on grounds of policy. Previous experience with similar cases offers the best chance of evaluation.

Table 1.1 Some causes of neonatal death

(1) CAUSE OF DEATH IS OBVIOUS, EXPECTED, AND TREATABLE
    (A) Extreme immaturity
    (B) Postmaturity
    (C) Placental insufficiency
    (D) Injury *in utero* – skiing, motor vehicle, gunshot wound, etc.
    (E) Co-existing teratoma, choriocarcinoma
    (F) Many genetic or congenital defects, including:
        (a) Hydrocephalus
        (b) Anencephalus
        (c) Absence of lungs
        (d) Absence of heart
    (G) Infection of mother – syphilis, gonorrhoea, tuberculosis

(2) INJURY DURING LABOUR OR DELIVERY
    (A) General
        (a) Feto-pelvic (cephalopelvic) disproportion
        (b) Amnionitis secondary to premature membrane rupture, iatrogenic or otherwise
        (c) Malposition (e.g. undiagnosed transverse lie)
        (d) Ruptured uterus
        (e) Aspiration by mother while drugged
        (f) Unattended precipitate delivery
    (B) Head
        (a) Dural laceration
        (b) Intraventricular haemorrhage
        (c) Skull fractures
    (C) Soft tissues
        (a) Subcapsular hepatic haematoma
        (b) Adrenal haemorrhage
        (c) Pulmonary haemorrhage
    (D) Specific respiratory lesions
        (a) Pneumothorax
        (b) Pneumomediastinum
        (c) Pneumothoromediastinum
        (d) Hyaline membrane disease
        (e) Aspiration
            (i) Amniotic fluid at birth: laryngospasm
            (ii) Pneumonia – amnionitis
            (iii) Poor gag reflex ('Gagenhalten') due to maternal sedation, anaesthesia, immaturity, or bronchotracheal fistula
    (E) Immunohaematological
        (a) ABO or CDE incompatibility: erythroblastosis
        (b) Haemoglobin disease: sickle cell, thalassaemia, etc.

The forensic pathologist is more likely to be the leading witness in the final act of these tragedies involving infants and children. Unfortunately, a shoddy autopsy – or a misinterpretation of the evidence – can ruin a family and may do incalculable harm to the innocent survivors. The autopsy must be carefully planned and documented. The importance of the history, and, particularly, of any discordance, is discussed in Chapter 14. Sometimes, the mode of death, which may be obscure on external examination, becomes readily apparent at internal autopsy:

Case 1.3

The mother of an 8-month-old male brought the child to the local hospital and stated that, when she went to pick him up for a feeding, she saw that he was not breathing. The local Coroner suspected 'sudden infant death syndrome' and ordered an autopsy as mandated by state law. The child appeared unremarkable on external examination (Fig. 1.1(a)), and the viscera exhibited minimal congestion. The scalp was peeled back, revealing the patterned lesion seen in Fig. 1.1(b). A hairline skull fracture was present and an acute epidural haemorrhage was found. The pattern of this was suggestive of a boot heel, and a boot of such shape was found in the house.

The following opinion was given: 'Based upon available history, gross and microscopic examination of the remains, Baby W, an 8-month-old male, died as a result of blunt force trauma to the head. The patterned contusion in the galea aponeurotica is consistent with the heel of a boot. The epidural haemorrhage does not exhibit any gross or microscopic evidence of healing or vital reaction, indicating that death occurred a short time after the child received the injuries'. [13]

Not every allegation of child abuse can be proved and some are unfounded. The following case has almost surrealistic overtones and the associated jurisdictional tangle complicated a bizarre situation:

Case 1.4

A 4-year-old boy lived with his parents in north-east Ohio and, because both parents worked, he spent the work week with his aunt and her family in West Virginia. He was an active youngster, and enjoyed using his bed at home as a trampoline, sometimes hitting his head on the nearby dresser. After one such incident, while at home with his parents, he was dropped off in West Virginia where he apparently tripped over a shoelace and fell with his forehead against the side of the kitchen counter. His screams brought his aunt who picked up the struggling child to take him to the bathroom to wash his head laceration but tripped on a loose bathmat, dropping the child into the bathtub. When she attempted to pick up the child a second time, her 9-year-old daughter came into the bathroom dragging a large towel on the floor. Her mother, with the boy in her arms, tripped over the towel and fell on top of the boy, now in the partially filled bathtub. When she finally got the child suitably wrapped to take to a paramedic neighbour, she tripped over a sheepdog, once again falling on top of the child.

The child was diagnosed at the local hospital in West Virginia as having a severe brain injury and was transferred across the state line into Pennsylvania where, after a brief comatose period and an attempt at decompression, he died. The local coroner released the body to West Virginia where allegations of child abuse were made by the treating neurosurgeon.

A county medical examiner, with little training in forensic pathology, performed an autopsy and concurred with the neurosurgeon that this was, indeed, a case of child abuse. The State of West Virginia held

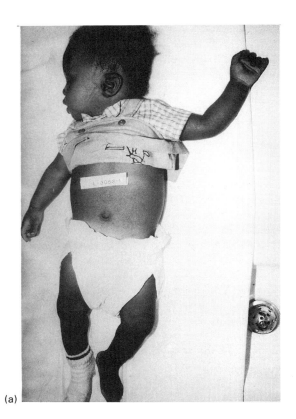

(a)

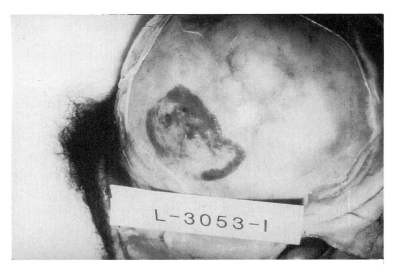

(b)

Fig. 1.1 (a) An 8-month-old child considered to be a death due to the sudden infant death syndrome ('cot death'). (b) Autopsy revealed a patterned lesion strongly suggestive of a heel mark. Fracture of the skull and epidural haemorrhage were present beneath the lesion.

the aunt on a general homicide charge and scheduled a hearing to take custody of her own children from her.

A forensic pathologist was called by the defence to evaluate the autopsy findings and other evidence. It turned out that the neurosurgeon had no knowledge of the previous trauma in Ohio; he had based his diagnosis on the presence of injury, associated with a garbled story from an hysterical aunt. The hospital pathologist who performed the rather inadequate autopsy did not attempt to analyse the brain lesion patterns or attempt to age the earliest subdural haemorrhage. It had a membrane around it, which indicated that it was older than the time required to fit the state's version of events [14].

A third example is more troublesome in that the pathologist was out of his element in an extremely complex case.

Case 1.5

A 2-year-old boy with a long history of gastrointestinal upset was brought to the emergency ward of a county hospital where he died. He had always been a poor eater and had been admitted to the hospital on several occasions because of diarrhoea and failure to thrive. The Coroner ordered and performed an autopsy because of the uncertain cause of death.

The major findings related to the abdomen where there was a segment of necrotic and perforated small bowel and florid peritonitis. He also noted several clots in the mesenteric 'vessels'. His conclusion was that the youngster had been hit in the abdomen, and had then developed multiple traumatic mesenteric thrombi, which in turn caused a necrotic bowel, ileus, perforation and sepsis. His response at a deposition totally confused both the defence and state's attorneys. In an unprecedented move, they jointly sought

out a forensic pathologist to attempt to determine the meaning of the coroner's arcane or nonsensical replies.

The autopsy descriptions and the pictures taken at the autopsy provided some of the answers sought by the lawyers. The child had a longstanding, chronic bowel inflammation, with extensive scar tissue formation and a necrotic perforation. However, the thrombi were found mostly in the tertiary arterial arcades, not in end-arteries, so that they could not have been the cause of the infarction [15].

No other medicolegal issue is more blurred by emotional involvement than alleged child molestation. False conviction is doubly tragic – to both the putative victim and the alleged perpetrator. A recent Texas case held that despite the doctor's findings of no injuries, the allegedly molested child's testimony constituted sufficient evidence for the jury to conclude there had been sodomy [16]. In a similar California case, rectal bleeding was present, but none of the deep lacerations that would be associated with the alleged acts performed on these children was present. The dilemma has recently reached new peaks in the United Kingdom where an escalation in the number of reported cases of child sexual abuse forced a judicial inquiry; the case is discussed further in Chapter 15.

Despite the legal problems relating to a child as young as 2 years old being placed on the witness stand and subjected to cross-examination, the public seems to be willing to accept this added psychological trauma to the alleged victim. Experiments are currently in train in England whereby a child is allowed to give evidence from behind a screen. Nevertheless, it is important that the rights of the accused are not compromised because, unfortunately, it is often impossible to distinguish between a legitimate victim and an overly imaginative, malevolent or improperly influenced child. In contrast to other criminal cases involving charges of physical assault by one individual against another, the conviction of an alleged sex molester or abuser of children solely on the basis of the victim's testimony has, traditionally, been disallowed. An eye-witness, the offender's confession or specific medical evidence has been required if prosecution was to be technically permitted. Now only Nebraska and the District of Columbia still require independent corroborating evidence to prosecute a case of child abuse in which the youthful victim has given testimony; a similar change will be introduced shortly in England. As in any criminal case, it will, of course, still be up to the judge and jury to weigh the credibility of conflicting witnesses.

The forensic pathologist must be able to recognize and evaluate any pattern of trauma due to deliberate injury and to differentiate it from that due to accident; he must satisfy himself that the injuries are the result of a specific type of action by another person and he must be able to exclude the less sinister explanations which are offered; he must accumulate data from a variety of sources, evaluate their authenticity and determine the mode of death after sifting fact from speculation and fantasy. Finally, he must not lose his objectivity – and this may be difficult in the emotionally charged atmosphere surrounding a battered baby.

Of course, the insoluble conflict between medical and legal causality hampers communication between the forensic pathologist and the attorney. The doctor sees an effect, such as a lacerated liver, which may result from several similar but not identical causes and he may not be able to testify 'beyond a reasonable doubt' that one particular mechanism, e.g. a 'punch in the belly', caused the liver laceration, to the exclusion of all other mechanisms. Since we are legally and morally forbidden to do controlled experiments on children to determine the mechanisms and forces involved in the creation of these fatal injuries, we can only infer how and with what force a specific injury is produced from animal experiments or from retrospective studies of victims. Therefore, the *certainty* of causality aimed at in the law is far from realized and the pathologist's *certainty* much diluted.

Once the cause and manner of death are certified by the Coroner as being of a criminal nature, a preliminary hearing and an indictment charging the implicated defendant with homicide usually follow. At this point, the pathologist must understand the legal procedures and must know what is expected of him.

In order to convict a person of any crime, the state must prove:

(i) the actus reus – that a crime was committed by the suspect;
(ii) the mens rea – that the defendant in committing the crime did so knowing that what he did was 'wrong';
(iii) the corpus delecti – that body of evidence required to prove the actus reus.

With a case of child abuse, the major portion of the corpus delecti is the victim's body, assuming that the pathologist can state without reservation that the child did, in fact, die from the actions of another person and not from an accident or disease. Other witnesses may give testimony concerning the circumstances of the death and the totality of the evidence will influence the trier of fact in reaching a verdict.

The current legal approach to the battered child syndrome is to adopt legislation which attempts to curb child abuse while, at the same time, having the best interests of the child at heart. Unfortunately, this has not always been the case. The child's interests were hardly acknowledged at common law; parental rights dominated all other concerns. Even during the twentieth century, it has been held that a parent's right over his child would 'transcend property rights' [17]. Only if the parent was found to grossly abuse his rights would the state intervene under the principle of *parens patriae* – a principle which is discussed in greater detail in Chapter 29. Not until 1972, did the court decide that a parent's right to care, custody and control over their children was no longer absolute [18].

In 1963, the United States Children's Bureau proposed a model reporting law [19] and all 50 states had laws mandating the reporting of child abuse by 1967. In an effort to encourage reporting, immunity from criminal or civil liability was provided for those whose reports were filed in good faith; penalties were set forth for those who 'knowingly and willfully' failed to report.

Despite the good intentions, these statutes failed, to an extent, in their purpose. Initially, not many physicians took them seriously. Others hesitated to report what they regarded as evidence of child abuse for fear of initiating criminal proceedings on the basis of little more than intuition. However, their attitudes shifted in 1976 as a result of the decision in *Londeros* v. *Flood* [20] in which the court decided that a physician who failed to report a suspected case of child abuse could be held liable at civil law for later damages to the same child.

This holding might have been more significant had the reporting statutes set forth explicit guidelines. However, it is difficult to find someone guilty of failing to report a nebulous disease. Originally, reports were required of children who suffered from 'non-accidental injury'. More recently, the court has recognized that child abuse may involve a series of unexplained injuries [21]. The Federal Child Abuse Prevention and Treatment Act, 42 U.S.C.§ 5103 [2] (1974) includes neglect, sexual molestation and mental injury in its definition of these injuries [22]. Realistically, however, there are no true guidelines to apply. The court in *In re Stacey* [23] declared that there is 'no fixed standard for neglect, so each case must be judged on its own particular facts ...'. It might be argued that a child who came in with non-accidental bruises sufficient to form blood clots had suffered from intentional physical abuse. However, the United States Supreme Court has held that physical beatings by public teachers, resulting in similar injury, are not constitutionally prohibited [24]. It is apparent that reporting is an unenforceable mandate in the absence of more specific guidelines.

The protective mechanisms in both the child custody and the criminal courts are discussed in detail in Chapter 29; here, we are concerned with the legal and medical interface. The prosecuting attorney's role in these cases is to determine whether sufficient evidence exists to enable him to meet his burden of proof. This is his most difficult task. The state must be able to establish by 'clear and convincing' evidence that harm to the child occurred as a direct result of parental unfitness.

Evidence is almost non-existent in many child abuse cases; other than the injury itself, most is circumstantial in nature. There are rarely witnesses, and those who do exist are often reluctant to tell their story. In addition, evidentiary rules tend to favour the suspect and hamper thorough investigation.

A protective custody hearing occurs in the civil court. Homicide, however, is a criminal matter; thus, child abuse cases which result in the death of the child must be brought in the criminal court. The more serious the offence, the more stringent becomes the burden of proof and, in order to convict someone of beating his child to death, the prosecution attorney must prove guilt beyond a reasonable doubt. It is apparent that much reliance must be placed on the pathologist's report which may or may not be as unequivocal as the prosecutor would wish.

The defence is on much firmer ground. Their main thrust, as in any criminal case, is to create doubt – any small amount of doubt – as to the guilt of the defendant. They may do this in several ways. First, they may argue that the child did not die as a result of being beaten – 'Those bruises all over the body are an external manifestation of leukaemia'. The child wasn't placed in a pot of boiling water, but 'accidentally spilled it on himself while the defendant-mother was chasing the younger brother'. He wasn't beaten by a wooden plank – instead, he 'fell down a flight of stairs'. Whatever the explanation, there is no child abuse if the cause of death can be attributed to an accident.

The defence attorney will usually try to prevent any gruesome details being introduced as evidence. The less the jury hears of torture and horror, the better. Evidentiary principles may be used to prevent photographs and colour slides being introduced into evidence; success will vary from one jurisdiction to another and from judge to judge.

The pathologist will be most helpful to the case if he can give a strong opinion backed by scientific conclusions. This is where a painstakingly detailed autopsy protocol will be of value. He may refresh his memory from his notes, so that he can deliver his opinion in an objective, concise fashion. Often, the strength of his testimony will be enhanced if he admits, when he lacks sufficient evidence, that he cannot answer a specific question. Above all, the pathologist's testimony will be most helpful if he can articulate his findings in a manner which is understandable to the layman jury.

While child abuse may provide the greatest challenge to the pathologist in his role of expert witness, his testimony may be required in many other paediatric deaths and, in particular, in the analysis of deaths apparently due to the sudden infant death syndrome (the epidemiology and pathology of this is discussed in Chapters 9 and 10). Most of these deaths occur at home and, therefore, fall into the medical examiner's jurisdiction in the United States; since such deaths are sudden

and unexpected, they are automatically the focus of inquiry by the coroner or procurator fiscal in the United Kingdom. Many of the United States mandate that all sudden infant deaths be autopsied. This may be as much in the interests of research as of anything else; nevertheless, it has to be admitted that evidence of child abuse is uncovered in a small minority of cases. Other forms of sudden natural death in childhood which may tax the pathologist's art are discussed in Chapter 11, while the role of the forensic pathological evidence in preventing future accidental deaths of children in, say, automobiles or in fires cannot be overemphasized.

The forensic pathologist also sees, all too often, the final effects of improper medical diagnosis and treatment. If he is able to present testimony that links a specific act or failure to act to the result, a legal action may be possible, either civil or criminal, and the responsible party held accountable. Equally importantly, he can help prevent a miscarriage of justice if he can state with the required degree of medical certainty that the putative act or failure to act was not the cause of the result – a matter which may be of particular importance in a case associated with product liability.

Expert evidence in relation to the living is also part of the forensic physician's spectrum of involvement; the development of the acquired immunodeficiency syndrome (AIDS), which is considered in detail in Chapter 23, provides a recent illustration. Several paediatric cases have been adjudicated involving transfusions of tainted blood to infants who have subsequently developed AIDS and have died from its effects. Such cases encapsulate a good portion of product liability litigation.

In *Kosop* v. *Georgetown University* [25], a premature infant was given a blood transfusion that was a life-saving procedure. The child subsequently developed AIDS and died from its effects at the age of 3 years. The parents sued both the hospital and the American Red Cross, the action being based on several legal theories:

(i) Lack of informed consent – failure to warn the parents of the potential danger of contracting AIDS via a blood transfusion.
(ii) Failure to let the parents know that they could have donated their blood to the infant.
(iii) Strict liability and breach of warranty by providing a contaminated product.

The court granted a summary judgement for the defendants, rejecting each of the plaintiffs' claims. It clearly rejected the theory that the American Red Cross was a 'merchant' of blood; it was further held that, because of the state of the art in 1983, the fact that AIDS was spread by infected blood could not have been known nor was there any way to test for the presence of human immunodeficiency virus. The court also rejected a theory of negligence to support liability on the same issues in this case. While other courts have exempted blood products from an implied warranty [26], they have only ruled on the theory of strict liability and not on the question of negligence.

Another aspect of product liability which is currently exercising the courts on both sides of the Atlantic is that of vaccine-related damage to children. Limited compensation from public funds without proof of negligence is admitted both in the United Kingdom and the United States [27], but this does not prevent parents, and children themselves, bringing individual actions in the tort of negligence. It is here that medical evidence is of supreme importance as to causality. Multi-million dollar awards have been made in the United States but the two United Kingdom courts to address the subject so far, one in Scotland and one in England, were not satisfied that pertussis vaccination had caused the plaintiff children's condition [28]; it is interesting to note that, so deeply ingrained is the adversarial system of justice, that experts who wished to give evidence in the latter case as *amici curiae*, or advisers to the court, were not permitted to do so. Such cases continue to be decided largely on the forensic performance of the expert witnesses.

So it is that the forensic expert bridges the gap between the hospital, the laboratory and the courtroom. Always mindful that he is first a physician, his objective is to make sense of the chaos caused by the ever-present, ever-active Fifth Horseman of the Apocalypse and his ubiquitous squires.

REFERENCES

1. Autopsy report: A1WE (Westmoreland County, Pa.).
2. Huser, C.J. and Smialek, J.E. (1986) Diagnosis of sudden death in infants due to acute dehydration. *Am. J. Forensic Med. Pathol.*, **7**, 278.
3. *Eyre* v. *Shaftesbury* (1722) 24 ER 659.
4. For a modern version of the historic case of *R.* v. *Brownrigg*, see Millet, K. (1979) *The Basement*, Simon and Schuster, New York.
5. For an example of a successful action for preconception tort, see *Jorgensen* v. *Meade Johnson Laboratories Inc.* 483 F 2d 237 (1973).
6. *Commonwealth of Pennsylvania* v. *Laufe* (1975) Allegheny County Coroner's Docket.
7. *Commonwealth of Pennsylvania* v. *Melnick* (1985) Court of Common Pleas of Philadelphia County, Trial Division, Criminal Section, February Term Nos 1611 and 1612 (case still pending).
8. Plank, J. (1965) Morphologische befunde in nicht beamten, nicht retrahierten lungen des neugenboren. *Virchows Arch. Pathol. Anat.*, **338**, 245.
9. Hirvonen, J., Tiisala, R., Uotila, U. *et al.* (1969) Roentgenological and autopsy studies on the gas content of the lungs and gastrointestinal tract in living and stillborn infants and sources of error in resuscitation. *Dtsch. Z. Gesamte Gerich. Med.*, **65**, 73.
10. Mityayeva, N.A. (1970) Discriminating live and stillborn infants according to histological features of the lungs. *Sud. Med. Ekspert.*, **13**, 15.

11. Prokop, O. (1971) Zur brauchbarkeit der elastichen fasern der lunge im rahmen der lebensproben. *Z. Rechtsmed.,* **69**, 177.
12. *Whitehouse* v. *Jordan* (1981) 1 All ER 267, HL.
13. Autopsy Report: 3051 (Iberia Parish, La.).
14. *State of West Virginia* v. *Hugi* (charges dropped).
15. *State of Ihio* v. *Bailey* (charges dropped).
16. *Villanueva* v. *State of Texas* 703 SW 2d 244 (Tex. 1985).
17. *Danton* v. *James* 107 Kan 729 (1920).
18. *Wisconsin* v. *Yoder* 407 US 205 (1972); *Poe* v. *Gerstein* 417 US 218 (1972).
19. US Children's Bureau (1963) *The Abused Child, Principles and Suggested Language for Legislation on Reporting of the Physically Abused Child.*
20. *Londeros* v. *Flood* 551 P 2d 389 (Cal., 1976).
21. *In re K D E* 210 NW 2d 907 (S D, 1973).
22. A recent government publication in England specifies five categories of abuse – neglect, physical abuse, sexual abuse, emotional abuse and 'grave concern': (1988) *Working Together,* HMSO, London, p. 26.
23. *In re Stacey* 365 NE 2d 634 (Ill., 1973).
24. *Ingraham* v. *Wright* 430 US 651 (1977); for England and Wales, see Education (No 2) Act 1986, ss. 47,48 which prohibits such punishment in State-run schools.
25. *Kosop* v. *Georgetown University* No. 86–0033 D C (July 7, 1987).
26. *Coffee* v. *Cutter Biological* 809 F 2d 191 (1987).
27. Vaccine Damage Payments Act 1979 (UK); National Childhood Vaccine Injury Act 1986 (US). For details of the latter, see Anonymous (1988) National Childhood Vaccine Injury Act: Requirements for permanent vaccination records and for reporting of selected events after vaccination. *JAMA,* **259**, 2527.
28. *Bonthrone* v. *Secretary of State for Scotland* (1987) SLT 34 (early stages of trial); *Loveday* v. *Renton and another (1988) The Times*, 31 March. For discussion see Dyer, C. (1988) Judge 'not satisfied' that whooping cough vaccine causes permanent brain damage. *Br. Med. J.,* **296**, 1189.

PART 2

Forensic medicine and pathology

CHAPTER 2

Genetic counselling and prenatal diagnosis

J.A. Raeburn

Technical developments in the field of medical genetics have expanded with unprecedented speed during the past 20 years and many area hospitals have established departments of medical genetics. There has been a strong tendency to direct the attention of such departments towards management of the family as a whole rather than to the treatment of individuals suffering from genetic disorder. The clinical descriptions and classifications of genetic diseases have also been extended – an aspect which is of great importance in providing accurate genetic counselling. Such counselling services have, at the same time, become available to more patients and families.

Medicolegal problems can occur easily in such a changing field, especially considering the individual choices which couples must make on matters such as contraception, sterilization or prenatal testing – with the possibility of considering a termination of the pregnancy. It is profitable, therefore, to summarize the recent history and to emphasize the developments which have led both to new approaches in management and to the reassessment of several legal and ethical dilemmas.

2.1 HISTORY

In 1955, after more than 30 years in which it was wrongly assumed that the human chromosomal complement was 48, two research groups simultaneously, but using quite different approaches, demonstrated that the correct number was 46 – 22 pairs of autosomes together with one pair of sex chromosomes. Knowledge of the correct chromosome number paved the way for descriptions of the cytogenetic abnormalities present in Down's, Turner's and Klinefelter's syndromes, all of which had been described previously as clinical entities. All three syndromes were shown to be associated with an abnormal number of chromosomes – either a chromosome in excess or one missing. Further studies showed that structural chromosome abnormalities occurred in a proportion of individuals who had congenital dysmorphic* syndromes, thus providing an explanation – and a diagnostic test – for other clinically recognizable entities such as the *cri du chat* syndrome – a condition in which part of the short arm of chromosome 5 is deleted and which contains several characteristic features as well as mental handicap [1].

* Dysmorphic means having abnormal external features, especially of the face.

Such cytogenetic research showed the value of studying individual cells from a patient and of analysing the genetic characteristics *in vitro*. In the late 1960s, biologists realized the importance of cell culture techniques which made more detailed study possible by increasing the yield of cells of a given genetic type. It was soon appreciated that amniotic cells, derived from the fetus and, therefore, sharing the fetal genotype, could be sampled at about the fifteenth week of gestation. These cells could be cultured until enough were available for biochemical measurements or for chromosomal analysis. The study of biochemical markers in the cell-free amniotic fluid was also initiated early in the 1970s. The most important of these markers was alpha-fetoprotein (AFP), the level of which was significantly elevated in the amniotic fluid if the pregnancy was complicated by a fetal neural tube defect such as anencephaly or spina bifida [2]: there was often, too, a degree of elevation in the maternal serum [3].

Thus, methods for prenatal diagnosis of genetic or partially genetic conditions were based on two principles: either that cultured cells from amniotic fluid, being derived from the skin of the fetus, were truly representative of the fetal genotype, or that abnormal fetuses could release substances into the amniotic fluid which caused measurable alterations from the normal. Fetal diagnosis could also be based on ultrasound imaging, a clinical investigation which has steadily improved in quality since its early development by Donald in 1967 [4]. In addition, there is a place for both fetal radiography and for fetoscopy – the direct visualization of the fetus by an instrument inserted through the uterine wall and into the amniotic sac. However, both these procedures carry a significant degree of risk to the fetus [5].

By the early 1980s, a new approach to the preclinical diagnosis of some conditions, mostly those due to the presence of a single abnormal gene, was being cautiously applied. This was founded on studies of genetic markers, which depend on variations of DNA throughout the genome and which were shown up by differing susceptibility to enzymic cleavage. There are thousands of such DNA variations and, since they are often close to genes responsible for specific diseases, they can be used to 'track' such genes in a family [6]. If a marker close to a disease gene is studied systematically in several people from an affected family, then the presence or absence of the abnormal gene in certain individuals can be inferred prior to there being any overt symptoms. This approach can be adopted to determine the status of the fetus by using cultured amniotic cells. Recently, however, it has been possible to sample chorionic membrane from the placental site at around 9–10 weeks' gestation. This tissue is also of fetal origin and can be utilized in the same way as can desquammated fetal cells for biochemical, cytogenetic or DNA studies of the embryo. In this way, a prenatal diagnosis can be carried out which provides the option of terminating an affected pregnancy before the twelfth week of gestation [7].

The ability to identify a severe genetic condition of the fetus before mid-pregnancy means that consideration can be given to the possibility of a termination of the pregnancy, particularly if the abnormality is one which is incompatible with extrauterine life. Such termination became legal in Great Britain following the passage of the Abortion Act 1967. The legislation stated (at s.1(1) (b)) that there were grounds for termination of a pregnancy provided 'there is a substantial risk that if the child were born it would suffer from such physical or mental abnormalities as to be severely handicapped'. However, the Act permitted other grounds for termination including where 'continuation of the pregnancy would involve risk of injury to the physical or mental health of the pregnant woman, greater than if the pregnancy was terminated'. This latter indication has been used to justify abortion carried out as a means of reducing social distress and 96.3% of abortions in Scotland in 1981 were for this indication [8] as were 97.4% in 1986 [9]. The same distribution was present in England and Wales where, in 1986, there were 153 857 abortions (89.7% of all legal terminations) because of risk to the physical or mental well-being of pregnant women and only 1234 abortions (0.7% of all legal terminations) by reason of genetic handicap [10].

The degree of public repugnance to 'social' abortions has led to simultaneous criticism of genetic reasons for termination of a pregnancy even though those comprise such a small proportion of all abortions. This public pressure has led to several unsuccessful reviews of the Abortion Act 1967. The most recent of these, represented by the Abortion (Amendment) Bill 1987, sought to reduce the legal limit for performing any termination of pregnancy – other than in a life-saving emergency – from 28 weeks to 18 weeks gestation. This would have serious implications for a couple who might consider any form of prenatal diagnosis based on amniocentesis and it would seem that, in practice, an 18-week limit would have a greater effect on terminations of pregnancy for fetal abnormalities than it would on the 'social' indications for abortion against which the Bill was mainly aimed; it was, in major part, for this reason that the Bill was rejected.

All of the prenatal diagnostic techniques summarized above require a great deal of skill and of exacting quality control on the part of the obstetrician and the ultrasonographer who collaborate in the collection of amniotic or chorion villus samples as well as by the laboratory scientists who process the tissue. The use of these procedures also demands that the patient and her spouse be fully informed of the options available, of the risks of the procedures and of the likelihood of incorrect or inconclusive results. This discussion is often best done by a medical geneticist who will investigate the family, list the options and help the couple to make their *own* decision. The medical model in which a patient gives trusting acquiescence to the advice of her physician, which was the norm in the 1960s, is no more appropriate nowadays than are old and outmoded laboratory techniques. Nor is it acceptable for the doctor, acting on his own ethical beliefs, either to recommend a procedure and to press the patient towards this or, by not mentioning an option, to deny it. There is a full discussion of this aspect, and of the overall ethical implications, in the monograph by Gillon [11]. As technology has improved, so has it created an urgent need for genetic counselling techniques to progress. A clinician who does not ensure that a family receive accurate genetic counselling is just as culpable in law as is the scientist who performs a laboratory examination incorrectly.

This brief history of the development of techniques involved in genetic counselling and prenatal diagnosis will emphasize how rapidly this subject has changed in just three decades – and especially in the past 5 years. The following paragraphs discuss the process of genetic counselling and describe the modes of inheritance of the more common genetic conditions. Later, there is a classification of prenatal diagnostic methods and descriptions of how these might be utilized, for example, in genetic screening.

2.2 WHAT IS GENETIC COUNSELLING?

Genetic counselling provides the means whereby a family, in which an inherited condition has occurred, is informed as to how likely it is that the condition will recur in other individuals. Thus, if a relative had Down's syndrome, then potential parents in the family would be told what risk there would be that other children would be affected. They would also be told the features of the condition, its severity and the availability and degree of success of treatments or of prenatal methods for identification. In the early stages of genetic counselling, it is helpful to write out a list of all the questions that the couple wish to have answered. Not only does this indicate their background knowledge about genetic matters but also their attitudes and, perhaps, their preconceived ideas about handicap. Then, specific questioning – and clinical examination – will accurately check the diagnosis in the probands and all relevant family members.

The next aspect of genetic counselling is most important. All possible options open to the couple must be listed so that they may come to their own decisions as to what to do. In this respect, genetic counselling epitomizes the doctrine of 'informed consent', which is developed particularly in the USA, in that the client, or patient, takes the major decisions, not the doctor. Genetic counselling is not the giving of advice based on the doctor's specialized knowledge. It is the giving of information about all the choices available, while understanding the emotional aspects in the family and ensuring that they realize that the choice must be the right one for them – not a decision made by professionals. Many of the medicolegal difficulties associated with genetic disease stem from failure to observe this rule. Clearly, the options presented to a couple must all be legal whether the situation arises after prenatal diagnosis has shown a specific condition, or following the birth of a handicapped baby or after a genetic handicap is identified later in life.

The need for sensitive counselling in all such situations is illustrated by two tragic situations, in both of which a neonate afflicted with Down's syndrome was either killed or was allowed to die [12, 13]. In the case of one of these Down's syndrome neonates, a senior paediatrician, after discussion with the baby's parents, decided to withhold adequate feeding unless the sedated infant demanded this. When the baby died, that doctor was tried for, and was later acquitted of, murder; this case, *R. v. Arthur*, is discussed also at pages 133 and 417. Not long after that a father of a Down's syndrome infant smothered the baby and was later tried and found guilty of manslaughter. He received the relatively short period of imprisonment of 5 years. In these two cases, it is reasonable to suggest that, if the parents' emotional state had been accurately assessed, if counselling support from a nearby self-help group had been requested and if all the *legal* options had been made clear, then the course of events might have been different – and parental guilt after the deaths might have been lessened. There are, now, economic pressures which might reduce the availability of genetic counselling; it is, nevertheless, especially important that the wishes of the individual members of a family are clearly identified and are followed despite the financial constraints which are being imposed on health services and the medical workloads which are, therefore, increasing. Here the voluntary sector wishes, and has the resources, to provide counselling.

2.3 THE DIFFERENT TYPES OF INHERITANCE

Although the information provided by genetic counselling will be different for each individual disease, the principles of inheritance can be summarized under three major categories:

(a) Single gene disorders.
(b) Chromosomal disorders.
(c) Multifactorial disorders.

(a) Single gene disorders

In these conditions the abnormality occurs at a specific genetic position (locus) either on one chromosome alone or at the same locus on both members of a pair of chromosomes.

Autosomal dominant disorders

These are due to abnormal genes which, sooner or later, can *dominate* the normal gene and lead to manifestations of disease. If a dominant gene is on an autosome – i.e. chromosomes number 1 to 22, the non-sex chromosomes – then the abnormality occurs with equal frequency in both males and females. Examples of dominant disorders are given in Table 2.1 which also notes the chromosomal location of the gene where this is known. These conditions are only examples; there are over 1150 autosomal dominant diseases listed in McKusick's catalogue [16]. The essential element in autosomal dominant disorders is that affected individuals have a 50% chance of passing the abnormal gene to their offspring.

Dominant disorders do not always show clear abnormal features in every individual who has the gene. The evidence that someone has the disorder may be very slight – for example, possession of the abnormal gene responsible for Marfan's syndrome, which, typically, demonstrates congenital heart disease, skeletal problems and dislocation of the lenses of the eye, may be manifested by no more than an excessive height. Another example is tuberous sclerosis in which an individual who has the abnormal gene might

Table 2.1 Examples of autosomal dominant disorders

Disorder	Chromosomal location
Marfan's syndrome	Not known
Huntington's disease	4
Adult polycystic kidney disease	16
Neurofibromatosis	17*
Tuberous sclerosis	9†
Achondroplasia	Not known
Polyposis coli	5

* Barker *et al.* [14].
† Fryer *et al.* [15].

escape the epilepsy or other mental features of the disease and have only minor skin manifestations. The occurrence of different manifestations of a condition in family members who have the same abnormal dominant gene is known as pleiotropy. The percentage of individuals who manifest the disorder when they have the abnormal gene is known as the penetrance. Unless the phenomenon of reduced penetrance is understood, and carefully allowed for, appropriate genetic counselling may be denied to a branch of the family who have quite a high risk of occurrence of severe disease. Such omissions might well lead to charges of medical negligence.

Some autosomal dominant disorders may not manifest in childhood, e.g. Huntington's disease in which over 30% of affected individuals show no symptoms or signs before the age of 50 years. The current view is that children who are at risk of inheriting such conditions should receive genetic counselling at around the ages of 14–16 years, depending on their degree of physical or social maturity. However, presymptomatic screening for the abnormal gene should not be undertaken in anyone under the age of 18 years even if they wish for such testing; this is because it is felt that the knowledge that he or she has inherited the Huntington's gene might be an impossible burden for a young person who has all the other 'normal' causes for an adolescent crisis.

Dominant genes can also be present on the X chromosome. Then, the female who is heterozygous – that is, she possesses the abnormal dominant gene as well as its normal counterpart – will manifest the disorder; her offspring are at 50% risk of inheriting the abnormal gene. The male is hemizygous with respect to all the genes of his X chromosome i.e. he only has one copy of them. A male who inherits a dominant gene on the X chromosome might be expected to have a more severe presentation of the disease than a female because he lacks the partial compensation of the normal gene. As an example, certain X-linked types of retinitis pigmentosa are more severe and have an earlier onset in the male but the daughters of a male with an X-linked dominant disorder will also inherit the abnormal gene and will manifest the condition, although possibly in a mild form; the sons of such an affected male will have inherited only the Y chromosome and will, therefore, be unaffected. A number of rare conditions of childhood are seen only in females, e.g. incontinentia pigmentii or the Aicardi syndrome. It is hypothesized, but not proven, that such conditions are lethal to the hemizygous male *in utero*.

Autosomal recessive disorders

An individual who has a recessive, abnormal gene present in a single dose will have no clinical sequelae because that abnormal gene is *recessive* to its normal homologue. However, if both members of a gene pair are abnormal, then the affected individual may have a combination of abnormalities which is often severe or even fatal. Affected individuals have inherited one abnormal gene from each parent, both of whom would have been carriers. If such a couple have further pregnancies the recurrence risk is 1 in 4 that the child is affected, 1 in 4 that the child is a normal homozygote and 1 in 2 that the child is a carrier. Table 2.2 lists the most commonly seen recessive disorders along with the available information as to chromosomal location of the abnormal gene and the possibility of antenatal diagnosis.

Since many recessive disorders are extremely severe, the affected person may die in early childhood but so far as common relatively easily diagnosed conditions, such as cystic fibrosis, are concerned, there is a further action to be taken so that subsequent genetic counselling is facilitated. Since DNA marker techniques may mean that future offspring can be tested prenatally for the condition

Table 2.2 Common autosomal recessive disorders

Condition	Chromosomal location	Prenatal diagnosis
Cystic fibrosis	7	Yes
Phenylketonuria	11	Yes
Hurler's syndrome	Not known	Yes
Other mental handicaps	Various sites	Sometimes
Sickle cell anaemia	Globin loci on 11 and 16	Yes
Thalassaemias	Globin loci on 11 and 16	Yes

provided a family linkage study has been carried out, it is essential that a source of DNA be established from the index child either by blood sampling or, perhaps, by post-mortem skin or other tissue biopsy. Families in which an affected child has died are most likely to request either prenatal diagnosis or testing of carrier status. As autosomal recessive genes are localized exactly on specific chromosomes, these tests will be feasible, but only if there has been the foresight to store DNA from the deceased child. There has not, so far, been litigation based on a negligent failure to test or store DNA but this development would be likely in the future. Therefore, it could be argued that blood for DNA studies should be taken and stored from any seriously ill individual with a recessive disorder.

X-linked disorders

The abnormal genes for these conditions lie on the X chromosome. We have already mentioned the rare possibility of X-linked dominant inheritance; the X-linked recessive disorders are more common by far. Here, the female carriers of an X-linked recessive disease carry the abnormal gene on *one* X chromosome and the normal homologue on the other. Carrier females are completely normal except for occasional minor clinical manifestations or certain laboratory abnormalities which may permit detection of carriers. This is because the normal X chromosome is able to programme appropriate functions despite the defect in its partner. At meiosis when reduction division takes place to form eggs, the separation of the two X chromosomes of a carrier female will result in half of the eggs having the abnormal X chromosome and half of them having the normal. Thus the sons of a carrier female have a 50% risk of being affected; half her daughters will be carriers and half will be normal.

The identification of female carriers is a significant element in the counselling of families in which there is an X-linked recessive disease. Identification is based, first, on recognizing those at risk by the analysis of pedigrees. Next, the possible carriers must be examined for any subclinical stigmata of the carrier state, e.g. minor muscle weaknesses in carriers of Duchenne muscular dystrophy. Tests may be available by which to measure the levels of certain proteins which are abnormal in carriers, such as the level of factor VIII, which is reduced in carriers of haemophilia, or of creatine kinase, which is increased in carriers of muscular dystrophies. Such methods will miss a significant proportion of carriers because the action of the normal X chromosome obscures any laboratory abnormality in about one-third of definite carriers.

Much more precise recognition of the carrier state is now becoming possible using molecular genetic techniques. The most common approach is to identify the marker patterns of DNA polymorphisms which are sited close to (or within) the disease gene. This can be achieved by testing relevant members of the family and thus identifying the 'phase' of markers which occur in association with the defective gene. Carrier females can then be identified if they are shown to have inherited the sequence of markers which 'flank' the abnormal gene (Fig. 2.1). Considerable experience is required to ensure that all relevant family members are sampled for DNA analysis including, particularly, the fathers of possible carrier females. As with recessive conditions, it is important that DNA is available from affected patients for later linkage analysis. The conditions in which this method of carrier detection is feasible include Duchenne and Becker muscular dystrophies, X-linked retinitis pigmentosa (two types), haemophilia and some disorders of immunity such as X-linked combined immunodeficiency or chronic granulomatous disease.

It will be appreciated that, in some families, there may be female carriers with an X-linked condition who do not know about the disorder or of the possible risks to their male offspring. This may be because communication in the family is poor or because the affected side of the family cannot bring themselves to talk about it – there is sometimes a feeling that the illness is their *fault* and is a matter which must be hushed up. There is a great need for sensitive collaboration between all medical specialists who deal with such families.

Medicolegal questions could arise if the doctor who diagnoses the X-linked condition does not refer the family to a service for genetic counselling and carrier detection. Or he may counsel the sisters and mother of the affected male and forget or ignore the maternal aunts and the female cousins. A full and careful pedigree must be elicited and follow-up must be offered to all individuals whose offspring could be at risk from X-linked disease.

The X chromosome can be the site of new mutations, causing any of the disorders which have just been discussed. In such cases, the mother of an unaffected male may not be a carrier as the mutation may have occurred for the first time in the relevant germ cells. Very meticulous examination and investigation of several members of a family are required

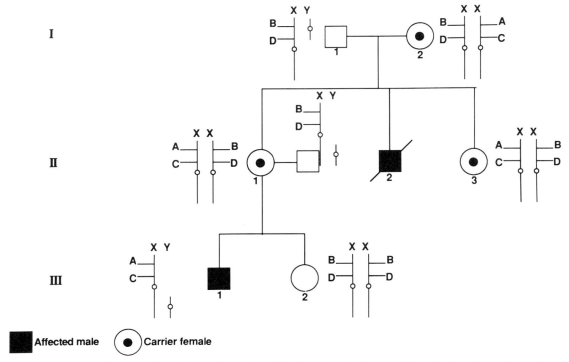

Fig. 2.1 Diagram showing the principle for using DNA-based techniques to identify female carriers of an X-linked recessive disorder. The three generations of the family are numbered I, II and III consecutively and the individuals in each generation of the affected side of the family are numbered 1, 2 and 3. After the male at III, 1, is diagnosed, the history of the maternal uncle II, 2, having died of the disease is discovered. DNA studies of polymorphisms on the X chromosome close to the disease locus show that the affected boy's mother is heterozygous for two marker systems which are both within 1% or so of the abnormal gene. These systems have been named the 'AB' system and the 'CD' system for simplicity, but often there are more than two possible alleles at the marker locus. Since the affected boy has the A marker and the C marker it can be assumed that these markers are both on the same X chromosome and that they are on the X chromosome that contains the defective gene. Further family studies show that the sister II, 3, of the carrier mother is also a carrier and that the sister of the affected boy is not.

before a single affected person can be proven to be a carrier or the reverse. It could be just as devastating to a woman to tell her wrongly that she is a carrier as it would be to miss or ignore the carrier state elsewhere in the kinship.

(b) Chromosome disorders

Diseases of single genes, as discussed above, occur at precise loci on a chromosome and are,

in a sense, defects within the structure of that chromosome. Conventionally, however, chromosome abnormalities are looked on as being defects which can be detected by microscopy after appropriate staining. These abnormalities are either of chromosome number (usually a single chromosome is present in excess or is deficient) or of chromosome structure (in which *part* of a chromosome is in excess or is missing). Twenty years ago, the methods used could identify abnormalities of chromosome number (Table 2.3 (A)) with ease but were less able to show abnormalities of structure (Table 2.3 (B)) unless these were very gross. In 1970, however, methods were developed for examining the substructure of chromosomes which made it possible to demonstrate duplications or deficiencies of chromosomal segments; more recently, high-resolution banding techniques have helped to identify still smaller deletions. Even so, chromosomal studies based on microscopy are presently limited to identifying defective chromosomal segments which are several thousand genes in length. Completely different techniques, based on the study of DNA variations at specific sites along all chromosomes, are required to pinpoint smaller deletions or duplications of groups of genes. A medico-legal implication here is that the methods which were used 20 years ago could not identify the type of chromosome abnormality

that can now be detected. Therefore, it is important to repeat the investigations using the best modern techniques if genetic counselling is undertaken in families in which a chromosome abnormality was suspected in the past but was not confirmed. A typical example is a lethal disorder occurring in one family which was described in 1974 under the label of 'Typus Edinburghensis' [17]. The author suspected, but could not then confirm, a chromosome anomaly; very recently, sadly because of the birth of a further affected baby, it has been shown that affected individuals in this family have an unbalanced translocation between the long arms of chromosomes 1 and 2 (Laing, I. and Ellis, P. 1988, personal communication).

As mentioned before, there are limits to the resolution possible even with the best cytogenetic techniques which could only detect defects of parts of chromosomes containing at least 1000 genes or thereabouts. It is clear that it will require a combination of cytogenetic and molecular genetic techniques to identify abnormalities of smaller parts of chromosomes and there is likely to be very rapid advance in this field over the next decade.

Table 2.3 Chromosomal defects

(A) DEFECTS OF CHROMOSOME NUMBER	
Down's syndrome	Trisomy of chromosome 21
Patau's syndrome	Trisomy of chromosome 13
Edward's syndrome	Trisomy of chromosome 18
Klinefelter's syndrome	XXY chromosome complement
XYY syndrome	Additional Y chromosome
Turner's syndrome	XO chromosome complement
(B) DEFECTS OF CHROMOSOME STRUCTURE	
(1) Deletion syndromes	e.g. *Cri du chat* syndrome or the Wolf–Hirschorn syndrome
(2) Ring chromosomes	Effects are due to deletion of chromosomal material
(3) Inversions	Effects are due to deletion of chromosomal material
(4) Insertions	Effects are due to trisomy of part of the chromosome

(c) Multifactorial disorders

These are abnormalities which involve either the interplay of several different genes or the interaction between a single important gene and certain environmental factors. Multi-factorial disorders include conditions that are very common such as ischaemic heart disease or neural tube defects, including spina bifida (Table 2.4). The greater complexity of this mode of inheritance should not be a deterrent to genetic studies or an excuse for nihilism as regards the approach to family management. On the contrary, if the family history is studied in a multifactorial condition which has a known environmental component, then the triggering factor in the environment could be

Table 2.4 Multifactorial disorders

Early-onset ischaemic heart disease
Peptic ulceration
Schizophrenia
Epilepsy
Diabetes mellitus
Neural tube defects
Rheumatoid arthritis
Asthma

avoided for those at highest risk. This might be true for heart disease where the environmental factor is still not fully understood but which might be a dietary constituent or one associated with smoking; genetic counselling may well become an important element in the prevention of heart disease in a few years time.

It has been suggested that the environmental factor in the aetiology of neural tube defects may be a relative vitamin deficiency [18]. If this is so, then identification of vitamin-deficient mothers prior to a pregnancy and the administration of replacement therapy would be an important health measure. For this reason a multicentre trial of vitamins in the prevention of neural tube defects is currently being conducted by the Medical Research

Table 2.5 Methods for prenatal diagnosis

Technique	Stage of gestation
Chorion villus sampling	9–11 weeks
Amniocentesis	15–18 weeks
Ultrasound	(i) 6–8 weeks (for determining gestational dates) (ii) 10 weeks onwards for diagnosis
Fetoscopy	18 weeks
Radiology	16 weeks
Fetal blood sampling	18 weeks

Council [19]. In order to evaluate preconception vitamin supplementation in an unbiased way, this trial has four subgroups for treatment, one of which consists of a vitamin-free regimen. Women taking part in the trial are given detailed explanations by a counsellor, and a printed booklet, to explain the purpose and structure of the investigation. However, it is the inclusion of a 'placebo' group which has attracted strong criticism including much from the medical profession. We cover the approaches towards screening for neural tube defects later in this chapter (p. 34).

2.4 PRENATAL DIAGNOSIS

Some principles of prenatal diagnosis have already been discussed. The main reason for considering such investigation is that it provides the grounds for terminating a pregnancy if the fetus is shown to be affected. Some couples, however, will not wish to take up this option and yet will request prenatal investigations. Every situation must be assessed in its own right but there are good reasons why prenatal diagnosis could be beneficial even if termination will not be considered, not least of which is the reassurance that can be given if the result is normal. The main approaches to prenatal diagnosis are listed in Table 2.5 which also indicates the stage of pregnancy when they can be useful.

As well as offering the possibility of prenatal diagnosis, the counsellor must inform the couple of the degree of risk inherent in the various procedures. There has been great experience of genetic amniocentesis over the past 15 years and the risk of the procedure causing an abortion is now less than 0.5 per cent [20]. However, the risk increases with repeat amniocenteses [20] or when there is a twin pregnancy [21]. In contrast, there is less experience of the chorionic villus sampling procedures and the risk of causing abortion is clearly higher. In an early study of 600 chorionic villus sampling procedures, Hogge *et al.* [7] showed that the overall risk of aborting due to the procedure was 6.3% but that this was lower if sampling was restricted to between 9 and 12 weeks' gestation. An international survey [22] recently reported an abortion risk of 2.5% if one sampling is carried out but of 8.6% if repeat testing is undertaken. A still more recent assessment quotes data on more than 30 000 chorionic villus samplings worldwide and reports a fetal loss of 3.7% [23]. Fetoscopy and fetal tissue sampling are high risk procedures; abortion rates of 6.8%, 7.9% and 16% have been observed following procedures for fetal blood sampling, for detailed visualization of external abnormalities and for fetal skin biopsy respectively [5]. It is for this reason that detailed ultrasound scanning is now the preferred method of identification of fetal abnormalities and is also the preferred ancillary technique for fetal blood sampling. Clearly, any couple who have procedures recommended as options must be told of, and must consider carefully, all of the risks. The situation in which a couple challenge a doctor's failure to offer prenatal diagnostic tests, say of chromosomes when the mother is aged 34, would be considerably influenced for the better if they were properly informed of the relative balance of risk.

The management of the couple who have chosen to have prenatal diagnosis carried out needs great sensitivity and it is important that the major issues have been discussed *prior to* the start of the pregnancy. If they have expressed a wish that the pregnancy be terminated in the event of the fetus being abnormal, then there is a great need for counselling and support both at the time of the termination and for a considerable time afterwards. It must not be forgotten that the estimated date of delivery of the baby, which would represent a fixed date in the parents'

calendar, will be a difficult landmark for the couple; counselling should be made available then.

Couples who do not wish an abnormal baby to be terminated are likely to need a great degree of further support, both in the pregnancy and afterwards. It may be that their wish to avoid termination was taken on religious grounds and that support and backup is, therefore, available from their church. Too often, however, the agencies that encourage couples against termination of an abnormal pregnancy are either unwilling or unable to provide support towards the care of a handicapped baby. In these circumstances, the couple will turn to the medical advisers who looked after the pregnancy, to paediatricians and to those who gave the genetic counselling information.

How can the doctor gain experience of counselling in such difficult situations? There are few opportunities to learn except by experience or by sharing sessions with those with counselling skills. Perhaps the doctor has experienced the sadness of having a handicapped baby, or has had to consider the question of terminating an abnormal pregnancy, and can, therefore, empathize with the couple and appreciate the long process involved in the recovery of psychological stability. The counsellor in these situations must not say 'I know how you feel' unless he or she has experienced exactly the same problems; otherwise that statement cannot really be truthful even though it was intended to be a kindly remark. Often, couples do not wish attempts at kindness. They want to make their own decision and they need professional advisers who can answer *their* own questions, not hypothetical ones. It is well to emphasize that couples often need emotional help over and above any that can be given by professionals. Timely referral to a 'self-help' group consisting of individuals who have themselves confronted similar options may be the most supportive decision that the genetic counsellor has made (see p. 24 and [12–14]).

Responsibility for genetic counselling does not end with a termination of pregnancy, or even with a further successful one. Future developments in genetic research may well lead to better ways of managing the high-risk family and, therefore, genetic records must be maintained in order to provide rapid recall of those families for whom the situation has changed. An inevitable result of this need has been the development of *genetic registers* which are updated and altered as families extend and as research techniques open new opportunities.

(a) Genetic registers

The first genetic registers were developed in the early 1970s so that families with high genetic risks could be recalled at appropriate times for updating the available genetic information [24]. The conditions most suitable for such approaches were the dominant conditions such as Huntington's disease or Marfan's syndrome or the X-linked recessives such as Duchenne muscular dystrophy. The parents of a boy who was diagnosed as having Duchenne muscular dystrophy might not be considering having any further family. However, such boys might well have young sisters who could be carriers of the Duchenne gene. By recording the family details so that the sister could be counselled when aged 15 years or so, it would be possible to ensure that the most up-to-date genetic information and investigations were available to the family. Such registers have become exceptionally important because there have been so many recent developments in Duchenne muscular dystrophy research. A family counselled 10 years ago could only have been told of the theoretical risks to sisters of affected boys with the possibility that measurement of creatine kinase levels could have detected some – but no means all – of the carriers. By using

molecular genetic techniques in several members of such families, it is now possible to identify or exclude those who are carriers with a much greater degree of certainty and, thus early prenatal diagnosis can often be offered.

Because of the nature of genetic information and the large numbers in the family that may be involved, it is likely that most genetic registers will be computerized. This will make recall of a family much simpler and speedier but clearly problems may arise when such sensitive information is on a computerized system. There must be great care to respect the confidentiality of each individual member of the affected family. The consultand (i.e. the individual who has come up for genetic counselling) may have given information about other family members who do not wish this to be discussed. How is such information confirmed? Should such information be stored in a computerized system? All such considerations must be tackled before a computerized genetic register is established. In the United Kingdom, the Data Protection Act 1984 has established, *inter alia*, that an individual must have access to information that is stored on a computer about himself or herself and this should ensure that care is taken in storing personal details of different members of a family. Full details about the practical implications of the Act can be obtained from the Data Protection Registrar (Springfield House, Water Lane, Wilmslow, Cheshire SK9 5AX, UK). However, the computer only provides a better way of storing data and it should be remembered that hospital records of one patient may contain information about other members of his/her family who are at risk from the same genetic disease.

The dilemma may be illustrated by considering a hypothetical example in the field of Huntington's disease. Although this condition rarely occurs in the paediatric years, it does have implications which must be considered by potential parents in affected

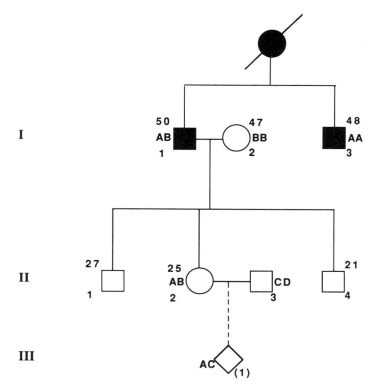

Fig. 2.2 Four generations of a family in which Huntington's disease occurs. The generations with living individuals are numbered I, II and III. Just above each symbol is the age of the subject. For convenience, individuals in a generation are numbered consecutively. Affected males are blacked in squares, affected females are blacked in circles. In this family II, 2, a female, has asked for both presymptomatic detection and prenatal diagnosis tests. To comply with her wish it is necessary to test the polymorphisms at the G8 locus, close to the Huntington's gene, in her father I, 1, and mother I, 2. In addition, her paternal uncle, I, 3, must be tested so that it is known whether the Huntington's gene is on the paternal chromosome with the 'A' or the 'B' form of the genetic marker (in this case it is on the chromosome with the A marker). Given all the information, it is shown here that the woman, II, 2, (and her fetus) both have a high probability of having the Huntington's gene – a situation that would only be changed if there had been a crossover between the HC locus and the G8 locus (a 5% risk). If the affected relative, I, 3, refused to be tested then the presymptomatic diagnosis of II, 2, would not be possible but prenatal testing to confirm a high risk of HC or to exclude it in the fetus would be an option.

families. If a 50-year-old man has the condition and is in hospital on a long-term basis, then a son or daughter might attend for genetic counselling. They might wish for both preclinical testing for themselves and for prenatal testing in any future pregnancies. Since the tests depend upon linkage analysis, the possibility of providing such testing might depend not only on the examination of blood from the affected man but also of that from a sibling of his who also has the condition. The sampling of the relative is not possible if he does not wish to be tested. However, confidential information about that affected person may be stored in the notes of the index consultand and this has been obtained without permission (Fig. 2.2 shows a worked example). After some consideration of these aspects, a Working Party on the Clinical Genetic Services in Scotland has decided that it is, for the present, preferable to have genetic registers stored on microcomputers in the four Scottish regional genetic centres rather than to have one centralized system containing data from the whole country [25]. There must be safeguards for the confidentiality of the individual at all levels. The person who controls a genetic register is responsible to all the families for maintaining correct information in a form which achieves this.

(b) Genetic screening

This term can be used in many different situations but generally implies the routine screening of high-risk groups for the most likely genetic conditions. For example, the risk of having a baby with Down's syndrome increases as the age of the mother increases (Table 2.6). Somewhere between age 35 and 40, the risk increases to above 1% and it is within these age limits that either amniocentesis or chorion villus sampling to detect the chromosome abnormality is considered.

Clearly, the decision to screen for Down's syndrome will depend, amongst other factors, on the attitude to that handicap in a

Table 2.6 Age-related risks of Down's syndrome

Maternal age (years)	Risk of Down's syndrome (rate per 1000 births)
<20	0.69
20–24	0.91
25–29	0.64
30–34	1.83
35–39	4.34
40–44	14.62

community and on the resources available for both obstetric and cytogenetic investigation. Some couples may be particularly anxious about the condition and may request prenatal testing when their risk is not as high as the usual level at which the tests are considered. The doctor involved in counselling must not, then, be authoritative and refuse testing. Rather he should appreciate that the request shows a need for counselling and he should either look into the family history himself or should refer the patient to a genetic centre. The doctor who finds this referral difficult should consider what he would do if the baby subsequently born did suffer from Down's syndrome – and he might further consider the legal implications which are discussed in Chapter 26.

Routine screening is often carried out to identify fetuses with neural tube defects in those areas of the world with a high incidence. Scotland and Northern Ireland are among such high-risk areas and both have programmes which screen for the disorders in pregnancy. The Scottish system is organized on an area basis and, in the south-east of the country, blood is taken from virtually all pregnant women at exactly 16 weeks' gestation. Information about the screening is made available in antenatal clinics so that women who wish to opt out of the service may do so. The blood sample taken at 16 weeks is tested for the level of alpha-fetoprotein and a repeat sample is taken at 17 weeks if a predetermined cut-off point is exceeded.

If both 16- and 17-week samples show abnormally high levels, then careful ultrasonography is undertaken to identify anencephaly or gross spina bifida, and this is followed by amniocentesis if necessary. The mothers of fetuses in whom an abnormality is discovered by these procedures can then be offered the option of a termination of the pregnancy. For a brief but informative review of the international workshop on the subject of maternal serum alpha-fetoprotein screening for neural tube defects, see Fuhrmann *et al.* [26]. These authors concluded that such screening can detect over 90% of babies with anencephaly and over 70% of cases of open spina bifida. They considered that screening should be undertaken if the birth prevalence of neural tube defects in a population exceeds 1 in 1000.

Some prenatal screening programmes now also take into account the recent observation that women carrying fetuses affected with Down's syndrome tend to have a lower level of alpha-fetoprotein than do the mothers of healthy babies. Clearly there is a great need for counselling at the time of these tests. It is most important that easily understandable information as to routine blood testing and the need for screening is presented to all pregnant women.

(c) Other causes of congenital handicap

When a baby is delivered with multiple congenital malformations, the cause may be genetic but the possibility of other causes must be considered. A variety of environmental factors may influence the fetus, especially if they operate very soon after conception. In general, the organs which are abnormal and the degree of abnormality will indicate the time of gestation and the agent responsible. For example, thalidomide treatment of the mother at around 20–30 days gestation will cause limb defects in around 20% of exposed pregnancies. Congenital rubella or other viral infections which may affect the fetus must also be considered. Therefore, genetic counselling must include a careful history to check for any teratogenic influences which may have been operating, especially in early pregnancy. Two further examples will indicate the wide range of adverse influences which may cause damage to the developing fetus. First, excessive exposure to X-rays during the pregnancy will increase the risk of microcephaly significantly and X-ray-exposed fetuses will have a higher incidence of acute leukaemia in childhood than will non-exposed individuals. Secondly, it has been shown that treatment of the mother's threatened abortion with diethyl stilboestrol in the first trimester of pregnancy will greatly increase the risk of adenocarcinoma of the vagina in teenage females who were thereby exposed *'in utero'*. Good counselling of couples who have had abnormal babies, thus, requires a sound genetic approach, careful attention to details of the history and an understanding of the fact that cause and effects may be widely separated in time.

2.5 SUMMARY

In a brief chapter it is impossible to summarize all the developments in medical genetics which have influenced present-day practice in genetic counselling and prenatal diagnosis; moreover, the rapid developments in this field indicate that present techniques and approaches will soon be superseded. It is essential that the doctor providing genetic counselling is up to date. It is equally important that the process of counselling be provided skilfully in the light of background knowledge of the emotional responses to handicap which prospective parents are likely to show. The decisions made by patients in whose families there is a genetic disease may not be the decisions that the doctor anticipated or wished – but they must be made from a position of information and understanding.

REFERENCES

1. Breg, W.R. and Ward, P.H. (1973) Chromosome five p-syndrome, in *Birth Defects Atlas and Compendium* (ed. D. Bergsma), Williams & Wilkins, Baltimore, p. 248.
2. Brock, D.J.H. and Sutcliffe, R.G. (1972) Alpha-fetoprotein in the antenatal diagnosis of anencephaly and spina bifida. *Lancet*, **ii**, 197.
3. Brock, D.J.H., Scrimgeour, J.B., Bolton, A.E. *et al.* (1975) Effect of gestational age on screening for neural tube defects by maternal plasma AFP measurements. *Lancet*, **ii**, 195.
4. Donald, I. and Abdulla, U. (1967) Ultrasonics in obstetrics and gynaecology. *Br. J. Radiol.*, **40**, 604.
5. Golbus, M., Antsaklis, A. and Bang, J. (1984) The status of fetoscopy and fetal tissue sampling. *Prenatal Diag.*, **4**, 79.
6. Ropers, H.H. (1987) Use of DNA probes for diagnosis and prevention of inherited disorders. *Eur. J. Clin. Invest.*, **17**, 475.
7. Hogge, W.A., Schonberg, S.A. and Golbus, M.S. (1985) Prenatal diagnosis by chorion villus sampling: lessons of the first 600 cases. *Prenatal Diag.*, **5**, 393.
8. Gibson, F.S. (ed.) (1987) *Abortion in Debate*, St Andrew Press, Edinburgh.
9. Scottish Home and Health Department (1987) Abortion statistics. *Health Bull. (Edinb.)*, **45**, 277.
10. OPCS (1987), *Abortion Statistics 1986*, Series AB, No. 13, HMSO, London.
11. Gillon, R. (1986) *Philosophical Medical Ethics*, John Wiley, Chichester.
12. Davis, J.A. (1985) The 'Baby Brown' case and Dr Arthur verdict. *J. Med. Ethics*, **11**, 159.
13. Kennedy, I. (1985) Response to Professor Davis. *J. Med. Ethics*, **11**, 159. See Pallister, D. (1985) Gaol for father of Down's baby. *The Guardian*, 16 March.
14. Barker, D., Wright, E., Nguyen, K. *et al.* (1987) Evidence that the gene for neurofibromatosis is in the pericentric region of chromosome 17. *Science*, **236**, 1100.
15. Fryer, A.E., Chalmers, A., Connor, J.M. *et al.* (1987) Evidence that the gene for tuberous sclerosis is on chromosome 9. *Lancet*, **i**, 659.
16. McKusick, V.A. (1988) *Mendelian Inheritance in Man – Catalogs of Autosomal Dominant, Autosomal Recessive, and X-linked Phenotypes*, 8th edn, Johns Hopkins University Press, Baltimore.
17. Habel, A. (1974) Typus Edinburgensis. *Pediatrics*, **53**, 288.
18. Smithells, R.W., Sheppard, S., Schorah, C.J. *et al.* (1981) Apparent prevention of neural tube defects by vitamin supplementation. *Arch. Dis. Child.*, **56**, 911.
19. Wald, N.J. and Polani, P.E. (1984) Neural tube defects and vitamins: the need for a randomised clinical trial. *Br. J. Obstet. Gynaecol.*, **91**, 516.
20. Simpson, N.E., Daltaire, L., Miller, J.R. *et al.* (1976) Prenatal diagnosis of genetic disease in Canada; report of a collaborative study. *Can. Med. Assoc. J.*, **115**, 739.
21. Palle, C., Anderson, J.W., Tabor, A. *et al.* (1983) Increased risk of abortion after genetic amniocentesis in twin pregnancies. *Prenatal Diag.*, **3**, 83.
22. Brombati, B., Kuliev, A., Jackson, L. *et al.* (1986) Risk evaluation in chorionic villus sampling. *Prenatal Diag.*, **6**, 451.
23. Jackson, L. (1987) *Chorionic Villus Sampling Newsletter*, 24 November.
24. Emery, A.E.H., Elliott, D., Moores, M. and Smith, C. (1974) A genetic register system (RAPID). *J. Med. Genet.*, **11**, 145.
25. Knox, J. (1987) *Clinical Genetic Services in Scotland: Report of a Working Party of the National Medical Consultative Committee*, Scottish Home and Health Department.
26. Fuhrmann, W., Boppart, I. and Brock, D. (1985) Maternal alphafetoprotein screening for neural tube defects. *Prenatal Diag.* **5**, 77.

FURTHER READING

Connor, J.M. and Ferguson-Smith, M.A. (1984) *Essential Medical Genetics*, Blackwell Scientific Publications, Oxford.

Emery, A.E.H. (1984) *An Introduction to Recombinant DNA*, John Wiley, Chichester.

Harper, P.S. (1988) *Practical Genetic Counselling*, 3rd edn, Wright, Guildford.

Winston, R.M.L. (1987) Why a ban on embryo research would be a tragedy. *Br. Med. J.*, **295**, 1501.

CHAPTER 3

Intoxication *in utero*

Eunice J. Larson

The effects of drug abuse on the developing fetus have been known since the time of Hippocrates, who wrote of 'uterine suffocation' caused by the use of opium [1]. The association between the symptoms of opium and of alcohol withdrawal and abnormal infants, including infant deaths, was well documented in the nineteenth century.

Most drug abusers use multiple drugs, and the majority of pregnant women have little insight into the extent or significance of their drug taking during early pregnancy. The organizers of a voluntary methadone programme involving 13 pregnant morphine addicts, who had a close relationship with their medical caretakers, tested urine samples from the patients during their treatment; the drug screens disclosed that four women were concomitantly using benzodiazepines and that one was positive for amphetamines [2]. It is often difficult to obtain a precise history – drug abusers are notorious for distortion of memory and prevarication. The obstetric history, including that of spontaneous abortions, is difficult to assess for the same reasons. Prospective studies are few; those that are undertaken are generally clinically orientated, dealing with drug-abusing mothers, their infants and their children to the age of 5 years. Deaths are documented but are generally not described in detail; autopsy data on the offspring of drug abusers are sparse.

The pattern of drug abuse is strongly influenced by the price and availability of drugs and by current fads or trends. In the early 1900s opium was replaced by morphine among the addicted. By the mid-1950s morphine was, in turn, replaced by heroin. At the present time, cocaine is becoming the most commonly abused drug followed by phencyclidine (PCP), heroin, marijuana, methadone, amphetamines, benzodiazepines and barbiturates. Alcohol and cigarettes generally have not been listed as drugs of abuse but their respective effects on offspring have been well documented. Table 3.1 lists the drugs which have been reported as being associated with withdrawal symptoms in neonates; the figures stem from child abuse report forms collected over a 6-month period in Los Angeles County, California, in 1986.

Experiments on laboratory animals have demonstrated a great deal of variation in the teratogenic effect of drugs on a fetus. Warkany described the problems as follows:

… The effects of a drug differ greatly before, during, and after organogenesis. A drug often adversely affects the embryo before organogenesis and leads to its death; in late pregnancy it may cause disease or death.

Table 3.1 Drugs associated with withdrawal symptoms in neonates

Drug used	Drug frequency (no. of cases)
Amphetamines	2
Cocaine	279
Codeine	9
Enobarbital	1
Heroin	29
Marijuana	22
Methadone	4
Morphine	5
Opiates	10
PCP	63
Phenobarbital	1
Thorazine	1
Alcohol	27
Unknown	44

Source: Los Angeles County Neonatal Withdrawal Reports, January to June 1986. Based on approximately 150 000 births per year.

Even within the period of organogenesis, different malformations are produced by administration of drug on different days of gestation, since the effects depend to a great extent on the developmental stage of the embryo ... Experiments in animals that carry more than one young demonstrate that a teratogen applied to the mother may produce different types of malformations in different members of the litter ... [3]

The subject of the pathology of the human offspring of drug abusers is similarly confusing. It is apparent that there are two types of abnormalities – morphological malformations and behavioural abnormalities. Periodic intoxication, followed by periods of withdrawal, occur *in utero* as a reflection of the mother's level of intoxication. The concentration of a given drug may be less than, equal to or higher than it is in the mother's bloodstream. Metabolic enzymes are produced in the fetal liver and drug metabolites are excreted by the fetus.

Alcohol has a unique distribution in the fetus. Alcohol (ethanol) crosses the placental bloodstream and gains access to the fetal circulation. So long as there is a measurable concentration of maternal blood alcohol, a relatively low concentration is present in the amniotic fluid. By contrast, a relatively high concentration of alcohol remains in the amniotic fluid following its elimination from the maternal bloodstream. The fetus, thus, remains exposed to alcohol for longer periods of time – and in potentially higher concentrations – than does the mother [4].

Drug-abusing mothers tend to have certain shared characteristics. Among these are the tendency to have received no prenatal care, to have had several spontaneous abortions, to have abused drugs for at least 5 years and to be in their mid-twenties. They have a higher incidence of anaemia and of infections and they run a higher risk of contracting hepatitis and the acquired immunodeficiency syndrome (AIDS). The onset of labour is premature and the babies are generally small for their gestational age.

There is a high incidence of meconium aspiration in the neonates and ventilatory patterns during sleep are abnormal [5]. Infants of addicted mothers may either have withdrawal symptoms at birth or the symptoms may be delayed as long as 14–21 days after delivery. The severity of the fetus' or infant's malformations or clinical course appears to be influenced by the concentration of the drug (or drugs) in the maternal bloodstream. Chromosomal abnormalities have not been identified as being associated with any of the drugs commonly abused.

Hospital personnel who are experienced in caring for babies with withdrawal symptoms are usually able to identify the drug causing withdrawal by the clinical signs and symptoms in the baby. The differences may be related to the time of onset after birth or there may be variations in the pattern of such

Table 3.2 Signs and symptoms of drug withdrawal in neonates

Symptom	Amphetamine	Alcohol	Cocaine	Cigarettes	Benzodiazipines	Barbiturates	Heroin	Methadone	Phencyclidine	Marijuana	Opium
Spontaneous abortions and stillbirths		+	+	+	+		+				+
Prematurity		+	+	+			+		+		+
In utero growth retardation		+	+	+			+		+	+	+
Low APGARS			+		+						
Growth retardation		+	+	+			+		+		+
Meconium aspiration			+				+				
Respiratory distress		+	+		+	+	+	+			+
Withdrawal	+	+	+			+	+		+		+
Lethargy	+		+		+				+		
Jittery	+	+	+			+			+	+	+
Hyperactivity							+		+		+
Tremulousness	+	+			+	+					
Tremors		+					+		+		
Poor fine motor coordination		+					+	+	+		+
Weak suck		+			+	+					+
Excessive crying		++	++			+	+				+
Sneezing							+				+
Poor feeding							+				
Gastrointestinal disturbance							V/D		V/D		
Sweating		+	+				+	+			
Sleep disorganization			+			+	+		+		
Developmental delays	+	+	+				+				
Seizures			+			+	+	+	+		+
Behavioural abnormalities		+	+		+		+				
Sudden infant death			+	+			+	+			+
Malformations		+	+				+		+		

V/D, vomiting/diarrhoea.

symptoms as staring, sneezing, excessive sweating, depressed respiratory status or miotic pupils. A comparison of the signs and symptoms provoked by the common drugs of abuse demonstrates similarities that are summarized in Table 3.2.

Death may be due to the damaging effects of drugs on the placenta, on the fetus or on the newborn infant. Premature birth, perinatal hypoxia and meconium aspiration are all recognized causes of death in these newborns. Respiratory distress occurs early in the presence of many of the abused drugs and may lead to death. The sudden infant death syndrome (SIDS) is estimated to be five to ten times greater in incidence in these babies [6]. Drug-addicted parents or other caretakers are reported as being responsible for an alarming numbers of deaths resulting from physical abuse or neglect [7]. In evaluating these data it is imperative that one takes into account the fact that prematurity requiring hospitalization for an extended period of time has been associated with respiratory distress syndrome, sudden infant death syndrome and with child abuse.

Urine drug screening is now ordered with greater frequency than was the case several years ago. The statutory indications in California include a maternal history of drug abuse, a mother having a positive toxicology screen during labour, an infant demonstrating a positive toxicology screen, an infant with symptoms consistent with drug withdrawal as well as a positive history or clinical findings and history indicating the diagnosis of fetal alcohol syndrome. Infants in any of these categories must be reported to the Department of Children's Services. During the postnatal period, a paediatrician must order a toxicological urine screen on any neonate that is born to a mother with an acknowledged history of drug or alcohol abuse, born to a mother with signs and symptoms suggestive of drug or alcohol abuse or one that demonstrates signs consistent with drug withdrawal. These are as follows:

(1) High pitched cry.
(2) Hyperactive Moro reflex.
(3) Poor sleeping.
(4) Tremors.
(5) Increased muscle tone.
(6) Generalized seizures.
(7) Frantic sucking of fists.
(8) Poor feeding.
(9) Regurgitation.
(10) Projectile vomiting.
(11) Loose or watery stools.
(12) Sneezing.
(13) Dehydration.
(14) Nasal stuffiness.
(15) Sweating.
(16) Excoriation of nose, knees or chin.

Health care team members must also notify the clinical social worker responsible for newborns in the hospital and must file California Department of Justice forms for suspected child abuse [8].

The analytical procedures most commonly used in the laboratory are the enzyme multiplied immunoassay technique (EMIT), radioimmunoassay (RIA), thin-layer chromatography (TLC), gas chromatography (GC), and gas chromatography/mass spectrometry (GC/MS) [9]. The drug groups sought in most laboratories routinely by these procedures are amphetamines, barbiturates, benzodiazepines, cannabinoids, cocaine, methaqualone, opiates and phencyclidine. A screen test is usually performed, and, when this is positive, a confirmatory test method follows. The methodology used will vary among laboratories. Tests are undertaken for alcohol and serum glucose in suspected alcohol intoxication.

A brief discussion of the effects of each of the drugs follows.

3.1 ALCOHOL

Alcohol is one of the most damaging teratogens and it is also the drug which is most widely used in the world. Its serious effects on newborns have been recognized since biblical times but the consequence of drinking during pregnancy were not fully appreciated until the early 1970s when studies by Jones, Smith and their colleagues began to appear in the English language literature [10–12].

Infants with the 'fetal alcohol syndrome' demonstrate a diagnostic triad of growth deficiency, mental retardation and facial abnormalities. These signs vary from mild to severe and they are found in the offspring of women who consume alcohol during pregnancy irrespective of whether the women are 'social drinkers' or chronic alcoholics. Table 3.3 summarizes the major features and associated features of the fetal alcohol syndrome.

Of the diagnostic triad, it is the facial features which are most commonly present; they may be recognized with a high degree of accuracy throughout childhood and, less often, in adult life. A study of photographs and morphometric analysis of a group of patients undertaken by judges from different training backgrounds located in two countries concluded that the facial features are recognizable and could be differentiated from a large group of age-matched patients suffering from other conditions. The alcoholic appearances include a short palpebral fissure, a long midface relative to an approximately normal nasal length, a long, flat philtrum, a thin upper lip and a flat midface [13].

All children suffering from the fetal alcohol syndrome show evidence of intrauterine growth retardation and of postnatal growth deficiency or 'failure to thrive'. The head circumference remains below the third percentile and their IQs are less than 70. Fine motor dysfunction – tremulousness, weak grasp and poor hand-eye coordination – are often seen and gross motor dysfunction is commonly present. They are irritable as babies and the children demonstrate hyperactivity as they grow older.

Spontaneous abortions occur early in gestation and the number of stillbirths is

Table 3.3 Signs and symptoms in the fetal alcohol syndrome

MAJOR FEATURES
Facial characteristics

Eyes:	Short palpebral fissures
Nose:	Short, upturned
	Hypoplastic philtrum
Mouth:	Thinned upper vermillion of lip
	Retrognathia in infancy
	Micrognathia or relative prognathia in adolescence
Maxilla:	Hypoplastic

Growth
  Intrauterine growth retardation
  Postnatal growth delay ('failure to thrive')

Central nervous system dysfunction
Neurological
  Microcephaly
  Poor coordination (fine motor and gross motor)
  Hypotonia
Intellectual
  IQ less than 70
Behavioural
  Irritability in infancy
  Hyperactivity in childhood

FREQUENT ASSOCIATED FEATURES

Eyes:	Ptosis, strabismus, epicanthal folds
Mouth:	Prominent lateral palatine ridges
Cardiac:	Murmurs, especially in early childhood, usually atrial septal defect
Genital:	Labial hypoplasia
Cutaneous:	Haemangiomas
Skeletal:	Aberrant palmar creases, pectus excavatum

OCCASIONAL ASSOCIATED FEATURES

Eyes:	Myopia, clinical microphthalmia, blepharophimosis
Ears:	Poor formed concha, posterior rotation
Mouth:	Cleft lip or cleft palate, small teeth with faulty enamel
Cardiac:	Ventricular septal defect, anomalies of great vessels, tetralogy of Fallot
Urogenital:	Hypospadias, renal anomalies
Cutaneous:	Hirsutism in infancy
Skeletal:	Limited joint movements of fingers and elbows, nail hypoplasia, radioulnar synostosis, pectus carinatum, bifid xiphoid, scoliosis
Muscular:	Hernias of diaphragm, umbilicus or inguinal region, diastasis recti

increased as compared with those born to non-drinking control mothers. The neonates show transient hypoglycaemia and hyperbilirubinaemia. They are tremulous and have a weak suck. Respiratory distress is a common problem in the neonatal period, and upper airway obstruction due either to choanal stenosis, to a small nasopharyngeal vault or to a laryngeal web has been described [14]. Neonatal mortality is estimated to be as much as eight times greater than that in a control group.

Central nervous system malformations have been identified at autopsy; these include absence of the corpus callosum, an incompletely developed cerebral cortex, aberrant neuronal migration resulting in multiple heterotopias, rudimentary cerebellum, dysplastic brainstem and hydrocephalus secondary to obstruction of the foramina of Lushka and Magendie by leptomeningeal neuroglial heterotopia [11, 15]. Atrial septal defect is the most common cardiac malformation followed by ventricular septal defect, anomalies of the great vessels and tetralogy of Fallot [11, 16]. Renal anomalies include unilateral hydronephrosis, renal hypoplasia and crossed fused ectopia [17]. One patient has been reported with sacral myelomeningocele additional to many of the other malformations which are common in the fetal alcohol syndrome.

3.2 COCAINE

Cocaine has become a serious problem in the USA in recent years. It is estimated that the incidence of withdrawal symptoms in neonates has increased by more than 400% in Los Angeles County and in New York City over the 1-year period between 1985 and 1986.

The drug is used intranasally, intravenously and in cigarette form. It is readily available, relatively inexpensive and highly addictive. Newer forms of cocaine are very concentrated and produce a 'high' (euphoria)

in less than a minute. The drug increases the pulse rate, blood pressure and oxygen consumption and has been associated with sudden death in adults. Myocardial toxicity and central nervous system haemorrhage secondary to sudden elevation of blood pressure are well-documented causes of death in adults [18].

Cocaine is used by all socioeconomic classes and it has rapidly become the most important of the drugs taken by polydrug users. It is as uncommon for abusers of cocaine to be using it solely as it is with any other drugs.

Experimental work involving lambs *in utero* has demonstrated that cocaine, like most other abused drugs, crosses the placenta readily and causes periods of intoxication and withdrawal in the fetus. High concentrations of cocaine can be identified in the brain [19].

Maternal abuse of cocaine results in a high incidence of spontaneous abortions, stillbirths and prematurity [20, 21]. Cocaine can precipitate labour and delivery within hours of being used; abruptio placenta is a common cause of premature delivery. The babies are small for their gestational age, they frequently aspirate meconium and often show respiratory distress. They are lethargic and catatonic at birth and demonstrate impaired visual attention.

A review of autopsies suggests that this form of respiratory distress is refractory to the usual ventilation therapy; a number of these patients have been treated with high-frequency jet ventilation therapy and many have been considered for extracorporeal membrane oxygenation therapy. An unusual autopsy finding reviewed by the author was that of a sterile, healed pulmonary abscess involving most of the right upper lobe of a 6-hour-old premature infant delivered by a mother without prenatal care. Several other cases in the author's experience have died as a result of overwhelming Gram-negative bacterial pneumonia despite intensive treatment with antibiotics. As many as 15% of the babies born to cocaine abusers succumb to the sudden infant death syndrome [22]. Abnormal ventilatory patterns during sleep have been demonstrated in a study of 27 infants of drug abusers [5] – prolonged apnoea is known to be associated with the sudden infant death syndrome.

Death has been documented following intracerebral haemorrhage in a baby whose mother had used a high dose of cocaine immediately before she delivered her baby precipitously and prematurely [22]. It is known that cocaine intoxication may cause microinfarcts in adult brains and it is speculated that fibrosis of the germinal matrix region of the brain of infants and children will be found in those born to mothers who have used high doses of cocaine periodically throughout pregnancy; episodes of high blood pressure associated with intrauterine cocaine intoxication may be the cause of seizures which are reported to occur after the newborn period.

A number of congenital malformations have been identified. These include two cases with renal anomalies, one demonstrating the 'prune belly' syndrome characterized by hydronephrosis, hydroureters, dilated bladder and abnormal, redundant abdominal skin [20] and one with a horseshoe kidney. Single cases of amniotic band syndrome, cerebro-hepato-renal syndrome (Zellweger) and generalized anasarca (hydrops) have been seen by the author. Congenital heart defects which have been described include transposition of the great vessels and a hypoplastic right heart. Skull defects – including exencephaly, parietal bone defects and ossification centre delays – and interparietal encephalocele occur in addition to intracerebral haemorrhage and infarction [21].

Some babies of cocaine-abusing mothers are asymptomatic during the neonatal period. Following discharge from the hospital, they become irritable, jittery and cry inconsolably, day and night, for weeks. This behaviour, coupled with the risk of infection with the virus of acquired immunodeficiency disease (AIDS), is making it increasingly difficult to provide foster care for these babies (see Chapter 23 for further discussion). Jitteriness persists and development delays are common. The children respond poorly to frustration and to stressful situations; their behaviour abnormalities continue into school age.

3.3 HEROIN

Until the 1970s, heroin was the drug most commonly used in pregnancy. Symptoms of withdrawal in the neonates have been well recognized and include coarse, flapping tremors, irritability, watery stools, a shrill cry, muscle rigidity of the extremities, skin abrasion, sneezing, hyperpyrexia, vomiting, hyperactivity, excessive sweating and yawning [1, 23].

Fetal death, stillbirths, neonatal death, intrauterine growth retardation, sudden infant death, meconium aspiration, respiratory depression and hyperventilation are described. Prior to modern ventilator therapy, as many as 25% of affected infants died as a result of the complications of respiratory distress. Respiratory distress continues to be a clinical management problem. The babies are poor feeders and have sleep disturbances. Seizures have been reported but are more common in cases of methadone withdrawal.

Congenital malformations are uncommon but have been reported. One case showing an umbilical hernia and severe divergent strabismus and a second, lethal case of a child appearing to have Down's syndrome with severe talipes equinovarus deformities and bilateral polycystic kidneys have been described [24]. Instances of cerebral atrophy, abnormal lamination of the lateral geniculate, hydrocephalus due to aqueductal stenosis, partial midline fusion of the cerebellum, polymicrogyria, coarctation of the aorta, persistent left superior vena cava draining into the coronary sinus, patent ductus arteriosus, hypertelorism, low-set ears, wide-spaced nipples, congenital dislocation of the hips and hydrops have also been seen by the author and her colleagues [25].

Children of heroin-abusing mothers are hyperactive, have temper tantrums and show a low tolerance to frustration. They have difficulty with fine motor coordination and suffer from speech and language delays, bilateral hearing deficits, attention deficits and learning disabilities. Impulsivity and the inability to interact socially lead to adolescent behavioural problems.

3.4 PHENCYCLIDINE

Phencyclidine (PCP) is inexpensive, is easy to manufacture and is a popular drug among pregnant teenagers. It is generally used in conjunction with other drugs, but there have been cases of phencyclidine being used solely or primarily.

Infants are not delivered prematurely and they are appropriate for gestational age in weight and height. Shortly after birth, they become jittery and hypotonic. They are irritable and have episodes of vomiting and diarrhoea. Attention spans are impaired and they have depressed grasp and rooting reflexes. Miotic pupils, decreased joint mobility and increased brachial reflexes are observed less frequently [4]. Fine motor coordination is poorly developed and affected infants often cannot say words at 20–24 months of age. While they grow in length, the development of their head circumference is severely delayed and more than 50% of these babies are microcephalic. Their IQ begins to fall at about 1 year; PCP babies have a larger proportion of low IQs than is found in exposure to other groups of drugs.

Four cases with congenital malformations had the following findings – one case with microcephaly [26], one patient with osteogenesis imperfecta, one infant who had unilateral renal dysplasia and a baby with Potter's facies, hydronephrosis and pulmonary hypoplasia [27].

PCP-abusing parents are difficult to manage in detoxification programmes; they have perpetrated a number of bizarre instances of child abuse and brutal murder.

3.5 THE RIGHTS OF THE FETUS AND THE ABUSED CHILD

Neonates exhibiting the signs of drug withdrawal become the ward of the legal enforcement system in the United States. A multi-disciplinary team of doctors, nurses, social workers and law enforcement officers is involved in the care and in the custodial planning for the child. The goal of the judicial system in the United States is evaluation of the home environment, provision of medical care, including detoxification, for the mother and the return of the infant or child to the nuclear family. Members of the multidisciplinary teams have been overwhelmed by the increasing numbers of cases of intrauterine intoxication and consequent withdrawal symptoms. Neither facilities nor funding appear to be adequate for an increase of 450% over a 2-year period (1984–86), especially if the estimate be accepted that as many as 50% of true cases are not being identified in the hospital.

'Boarder babies' are becoming a relatively new custodial problem for hospitals in New York City. Most are the offspring of cocaine-abusing mothers, and a significant number have been abandoned in the hospital for as long as 5 months [28]. Foster parents are less inclined to accept known drug abusers' babies because of the high incidence – approximately 50% – of AIDS and because they are difficult babies to care for. Babies of drug-abusing mothers on the West coast of the United States develop AIDS less frequently than do those in the East.

There is virtually nothing the law enforcement agency is able to do in cases of babies born 'under the influence' of drugs of abuse. The courts have decided that intoxication does not constitute a criminal act on the parent's part. In a 1986 case in San Diego, California, a 27-year-old indigent woman faced criminal prosecution for wilfully failing to provide adequate medical care for her fetus and for being responsible for the infant's later death. She had ignored a physician's warning earlier in her pregnancy to seek medical aid immediately if she began haemorrhaging. Diagnosed as having placenta praevia, she had been told to abstain from illegal drugs. Her baby was born with no brain function and expired a few weeks after birth from bronchial pneumonia. The infant's blood contained amphetamines and THC (cannabinoids) at the time of birth. The case was dismissed by the Court on the grounds that there was no statutory basis for the charge; it was, therefore, never reported officially but caused widespread anxiety for those concerned for the civil liberties of women [29] (see also Chapter 1).

Section 273-A of the California Penal code prohibits child endangering, but Appellate Court decisions have consistently required law enforcement officials to prove that a woman who was pregnant and who continued to use drugs knew of the possible effects of these drugs. Parents claim they are 'not responsible for their acts' and are almost invariably released by the judicial system.

No comparable case in criminal law has been taken in the United Kingdom; a prosecution, say, under the Infant Life (Preservation) Act 1929, would be difficult, if not impossible, on the grounds of proving intention (see Chapter 5). The problem has, however, been addressed under the Children and Young Persons Act 1969, s.1. In this important case [30], the local authority sought to remove a child, who was the victim of narcotic withdrawal, from her heroin-addicted mother at birth. The House of Lords had no difficulty in deciding that, for the purposes of interpreting the statute, the words 'is being … neglected … or ill-treated' included the intrauterine phase of life; child care was a continuum and, so long as the neglect was part of that continuum, there was no reason why the juvenile court should not look back at the conditions pertaining before the child was born.

A very similar position has been adopted in Canada where the concept of a fetal right to protection and to continuing protection after birth appears to be gaining ground – it may well be that fetal abuse will become reportable under the universal child abuse reporting statutes which exist in the Canadian Provinces. Instances of judicial protection of the fetus have included cases where the mother was addicted to alcohol [31] and to drugs [32]. In the latter case, it was stated that:

> It would be incredible to come to any other conclusion than that a drug-addicted baby is born abused. The abuse has occurred during the gestation period.

PCP-intoxicated parents have been responsible for an increasing proportion of the more than 600 child abuse cases that are seen each year at the Childrens Hospital National Medical Center in Washington, DC. Examples are a mother who had attempted suicide and mutilated her infant while intoxicated with PCP; another mother who gave her 2-month-old baby an overdose of cough medication; PCP parents who dropped a television set on their 2-week-old infant during a fight; and a 21-day-old premature infant who stopped breathing after her intoxicated father held her upside down. Between 1983 and 1986, there were 12 cases in Los Angeles County in which babies were decapitated by PCP-intoxicated parents, each with a serrated bread knife.

The solution of the question of fetal abuse by virtue of giving drugs to a viable fetus has been considered by the United States Federal Court of Appeals. The early decisions in, for example, *Re Vanessa F* [33] and *Grodin* v. *Grodin* [34] appeared to have been overruled in that the court decided that the fetus is not a person and thus does not fall under the child abuse reporting laws. Fetal deaths do not have to be reported to any of the legal enforcement agencies and this is also true in the United Kingdom. In both the United States and the United Kingdom, a certificate of stillbirth is issued in the case of a mature fetus – 28 weeks in the UK and 20 weeks in, for example, California. The English coroner would still not be involved even were the fetal death thought to be due to maternal drug abuse – he would have no jurisdiction for the stillbirth has never been alive.

REFERENCES

1. Zagon, I.S. (1985) Opioids and development: new lesions from old problems, in *Prenatal Drug Exposure: Kinetics and Dynamics* (eds C.N. Chiang and C.C. Lee), National Institute on Drug Abuse, Rockville, Md.
2. Offidani, C., Chiarotti, M. and de Giovanni, M. (1986) Methadone in pregnancy: clinical-toxicological aspects. *Clin. Toxicol.*, **24**, 295.
3. Warkany, J. (1971) Experimental teratology and drug testing, in *Congenital Malformations* (ed J. Warkany), Year Book Medical Publishers, Chicago.
4. Kuhnert, B.R. and Kuhnert, P.M. (1985) Placental transfer of drugs, alcohol, and components of cigarette smoke and their effects on the human fetus, in *Prenatal Drug Exposure: Kinetics and Dynamics* (eds C.N. Chiang and C.C. Lee), National Institute on Drug Abuse, Rockville, Md.
5. Davidson-Ward, S.L., Schuetz, S., Krishna, V. *et al.* (1986) Abnormal sleeping ventilatory pattern in infants of substance-abusing mothers. *Am. J. Dis. Child.*, **140**, 1015.
6. Chaves, C.J., Ostrea, E.M., Stryker, J.C. *et al.* (1979) Sudden infant death syndrome among infants of drug-dependent mothers. *J. Pediatr.*, **95**, 407; Pierson, P.S., Howard, P. and Kleber, H.D. (1972) Sudden death in infants born to methadone-maintained addicts. *JAMA*, **220**, 1733.
7. Mayor's Task Force on Child Abuse and Neglect (1985) *Executive Summary*, New York City Department of Health.
8. A Review and Evaluation of Existing Data on Perinatal Substance Abuse in Los Angeles County (1986) Prepared by The Council on Perinatal Substance Abuse of Los Angeles County.
9. Council on Scientific Affairs (1987) Scientific issues in drug testing. *JAMA*, **257**, 3110.
10. Jones, K.L. and Smith, D.W. (1973) Recognition of the fetal alcohol syndrome in early infancy. *Lancet*, **ii**, 999.
11. Smith, D.W. (1979) The fetal alcohol syndrome. *Hosp. Pract.*, **14**, 121.
12. Clarren, S.K. and Smith, D.W. (1978) The fetal alcohol syndrome. *New Engl. J. Med.*, **298**, 1063.
13. Clarren, S.K., Sampson, P.D., Larsen, J. *et al.* (1987) Facial effects of fetal alcohol exposure: assessment by photographs and morphometric analysis. *Am. J. Med. Genet.*, **26**, 651.
14. Usowics, A.G., Solabi, M. and Curry, C. (1986) Upper airway obstruction in infants with fetal alcohol syndrome. *Am. J. Dis. Child.*, **140**, 1039.
15. Clarren, S.K. Alvord, E.C., Sumi, S.M. *et al.* (1978) Brain malformations related to prenatal exposure to ethanol. *J. Pediatr.*, **92**, 64.
16. Danis, R.P., Newton, N. and Keith, L. (1981) Pregnancy and alcohol. *Curr. Probl. Obstet. Gynecol.*, **4**, 1.
17. DeBukelaer, M.M. and Randall, C.L. (1977) Renal anomalies in the fetal alcohol syndrome. *J. Pediatr.*, **91**, 759.
18. Tazelaar, H.D., Karch, S.B., Stephens, B.G. and Billingham, M.E. (1987) Cocaine and the heart. *Hum. Pathol.*, **18**, 195.
19. Woods, J.R., Plessinger, M.A. and Clark, K.E. (1987) Effect of cocaine on uterine blood flow and fetal oxygenation. *JAMA*, **257**, 957.
20. Chasnoff, I.R., Burns, W.J., Schnoll, S.H. and Burns, K.A. (1985) Cocaine use in pregnancy. *New Engl. J. Med.*, **313**, 666.
21. Bignol, N., Fuchs, M., Diaz, V. *et al.* (1987)

Teratogenicity of cocaine in humans. *J. Pediatr.,* **110**, 93.

22. Chasnoff, R.I., Bussey, M.E., Savich, R. and Stack, C.M. (1986) Perinatal cerebral infarction and maternal cocaine use. *J. Pediatr.,* **108**, 456.

23. Kahn, E.J., Neumann, L.L. and Polk, G.-A. (1969) The course of heroin withdrawal syndrome in newborn infants treated with phenobarbital and chlorpromazine. *J. Pediatr.,* **75**, 495.

24. Krause, S.O., Murray, P.M., Holmes, J.B. and Burch, R.E. (1958) Heroin addiction among pregnant women and their newborn babies. *Am. J. Obstet. Gynecol.,* **75**, 745. For a UK overview, see Caviston, P. (1987) Pregnancy and opiate addiction. *Br. Med. J.,* **295**, 285.

25. Landing, B.H., personal experience; Larson, E.J., personal experience.

26. Strauss, A.A., Mondanlou, H.D. and Bosu, S.K. (1981) Neonatal manifestations of maternal phencyclidine (PCP) abuse. *Pediatrics,* **68**, 550.

27. Larson, E.J., personal experience.

28. Courts face questions on legal status of fetus (1987). From *American Medical News,* 2 January, p. 23.

29. See, for example, Bonavoglia, A. (1987) The ordeal of Pamela Rae Steward. *Ms,* **16**, 92; Chambers, M. (1986) Are fetal rights equal to infants. *New York Times,* 16 November. For UK newspaper comment, see Editorial (1986) A pregnant pause. *The Independent,* 9 October.

30. *D (a minor)* v. *Berkshire County Council* [1987] 1 All ER 20.

31. *Re Children's Aid Society of Kenora and J L* (1982) 134 DLR (3d) 249.

32. *Superintendent of Family and Child Service and McDonald* (1982) 135 DLR (3d) 330.

33. *In re Vanessa F* 76 Misc 2d 617 (NY, 1974).

34. *Grodin* v. *Grodin* 301 NW 2d 869 (Mich., 1981).

CHAPTER 4

The examination of stillbirths

W.J.A. Patrick

In recent years stillbirth rates have fallen progressively throughout the world as a result of improved obstetric care, generally improved living standards and falling birth rates. Fetal loss is, however, still appreciable in many countries (Table 4.1), and up to 40% of cases remain of unknown aetiology.

The accurate analysis of stillbirth rates is not entirely straightforward because definitions vary. The United Nations returns, for example, relate to *live* births while, in Britain, the stillbirth rates are given per 1000 *total* births. Furthermore, there seems to be no standardization of reporting so that figures from different areas of the world cannot necessarily be compared directly. In the United Kingdom, and for the purposes of this Chapter, stillbirths are defined as infants born after the 28th week of gestation who do not breathe or show any other signs of life after complete separation from the mother. The current stillbirth rate in the UK – at 5.9/1000 total births – is similar to the postperinatal infant death rate (the number of deaths from the end of the first week to the end of the first year/1000 live births) and makes up approximately half the perinatal mortality rate (stillbirths + deaths in the first week/1000 total births) (Table 4.2).

The post-mortem examination of stillbirths aims to determine the cause of death and, thereby, to provide an estimate of the likelihood of recurrence. In addition to the post-mortem examination, most specialist centres will attempt to include histological, photographic, radiological, microbiological and chromosomal studies in order to delineate causes as accurately as possible and to provide the information needed which may further our understanding of the mechanisms of fetal loss. However, it is the gross post-mortem findings which will provide the most useful amount of information in most cases and it is reasonable to be selective in the use of supportive investigations. For example, relevant tissue samples can be taken for chromosomal analysis where there is a family history of abnormal children or a history of recurrent fetal loss. Karyotyping would also be essential in cases of idiopathic hydrops fetalis and in renal cystic disease because of their recognized association with aneuploidy [1]. Histopathological examination can provide a definite diagnosis of most renal abnormalities and should be routine even in the absence of gross disease. Nevertheless, it will be necessary, in a proportion of cases, to support the gross post-mortem dissection with all the associated investigative procedures which have been quoted since the underlying cause may well be multifactorial. At all events, the protocol must be systematic

Table 4.1 Late fetal (stillbirth) mortality rates per 1000 *live* births in various countries (Demographic Year Books of the United Nations)

Country	Year					
	1956–60	1961–65	1966–70	1971–75	1976–80	1981–85
Africa						
Tunisia	—	—	14.4	13.3	—	—
America (North)						
Canada	14.3	12.3	10.7	8.1	5.9	4.8
Cuba	—	22.0	—	13.4	11.1	11.6
Mexico	16.8	—	17.1	—	12.5	—
USA	12.7	12.5	—	9.2	7.7	—
Asia						
Japan	—	—	18.0	12.2	8.7	6.3
Hong Kong	—	14.1	10.5	—	—	—
Singapore	—	12.3	10.5	—	—	—
Europe						
Austria	16.6	13.1	10.8	—	—	—
Belgium	16.1	14.5	12.3	—	—	—
Bulgaria	12.2	11.0	9.8	9.0	—	—
Czechoslovakia	11.1	9.0	7.6	6.8	6.3	—
Denmark	15.3	11.6	8.9	—	—	—
East Germany	16.8	14.3	11.4	8.9	7.2	5.8
England and Wales	22.0	17.6	14.3	11.6	8.6	6.0
Finland	13.9	11.0	—	—	—	—
France	17.3	16.1	14.4	12.1	10.0	7.8
Greece	13.4	14.9	14.6	12.6	10.0	—
Hungary	14.5	12.1	10.3	9.1	8.2	—
Italy	26.7	22.2	17.5	13.0	9.4	—
Netherlands	16.5	14.3	11.7	9.1	7.3	6.0
Norway	14.4	12.6	11.3	—	—	—
Poland	13.0	11.4	10.6	8.6	7.1	6.1
Portugal	32.3	27.9	25.4	19.0	14.0	10.4
Rumania	17.1	15.5	15.6	11.1	9.4	—
Scotland	23.4	19.5	15.1	—	—	—
Spain	28.9	24.7	19.6	14.7	8.4	—
Sweden	15.5	11.8	9.0	—	—	—
Switzerland	12.8	11.5	9.7	—	—	—
West Germany	16.9	13.4	11.0	8.9	6.2	4.6
Yugoslavia	10.5	10.1	9.7	8.1	7.2	—
Oceania						
Australia*	14.8	12.6	10.7	—	6.6	5.1

* Excludes full-blooded Aborigines.

Table 4.2 Stillbirth rates (SBR), perinatal mortality rates (PMR), infant mortality rates (IMR) and post-perinatal mortality rates (PPMR) in Scotland, and England and Wales (stillbirths and deaths in the first week/1000 live births). (Annual Report of the Registrar General for Scotland; Childhood Mortality Statistics, Office of Population Censuses and Surveys)

Year	Scotland				England and Wales			
	SBR	*PMR*	*IMR*	*PPMR*	*SBR*	*PMR*	*IMR*	*PPMR*
1931–35	—	—	—	—	41.0	62.5	59.6	38.1
1936–40	—	—	—	—	38.5	59.2	53.3	32.6
1941–45	35.7	57.6	67.7	45.6	30.7	48.6	48.8	30.9
1946–50	29.2	48.3	47.3	28.2	23.9	39.8	35.1	19.2
1951–55	25.5	42.4	32.9	16.0	23.0	37.6	26.3	11.7
1956–60	22.8	38.8	27.9	11.9	21.5	34.9	22.2	8.8
1961–65	19.1	33.6	25.0	10.5	17.3	29.4	20.3	8.2
1966–70	15.0	26.6	21.2	9.6	14.1	24.7	18.1	7.5
1971–75	12.3	23.0	18.8	8.1	11.6	21.0	16.6	7.2
1976–80	8.0	15.8	13.7	5.9	8.6	15.6	13.1	6.1
1981–85	5.8	10.9	10.5	5.4	5.9	10.7	9.3	4.5

and as detailed as is possible. The purpose of this Chapter is to describe a comprehensive but manageable approach to the routine examination of the stillborn fetus.

4.1 THE EXTERNAL EXAMINATION

Standard weights and measurements are taken before any examination of the internal structure is carried out. These include the total bodyweight, the crown–heel (CH) length, the crown–rump (CR) length, the occipito-frontal circumference (OFC) and the length of the foot from the heel to the tip of the great toe. The figures are compared with standard charts of weight and length related to gestational age [2]. The crown–rump length should equal the circumference of the head and any reduction of the OFC measurement suggests a degree of microcephaly.

Many conditions are associated with external abnormalities which may be diagnostic instantly, but this is the exception rather than the rule; it is usually necessary to document abnormalities and specific stigmata

quite systematically to help to determine whether ancillary investigations, such as chromosomal analysis, are required. Careful note should be taken of the position, shape and size of the eyes, ears, mouth and general bone structure. Low-set ears are, by definition, ears that lie entirely below a horizontal line drawn from the outer canthus of the eye. However, a more practical measure that is less liable to observer error is a line drawn from the point of the chin to the posterior fontanelle, which should pass through the tragus. The external structure of the ear may be visibly abnormal, the auditory meatus may be non-patent and there may be accessory auricles or preauricular sinuses.

The distance apart of the eyes is usually measured with reference to the inner and outer canthal, the midpupillary and the outer orbital distances; they can be compared with standard measurements [3]. Racial differences occur and can be taken into account by using the canthal index ((inner canthal distance/outer canthal distance × 100). The various conditions in which the eyes are widely spaced include Apert's syndrome, Cruzen's syndrome and some drug-induced syndromes. The size of the palpebral fissure can be measured. A narrow palpebral fissure occurs when the inner canthus is displaced laterally and partially obscures the medial part of the eye. It may be associated with gross ocular developmental abnormalities including, in its most severe form, anophthalmos.

The overall facial structure can give specific evidence of a number of diseases such as renal agenesis, trisomy 18 and the Pierre–Robin syndrome. Note should be taken of any midfacial abnormalities and of any underdevelopment of the midline structures. There may be obvious facial clefts which are due to failure of development or of incomplete fusion of the mesenchymal swellings that form the facial structures [4]. The commonest facial cleft is the classic cleft lip and palate which is due to a failure of fusion of the medial nasal and maxillary swellings. It can be of varying severity, ranging from a barely visible notch in the vermillion border of the upper lip to a complete bilateral cleft involving both lip and palate. Median clefts, similarly, arise from failure of fusion of the medial nasal swellings in the midline, thus causing a deep groove between the right and left sides of the nose. The most extreme form of median cleft is seen when the nasal swellings fail to develop at all; this results in a central upper lip defect with total absence of the nose and is usually associated with arrhinencephaly and holoprosencephaly (Fig. 4.1). Lateral or oblique facial clefts stem from a failure of the maxillary and lateral nasal swelling to fuse and form the nasolachrymal duct; the maxillary and mandibular swellings may fail to merge on one or both sides, resulting in macrostomia.

Different shapes of head may be of some diagnostic significance and this is particularly so of microcephaly which is a feature of a number of different syndromes. In broad terms, the shape of the head is influenced

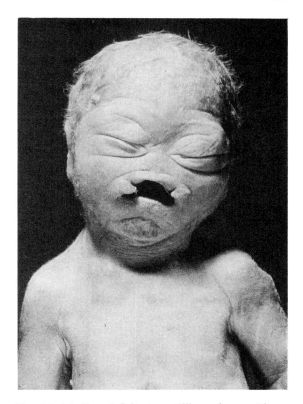

Fig. 4.1 Median cleft lip in a stillborn fetus with arrhinencephaly and holoprosencephaly.

either by the size of the developing brain, and any abnormalities of cerebrospinal fluid flow, or by irregular fusion of particular sutures.

Note should be taken of obvious gross defects of limb size and structure and this should be supported by detailed radiology, especially in any case of short-limbed dwarfism.

Useful information may be obtained by looking carefully at the palmar skin creases. The normal pattern is so familiar that abnormal creases will be obvious immediately. The single transverse (simian) crease occurs in a very small proportion of normal persons but is particularly common in Down's syndrome and other autosomal trisomies. The Sidney crease is a variant of the simian and is a small distal transverse crease which extends for a short distance across the palm from the ulnar aspect. Excessive incurving of the digits (clinodactyly) is most commonly seen in the fifth finger and is a particularly common feature of trisomy 18 although it is not exclusive to this condition. Syndactyly usually involves the third and fourth fingers and the second and third toes; again, this finding is non-specific and occurs in a wide variety of conditions including Apert's syndrome and triploidy. Many other minor malformations of the digits – including hypoplasia, poly-dactyly, hypoplasia of the distal phalanges and small nails – may offer clues to specific syndromes but are not diagnostic in them-selves.

4.2 RADIOLOGY

A radiological skeletal survey may provide useful additional information in stillborn fetuses. It may disclose abnormalities which might not otherwise be detected as well as clearly defining major skeletal anomalies. A further point, which is not often realized, is that it can be used as a non-intrusive investi-gation should permission for a post-mortem examination be refused. It also provides useful material for teaching and research purposes [5].

Anteroposterior and lateral projections are used routinely; care must be taken in pos-itioning the fetus so that overlap of the limb bones is avoided so far as is possible. Fetuses can be accommodated on one film and optimal results will be obtained if the radiological examination is carried out before the autopsy.

Post-mortem radiology is most useful in the assessment of fetal maturity. This can be determined either by identifying epiphyseal centres of ossification around the knee and ankle joints or by direct measurement of the biparietal diameter, the height of thoracic and lumbar vertebrae, the femoral length or the femoral length/midshaft ratio [6]. The centres

of ossification provide only a rough guide to maturity as they may be delayed in a number of conditions – for example, small for date babies, congenital rubella, Zellweger's cerebrohepatorenal syndrome, Down's syndrome, achondroplasia and thanatophoric dwarfism [7]. Allowing for individual variations, they appear, on average, in the calcaneum at 24 weeks, the talus at 28 weeks, the distal femoral epiphysis at 36 weeks and the proximal tibial epiphysis at 40 weeks' gestation. There is little difference between males and females of similar gestational age. Centres of ossification can be seen by the naked eye at post-mortem dissection should radiological facilities not be available. The most accurate and eminently practical means of assessing fetal maturity is by direct measurement of the overall length of the femur in either the anteroposterior or lateral projections; the femur with the least distortion of the metaphysis should be selected [8].

Bone changes tend to be non-specific in stillbirths. Congenital syphilis, for example, has features in common with rubella and with cytomegalovirus disease [9]. However, at the present time, a complete radiological skeletal survey provides the only means of differen-tiating the skeletal dysplasias, a number of which are lethal in the neonatal period [10].

4.3 DISSECTION TECHNIQUE

After routine weights and measurements have been recorded and the maturity of the fetus calculated, all the external orifices are examined so as to exclude choanal, urethral and anal atresia.

Formal dissection begins with an incision which passes to the left of the umbilicus so as to avoid the umbilical vein. The thoracic organs are exposed by removing the sternum carefully and both sides and the central part of the diaphragm are inspected for diaphragmatic herniae. The innominate vein, which lies immediately behind the thymus, is identified by dissecting off the thymus gland. A persistent left superior vena cava is excluded by passing a probe through an opening in the left internal jugular vein; when one is present, the probe passes directly downwards into the left side of the coronary sinus instead of crossing the midline to the right atrium. The pericardial sac is now opened and the probe is inserted through an incision in the left atrial appendage to enter the pulmonary veins on each side. Large venous channels frequently pass down below the diaphragm in the presence of anomalous pulmonary venous drainage and are an indication for removal of the thoracic and abdominal viscera *en bloc*. The thoracic viscera may be more conveniently removed separately in the absence of this anomaly.

A probe is passed into the oesophagus without force and, then, into the larynx and trachea to exclude atresia. Care must be taken when manoeuvering the probe into the larynx to avoid rupturing by undue force the uncommon membranous or web-like type of atresia which passes across between the vocal cords. The pathologist is often alerted to this condition by the presence of voluminous, rather mucoid lungs and by the presence of prominent rib markings. If laryngeal atresia is suspected, it is prudent to fix the upper respiratory tract without further dissection so that adequate histological blocks can be taken at several levels by which to define the extent and the morphological details of the atretic segment. In the commonest form of oesophageal atresia, there is a blind upper pouch and a tracheo-oesophageal fistula is present at the carina.

The dissection of the heart is continued by reflecting the pericardium from the base so as to display the pulmonary artery, the ductus arteriosus, the arch of the aorta and the innominate, left common carotid and left subclavian arch arteries. The probe is then passed into the inferior vena cava from below

and is lodged in the superior vena cava. The inside of the right atrium is exposed by cutting along the probe with coronary artery scissors. The foramen ovale lies slightly below the midpart of the atrial septum and the opening of the coronary sinus is placed posteriorly between it and the tricuspid valve. The valvular mechanism of the foramen ovale can be demonstrated by gentle pressure on the septum. A persistent left superior vena cava can be confirmed at this stage by passing the probe directly through the coronary sinus to emerge at the left lateral border of the heart.

A small incision is now made in the outflow tract of the right ventricle and the probe is inserted into the pulmonary artery and the ductus arteriosus. The incision is enlarged upwards by cutting along the probe so that the outflow tract, pulmonary vessels and ductus can be visualized. Finally, the probe is inserted into the opening already made in the left atrial appendage for inspection of the pulmonary veins and is passed through the mitral valve. Holding the left ventricle with the probe *in situ* between the thumb and index finger of the opposite hand, an incision is made in the left lateral ventricular wall by cutting down on the probe. The probe is removed, re-inserted into the opening in the left ventricle and passed into the aortic trunk. As before, the incision is extended along the probe, passing vertically at first towards the atrioventricular groove and, then, in a curve along the groove into the proximal part of the aorta immediately above the coronary ostia. Care must be taken to avoid transecting the main pulmonary trunk. The final incision facilitates inspection of the interventricular septum in the upper membranous part of which interventricular septal defects are most commonly seen. It will be appreciated that, in this way, a complete assessment of the heart and great vessels can be made with a limited number of incisions and that, as a result, the heart can easily be reconstructed in order to demonstrate any anomaly.

Access to the abdomen is improved by dividing the umbilical vein before transecting the rectum and removing the alimentary tract in one piece by reflecting it upwards towards the diaphragm. Removal of the retro-peritoneal and pelvic organs is facilitated by separating the hypogastric arteries and urachal remnant together as a pedicle from behind the anterior abdominal wall below the umbilicus. The pedicle is useful for traction and the manoeuvre ensures positive identi-fication of the hypogastric arteries. A gonad can be taken for histology at this stage.

The gastrointestinal tract is inspected for diverticulae and duplication by passing the loops of bowel through the finger and thumb of one hand using toothed forceps in the other. A persistent vitello-intestinal remnant in the form of a Meckel's diverticulum is the most commonly observed anomaly and is present in about 2% of the population. It arises from the antimesenteric aspect of the proximal ileum and can be seen lying anteriorly in the abdomen when the cavity is first opened. The diverticulum is fre-quently the site of heterotopic pancreas or of acid-secreting gastric mucosa. Again, the minimum amount of dissection allows reconstitution of the anatomical relationship of the various organs for the demonstration of any anomalies.

Any enlargement of the organ or loss of corticomedullary definition in the kidney may be a sign of renal cystic disease. Absence of the kidneys is associated with large discoid adrenals which can be mistaken for kidneys in prenatal ultrasound examinations.

A small posterior cranial fossa – with associated Arnold–Chiari malformation – is almost invariable in the severe cystic forms of spina bifida. This is best demonstrated before opening the skull by extending the initial skin incision as described in Chapter 5. The neck muscles are dissected off and the spinal arches removed to show the downward protrusion of

cerebellum and medulla into the cervical canal on opening the dura.

Removal of the fetal brain is most easily achieved by cutting along the suture lines with sharp pointed scissors having reflected the scalp. The points of the scissors are inserted through small incisions in the lateral angles of the anterior fontanelle; the frontal and parietal bones are separated and reflected outwards by cutting through the sutures on either side of the midline, thus exposing the cerebral hemispheres and avoiding injury to the venous sinuses and the dural folds.

The fetal brain is displaced very gently so as to inspect the falx tentorium and great cerebral vein for any tears that might be the source of subdural haemorrhage. The olfactory bulbs are firmly attached to the cribriform plate in the fetus and can be left behind inadvertently when the brain is removed. Specific identi-fication is necessary to avoid the mistaken diagnosis of arrhinencephaly.

The final removal of the brain follows the conventional method with division of the falx at its attachment to the crista galli, incision of the outer part of the tentorium where it is attached to the petrous temporal bone and transection of the brain stem in the base of the skull. These recommendations for dealing with the small fetal brain may be contrasted with those suggested for the post-mortem examination of the baby in Chapter 5.

4.4 THE PLACENTA

The placenta should be examined routinely in all stillbirths as it may give clues to the likely cause of death. Placental 'weights' usually include the placenta together with the membranes and the umbilical cord attached; the trimmed weight following removal of the membranes and cord is more accurate.

Complications related to the placenta and umbilical cord may occur in up to 75% of stillbirths. In only about 40% may there be an organic abnormality significant enough to have caused death. A breakdown of these abnormalities shows that they include placental infarcts, chorioamnionitis, feto-maternal haemorrhage and cord complications.

Routine macroscopic examination of the placenta may show some irregularity of outline and accessory (succinturiate) lobes which, as such, are of little importance. The maternal surface is frequently ragged and postpartum haemorrhage can result from retention *in utero* of part of the basal plate. The placenta is likely to be disrupted if it has been removed manually. In monovular multiple (twin/triplet) pregnancies the placenta is monochorionic with no chorionic ridges or division on separating the membranes from the fetal surface.

The placenta is lobulated with some 15–20 cotyledons which usually, but not invariably, correspond with the distribution of the fetal vessels [11]. They are unusually bulky and oedematous in conditions such as diabetes or Rhesus isoimmunization. The frequent finding of blood clot on the maternal surface of the placenta has little significance in relation to fetal mortality. Large haematomas which indent the surface and commonly overlie a significant area of infarction are the most reliable evidence of abruption. Minor bleeding from the fetal to the maternal circulation occurs in up to 50% of pregnancies, reaching a maximum during labour [12]. Significant fetomaternal haemorrhage can result in exsanguination of the fetus. The most accurate method of detecting fetal cells in maternal blood is by means of a simple staining technique (Kleihauer-Betke test). It is possible that the areas of fibrinoid degeneration which are seen routinely in histology sections may be an attempt by the body to prevent loss of fetal blood into the maternal circulation.

At least 20% of stillbirths are thought to result from acute amnionitis [13], which is a common complication of prolonged rupture of the membranes. Amnionitis manifests itself

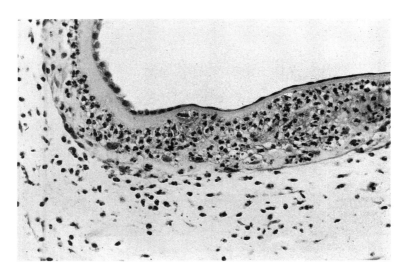

Fig. 4.2 Acute amnionitis with an intense inflammatory cell reaction in the loose supporting connective tissue of the amniotic epithelium (× 25 obj.).

as thickening and opacity of the membranes with a dry lustreless surface akin to that seen in pleurisy or fibrinous pericarditis. Histologically, there is an inflammatory cell reaction in the loose connective tissue immediately underlying the thick basement membrane of the amnion (Fig. 4.2) and, in some cases, this is associated with migration of acute inflammatory cells through the walls of the umbilical cord vessels (funitis). The condition is primarily an infection of amnion and, in its pure form, is confined to that structure – it should, therefore, properly be designated 'amnionitis', not the more commonly used 'chorioamnionitis'. There is a risk of intrauterine pneumonia due to infected amniotic fluid circulating through the fetal lungs when amnionitis is present. There may be no gross sign of fetal pneumonia and the diagnosis depends on the histological definition of inflammatory cells in the alveolar ducts (Fig. 4.3).

Amniotic bands are a common cause of limb deformities and amputations and occur in 1–2% of malformed fetuses [14]. Severe malformations may result from adhesions between the placenta and the cranial vault, and the fetus may die as a result of constriction of the umbilical cord (Fig. 4.4). A reasonable explanation for the formation of amniotic bands is that they arise from defective separation of the amnion from the upper surface of the embryo during the early stages of development of the amniotic sac.

Amnion nodosum is a specific condition secondary to renal agenesis, dysplastic kidneys or urethral atresia. The normal circulation of amniotic fluid through the fetus is impaired and this gives rise to oligohydramnios. As a result of oligohydramnios, the uterine wall becomes closely applied to the fetus and fetal squames adhere to the surface of the amnion. The characteristic manifestation of the condition is seen in the presence of smooth, light brown or yellow nodules on the surface of the amnion (Fig. 4.5); these consist of fetal squames embedded in an amorphous matrix with some underlying

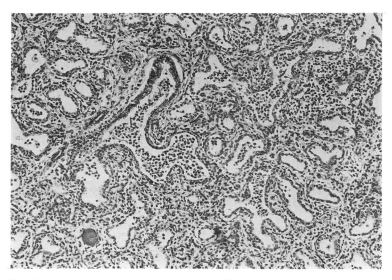

Fig. 4.3 Intrauterine pneumonia with inflammatory exudate in the alveolar ducts of immature fetal lung (× 10 obj.).

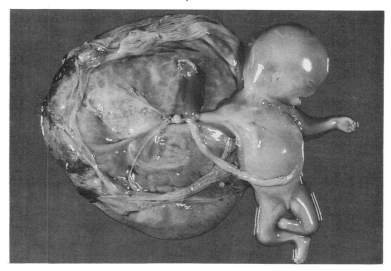

Fig. 4.4 Amniotic bands constricting the umbilical cord and the right forearm of a macerated fetus with intrauterine amputation of the left leg.

fibroblastic proliferation. A fetus with renal agenesis is usually stillborn and has a typically squashed appearance with varus deformity of the feet (Fig. 4.6).

A circumvallate placenta is one in which the fetal surface is surrounded by a double layer of pale membranes, thought to be formed by separation of the parietal decidua around the margin of the placenta, thereby exposing a rim of chorion (placenta extrachorialis). It is of

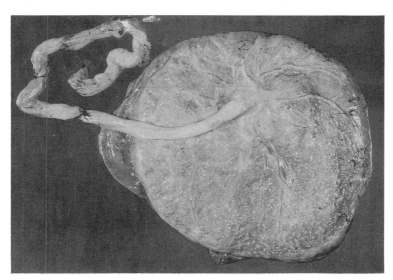

Fig. 4.5 Amnion nodosum with raised discrete nodules on the (fetal) surface of the amnion.

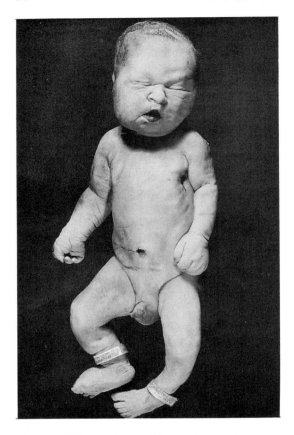

Fig. 4.6 Stillborn fetus with renal agenesis showing the squashed features, redundant skin on the back of the hands and varus deformity of the feet.

little significance in its minor form but, occasionally, the membranes form a tight ring close to the centre of the placenta, drawing it inwards and restricting the fetal vessels.

The umbilical cord is normally attached near the centre of the placenta. Occasionally it is attached more peripherally or it may even have a velamentous attachment in the membranes at some distance from the placental surface. In the latter situation, the vessels run unsupported to the placenta and, thus, may be damaged during delivery or may cause vasa praevia if they cross the internal os.

The average length of the umbilical cord is about 50 cm. An excessively long cord is liable to become wound around the fetus and cause fetal deformity (Fig. 4.7). One that is too short can cause premature separation of the placenta during delivery and endanger the fetus. A true knot in the cord is quite a common finding but is unlikely to obstruct the fetal blood flow in the fluid medium of the amniotic cavity or because of the physical nature of its structure. False knots are varicosities of little significance. In congenital syphilis, the cord vessels may show a perivascular lymphocytic infiltrate and endarteritis [15].

A single umbilical artery occurs in about 0.45% of pregnancies and is associated with other fetal malformations in 22% of cases [16]. It is common in sirenomelia (mermaid syndrome) and in the VATER association

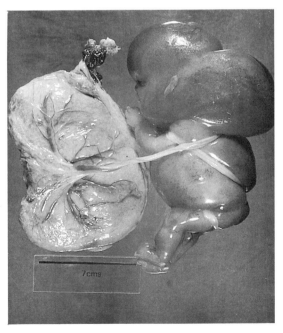

Fig. 4.7 Umbilical cord wound several times around a fetus with subcutaneous oedema.

(a non-random association of vertebral anomalies, imperforate anus, oesophageal atresia, tracheo-oesophageal fistula, radial dysplasia and renal anomalies) and is seen not uncommonly in association with chromosomal abnormalities.

Dystrophic calcification frequently occurs in areas of fibrinoid degeneration and is manifest in the gross specimen as flecks of calcification on the maternal surface of the placenta. Such calcification is said to be more common in first pregnancies and may impart a feeling of grittiness when the placenta is sectioned. Another degenerative change of uncertain significance is the punctate basophilic ferocalcific material seen in the outer layers of chorionic villi in the placentas of macerated stillbirths.

Routine histology of the placenta is of limited value as most of the changes seen are of a non-specific nature and their significance not fully understood. A chronic inflammatory cell infiltrate in individual villi or groups of villi (villitis or placentitis) supports the concept of haematogenous as opposed to ascending infection but it is an incidental finding in most instances and cannot be related to a specific infection. Histological techniques are, however, becoming progressively more sophisticated and, ultimately, definitive diagnoses, based, for example, on specific immunohistochemical findings, may be achieved in most cases.

4.5 MACERATED STILLBIRTHS

Maceration is the term used for the autolytic process which the fetal body undergoes when death occurs *in utero* [17]. Over 40% of stillbirths show some degree of maceration. Putrefaction will not occur if the membranes are intact. The earliest sign of maceration is generalized dusky discoloration of the skin in which desquamation can be demonstrated, if it is not already obvious, by rubbing the surface. This is followed in 24–48 hours by uniform dark red haemic discoloration, laxity of the tissues, separation of the skull bones, and accumulation of excess fluid in the body cavities. If the pregnancy continues, which it is more likely to do in second trimester missed abortions than in stillbirths, the blood pigment and fluid are gradually absorbed, and the fetus becomes increasingly pale, shrunken and papyraceous in the ensuing weeks. The timing of the events is arbitrary but serves as a useful means of correlating the degree of maceration with the loss of fetal movements.

The weight and measurements of a macerated fetus are inaccurate and will not necessarily correspond to the standard weights and measurements for gestational age. The processes that result in fetal loss *in utero* may also cause some slowing of fetal growth during the last few weeks of pregnancy and a radiological skeletal survey is of particular value in assessing the maturity of the fetus in relation to the gestational age at the time of delivery.

Dysmorphic features are difficult to recognize in a macerated fetus and the postmortem examination is made more difficult by the uniform discoloration of the tissues. Developmental anomalies can usually be identified and the variable loss of cellular detail does not preclude the histological recognition of the structural outline of the tissues and assessment of the maturity of the individual organs. A diagnosis of unsuspected diseases such as cytomegalovirus disease and human parvovirus infection can be made in some cases.

Excess amniotic aspirate in the form of keratin or fetal squames is almost invariably present to some degree in the periphery of the lungs of macerated stillbirths (Fig. 4.8). It is evidence of fetal distress and is frequently referred to as 'meconium aspiration', although it rarely contains bile pigment even when meconium or meconium-stained liquor is present in the larynx or trachea.

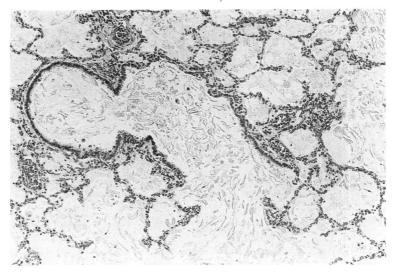

Fig. 4.8 Amniotic aspirate in peripheral airways of mature fetal lung as a result of intrauterine hypoxia (× 10 obj.).

Some assessment of fetal maturity can be made from the histological sections of the kidney where the nephrogenic zone becomes discontinuous after 36 weeks gestation as the kidney acquires a full complement of nephrons. Alveolar development in the lungs is not obvious until about the 28th week of gestation. Interstitial cells are prominent in the fetal testis and the ovary may show some follicular development. Changes of cystic fibrosis can occur in stillbirths and histological sections of the pancreas should be examined routinely even in a macerated fetus.

Human parvovirus affects the progenitor cells of the erythroid series. Affected fetuses are unusually pale and hydropic, and the typical eosinophilic nuclear inclusion bodies [18] in circulating red cells and erythropoietic elements in fetal liver or bone marrow can be readily seen, as in the case of cytomegalovirus disease, in autolysed tissues. The changes of parvovirus infections and cytomegalovirus disease are fully described in Section 4.6 below.

Karyotyping is successful only in some 20% of macerated stillbirths. It should be attempted in all cases but is particularly important in the case of macerated fetuses with dysmorphic features or with fetal hydrops. Amnion is preferred for tissue culture purposes as the viability of fascia lata may be in doubt but care should be taken not to include chorion as this may give rise to maternal contamination.

4.6 INTRAUTERINE INFECTIONS

Intrauterine infections, which may be acquired across the placenta or by ascending infection, are a relatively frequent cause of intrauterine fetal loss, although the precise mechanism by which infection overwhelms the fetus is not understood. Acute amnionitis with associated intrauterine pneumonia has already been discussed and can result from infection by many bacterial pathogens.

Cytomegalovirus disease is endemic in the community and about 2% of fetuses infected

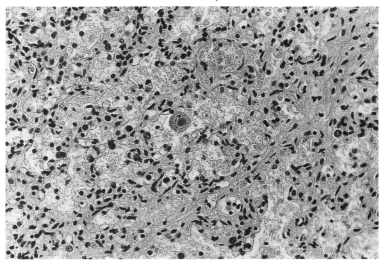

Fig. 4.9 Cytomegalovirus infection of the lung of a macerated stillbirth
(× 25 obj.).

with cytomegalovirus are stillborn [19]. Epithelial structures are most commonly involved and the fetuses usually have gross ascites and splenomegaly. Infected cells are greatly enlarged and contain large rounded dense eosinophilic nuclear inclusion bodies and coarsely granular cytoplasm (Fig. 4.9). The changes are most readily seen in the kidney and pancreas and may still be evident in severely autolysed tissues (Fig. 4.10); both

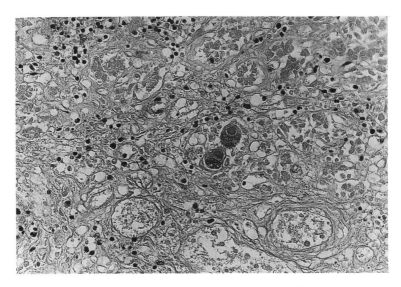

Fig. 4.10 Cytomegalovirus disease of the pancreas of a macerated
stillbirth (× 25 obj.).

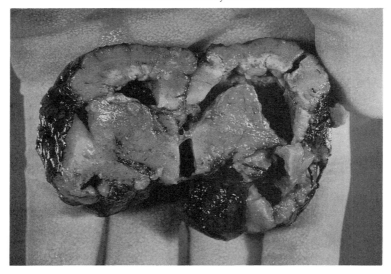

Fig. 4.11 Severe microcephaly in congenital cytomegalovirus disease with calcification around the laternal ventricles and in the outer layers of the cerebral cortex.

the exocrine and endocrine parts of the pancreas can be involved and diabetes mellitus has been reported in congenitally infected infants [20]. Microcephaly is a common feature; dystrophic calcification is seen around the lateral ventricles and in the outer cortical layers (Fig. 4.11). Similar changes may occur in the brain in toxoplasmosis.

Human parvovirus infections have recently

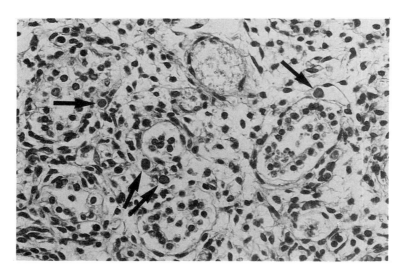

Fig. 4.12 Human parvovirus inclusion bodies in the nucleus of circulating red cell precursors in fetal lung ($\times$ 25 obj.).

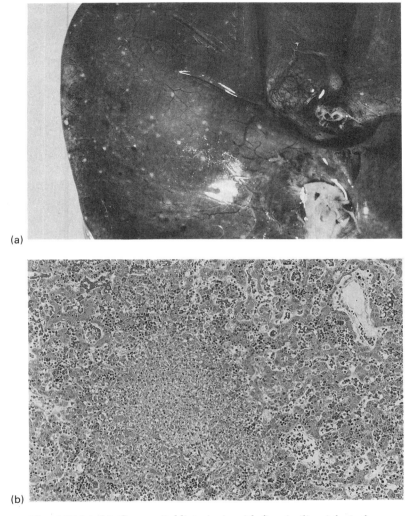

(a)

(b)

Fig. 4.13 (a),(b) Congenital listeriosis with fine (miliary) foci of necrosis in the liver of a 2-day-old preterm infant.

been described as a cause of mid-trimester abortions and stillbirths. The virus appears to affect principally the pronormoblasts in the fetal bone marrow resulting often in severe anaemia and hydrops fetalis. Maternal serum alpha-fetoprotein levels can be raised and histology may show brick red nuclear inclusion bodies in the precursor cells of the erythroid series (Fig. 4.12); these bodies have been shown to contain human parvovirus by DNA hybridization techniques [18, 21, 22]. Cases diagnosed as idopathic hydrops fetalis and polyserositis in the past may well have been due to parvovirus infections.

Several infective agents are known to cause patterns of disease in both man and animals and can occasionally be transmitted from one to the other, for example, *Toxocara canis* and

Chlamydia psittaci. Some mammalian strains of *C. psittaci* are an important cause of stillbirth and abortion in sheep. Recently, cases have been reported in which severe chlamydial sepsis in mothers was accompanied by intrauterine death and premature labour [23]. Gross post-mortem examination of the stillborn fetus and placenta may not show any macroscopic abnormality but, histologically, large dense intracytoplasmic inclusion bodies characteristic of *C. psittaci* can be demonstrated in the cells of the syncytiotrophoblastic and cytotrophoblastic cells using both standard staining methods and immunohistochemical techniques. The organism tends to localize in the placenta and has been isolated from human placental tissue.

Mycoplasma infections can cause abortions and stillbirths in undernourished populations. The mycoplasma gives rise to an acute amnionitis and intrauterine fetal pneumonia – often through apparently intact membranes [24].

Syphilis is now a very uncommon cause of fetal loss in this country, but may well cause appreciable mortality in countries where the disease in still endemic. The fetus is rarely affected during the first half of pregnancy so abortion is rare; those affected early in the second part of pregnancy are often stillborn. The fetuses of untreated syphilitic mothers die of septicaemia; a characteristic feature is syphilitic inflammation of the lungs (pneumonia alba) with macrophages in the alveolar spaces and an increase in the connective tissues in the intra-alveolar septae. There may be no diagnostic external stigmata.

Viral disease in the mother may cause stillbirth without any manifest evidence of infection in the fetus; death may be caused directly or result from associated malformations. Included in viral diseases which are capable of producing death and congenital infection are chickenpox, herpes simplex, poliomyelitis, measles, rubella, smallpox, hepatitis B, Coxsackie B infection, vaccinia and equine encephalitis.

Listeriosis is a bacterial infection that may be acquired transplacentally or via the amniotic cavity. There will usually be an amnionitis in fatal cases and *Listeria* organisms will be present on the surface of the amnion. The presence of fine scattered necrotic lesions in many of the organs is a characteristic septicaemic appearance (Fig. 4.13).

Candidiasis affects a large number of women in pregnancy and candidial infections of the amnion may occasionally give rise to intrauterine pneumonia.

4.7 CHROMOSOMAL ANOMALIES

The commonest chromosomal anomalies in midtrimester abortions and stillbirths are trisomy 21, trisomy 18, trisomy 13, triploidy and Turner's syndrome. Physical stigmata may be specific, allowing for instant diagnosis, but chromosome analysis should be carried out in any case in which developmental anomalies are present or dysmorphic features are suspected.

The incidence of trisomy 21 (Down's syndrome) is approximately 1 in 600 pregnancies. More than 60% of these abort spontaneously and 20% are stillborn. The condition is usually due to non-dysjunction of the chromosomes during reduction division but can arise from translocation or mosaicism in younger women. The overall risk of recurrence in families with a previously affected child is 1–2%; it is greater with translocation or mosaicism than with non-dysjunction so that it is imperative that the carrier status of the parents should be determined in these situations. Down's syndrome (Fig. 4.14) is characterized by a flat facies, slightly protuberant and thickened tongue, a small, rounded brachycephalic head, upward slanting eyes, prominent epicanthic folds, small ears, abnormal palmar

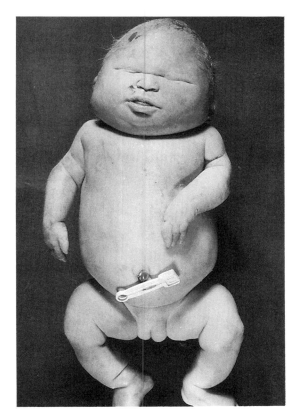

Fig. 4.14 Trisomy 21 (Down's syndrome) with small head, flat facies, upward slanting eyes and protuberant tongue.

Primary ventricular septal defects arise less frequently. It is, perhaps, surprising that the cardiac defect seen most commonly in Down's syndrome is one of the most severe. Other frequently associated anomalies include duodenal atresia and Hirschsprung's disease (megacolon). Children with Down's syndrome are all mentally retarded to some degree. The frontal lobes are foreshortened and neurofibrillary tangles, similar to those seen in Alzheimer's disease, develop at an early age. A major advance in our understanding of Down's syndrome and its link with Alzheimer's disease has been the localization on chromosome 21 of the gene

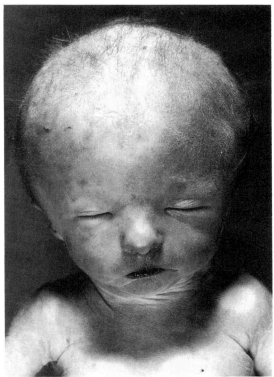

Fig. 4.15 Trisomy 18 (Edward's syndrome) showing the characteristic small mouth and chin, and short palpebral fissures.

skin creases, broad spatulate hands and wide spacing between the fourth and fifth digits. Up to 40% of cases have cardiac anomalies, the most frequent of which is a persistent atrioventricular canal due to failure of endocardial cushion development. In this situation, the atrio-ventricular canal is not divided in right and left parts during development and there is, thus, a large central defect with low atrial and high ventricular septal components; large valve leaflets, formed by fusion of the anterior and posterior parts of split septal tricuspid and anterior mitral valve leaflets, pass through the defect.

sequence at the A4 polypeptide subunit of the amyloid fibril in the neurofibrillary tangles [25].

Trisomy 18 (Edward's syndrome) has facial characteristics which are also unmistakeable (Figs 4.15 and 4.16). It is the second most common chromosomal syndrome; there is a preponderance of females over males and few infants survive the first few weeks or months of life. Infants with trisomy 18 have a small mouth and chin, short palpebral fissures, low-set malformed ears and marked incurving of the index and fifth fingers. The internal anomalies are less specific and, most frequently, include incompletely lobated lungs, ventricular septal defect, Meckel's

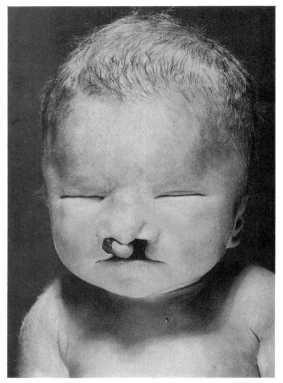

Fig. 4.17 Trisomy 13 (Patau's syndrome) with bilateral complete cleft lip and palate, and broad-based nose.

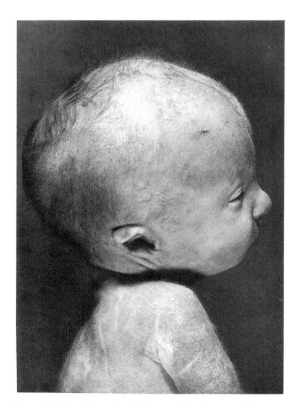

Fig. 4.16 Profile of an infant with trisomy 18 showing the low-set malformed ears.

diverticulum, bicornuate uterus in females and a single hypogastric artery.

Facial clefts are a more characteristic feature of trisomy 13 (Patau's syndrome) than of the other two major syndromes (Fig. 4.17). Most infants with trisomy 13 die within a short time of birth and survivors have severe mental retardation. A ventricular septal defect is present in 80% of cases [3]. Associated central nervous system defects include microcephaly, holoprosencephaly, arrhinencephaly and agenesis at the corpus callosum.

The triploidy syndrome, in which the fetus has a complete set of extra chromosomes probably resulting from double fertilization, is frequently encountered in midtrimester abortions. Infants surviving after 28 weeks' gestation usually die in the early neonatal period. It is estimated that it occurs in about 2% of pregnancies and that only about 3% of affected fetuses survive beyond the first trimester. Fetuses with triploidy have large heads relative to the size of the face with syndactyly and hydatidiform change in the placenta. Internal anomalies may include hydrocephalus or holoprosencephaly, cardiac septal defects and, in males, hypospadias and cryptorchidism.

Turner's syndrome is more common in first and second trimester abortions than in stillbirths. The cases have an X0 chromosome constitution, soft-tissue swelling and webbing of the neck or more generalized oedema, and dysplastic ovaries.

Many chromosomal anomalies which may predispose the fetus to early death demonstrate less obvious features than the listed examples. Careful recording of any abnormal stigmata is, therefore, essential and, ideally, routine chromosome analysis should be carried out on all abortions and stillborn fetuses in order to define syndromes and to help identify the familial pattern of disease.

Karyotyping is usually performed using cord or heart blood and fascia lata; amnion can be used instead should the viability of the fascia lata be in doubt, as, for example, in the macerated fetus, but, as mentioned above, chorionic tissue must not be included if contamination with maternal blood is to be avoided. Cell lines for *in vitro* studies are also necessary if there is any question of an underlying metabolic disorder.

4.8 CONGENITAL TUMOURS

Congenital tumours are usually an incidental finding at post-mortem in the stillborn fetus. The congenital rhabdomyoma of the heart, although rare in itself, is one of the most frequently encountered cardiac tumours of infancy and may present with fetal hydrops and polyhydramnios [26]. It is a reasonably well demarcated greyish white tumour composed of large vacuolated pleomorphic cells with spidery strands of cytoplasm extending outward from a relatively small centrally placed nucleus. The tumour can arise in any part of the myocardium and may obstruct the ventricular outflow tracts or involve the conducting system [27].

Congenital leukaemia is also rare but may present in stillborn fetuses as deeply congested haemorrhagic subcutaneous nodules and widespread involvement of internal organs (Figs 4.18 and 4.19). It can be

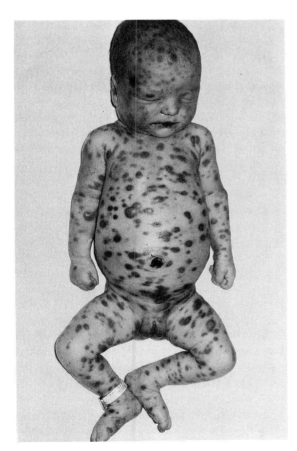

Fig. 4.18 Stillborn fetus with congenital leukaemia.

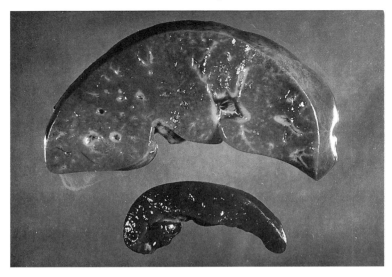

Fig. 4.19 Thickening and opacity of connective-tissue septae of the liver and spleen due to the leukaemic infiltrate in congenital leukaemia.

associated with Down's syndrome and has been reported in infants of mothers suffering from leukaemia during pregnancy.

Congenital neuroblastomas are more frequent. Massive liver involvement (and ascites) is a particular feature of this tumour and results in severe respiratory embarrassment in the newborn infant due to splinting of the diaphragm. In most instances, however, the tumour has a benign outcome, regressing spontaneously with only supportive therapeutic measures.

Sacrococcygeal teratoma is the most common congenital tumour – 45–60% of all germ cell tumours in children occur in this site. Other extragonadal sites include the retroperitoneum, mediastinum and the head and neck region. Only a small proportion of congenital teratomas diagnosed in the neonatal period are malignant and the presence of embryonic tissues in these tumours should not necessarily be regarded as evidence of malignancy. The only renal tumour that occurs in the neonate is the mesoblastic nephroma, a hamartomatous

tumour with a trabeculated structure consisting of interweaving strands of fine spindle-shaped cells. Mesoblastic nephromas are entirely benign and any deaths associated with them have been due to complications of chemotherapy.

Renal blastema persisting in the subcapsular cortex of the kidney after completion of normal nephrogenic activity at 36 weeks' gestation resembles the structure of a Wilms' tumour. This may be present in a kidney which also contains a Wilms' tumour but nephroblastomas are rare before 6 months of age. Isolated renal blastema may be associated with congenital abnormalities.

In the liver, the commonest congenital tumours seen incidentally in this age-group are vascular tumours (haemangiomas) and hepatoblastoma [28]. The latter is usually located in the right lobe and tends to merge with the surrounding normal parenchyma. Some have a fetal pattern which can closely resemble the trabecular structure of the liver, others are more embryonal showing ribbons or sheets of cells and some pseudorosette and acinar formation. Extramedullary haemo-poiesis is usually a prominent feature. Hepatocellular carcinomas usually occur in older children but may also present in early infancy and, presumably, are of congenital origin in this age-group.

4.9 POSTMATURITY

A postmature fetus is defined as one that is born after 42 weeks' gestation irrespective of weight. The definition, however, is often used synonymously for pregnancies that continue beyond 40 weeks' gestation and approximately 5–10% of pregnancies fall into this broader category.

Stillbirth and perinatal mortality rates increase with postmaturity and the risk to the postmature fetus appears to be greater in primigravid women and mothers who are over 35 years of age. It is estimated that some 200 stillbirths occur in the 41 weeks and over gestational age-group in England and Wales each year [28].

The majority of the fetal deaths in this group are unexplained. The postmature fetus can be recognized by the decrease or absence of vernix caseosa, loss of lanugo, dry flakey skin, long nails and hardness of the skull bones – but it may be indistinguishable from one born at term. Nor are there any consistent placental changes attributable to postmaturity; it is to be assumed that the placenta has reached physiological limits which cannot be recognized either at a macroscopic or micro-scopic level.

4.10 DRUGS AND DRUG ABUSE

Any drug which crosses the placental barrier is potentially able to influence or damage the fetus and, since the early 1960s when the thalidomide tragedy hit the headlines, aware-ness of the possible teratogenic effects of drugs has been high.

The literature continues to identify isolated cases or groups of cases where a teratogenic effect of drug therapy is implicated in fetal loss or malformation, but there have been few major surveys reviewing drug ingestion in a population of young pregnant women. A recent prospective survey from Glasgow (1982–84) identifies a trend – at least in the United Kingdom – of a significant reduction in the ingestion during pregnancy of pre-scribed and self-administered drugs. Over 90% of the mothers avoided drugs during the first trimester and 65% avoided drugs at any stage in the pregnancy; a 16% incidence of self-administration of drugs at some stage of pregnancy which was discovered in a previous Edinburgh series (1963–65) was reduced to 8% in the Glasgow series [29]. Only those drugs which have been associated with a definitive diagnostic pattern of malformation will be referred to in this chapter. (See also Chapter 3.)

Phenytoin has been associated with a number of stillbirths and neonatal deaths [30]. Affected infants have coarse features, a broad depressed nasal bridge, wide-set eyes, prominent inner epicanthic folds, broad upper lip, wide mouth, a short neck, low posterior hair-line, prominently ridged metopic sutures, hypoplastic distal phalanges and small nails. Fetal weights may be less than expected for gestational age and the infants frequently show some degree of microcephaly [31, 32, 33]. Up to 40% of fetuses of mothers treated with phenytoin in the first trimester may be affected. The phenytoin syndrome has some similarities to the Coffin–Siris and Noonan syndromes for which it is often mis-taken; it has been postulated that affected infants may be genetically predisposed to the teratogenic effects of the drug [34].

Trimethadione, used in the treatment of petit mal, has also been associated with characteristic stigmata. It is rarely used in women of child-bearing age but, when it is, it can cause spontaneous abortion, stillbirth and neonatal death in addition to a recognizable pattern of defect which includes V-shaped eyebrows, a broad upturned nose with a low nasal bridge, a large mouth with high arched palate and low-set, backwardly rotated ears with a poorly developed anteriorly folded helix. Some infants have cardiac defects and most are mentally retarded [35].

Sodium valproate, previously thought not to have teratogenic effects, has since been specifically implicated and shown to be associated with an increased incidence of spina bifida. Other associated anomalies include hydrocephalus, facial dysmorphism and hypospadias [36].

The anticoagulant warfarin has also been implicated in the production of teratogenic effects when used in the first trimester. Affected infants show a typical under-development of midfacial structures and stippling of bone epiphyses. Other features, including optic atrophy, microcephaly and agenesis of the corpus callosum, are more specifically associated with exposure in the second and third trimester of pregnancy and may be the result of intracerebral haemor-rhage [37]. Twenty eight per cent of fetuses exposed to warfarin are either abnormal or die *in utero* [38].

Alcohol is the commonest cause of fetal malformation and accounts for a large pro-portion of cases of growth deficiency or mental handicap. A variety of anomalies occur [3, 39] which are described in detail in Chapter 3. Cigarette smoking has not, so far, been equated with fetal abnormality or a clearly defined syndrome. It is, nevertheless, associated with low birth weight infants and the implication is that the effect on birth weight is dose-related [40].

There is no doubt that there are increased stillbirth and neonatal mortality rates in the drug-addicted population, although the figures vary in different series from near normal stillbirth rates to those approaching 71/1000 live births [41]; it has been suggested that, in some cases, the cause of stillbirths may

be the actual withdrawal of narcotics [41, 42]. The subject is, again, addressed more fully in Chapter 3.

REFERENCES

1. Mueller, R.F., Sybert, V.P., Johnson, J. *et al.* (1983) Evaluation of a protocol for post-mortem examination of stillbirths. *New Engl. J. Med.,* **309**, 586.
2. Gruenwald, P. and Minh, H.N. (1960) Evaluation of body and organ weights in perinatal pathology. *Am. J. Clin. Pathol.,* **34**, 247.
3. Smith, D.E. (1982) *Recognisable Patterns of Human Malformation,* 3rd edn, W.B. Saunders, Philadelphia.
4. Langman, J. (1963) *Medical Embryology,* Williams and Wilkins, Baltimore.
5. Foote, G.A., Wilson, A.J. and Stewart, J.H. (1978) Perinatal post-mortem radiology – experience with 2500 cases. *Br. J. Radiol.,* **51**, 351.
6. Seppanen, U. (1985) The value of perinatal post-mortem radiography. Experience of 514 cases. *Ann. Clin. Res.,* **17**, Suppl. 44.
7. Kuhns, L.R. and Finstrom, O. (1976) New standards of ossification of the newborn. *Radiology,* **119**, 655.
8. Barnett, E. (1970) Foetal maturity, in *A Textbook of X-ray Diagnosis,* 4th edn. (eds S.C. Shanks and P. Kerley), H.K. Lewis, London.
9. Cremin, B.J. and Fisher, P.M. (1970) The lesions of congenital syphilis. *Br. J. Radiol.,* **43**, 333.
10. Connor, J.M., Connor, R.A.C., Sweet, E.M. *et al.* (1985) Lethal neonatal chondrodysplasias in the West of Scotland 1970–1983 with a description of a thanatomorphic dysplasia-like autosomal recessive disorder, Glasgow variant. *Am. J. Med. Genet.,* **22**, 243.
11. Benirscke, K. (1961) Examination of the placenta. *Obstet. Gynecol.,* **18**, 309.
12. Saber, R.S. (1977) Stillbirth due to extensive feto-maternal transfusion. *NY State J. Med.,* **14**, 2249.
13. Hovatta, O., Lipasti, A., Rapola, J. and Karjalainen, O. (1983) Causes of stillbirth: a clinicopathological study of 243 patients. *Br. J. Obstet. Gynaecol.,* **90**, 691.

14. Heifetz, S.A. (1984) Strangulation of the umbilical cord by amniotic bands: report of 6 cases and literature review. *Pediatr. Pathol.*, **2**, 285.

15. Macgregor, A.R. (1960) *Pathology of Infancy and Childhood*, E. & S. Livingstone, Edinburgh.

16. Grall, J.Y., Coudrais, C., Jouan, H. *et al.* (1983) L'artère ombilicale unique: à propos de 194 observations. *Arch. Anat. Cytol. Pathol.*, **31**, 111.

17. Ballantyne, J.W. (1902) *Manual of Antenatal Pathology and Hygiene – The Foetus*, W. Green, Edinburgh.

18. Carrington, D., Gilmore, D.H., Whittle, M.J. *et al.* (1987) Maternal serum alphafetoprotein – a marker of fetal aplastic crisis during intrauterine human parvovirus infection. *Lancet*, **i**, 433.

19. McDonald, H. and Tobin, J.O'H. (1978) Congenital cytomegalovirus infection: a collaborative study on epidemiological, clinical and laboratory findings. *Dev. Med. Child Neurol.*, **20**, 471.

20. Ward, K.P., Galloway, W.H. and Achterlonie, I.A. (1979) Congenital cytomegalovirus infection and diabetes. *Lancet*, **i**, 497.

21. Anand, A., Gray, E.S., Brown, T. *et al.* (1987) Human parvovirus infection in pregnancy and hydrops fetalis. *New Engl. J. Med.*, **316**, 183.

22. Clewley, J.P. (1985) Detection of human parvovirus using a molecularly cloned probe. *J. Med. Virol.*, **15**, 173.

23. Johnson, F.W.A., Matheson, B.A., Williams, H. *et al.* (1985) Abortion due to infection with *Chlamydia psittaci* in a sheep farmer's wife. *Br. Med. J.*, **290**, 592.

24. Tafari, N., Ross, S., Naeye, R.L. *et al.* (1976) Mycoplasma strains and perinatal death. *Lancet*, **i**, 108.

25. Kang, J., Lemaire, H.-G., Unterbeck, A. *et al.* (1987) The precursor of Alzheimer's disease amyloid A4 protein resembles a cell-surface receptor. *Nature*, **325**, 733.

26. Soltan, M.H. and Keohane, C. (1981) Hydrops fetalis due to congenital cardiac rhabdomyoma. Case report. *Br. J. Obstet. Gynaecol.*, **88**, 771.

27. Dubois, R.W., Neill, C.A. and Hutchins, G.M. (1983) Rhabdomyoma of the heart producing right bundle branch block. *Pediatr. Pathol.*, **1**, 435.

28. Benjamin, E., Lendon, M. and Marsdon, H.B. (1981) Hepatoblastoma as a cause of intrauterine fetal death. Case report. *Br. J. Obstet. Gynaecol.*, **88**, 329.

29. Yudkin, P.L., Wood, L. and Redman, C.W.G. (1987) Risk of unexplained stillbirth at different gestational ages. *Lancet*, **i**, 1192.

30. Rubin, P.C., Craig, G.F., Gavin, K. and Sumner, D. (1986) Prospective survey of use of therapeutic drugs, alcohol and cigarettes during pregnancy. *Br. Med. J.*, **292**, 81.

31. Hiilesmaa, V.K., Bardy, A. and Terama, K. (1985) Obstetric outcome in women with epilepsy. *Am. J. Obstet. Gynecol.*, **152**, 499.

32. Meadow, S.R. (1968) Anticonvulsant drugs and congenital abnormalities. *Lancet*, **ii**, 1296.

33. Hanson, J.W. and Smith, D.W. (1975) The fetal hydantoin syndrome. *J. Pediatr.*, **87**, 285.

34. Strickler, S.M., Dansky, L.V., Miller, M.A. *et al.* (1985) Genetic predisposition to phenytoin-induced birth defects. *Lancet*, **ii**, 746.

35. Zackai, E.H., Mellman, W.J., Neiderer, B. and Hanson, J.W. (1975) The fetal trimethadione syndrome. *J. Pediatr.*, **87**, 280.

36. Bjerkedal, T., Czeizel, A., Goujard, J. *et al.* (1982) Valproic acid and spina bifida. *Lancet*, **ii**, 1096; Lindhout, D. and Meinardi, H. (1984) Spina bifida and *in-utero* exposure to valproate. *Lancet*, **ii**, 396.

37. Stevenson, R.E., Burton, O.M., Ferlauto, G.J. and Taylor, H.A. (1980) Hazards of oral anticoagulants during pregnancy. *JAMA*, **243**, 1549.

38. Holzgreve, W., Carey, J.C. and Hall, B.D. (1976) Warfarin-induced fetal abnormalities. *Lancet*, **ii**, 914.

39. Jones, K.L., Smith, D.W., Ulleland, C.N. and Streissguth, A.P. (1973) Pattern of malformation in offspring of chronic alcoholic mothers. *Lancet*, **i**, 1268.

40. Abel, E.L. (1980) Smoking during pregnancy: a review of effects on growth and development of offspring. *Hum. Biol.*, **52**, 593.

41. Rumenteria, J.L. and Nunag, N.N. (1973) Narcotic withdrawal in pregnancy: stillbirth incidence with a case report. *Am. J. Obstet. Gynecol.*, **116**, 1152.

42. Sutherland, J.M. and Light, I.J. (1965) The effects of drugs upon the developing fetus. *Pediatr. Clin. North Am.*, **12**, 781.

CHAPTER 5

The post-mortem examination of a baby

John L. Emery

Learning the technique of dissecting a baby so as to gain most knowledge about diseases and death is like learning to play a piano – there is a technique that you can learn but making music depends on something else. A lack of technique, however, limits one's findings.

There is a primary rule – do the whole examination yourself. To let a technician remove the viscera in a baby will mean that vascular anomalies will often be overlooked and those minute hair-like flecks of fibrin in the serous cavities that may be the only findings of a septicaemia will be missed. The conventional opening of the skull from the crown also prevents the diagnosis of many instances of cerebral oedema.

There is also a concept of doing a 'routine necropsy' which is a relative concept. A routine necropsy on a hospital patient could be simply to confirm or disprove a clinical diagnosis; one on a road accident could be to determine the extent and direction of the lethal trauma and to exclude other natural causes of death; and, on a cot death, to exclude trauma or some gross natural disease such as pneumonia or meningitis. But a routine necropsy in a research department would involve histology of all tissues, multiple cultures, immunochemistry, tissue cultures, chemistry of a variety of fluids and tissues, a developmental assessment of all organs and even an extensive study of the background of the baby. A necropsy technique is only valid for the type of necropsy to which it applies; to set about a necropsy on a baby without knowing what questions are being asked will only lead to frustration and confusion.

The technique described here is one that we have developed and used over 40 years as a basic procedure onto which special techniques such as in-situ brain fixation can be grafted. In this description, it will be assumed that the pathologist is already familiar with standard techniques used on adults. The method described is applicable to babies of between 15 weeks' gestation and 5 years of age. Modifications are needed for smaller babies and techniques used on adults are directly applicable for children approaching puberty.

5.1 HISTORY

A good history is essential prior to some types of necropsy; this applies particularly to deaths where parents or others have made statements about the child that need to be confirmed or refuted or where the child was reported to have had particular symptoms or eaten particularly abnormal foods. The history in children needs to be interpreted in a different manner from that in adults: first, most of the reported symptoms and signs are being interpreted by adults and, secondly, the persons reporting the history are usually deeply emotionally involved with the child. Although the baby becomes physically detached from the mother at birth, it is not psychologically detached for months; confusion often arises because people take 'histories' from parents before the mother, in particular, has accepted that the child is dead. Negative histories have almost no value and should never be treated as such – and this applies particularly to cot deaths. I have often felt that it is best to have no history at all when dealing with unexpected deaths so that all avenues of exploration are open – it is too easy to concentrate on one system and miss something in another in a history-directed necropsy.

5.2 PERMISSION FOR NECROPSY

The examination of most deaths referred to the forensic pathologist is directed by the medicolegal authorities but their keenness to do so varies greatly. It would be unexceptionable for a cot death to be certified in Scotland without necropsy and there have been instances in England and Wales where this has been so. A coroner once remarked to me: 'If the pathologist is not going to find anything, why pay him to do it?' A recent survey of cot deaths undertaken by Huber in Utrecht, Holland, indicates that a quarter of the babies so certified in that country are not examined by necropsy and this practice is also prevalent in the United States (see Chapter 27B).

The medical attendants will seek permission for necropsy so as to satisfy a general interest in establishing why a particular child died; the parent, however, is usually more motivated by a desire to ensure that the baby had no concealed condition that might affect future or existing members of the family. Consent then represents an attempt to rationalize the baby's natural death as something that will lead to the prevention of deaths of other children.

5.3 PROCEDURES BEFORE NECROPSY

Upon receipt of the baby into the mortuary:

(1) Take the temperature subject to the precautions outlined in Chapter 18.
(2) Extract vitreous fluid from one eye. This may be done by trained mortuary staff at any time of the day or night.
(3) Examine all the clothes in which the baby was dressed, including the pillow, mattress and sheets if possible.
(4) Retain any wet nappy or urine.
(5) Ideally, take an X-ray picture of the whole body and limbs in standard position. This should be insisted upon but it usually requires that the mortuary porter handles and positions the body as many radiographers are disinclined to touch a dead body.

5.4 EXTERNAL EXAMINATION

If possible, start your examination with the baby as nearly as possible in the situation in which it was found dead. Undress the child yourself – this will assist considerably in the interpretation of hypostatic marks. When the baby is fully naked, use some form of dissecting block so that the child's body is lifted an inch or two from the level of the dissection bench (Fig. 5.1); this makes it much easier to inspect and control the body for dissection than is possible on any flat surface.

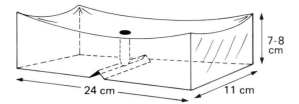

Fig. 5.1 Block for stabilizing the infant's body during dissection.

(a) Hypostasis

This must be interpreted with care as the posture of the baby in the mortuary refrigerator is often the most obvious feature. When that position is known and described, it is often possible to find other features – such as palor at the nosetip or back of the head – that give an indication of body position at death. A double pattern is sometimes clearly discernible. The search for signs of child abuse (see Chapter 18) should not be omitted, even in hospital deaths.

(b) Facies

The number of syndromes being recounted by paediatricians as being associated with abnormal facies seems to grow daily. If there is any suspicion that the face is 'slightly queer', have true anteroposterior and lateral photographs taken of the face with a scale included. Such photographs can be of vital importance later – for example, when questions related to 'fetal alcoholism' are raised.

(c) Weight

The baby needs to be weighed naked and the weight related not only to the age of the child and its length but also to its previous weights. It will be of little significance if a child with weight on the 10th centile has been on that centile line since birth; on the other hand, the

weight of a child which is on the 50th centile could represent a significant reduction if it had been on the 90th centile for several months. Babies are now being weighed more frequently than in the past and the health visitors' records of weights are easily obtained and charted.

(d) Lengths

Measurements of the child are often of more value than weight as related to the long-term effects of disease. The most useful measurements are crown/heel, crown/rump (sitting length), foot length and skull circumference. The circumferential lengths around the body are best done at the level of the nipples and at the umbilicus. The body length measurements must be taken using a solid rule with rigid vertical planes placed firmly either against the buttocks or against the base of the feet with ankles flexed.

(e) Skin

The cleanliness of the skin, particularly behind the ears and in body folds, and the lengths of finger and toe nails should be noted, together with the extent and type of napkin reaction. Care must be taken in interpreting napkin reactions because severe reddening and blistering of the skin can occur post-mortem when a wet napkin is left in place and is confined by an impervious cover. The minutest amount of urine is worth retaining, even from a napkin if it is not contaminated by faeces, as some inborn errors of metabolism may still be diagnosable (a piece of urine-wet napkin put into a small plastic container can often suffice).

(f) The skin incision

The traditional midline, neck to pubis incision is contraindicated in a young child for two reasons. First, the skin of a baby is less fibrous

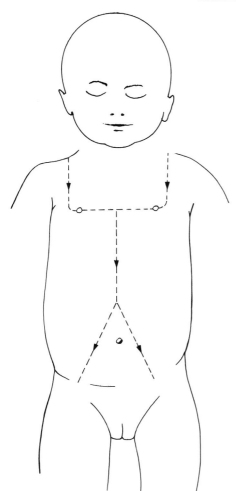

Fig. 5.2 Lines of incision for opening the body.

The skin of the baby is more easily separated from the underlying tissues than is the case in an adult and this can be done by blunt dissection using a finger or the handle of the forceps. To expose the neck, it is easiest to discard the knife and to use both hands, dissecting with the thumbs; the skin can easily be freed up to the chin and base of tongue by this means. Difficulty in exposure of the base of the tongue at the front is usually due to the incision not being extended far enough backwards over the shoulders. The incision is extended caudally in the midline to about 1 cm above the umbilicus where it is divided and extended to the inguinal canals on both sides. When this has been done, the umbilical vein needs to be cut; the lower skin flap is then lifted downwards to expose the lower anterior abdominal wall and the bladder.

(g) The abdomen

The abdomen must be examined before the intestines are disturbed. The caecum and appendix are sought and their position identified. If this is not done immediately and there is imperfect lateral attachment of the mesentery, it is often not possible to be certain later as to the presence or absence of any degree of volvulus.

(h) The thorax

If the child has been X-rayed, the plates should be examined and the presence or absence of pneumothorax (or pneumo-peritoneum) determined before opening the body cavities. Otherwise the whole child can be immersed in a bowl of saline or a small pool of saline may be made in a fold of skin in the region of the axilla; a small incision in the intercostal space under saline reveals the presence or absence of gas.

Care is needed in removing the sternum to avoid cutting the veins at the base of the neck

than that of an adult; the skin can easily split and a neck incision can extend to and over the chin if it is put under tension. Secondly, at the pubic end, the urinary bladder is usually an abdominal organ and often extends to the umbilicus; the urachus and hypogastric arteries and bladder need to be exposed (Fig. 5.2).

The most convenient incision commences over the shoulder, runs down to and across the nipple line and back up to the shoulder.

and near the thymus. It is simplest to lift the costochondral diaphragmatic edge of the thorax slightly on the left side and to cut through the cartilage of the lower ribs about 1 cm from the bone. Having opened the left pleura, lift the cartilage on the sternal side and, holding the ribs away from the lung, continue cutting the cartilages up to the first rib. Still holding the sternum to the right, separate the pericardium from the sternum and continue into the right chest; then cut up the right ribs as on the left side. Keep the sternum clear of the thymus as the ribs are freed. Hold the sternum forward and separate the manubrium from the thymus. Then cut through the joints betwen the manubrium and the clavicles and first rib leaving the sternocleidomastoid muscles attached to the sternum but freeing them from the clavicles. Lift the sternum with the muscles attached and gently dissect them free on both sides; this gives a controlled exposure of the vessels at the base of the neck and of the thymus up to the thyroid. The sternum can now be detached with the sternocleidomastoid muscles at their mastoid ends.

Until this time no large blood vessels have been opened but the next step, which involves removing the thymus, will result in spilling blood as a large vein runs across the thymus; now is the time to take blood samples from the left and right heart and from the right jugular vein. If desired, the body can be almost exsanguinated from the right superior vena cava; this is facilitated by lifting the child's legs and, thus, emptying the inferior vena cava and hepatic veins.

(i) Removal of the thymus

The thymus is dissected free from the anterior pericardium and the vessels at the base of the heart are exposed. The innominate vein runs across the thymus but need not be cut if the gland is handled gently. Dissect the thymus off up to the thyroid gland and, at this time,

note the presence or absence of other nodules of thymic tissue in that area.

(j) Neck tissues

The sternocleidomastoid muscles have been removed and the carotid and jugular vessels are now identifiable; if necessary, the internal carotids are now ligated. The carotid bodies are best identified at this time.

(k) Removal of the tongue

The lower margins of the jaw have been exposed. Pass the point of a scalpel behind the jaw into the mouth in front of the tongue and cut back on both sides against the bone to the angles of the jaw. This frees the tongue which is then delivered below the jaw into the neck. At this time it is useful to put a pair of tongue forceps on the tongue.

(l) Nasopharynx and nose

There are several approaches to the naso-pharynx. I have found it most convenient to remove the tongue and larynx first. To do this, carry the lateral cuts behind the jaw backwards between the tongue and the tonsils and take the incision around to the upper oesophagus below the adenoids. This is facilitated by gentle forward tension on the tongue. The nasopharynx can be dissected at this time or left until after the thoracic and abdominal viscera have been removed.

Viewed from below, the pharyngeal ring with the uvula is apparent and the size can be measured. The pharyngeal ring is removed in one piece. This is done by cutting across the palate into the nose immediately behind the hard palate. Continue the incision laterally to the eustachian tubes and around the base of the skull, freeing the adenoids. When this is done on both sides, Waldeyer's ring is complete and, after fixation, a single block that contains both surfaces of the soft palate, the tonsils and the adenoids may be taken for histology.

(m) Nasal mucosa

The most convenient histology of the nasal mucosa comes from the nasal septum. This is obtained by using a strong pair of scissors to cut forward through the hard palate on each side of the septum. Then, using a solid metal scalpel, cut the palate across as near the front as possible and take this cut up across the septum to the base of the nose. Withdraw the scalpel and insert it from behind, first on one side then the other, and cut the septum to the base of the nose from as far up the posterior septum as is convenient. A keel-shaped piece of septum together with the centre of the hard palate is obtained which includes the posterior end of the septum (Fig. 5.3). This is fixed before being handled further. Then an oblique 'tuning fork' block for histology is taken after dissecting the mucosa from the underlying nasal-septal bone. The turbinates can be inspected after the nasal septum has been removed.

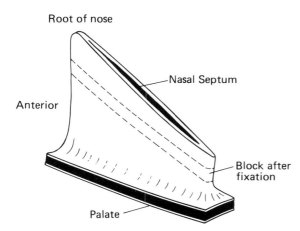

Fig. 5.3 Keel-shaped piece of nasal septum and palate. Dotted lines show the site of the 'tuning fork block' tissue taken after fixation.

5.5 THE VISCERA

Before the viscera are touched it is essential to identify the blood vessels, including the subclavian leaving and entering the heart, and to confirm the normality or otherwise of the aortic arch and main vessels. While it is not difficult to remove the whole of the viscera from pharynx to anus in one piece, it is often better to dissect the organs in stages; the technique may, however, require modification in the event of a violent death (c.f. Chapter 18).

(a) The intestines

Before touching, confirm the normality of the situation of the caecum and appendix. Identify the junction of the sigmoid with the rectum and, depending on the content of the bowel, either ligate and cut or, simply, cut. Then, starting with the sigmoid, dissect the large bowel free of the mesentery, inspecting the viscus as this is done. Continue to the ileocoecal valve and, then, dissect the small bowel away, cutting the mesentery as near to the bowel as possible; continue this to the jejuno-duodenal junction, at which point, either ligate and cut or cut direct if the bowel is empty. Then free the spleen from the posterior abdominal wall and bring it forward with the pancreas and duodenum so that the mesenteric arteries and root of the mesentery can be cut.

(b) Heart, lungs and liver

Open the pericardium, inspect the heart and confirm its general normality (the heart will have been exposed earlier if cardiac cultures have been taken). Starting from the top, dissect the oesophagus away from the cervical spine and, taking deep sweeps laterally, cut through the subclavian arteries. Holding the heart and lungs by the larynx, dissect the oesophagus and aorta away from the thoracic spine as far as the insertion of the crura of the diaphragm. Replace the heart and lungs in the thorax. Then free each lobe of the diaphragm from the chest wall and bring this dissection in to the midline first on the left side taking care to avoid the adrenal and kidney. Then do the same on the right side but, while doing so, lift the liver forward and separate the liver from the adrenal. When this has been done, cut across the aorta and inferior vena cava with scissors below the liver but above the renal vessels. This frees the block of tongue, heart, lungs, liver, spleen, stomach, pancreas and mesentery in one piece.

(c) Urinogenital tract

The kidneys are now clearly displayed. The adrenals need careful handling and should be removed before the kidneys are manipulated. They are best removed with their surrounding fat and dissected with blunt-ended scissors with the hilar vessels firmly held but without touching the cortex; the body of the adrenal should not be grasped. The kidneys, ureter, bladder and urinogenital tract are removed much more easily in a baby than in an adult if the child's legs are held apart and the cartilage of the symphysis pubis is cut in the midline. This opens the pelvis so that the necks of the bladder and of the penis are easily exposed. The vagina, urethra and anus can be removed easily through a circular incision in the skin. Child abuse is believed by some to occur in many children; an examination for sexual abuse needs to be part of every necropsy (see Chapter 18).

5.6 SKULL AND BRAIN

The brain of a baby has a much higher water content than that of an adult and its general structure is not held fixed by a vast network of myelinated nerves; the essence of a baby's brain is its fluidity. The conventional opening of the skull from the vertex, cutting the margins of the frontal and parietal bones and folding them back like the leaves of a flower, frequently results in a flattened, sagging mass which all too easily breaks and which, particularly later, breaks at the brain stem. Using that method, the only way of measuring cerebral oedema is through assessment of the superficial wetness of the brain as the skull is cut and an estimate of flattening of its convolutions. The major importance of cerebral oedema probably lies in the way it affects the vital centres within the brain stem; thus, from a functional point of view, the brain stem is of greater importance than is the cortex.

For this reason we have, for many years, inspected the brain through the foramen magnum before opening the cranial cavity. To do this, place the child face down with the body mass supported on a block and open the skin at the back of the head and skull using a 'question-mark' incision (Fig. 5.4). It is important that the incision is carried fairly well back behind the ears and over the back of the skull; the line of the incision must be out of sight when the skin is replaced after the necropsy but, at the same time, the line across the skull must be far enough forward to enable the scalp to be pulled forward. Having produced the skin flap, remove the muscles attached to the occiput and clean the rami of the upper cervical vertebrae. Then, using small bone forceps, snip off the back of the atlas and, possibly, of the second or third cervical vertebrae leaving the dura exposed beneath. Make sure that the area is free of blood, hold the skull level with the body and incise the dura at the level of the foramen magnum. If this is done carefully, the dura can be incised without cutting the arachnoid so that the cerebral spinal fluid does not escape. At this point, perforate the arachnoid using an ordinary glass pipette with a rubber teat and remove a sample of cerebral spinal fluid. Then, extend the dural incision, expose the cervical cord and foramen magnum and

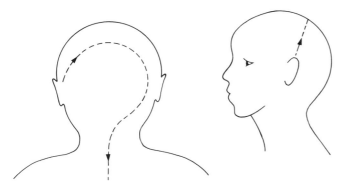

Fig. 5.4 The 'question-mark' incision across the back of the skull and into the nape of the neck for exposing the foramen magnum.

observe the position of the cerebellar tonsils. In the normal child's brain, with no cerebral oedema, the cavity of the fourth ventricle is immediately apparent and the tonsils can just be visualized by looking at the lateral surfaces through the foramen magnum. But any degree of cerebral oedema induces a variety of positions of the cerebellar tonsils – first approximating, then presenting and, then, herniating into the cervical canal. This caudal displacement of the cerebellum is usually accompanied by a lesser displacement of the brain stem, but this is not easy to estimate from the back. To measure this, it is necessary, at this time, to take the knife and cut at right angles through the brain stem exactly at the level of the foramen magnum. The position of the brain stem related to the foramen magnum can be measured later when the brain stem has been removed, the critical distance being from this cut to the lower edge of the inferior olives which, in most children, is between 8 and 10 mm. If this distance is reduced, there has been some movement of the brain stem which is almost invariably due to cerebral oedema pushing the brain stem downwards.

The skull can now be opened from above. The cranial cavities can be opened on both sides but there are advantages in doing so from one side only. After folding the scalp forward, inspect the cranial bones. It is usually possible to identify the birth presentation in a child dying within a month of birth and, in a newborn child, it is important to look at the skull bones from the point of view of locking and overriding. Cut around one frontal and one parietal bone, avoiding the longitudinal sinus and leaving the lateral edge attached; this can usually be done in the younger child by means of a scalpel and, in the slightly older child, with a pair of strong scissors (Fig. 5.5). When this has been done, the frontal and parietal bones can be folded out while the head is suspended in the palm of the hand.

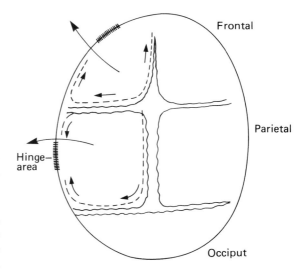

Fig. 5.5 Diagram showing the directions of cutting and hinge areas for opening the skull.

It is our technique to remove the brain in three separate pieces. This has the advantages over the classic suspension of the whole brain in that it enables the individual parts of the brain to be removed with less trauma and, at the same time, allows for critical and detailed inspection of the major intracranial contents as the brain is dissected; it also facilitates fixation of the brain. When the single side of a hemisphere has been exposed, dislocate the back end of the hemisphere from its pocket beneath the parietal bones with your finger or back of a scalpel and cut the vessels running from the surface of the hemisphere to the longitudinal sinus. This opens up the whole length of the corpus callosum which is then cut in the midline throughout its entire length, thus exposing the third ventricle; distortion and asymmetries of the third ventricle and thalamus are noted. The great veins running into the falx and tentorium are also exposed. When these have been inspected, continue the incision anteriorly so that the frontal lobes are completely separated; they are frequently partially interdigitated if there is some slight defect in the anterior aspect of the falx. Cut through the cerebral peduncle, attempting to do this at right angles and cutting so that the infundibulum and optic nerves are not touched. This completely frees the lateral hemisphere which slides easily onto the palm of the hand when the skull is tilted; the hemisphere can be placed immediately into fixature. Removing one lateral hemisphere exposes the whole of the falx and one leaf of the tentorium, the great sinuses and also the position of the infundibulum but, in particular, the presence or absence of any herniation of the cerebellum through the tentorial opening can be visualized. Then, open the length of the longitudinal sinus, the straight sinus and the exposed lateral sinus with a scalpel. The falx is then cut radially in three or four cuts so that the cerebral hemisphere of the opposite side is exposed. This hemisphere is then removed as was the first. The whole of the cranial cavity and the upper surface of the tentorium are now exposed and the opposite lateral sinus can be explored for clots.

At this time, the pituitary, infundibulum and optic nerves can be inspected, as can the cranial nerves. These are cut and an incision is made around the posterior aspect of the tentorium exposing the upper surface of the cerebellum behind the pineal. The brain stem and cerebellum are now free and this mass of brain tissue will slide into the waiting hand on tilting the skull. Before placing it in fixative, the distance of the inferior olives from the transected cervical spine can be measured but it is probably more important at the time to note the degree of swelling of the brain stem tissue through the pia at the point where the foramen magnum cut was made (Fig. 5.6). Oedema of the brain stem is probably best estimated from the relative tension with which the brain tissue is held within its pial membrane. The cervical cord tissue usually does not pout in the adult and the same applies to a child that does not have brain oedema; if, however, the tissue in the cord is under tension, there will have been time while the cerebral hemispheres were being dissected for a definite pouting of the tissue through the cervical incision. This is a good guide which should be assessed at this time as

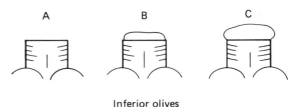

Inferior olives

Fig. 5.6 Diagrammatic representation of the medulla showing different degrees of brainstem oedema observed to have occurred during the time that the brain has been dissected. A, Normal; B, minor oedema; C, gross oedema as is likely to be seen after a child has been resuscitated for several hours.

the swelling can disappear during fixation. Distortion of the cerebellum due to herniation may be apparent at this time but this can also disappear rapidly when the brain is put into fixative or even after the brain has been left exposed for half an hour or so to demonstrate to students.

The brain can be weighed in its three parts, or the parts separated still further by cutting off the cerebellum at its peduncles. The weight of the brain, however, is not very important in assessing cerebral oedema due to variability in its size and weight and in the size of the skulls and heads of children. It is the volume of the brain within its own cavity that is important and the pouting of the brain tissue through the cervical incision is much more important than its weight. The brain needs to be related to its own skull.

(a) Removal of the pituitary

Attempted dissection of the body of a baby's pituitary from the dural capsule in its fossa usually results in damage to the gland; it is our practice to remove the whole pituitary fossa intact and to fix this before secondary dissection. This is carried out simply by cutting the dura on both sides and making a flat cut through the base of the skull.

(b) Ears and mastoids

The middle ears and mastoids should be inspected at all necropsies as quite surprising results are frequently found. In the child, the dura is not easily stripped over the mastoid cavities and middle ears and, thus, needs to be cut *in situ* along the lines where the bone incisions will be made. The middle ears and mastoid cavities in the baby can easily be removed using a pair of bone forceps to make the incisions; practice is probably more important than anything else in learning exactly where to make the cuts. The most useful tip is to stabilize the posterior tip of the bone forceps in one of the cranial nerve apertures when making these cuts.

(c) The parotids

It is usually convenient to take a sample of the parotid glands while dealing with the skull. These are probably the best samples to take for identifying the presence of cytomegalic disease in the baby. The parotid is most easily exposed from behind by making an incision across the ear at the level of the external auditory meatus of the skull and dissecting forward to expose the parotid gland. By this means there is no external evidence of any dissection and a good sample of parotid can be easily removed; scissor dissection is easier than with a knife.

5.7 REMOVAL OF THE SPINAL CORD

Our experience has been that the spinal cord of a baby is much more easily removed from the front than the back. The simplest way to do this is to place the child on its back and to hold the body supporting the lumbar region with the hand, slightly lifting it; the fibro-cartilaginous material between two of the most prominent lumbar vertebral bodies is then cut through. When this has been done, it is then easy to cut the rami systematically on alternate sides using a strong pair of scissors. The whole length of the spinal cord in its dura is exposed up to the cervical region; this, incidentally, gives a clear display of the cervical plexus and exposes the dorsal root ganglia. This incision can be taken down through the pelvis to expose the lumbar plexus and filum in a similar way. Care must be taken not to press on the cord as it is much softer and labile than that of the adult. The cord is surrounded by red and yellow fat pannicles and you can be confident of there being no trauma to the cord if these are undisturbed. The spinal cord has already been cut at the level of the foramen magnum and it is now relatively easy to cut through the spinal nerves and to remove the whole length of the cord within its dura. It is our procedure to fix the cord in the dura before dissecting any further – an attempt to cut it before fixation usually results in artefacts.

5.8 TISSUE SAMPLING

The most important samples to be taken at the time of the necropsy dissection are those required for a variety of cultures and chemical analyses.

(a) Bacterial and viral cultures

Most children who die today have been subjected to a variety of resuscitation procedures, both mouth to mouth and instrumental; a growth of organisms from any part of the respiratory tract therefore needs to be interpreted very carefully. However, cultures derived from the cerebrospinal fluid taken via the foramen magnum, from the cerebral sinuses or from heart blood collected before dissection will have different credence. Bacterial, viral and fungal cultures require histological and/or immunological backing and the appropriate tissues need to be taken.

(b) Tissue cultures

The cells of infants seem to have greater autonomy than do those of adults and it is possible to make successful tissue cultures from a child that has been dead, in the general sense, for 3 or 4 days; cartilage cells can remain viable even longer. Thus tissue cultures involving carrier media and refrigeration should always be attempted in any child death where there is any probability of familial disease and, in particular, when there has been a history of a similar death among siblings.

(c) Chemical studies

There are three basic chemical possibilities to be explored in all unexpected child deaths. These are:

(1) Possible poisoning (see Chapter 17).
(2) The biochemical state of the child – hypoglycaemic, hypernatraemic, etc.
(3) The presence of an inborn error of metabolism which, according to some studies, may account for up to 1 in 10 cot deaths.

The forensic pathologist will already be skilled in the first category. The second will be covered by examination of the vitreous humour and cerebrospinal fluid (see Chapter 13), but inborn errors of metabolism are not currently investigable everywhere. The requirements of the local experts in these fields should be known and tissues retained in the frozen state from the liver, heart, kidneys, muscles and brain for possible future study.

5.9 DISSECTING AND HANDLING THE VISCERA

(a) Naked-eye dissection

The extent of immediate naked eye dissection carried out prior to fixation will depend on the questions being asked of the necropsy and on the urgency of the answer.

The general or forensic pathologist who feels that the case is likely to be complicated involving aspects of maturity of fetal growth, insults to the child around the time of labour or related to therapeutic procedures, and is likely to lead to legal proceedings, would be wise to pause before dealing with the viscera and to invoke the assistance of a specialist paediatric pathologist at the earliest possible moment – not with the aim of handing the case over, but of making a joint investigation. The paediatric pathologist will be able to be of greatest assistance if this is done before the fresh viscera have been dissected and tissues have been taken for histology. To answer some questions such as those relating to tissue maturity, very standarized blocking of tissues is necessary – this applies particularly to organs such as the brain and kidneys. Any conscientious paediatric pathologist would much prefer to do his own dissection of tissues and do his own blocking rather than be presented with a series of sections for an opinion.

Nothing, other than some time, is lost by delaying the dissection of the viscera until after fixation and very much may be gained, remembering that this applies only after collection of fresh tissues for culture as mentioned above. If in doubt, fix the tissues and consult. If everything is straightforward, the dissection of the organs can continue along the same lines as in the adult. There are a few special points that need to be made:

(1) Most critical diagnoses in infants are made with the microscope.
(2) It is easy to misinterpret the naked-eye appearance of fluids in the respiratory passages, e.g. between milky foods and pus; do not open all the air tubes, take complete cross-sections of some for microscopy.
(3) Pneumonia cannot be diagnosed by the naked eye in the absence of pleurisy; always take blocks for microscopy before making a firm diagnosis.
(4) Perhaps the still most lethal pulmonary infection in a child is capilliary bronchitis and bronchiolitis. Manipulating unfixed lungs can move material about in the air passages; handle the lungs very carefully.
(5) The wall of the intestines of the infant will fix easily from the outside provided enough fixative is used; block the gut uncut. The form of the villi can often be made out in autolysed material.
(6) In the kidneys, early growth activity takes place at the capsule level. Stripping the

Table 5.1 Summary of paraffin blocks

	Blocks (no.)	
Tissue/organ		
Respiratory tract		
Nasal mucosa	1	
Palate, tonsils and adenoids	1	
Vocal cord	1	
Trachea	1	(R)
Lungs	4	(R)
CNS		
Cortex (motor)	1	
Caudate nucleus and germinal plate	1	(R)
Ammon's horn	1	
Cerebellum	2	
Aqueduct	1	
Pons	1	
Inferior olives	1	
Spinal cord	3	
Heart	2	(R)
Liver (L and R)	2	(R)
Spleen	1	
Kidneys	2	(R)
Pancreas	1	
Parotid	1	
Intestines	5	(R)
Thymus	1	(R)
Thyroid	1	
Ovary/testis	1	
Pituitary	1	
Adrenals	2	(See frozen section)
Mesenteric } lymph nodes	1	
Cervical }	1	
Rib	1	
Frozen section for fat		
Liver (L and R) Oil red O	2	(R)
Adrenal (a) Oil red O	1	
(b) Unstained for polarization	1	(R)
Heart Oil red O	1	

(R), most useful blocks in routine necropsy diagnosis.

capsule as in an adult necropsy does not help; the capsule must be kept *in situ* for critical blocking.

(7) Many severely autolysed tissues can often reveal surprises if histology is attempted.

(b) What tissues to block

My own necropsies entail about 40 completely standardized blocks that include all organs and tissues and then *extra* blocks taken as related to any lesions seen naked eye. A further seven blocks are used for frozen sectioning (brain two blocks, liver right and left, heart, kidney, adrenals). The cost and time involved in such studies is impractical in all but a very few centres.

The standard blocks that were taken and used by the panel of paediatric pathologists taking part in the recent DHSS 'Thousand Baby Death Study in the UK' are set out in Table 5.1. These are the blocks that it was thought were needed to be looked at in order to exclude disease that would prevent the death of a child being called a true unexpected 'Cot Death'. This was addressing the topic at a research level; in Table 5.1 I have marked with '(R)' the 10 blocks that I consider to be most useful for use in routine necropsy diagnoses. At a practical, clinical level, baby deaths can be – and are – labelled cot deaths following much less intense study to the apparent benefit of parents. However, much of the confusion in the literature on cot deaths has resulted from studies in which cases registered at many levels of necropsy have been used; it is important that the deaths subject to more limited study, e.g. those in which metabolic errors or the possibility of filicide have not been investigated, should not be used for research purposes.

To the paediatric pathologist, there are very few routine necropsies that yield completely negative findings. The problems lie in the interpretation of the findings present – which is an even more fascinating subject!

CHAPTER 6

The identification of the dead, abandoned baby

Richard C. Froede and Thomas E. Henry

The identification of the dead, abandoned baby is often difficult and, at times, may be an impossible task. This medicolegal procedure must be based primarily on physical or genetic characteristics although, with certain fortuity, a few items of an evidentiary nature may be found with the body. In many cases, the body may exhibit varying degrees of post-mortem decomposition or may be partially or completely skeletonized.

Most jurisdictions define the primary goals of a medicolegal investigation as the determinations of the cause and manner of death [1]. These determinations, although having certain probative value, are meaningless in criminal or civil actions if a positive identification is not made. Misidentification may result in injustice for an accused person, tragedy for the next-of-kin or possible tort action for a medical negligence charge against the physician performing the procedure [1].

6.1 PROBLEMS AND CIRCUMSTANCES

The paucity of information available at the time the baby is discovered complicates the handling of the situation. For this reason, each case should be treated, at least initially, as a homicide with appropriate documentation of all evidentiary material. As with any death investigation, but especially in these circumstances, no finding should be considered insignificant or superfluous.

Consideration should be given to consulting an obstetrician if the infant has the appearance of a stillborn or newborn. The obstetrician's experience with birth injuries, clamping and cutting of the cord, moulding of fetal parts, local customs, etc. may give some information regarding labour and delivery, the possibility of a hospital birth and/or medical involvement (i.e. midwife), and the potential for maternal complications following delivery (see Case 6.1 below).

6.2 SCENE INVESTIGATION

The scene can contribute significantly to the eventual identification of the baby. The location may provide a geographical centre for the initial search area. A scene may have limited access (e.g. the basement of an apartment house) which will also aid in narrowing the maternal possibilities. Once the child is found, the processing of the scene should proceed from the periphery to the body. In a secluded area, this may involve a wide area in which footprints or trace evidence will have significant value. In an area to which there is easy access and where there is abundant traffic (e.g. a community rubbish dump), significant material may be limited to the infant and its immediate surroundings. This can be something of an advantage since the relevant 'scene' can be moved intact to a more controlled environment to facilitate processing for evidentiary material (Case 6.2).

Special care should be taken with any container in which the body is found. Fingerprints, hairs, or other trace evidence can be left on the container by the individual disposing of the body. Rarely, the type of container (e.g. a laundry or garment bag) may serve as a starting point in attempting to establish identity.

Such clothing as is present may prove useful in indicating the socioeconomic status of the parent. Hospital clothing might allow the identification of a hospital where birth records are available for comparison. Sometimes religious articles, alteration of the body (e.g. pierced ears) or post-mortem prep-aration of the body will indicate that a particular group or sect is involved.

Estimation of the time of death will clarify who had access to the scene. All available parameters such as rigor mortis, post-mortem lividity (livor mortis), temperature of the body, etc. should be used. In addition, an entomologist may be valuable in attempting to fix an approximate time of death when the remains are decomposed and there is insect activity.

The placenta should also be carefully studied if it is recovered. Valuable information may be given relative to the cause of death (e.g. abruptio placenta) as well as to the maternal history (e.g. diabetes mellitus, erythroblastosis fetalis). Placental tissue may also be utilized for further genetic studies.

6.3 CASE STUDIES

Case 6.1
Fig. 6.1 illustrates the mutilation and partial dismemberment of a body that may occur

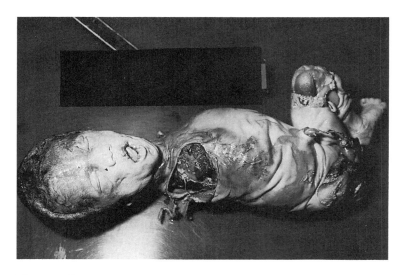

Fig. 6.1 The remains of a surgically removed dead fetus show mutilation and dismemberment which may be confused with homicidal dismemberment if not properly disposed.

during the delivery of a dead fetus. This can easily be confused with a homicidal dismemberment for disposal.

Case 6.2
The commingled fetal remains shown in Fig. 6.2 illustrate some of the problems facing the investigator. The placental fragments and fetal parts were removed from a rubbish truck and were identified by number (three fetuses) and lunar age (4–5 months gestation). Investigation showed them to have been placed there without authorization by a technician from an

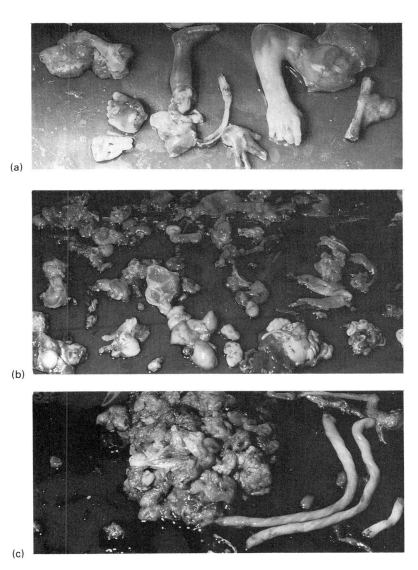

(a)

(b)

(c)

Fig. 6.2 (a),(b),(c) Commingling fetal remains from an abortion service that were improperly disposed.

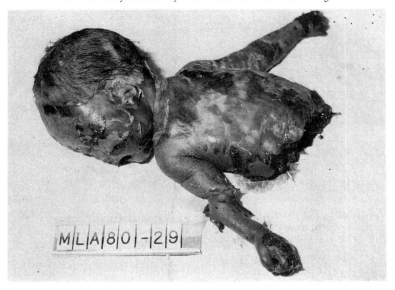

Fig. 6.3 These partial human remains were found in a yard. The remains had canine teeth marks and were obviously dragged to the site by a dog. No identification was made.

abortion service where legal abortions were performed.

Case 6.3

The partial remains of a fetus were found in the front yard of a home in Southern Arizona. Later the same day a dog was observed dragging an umbilical cord into the same yard. The fetal remains weighed 950 g. Canine teeth-marks were observed but there were no other traumatic lesions. Toxicological studies were negative. The upper torso was identified as female by histological studies (see below). The gestational age was estimated as being 7.5–9.0 months, based on a body length of 40.86 ± 1.8 cm (derived from the humerus) and 57.87 ± 1.6 cm (from the radius) (see below). The blood group was O. No suspects were found and no specific identification was possible (Fig. 6.3).

Case 6.4

The remains of a fire-damaged fetus were found in a rubbish dump near a residential area. Toxicological studies were negative. The blood group was A Rh+. The estimated gestational age was 8–9 months. The body of this male baby was eventually identified as being that of an infant prematurely delivered from a 14-year-old neighbourhood girl who had tried to destroy the body by burning it in a dustbin. Identification was made by law enforcement officers who located the mother (Fig. 6.4).

6.4 POST-MORTEM EXAMINATION

(a) Authorization

The medicolegal post-mortem examination or autopsy is generally authorized by a coroner, medical examiner or other legal agency,

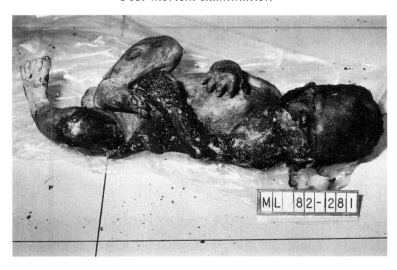

Fig. 6.4 The remains of a fire-damaged fetus were found in a rubbish dump near a residential area. Positive identification was made by the investigating team.

judiciary officer, or law enforcement agency. Knowledge of the required authorization is mandatory prior to any investigative procedure involving a dead abandoned baby since this authority may vary from jurisdiction to jurisdiction depending upon the country or its legal subdivisions.

In general, in the United States, the post-mortem examination will be performed by the medical examiner or by a fellow-in-training with the medical examiner. In most jurisdictions, the coroner, if not, himself, a physician-pathologist, will designate a forensic or anatomic pathologist to perform the post-mortem examination if this type of examination is required. The trend in the United States is to appoint medical examiners and move away from the elected coroner's system. About half of the states now have a medical examiner's system and about half have coroner's positions; six of the latter states have coroner-medical examiners. In England and Wales, the finding of a dead abandoned baby would be reportable to the coroner if for

no other reason than that no registered medical practitioner would be able to sign a certificate of cause of death 'having been in medical attendance during the deceased's last illness'; in Scotland, the death of a newborn child whose body is found is specifically reportable to the procurator fiscal. The English coroner may – and certainly would – authorize a full post-mortem examination; the Scottish fiscal must petition the sheriff to authorize an autopsy although it is inconceivable that the sheriff would refuse permission in such circumstances.

(b) External examination

The identification procedure begins with a meticulous external examination with documentation of all findings including photographs, radiographs, diagrams and detailed written description. The usual observations are made if they are obtainable. These include: sex, race, body measurements, weight, eye colour, hair colour and distribution, size of fontanelles, scars and marks. Careful documentation of congenital defects and traumatic injuries is imperative. Descriptions of blunt force injury – with specific attention to patterned injuries – and of trauma resulting from instrumentation, sharp force injury, gunshot wounds and burns, whether due to chemical or heat, must be detailed. Evidence of asphyxiation by strangulation, suffocation or choking must be looked for during careful examination of the neck, mouth – including, especially, the lips and buccal mucosa – and nose. The umbilical area must be carefully examined for cord remnants and signs of instrumentation or ligatures. If the placenta is present, the examination must include retention of tissue or blood and preservation by freezing or fixation. Evidence of hospitalization, such as needle punctures, heel sticks and ink on the soles resulting from footprinting must be documented.

(c) Internal examination

The external examination must be followed by careful and systematic evaluation of all the organ systems. The examination of the internal organs may reveal congenital defects or trauma even when decomposition is present. The gastrointestinal system must be evaluated for the presence and nature of its contents. If only skeletal material remains, the careful examination of the bony structures may reveal physical characteristics such as congenital defects or sharp or blunt force trauma. Adequate radiography is important. The radiographs should be interpreted by a well-trained and experienced radiologist or anthropologist. In general, little additional information concerning race or sex is obtained but the radiographs are important for the possible determination of age and the demonstration of congenital malformations and trauma.

(d) Toxicological evaluation

The value of toxicological analyses in the identification procedure is limited [2]. The results of the gross inspection of the body may narrow the parameters in ascertaining the cause of death; e.g. cherry-red colour in carbon monoxide poisoning, pink in hypothermia, brown in nitrate poisoning. The results of toxicological studies could also narrow the parameters for ascertaining parentage because of the presence of certain types of therapeutic or abused substances that might be present within certain households. The demonstration of other therapeutic or abortifacient drugs may also be of evidentiary value.

The best specimens to be collected are vitreous humour, blood, urine, bile, liver and gastric contents. Vitreous and bile may still provide possibly valid results even in the decomposed body. Lung and brain tissue may be useful if volatiles are suspected. All specimens should be collected in separate containers. Duplicate samples for subsequent analysis may be very helpful. Decomposed muscle, nails, hair or bone marrow may still be of value if the body is so decomposed that no organ or body fluids remain. The results of all screening procedures must be confirmed by an alternate more specific method. Samples of earth or materials surrounding the body at the scene must be obtained and tested if the presence of heavy metals is suspected [2]. Care must be taken when decomposed tissues are analysed since putrefactive bases may be interpreted as specific drugs.

6.5 SYSTEMS FOR IDENTIFICATION

(a) Physical traits

There is little doubt that physical characteristics are, in some cases, passed on directly from parent to child [3]. The unfortunate aspect of the evaluation of such traits is that they are so poorly developed in the newborn and in the early months and years of the infant's life.

The physical traits to be considered are skin colour; hair colour, form and structure; eye colour and structure; facial features, e.g. nose, mouth and eyes. The mouth should be examined for the size and shape of the lips and jaw together with dimpling of the chin or cheeks and teeth. Body build is of little value.

The following physical characteristics, extracted from Bryant's *Disputed Paternity*, Table 3.13 [3], may be among the most valuable findings in this context:

Characteristic	Usual inheritance
(i) Adherent ear lobes	Recessive
(ii) Ear pits	Recessive
(iii) 'Hitch-hiker's thumb'	Recessive
(iv) Webbed toes	Dominant
(v) Brittle bones	Dominant
(vi) Cleft spine	Dominant
(vii) Cleidocranial dysostosis	Dominant
(viii) Drooping eyelids	Dominant
(ix) Missing muscles	Dominant
(x) Birthmarks	Dominant
(xi) Absence of nails	Dominant
(xii) Thick nails	Dominant
(xiii) Milky white nails	Dominant
(xiv) Bluish-white spots on nails	Dominant

Histologically, the presence of Barr bodies on the nuclear membrane are helpful in determining female sex when external sexual characteristics are missing – as, for example, when the body has been severely mutilated. The epithelial cells from the buccal mucosa are the best cells in which to visualize Barr bodies; the remains would be classified as female if 25–30% of these cells show their presence. If Barr bodies are present in less than 25%, the body would be classified under the term of mosaicism. This determination must be performed by counting 100 or more cells. Barr bodies can also be found in other species, e.g. swine.

The Y chromosome for determination of male sex is best demonstrated on lymphocytes on a blood smear. This technique can be performed even after death if it is done early enough and prior to the onset of decomposition. The best post-mortem sample to use is heart blood. Other tissues may be used provided that bacterial growth or invasion has not taken place. False-positives will occur when the bacteria pick up the fluorochrome which is used to identify and demonstrate the Y chromosome. Once decomposition processes have begun this procedure is of negative value.

(b) Body and skeletal traits

The skeletal age during the years from birth to pre-adult development is estimated by comparisons with standards derived from living populations. In general, the only useful information as to age is based on the appearance of the centres of ossification and on tooth formation and eruption.

The basis of the age identification process using the skeleton or skeletal remains is that the ossification and growth centres show a variable development with time which evolves in a relatively constant order. The centres of primary ossification generally appear first in the areas of the hand, wrist and knee. Radiographic atlases are best referred to for identification of small bony structures [4–6]. The union of these centres can be used to estimate the skeletal age of infants and children. The development of ossification centres differs not only by age but also by sex, as is indicated in Tables 6.1 and 6.2.

Tooth eruptions in the unidentified child may be compared to documented stages of dental development to determine age. Several charts are available including those published by Schour and Massler [7] and Stewart [8] (Table 6.3). In addition to eruption, use can be made of mineralization of the crowns of the deciduous teeth and of the development of

Table 6.1 Age order of appearance of ossification centres: superior white males*

Birth	14 months	2 years, 2 months
Calcaneus	4 T– ⎫ 1 phalanx	2 metatarsal
Talus	2 T– ⎭	2 years, 5 months
Femur, distal	3 T – 2 phalanx	2 F– ⎫ 3 phalanx
Tibia, proximal	15 months	5 F– ⎭
Cuboid	3 metacarpal	2 years, 11 months
Humerus, head	2 T – 2 phalanx	3 metatarsal
2 months	5 F – 1 phalanx	Fibula, proximal
Capitate	16 months	3 years, 1 month
Hamate	4 T – 2 phalanx	Femur, greater trochanter
Lateral cuneiform	4 metacarpal	Patella
3 months	18 months	3 years, 3 months
Femur head	2 F– ⎫	4 metatarsal
Capitulum	3 F– ⎬ 2 phalanx	3 years, 4 months
Tibia, distal	4 F– ⎭	5 T – 3 phalanx
6 months	5 metacarpal	3 years, 7 months
Fibula, distal	20 months	3 T– ⎫ 3 phalanx
7 months	1 T – 1 phalanx	4 T– ⎭
Humerus, greater tuberosity	Middle cuneiform	3 years, 8 months
Radius, distal	21 months	5 metatarsal
10 months	3 F– ⎫ 3 phalanx	2 T – 3 phalanx
Triquetrum	4 F– ⎭	3 years, 10 months
11 months	Navicular of foot	Radius, proximal
3 F – 1 phalanx	5 T – 1 phalanx	4 years, 2 months
1 T – 2 phalanx	22 months	Multangulum majus
12 months	1 metacarpal	4 years, 4 months
2 F– ⎫ 1 phalanx	1 metatarsal	Navicular, hand
4 F– ⎭	23 months	4 years, 8 months
1 F – 2 phalanx	1 F – 1 phalanx	Multangulum minus
13 months	2 years	5 years +
3 T – 1 phalanx	5 F – 2 phalanx	Humerus, medial epicondyle
2 metacarpal	Lunate	Ulna, distal
Medial cuneiform		5 T – 2 phalanx

Note: T, toe; F, finger. The columns should be read as a continuum from birth to 5 years, 1st column then 2nd column and lastly the 3rd column.
* From Francis, Werle, Behm, 1939; Table 1 in [13].

their roots. Ashley [9] described an ingenious method for estimating the dental age of infants based on these factors. His practical work related to infants of Asian origin; Gustafson [10] has pointed out that the eruption of the deciduous teeth is only very slightly influenced by external factors, since children of the same age in different countries have practically identical eruption times. The subject of dental identification is discussed in greater detail in Chapter 7.

The problem of estimating the age of immature skeletons is best accomplished by using all age indicators, special attention being given to dental formation and other processes which show the highest correlation with chronological age at death [11]. At best this will still result in an estimation.

Table 6.2 Age order of appearance of ossification centres: superior white females*

Birth	10 months	21 months
Calcaneus	2 metacarpal	5 T – 3 phalanx
Talus	2 T – ⎱ 2 phalanx	22 months
Femur, distal	4 T – ⎰	3 metatarsal
Tibia, proximal	3 metacarpal	23 months
Cuboid	2 T – 1 phalanx	Patella
Humerus, head	Triquetrum	2 years
2 months	11 months	Lunate
Capitate	4 metacarpal	3 T – ⎱ 3 phalanx
Hamate	5 F – 1 phalanx	4 T – ⎰
Lateral cuneiform	12 months	Fibula, proximal
3 months	4 F – ⎱ 2 phalanx	Femur, greater trochanter
Femur head	3 F – ⎰	2 years, 2 months
Capitulum	13 months	2 T – 3 phalanx
Tibia, distal	5 metacarpal	4 metatarsal
4 months	2 F – 2 phalanx	2 years, 5 months
Humerus, greater tuberosity	14 months	5 metatarsal
6 months	1 metacarpal	2 years, 8 months
Fibula, distal	1 T – ⎱ 1 phalanx	Multangulum majus
Radius, distal	5 F – ⎰	2 years, 9 months
7 months	3 F – ⎱ 3 phalanx	Humerus, medial epicondyle
1 T – 2 phalanx	4 F – ⎰	3 years
3 F – ⎱ 1 phalanx	Navicular of foot	Radius, proximal
4 F – ⎰	Middle cuneiform	Multangulum minus
8 months	1 metatarsal	3 years, 2 months
2 F – 1 phalanx	15 months	Navicular, hand
1 F – 2 phalanx	1 F – 1 phalanx	4 years, 6 months
3 T – 1 phalanx	5 F – 2 phalanx	Ulna, distal
9 months	17 months	5 years +
3 T – 2 phalanx	2 F – ⎱ 3 phalanx	5 T – 2 phalanx
4 T – 1 phalanx	5 F – ⎰	
Medial cuneiform	19 months	
	2 metatarsal	

Note: T, toe; F, finger. The columns should be read as a continuum from birth to 5 years, 1st column then 2nd column and lastly the 3rd column.
* From Francis, Werle, Behm, 1939; Table 1 in [13].

The determinations of skeletal, racial and sexual differences are difficult. True sex differences appear in skeletal material at the time of puberty but an anthropological and odontological method is available by which to determine the sex of pre-adolescent material. This method, developed by Hunt, uses dental maturation and the presence of centres of ossification standardized for both males and females [12]. If both sets of criteria agree with the male or female standard, then the skeleton is classified accordingly. Racial characteristics may be more difficult to determine in the developing skeleton until the bones are in a greater stage of maturity.

The crown–rump length is also useful for estimating fetal age (Table 6.4) [13]. Weights of the organs of children may also be of some

Table 6.3 Usual order and typical rate of eruption of the deciduous dentition in the United States*

Order of eruption	Rate of eruption			
	7.5 months	1 year	2 years	3 years
i_1	+	+	+	+
i^1		+	+	+
i^2		+	+	+
i_2			+	+
m^1 and m_1			+	+
c (upper and lower)			+	+
m^2 and m_2				+

* Modified from Meredith [20, 21].

Table 6.4 Fetal age by crown–rump length

Lunar month	C–R length (mm) (with range)
2	69 (up to 80)
3	115 (81–135)
4	157 (136–175)
5	194 (176–215)
6	233 (216–255)
7 male	274 ⎫ (256–285)
7 female	268 ⎭
8 male	298 ⎫ (286–315)
8 female	298 ⎭
9 male	332 ⎫ (316–340)
9 female	333 ⎭
10 male	348 ⎫ 341 plus
10 female	349 ⎭

value (Table 6.5) [14]. Such data are, clearly, not decisive for identification but they allow the investigative parameters to be narrowed.

(c) Finger and footprints

This system of identification is based on the friction ridges on the fingertips and on the soles of the feet. As growth occurs in the hands and feet there are changes in scale but not in consistency. The basic pattern of whorls, loops, and arches on the fingertips have a number of subgroups that may be useful. Photographic techniques with one-to-one comparison are very helpful if a previous pattern is available. Latent prints from likely infants should be obtained if possible. Footprints recorded in hospitals can be used for comparison with the footprints of the unidentified body (Fig. 6.5). The patterns can be magnified by photographic techniques including electronic image enhancement, but hospital records are often unsatisfactory, largely because they are taken as a 'routine' and the possibility that they will be needed in a criminal context is not envisaged.

Fingerprints or footprints may be taken from mummified bodies using Ruffer's solution [15]. Care should be taken to clean the hands or feet with detergent or cleaning solution to remove all debris, blood, oil, grease or other contaminating matter.

Table 6.5 Weight of organs of children

Age	Body length (cm)	Heart (g)	Lungs		Spleen (g)	Liver (g)	Kidneys		Brain (g)
			Right (g)	Left (g)			Right (g)	Left (g)	
Birth–3 days	49	17	21	18	8	78	13	14	335
3–7 days	49	18	24	22	9	96	14	14	358
1–3 weeks	52	19	29	26	10	123	15	15	382
3–5 weeks	52	20	31	27	12	127	16	16	413
5–7 weeks	53	21	32	28	13	133	19	18	422
7–9 weeks	55	23	32	29	13	136	19	18	489

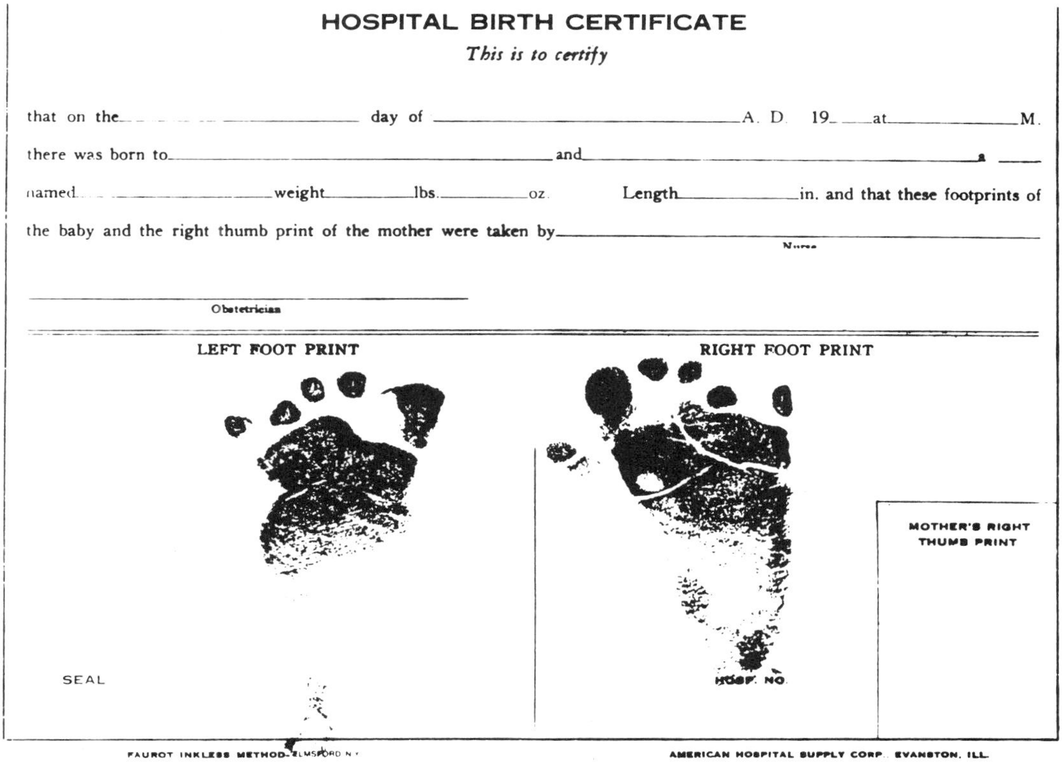

HOSPITAL BIRTH CERTIFICATE

This is to certify

that on the_____ day of _____A. D. 19____at_____M.

there was born to_____and_____ᵃ_____

named_____weight_____lbs._____oz.   Length_____in. and that these footprints of

the baby and the right thumb print of the mother were taken by_____
Nurse

_____
Obstetrician

LEFT FOOT PRINT	RIGHT FOOT PRINT

MOTHER'S RIGHT THUMB PRINT

SEAL

HOSP. NO.

FAUROT INKLESS METHOD—ELMSFORD N Y   AMERICAN HOSPITAL SUPPLY CORP. EVANSTON, ILL.

Fig. 6.5 This case illustrates the need for good footprints. These prints were extremely difficult to interpret (AFIP study set).

(d) Hair

The recovery of hair or even fibres from the human remains can be used to help narrow the field of identification. Body hair may suggest a racial affinity within the broad categories of Caucasian, Negroid or Mongoloid, the distinction being made on the distribution of pigment granules or through the cross-sectional appearances. In general, Caucasian hairs are oval, Negroid are flattened or triangular and Mongoloid are round to oval.

The human hair is composed of three layers – medulla, cortex and cuticle. These are best observed longitudinally rather than in cross-section. The outer or cuticular portion (the scale) shows a variable pattern of overlapping cells. The cortex is made up of keratin fibrils and the medulla commonly contains pigment granules. Infants' head hairs show a somewhat characteristic pigment distribution according to race [1]. Caucasian hair shows a sparse to moderately dense distribution pattern of the pigment granules; Negroid head hair is characterized by an uneven medullary pigment pattern with clumping of the granules; Mongoloid hairs, including those from American Indians, orientals and most Caucasian-Mongoloid admixtures (Hispanics), contain more dense pigment granules exhibiting a streaking rather than clumping pattern (Figs 6.6 and 6.7). Some

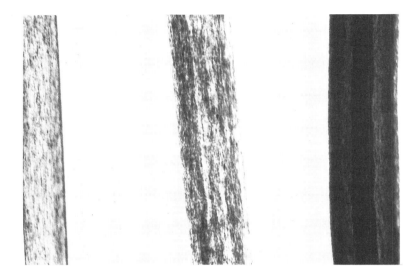

Fig. 6.6 Composite photograph of three human head hairs, Caucasoid, Mongoloid and Negroid (× 100).

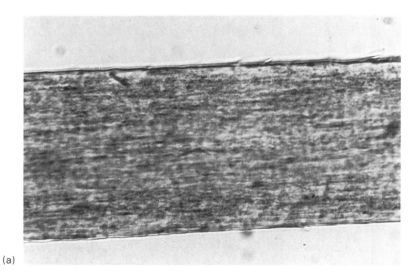

(a)

Fig. 6.7 (a) Caucasoid human hair: oval with evenly distributed pigment, medium cuticle and uncommon undulation (× 400). (b) Mongoloid human head hair: round with dense auburn pigment, thick cuticle and no undulation (× 400). (c) Negroid human head hair: flat with densely clumped pigment action and prevalent undulation (× 400).

variations depend upon the location of the hair on the body [16], but they are of little significance in paediatric work.

Samples can even be obtained from a decomposed, burned or skeletonized body. Hairs from a skeletonized body may sometimes be found in bony crevices in the skull, in the orbital areas and in other apertures. The best way of detecting and collecting these samples is by use of a variable magnification microscope (7× to 15×) with a good light source. Debris may be removed with a mild soap solution followed by degreasing in methyl alcohol; the length of the specimen

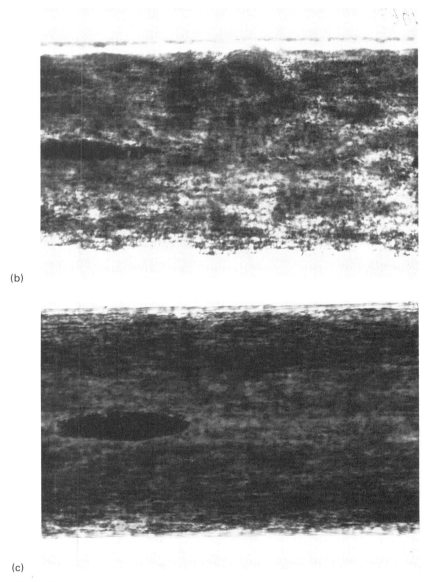

(b)

(c)

Fig. 6.7 *continued*

should be determined before mounting on a microscope slide [1].

Non-attached hairs found on a body may be valuable as evidentiary material as they may be human or non-human and, perhaps, indicate a secondary source. Non-human hairs can be distinguished microscopically through their characteristic medullary diameter, pigment granules, scales and root variations [1]. Any fibres removed may be useful for comparison with materials from the supposed source of the body – home or hospital – or from persons who may have transported the body. All samples should be placed in separate containers marked with the source of the specimen, date and time of collection and name of collector.

(e) Blood groups – marker systems

The distribution of red blood cell antigen markers varies in different populations [1]. Table 6.6, for example, shows the distribution of ABO blood groups in the two major ethnic populations of the United States.

The simpler procedures developed for identifying the blood group marker systems require the use of fresh or unhaemolysed blood. Unfortunately, in most cases of the type under consideration, only haemolysed or dried blood or decomposing bone marrow is available to the forensic investigator. In instances of badly decomposed bodies or skeletonized remains from which no form of

Table 6.6 Distribution of blood groups in the United States*

Ethnic group	Blood groups (%)			
	A	B	AB	O
White	40	11	4	45
Black	25	21	5	49

* After Gaensslen [17].

blood is available, attempts can be made to determine the ABO group systems from skin, dandruff, hair or nails [18].

The use of blood group antigens and other polymorphisms in determining parentage is discussed in Chapter 22. Samples of blood for testing may be obtained from suspected parents or assailants by way of consent or by court order.

(f) DNA identification

The new technology involving the use of nuclear rather than mitochondrial DNA is useful in paternity testing, in the solution of immigration problems and in the identification of missing children. The analytical procedure is described in Chapter 22; a genetic pattern may be obtained from blood, semen, saliva, vaginal secretions, faeces, urine and body tissues including hair and nails.

This technique circumvents the usual problems encountered in protein analyses using decomposed post-mortem fluids or tissues, since the DNA molecule is highly resistant to drying and to bacterial or chemical contamination. The technique when properly used is alleged to give no false-positives – it will give the correct answer or none at all.

(g) Miscellaneous assistance

Photographs

Birth or family photographs can be used for comparative purposes. Occasionally the investigator may have to resort to electronic image enhancement techniques which have been used for a number of years by engineers, astronomers, archeologists, law enforcement officers and physicians for evaluating diverse images ranging from the results of non-invasive body tests to photographs of the universe. One of the instruments used is a closed-circuit video device which allows the simplification of analogue-imaged data. Photographs of the video output, in black and white or in colour, can be taken for permanent record [19].

Clothing

Any clothing found with the body may provide the investigator with clues as to the hospital or family from which it originated.

6.6 SUMMARY

It must be remembered that a positive identification is accomplished only by comparison with a known sample whether that sample be a fingerprint, radiograph or genetic fingerprint. The thrust of the investigation is to arrive at a highly probable identity before attempting comparative methods. Since what will eventually be available for comparison is unknown, it follows that the investigator should compile all the available data from which positive identity could, ultimately, be determined.

REFERENCES

1. Froede, R., Froede, S. and Birkby, W.H. (1981) Systems for human identification. *Pathol. Annu.*, **16**, (I), 337.
2. McBay, A. (1986) *CAP Handbook for Postmortem Examination of Unidentified Remains*, College of American Pathologists, Skokie, p. 78.
3. Bryant, N.J. (1980) *Disputed Paternity*, B.C. Decke, New York, p. 18.
4. Flecker, H. (1942) Time of appearance and fusion of ossification centers as observed by roentgenographic methods. *Am. J. Roentgenol.*, **47**, 97.
5. Greulich, W.W. and Pyle, S.I. (1959) *Radiographic Atlas of Skeletal Development of the Hand and Wrist*, 2nd edn, University Press, Stanford.
6. Pyle, S.I. and Hoerr, N.L. (1959) *Radiographic Atlas of Skeletal Development of the Knee*, Thomas, Springfield.
7. Schour, I. and Massler, M. (1944) *Development of the Human Dentition* (chart), 2nd edn, American Dental Association, Chicago.
8. Stewart, T.D. (1979) *Essentials of Forensic Anthropology*, Thomas, Springfield, pp. 140–9.
9. Ashley, K.F. (1970) Identification of children in a mass disaster by estimation of dental age. *Br. Dent. J.*, **129**, 167.
10. Gustafson, G. (1966) *Forensic Odontology*, Staples Press, London, p. 112.
11. Ubelaker, D.H. (1987) Estimating age at death from immature human skeletons: an overview. *J. Forensic Sci.*, **32**, 1245.
12. Hunt, E.E. and Gleiser, I. (1955) The estimation of age and sex of preadolescent children from bones and teeth. *Am. J. Phys. Anthropol.*, **13**, 470.
13. Krogman, W.M. (1978) *The Human Skeleton in Forensic Medicine*, 3rd edn, Thomas, Springfield, pp. 24, 25, 56.
14. Saphir, O. (1958) *Autopsy Diagnosis and Technic*, 4th edn, Hoeber, New York.
15. Allison, M.J. and Gerstzen, E.L. (1977) *Paleopathology in Peruvian Mummies: Application of Modern Techniques*, Department of Pathology, Medical College of Virginia.
16. Collom, W.D. (1980) Microscopic diagnosis of hairs and fibers, in *Microscopic Diagnosis in Forensic Pathology* (eds J.A. Perper and C.H. Wecht), Thomas, Springfield, Ch. 13.
17. Gaensslen, R.E. (1980) Blood, sweat, tears, saliva, and semen. *Law Enforcement*, 23 February.
18. Moenssens, A.A., Inbau, F.E. and Starr, J.E. (1986) *Scientific Evidence in Criminal Cases*, 3rd edn, Foundation Press, Mineola, pp. 352–9.
19. Campbell, H.R., personal communication.
20. Meredith, H.V. (1946) Order and age of eruption for the deciduous dentition. *J. Dent. Res.*, **25**, 43.
21. Meredith, H.V. (1951) A chart on eruption of the deciduous teeth for the paediatrician's office. *J. Pediatr.*, **38**, 483.

CHAPTER 7

Paediatric forensic odontology

(A) Introduction and identification

Bernard G. Sims

The application of odontology, odonto-stomatology or dentistry to forensic problems has been well recognized for nearly half a century. Whichever terminology is used, the subject is defined as 'that branch of forensic medicine which, in the interests of justice, deals with the proper evaluation and presentation of the dental findings' [1]. It requires a trained dental expert to handle and examine any dental evidence with the degree of accuracy that law enforcement authorities and the legal profession expect and to apply his or her additional knowledge and experience to objectives which differ considerably from conventional dental education and the routine pursuit of dental practice [2].

The scope of this forensic speciality has been expanded considerably over the years through the increasing use of dental methods of identification in circumstances which preclude the routine visual means of recognition and in situations where other methods of identification are not applicable. The burgeoning of interest in the subject has promoted the desire to carry out research in response to the various problems that have

been encountered, although there are many who believe the subject still to lie within the state of the art rather than the science.

The value of dental methods of identification depends on the facts that the hard dental tissues and dental restorations tend to be extremely resistant to fire, trauma and immersion – which the rest of the body is not – and that the hard dental tissues may remain intact long after the rest of the body has been destroyed. These properties have been well used in relation to an increasing number of air disasters and to single cases of identification in deaths resulting from criminal acts.

Article 6 of the United Nations' Universal Declaration of Human Rights issued in 1948 states that 'everyone has the right to recognition everywhere as a person before the law'. This has been held to imply that the citizen of a United Nations member state has a right 'to possess his personal identity unquestioned even after death', and the article prescribes that the identification of the dead must be carried out whenever possible [3]. This chapter, therefore applies equally to children and minors as to adults and there are specific aspects of methods of dental identi-fication which are applicable to particular age-groups.

7.1 SCOPE OF THE DISCIPLINE

Forensic odontology may be divided into three sections of study – civil and non-criminal, criminal and research. The civil element includes:

(A) *Identification of an individual's remains* where death is not due to suspicious circumstances. This includes recon-structive and comparative studies.
(B) *Identification of victims* in natural disasters and in other mass disasters which involve travel by land, sea and air and others due to fires and destruction of buildings. These also rely upon reconstruction and comparisons.
(C) *Identification of living persons* by reason of loss of memory or coma.
(D) *Aspects of malpractice* including fraud which may lead to criminal charges.
(E) *Neglect* – which may also result in criminal investigation.

Criminal responsibilities include:

(A) *The identification of individuals* from reconstructive and comparative studies of the teeth, either in the living or the dead.
(B) *The study of bite-marks*:
  (1) Agents producing bite-marks and teeth-marks:
    (i) Human – adults and children.
    (ii) Animals.
    (iii) Mechanical.
  (2) Materials and substances exhibiting teeth-marks:
    (i) Skin and body tissues.
    (ii) Foodstuffs.
    (iii) Other materials and substances.

Research in forensic odontology involves:

(A) *Research* based on the examination of evidence derived from cases outlined above, ongoing research into develop-ment and growth, maintaining obser-vation of progress and innovations in clinical dentistry, and consideration of the medicolegal and social aspects of the subject.
(B) *Academic courses and postgraduate training*.

7.2 DENTAL IDENTIFICATION IN PRACTICE

Many unreliable identifications are made by visual recognition by relatives or associates in a shocked or distressed state. It has been found that there are occasions when relatives are even unable to recognize their loved-ones when asleep – the facial expression of animation is lost and the normal identi-fying features are not there for relatives to appreciate when facial features are in repose. If mistakes in visual identification can be made under the duress of grief and distress in viewing an intact body, this will be even more the case in circumstances involving major incidents and mass disasters where the emotional stress of relatives is at a higher level. Visual means of identification are untenable in such circumstances and one advantage of the dental means of identi-fication is that it obviates the necessity of relatives viewing a body, which may be frag-mented or mutilated, in these circumstances. Even so, visual means of recognition are used in approximately 90% of cases in which identification is required in the United Kingdom and this is possibly so on a worldwide basis.

Once a body is positively identified, the deceased may be disposed of appropriately according to religion, tradition and custom. The period of grief is prolonged beyond the natural period if identity is delayed and the psychological effects are well documented in such an event. During this grief period relatives will either try to identify any other body, however poor the resemblance, or maintain that their loved-one is not part of the incident and is 'missing' and will return home one day. This is a most common occurrence involving the death of children when identity is based on an age assessment alone. In such circumstances, not even confirmatory evidence by other methods of identification will convince a mother of the death of her child, although other members of the family will accept the tragedy and will carry through the appropriate funeral arrangements.

7.3 SEX, AGE AND RACE DETERMINATION

Any identification procedure requires the recording of the physical attributes of the unknown individual with accuracy and of the associated personal effects, and these are then compared with details of relevant missing persons; the general methods involved have been described in Chapter 6. The assessment of such data is reasonably simple if bodies are intact but, in cases of decomposition or when skeletal remains only are available, the important characteristics to be determined are sex, race and age.

The accuracy of sex determination and that of race depends on the completeness of the skeletal remains and whether the remains are adult or immature. This is the particular field of the anatomist or forensic anthropologist – and especially so when the remains of children are recovered. An intact adult skeleton can be accurately sexed in 98% of cases. The adult pelvis alone provides an accuracy of 95%, the skull of 90% and the long bones of 80%. The distinguishing features of sex and race in fetal and immature bones are, however, not particularly evident other than to the expert. Much anthropological research at the present time is involved with computer-assisted studies and the production of microcomputer programs which can perform the required calculations for the discriminant factors of sex, race, ageing, etc. with little delay [2].

7.4 AGE ASSESSMENT

The assessment of age has great historical interest to the forensic odontologist. Throughout the nineteenth century, children were exploited as cheap labour due to the demands of the industrial revolution. At that time, the age of a child for employment purposes was assessed by his or her height. If the child was more than 51½ inches (130 cm) tall, he or she was considered to be 13 years of age and was allowed to work to a maximum of 69 hours per week. Needless to say, there was even a 'black market' in doctors' certificates attesting to 'age over 13' for those who wished to obtain increased wages in a poor family. This situation was eased when Edwin Saunders published his findings in 1837 to the effect that the teeth provided the most reliable guide to age. Thus, forensic odontology can be said to have been applied in the United Kingdom for one and a half centuries [4].

It has been found that chronological age does not always coincide with that assessed from physical, bone or dental development but, in practice, it has been found that dental development varies less than does that of bone and that different methods of ageing provide more accurate indications at particular periods of life. The three periods generally referred to are '*in utero*', from birth to the age of 14 years during which the dentition progresses from deciduous to mixed, and, finally, the adult years; the last period is irrelevant to this book.

The assessment of age is interrelated with the sex and race of the individual. If one compares the osseous development of the hand with dental development and finds it similar, the individual is likely to be male; if the osseous development is in advance of that of the teeth, then the individual is most likely female. The skeletal development of females may be 1 year in advance of that of males while their dental development may differ only from 1 to 4 months.

It may be possible to estimate the approximate age at the site when adult human remains are found but, when dealing with the remains of fetuses or children, it is advisable to apply the particular methods at a more central place of study. It is of prime importance to complete a full radiographic survey of fetal or children's remains prior to commencement of the autopsy in order to locate and maintain the minute dental structures, to prevent their loss during dissection and to ensure their complete removal for histological study. This procedure is especially important when the remains are decomposed.

Many studies in the chronology of tooth development have been published which present the extent of calcification and state of eruption of the deciduous and permanent teeth of children and young persons at given ages. One of the first tables to be taken into common use was that of Schour and Massler in 1941 [5]; it is still popular because its pictorial representation of tooth development and eruption has been found to be most convenient for instant use in field-work but its accuracy is limited, the details having been derived from a study of a few individuals of one race. The charts published in 1963 by Moorress, Fanning and Hunt [6, 7] are derived from a radiographic survey of the deciduous and permanent teeth of a large number of American schoolchildren; they present the progress of tooth formation as a series of radiographic landmarks with a standard deviation either side of the average age. The limitation of these charts is the absence of information related to the posterior teeth because the radiographic appearance of the bone structure in the posterior part of

the upper jaw masks the relevant tooth formation. The chart of Gustafson and Koch cited by Johanson in 1971 [8] covers the period of tooth development from 8 months prior to birth up to the age of 16 years; it was derived from 19 sources over a period of 60 years. Four developmental landmarks are recorded: commencement of mineralization, completion of crown formation, completion of tooth eruption and completion of root formation (Fig. 7.1). Each landmark is represented by a triangle with the apex indicating the average age and the angles at the base indicating the earliest and latest time limit for each of the four landmarks. Johanson's critical evaluation of the various authors' methods for age determination up to 1971, which pays special attention to the age-groups above 14 years of age where forensic age assessments are not very accurate, provides a valuable source of information which has not yet been supplanted. Recently, an assessment of the dental age of Essex schoolchildren was undertaken using panoral radiographs with the intention of providing an up-to-date flexible and easily referenced 'field-chart' for forensic needs (Fig. 7.2). Some 255 girls and boys of ages ranging from 4 years to 16 years were examined and the findings were compared with those of previous authors. It was found that the Essex children's dental development lagged behind that of their American counterparts but that developmental variations were greater within their groups. In view of the variations which occur worldwide, it is well to remember Altini's conclusion in 1983 [10] that: 'Each forensic odontologist should have a reference data base peculiar to the population he serves'. In addition, each method of age assessment has its own disadvantages of which any dental expert should be aware in making the relevant choice to fit the particular circumstances – it may, perhaps, be necessary to apply a number of methods in combination in order to achieve an identification.

The age of young individuals has frequently

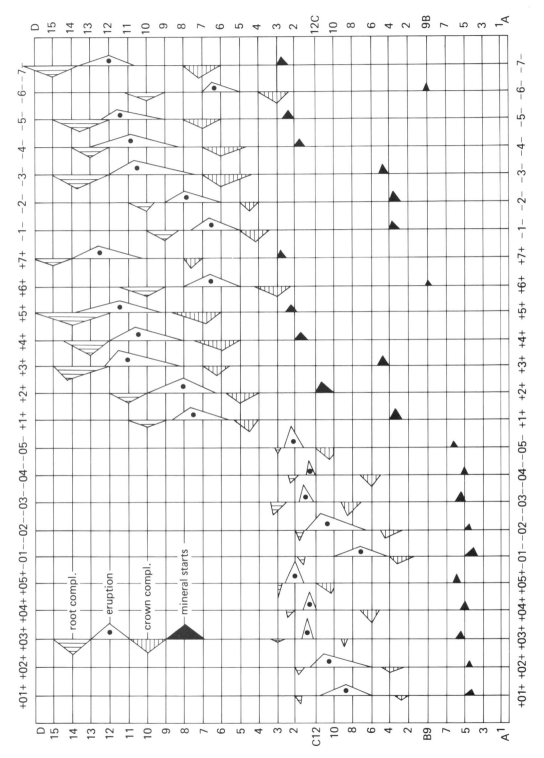

Fig. 7.1 Diagrammatic representation of dental development originally by Gustafson, G. (1966) *Forensic Odontology*, London Staples Press, reproduced from Cameron, J.M. and Sims, B.G. (1973) *Forensic Dentistry*, Edinburgh: Churchill Livingstone (with permission of the publishers).

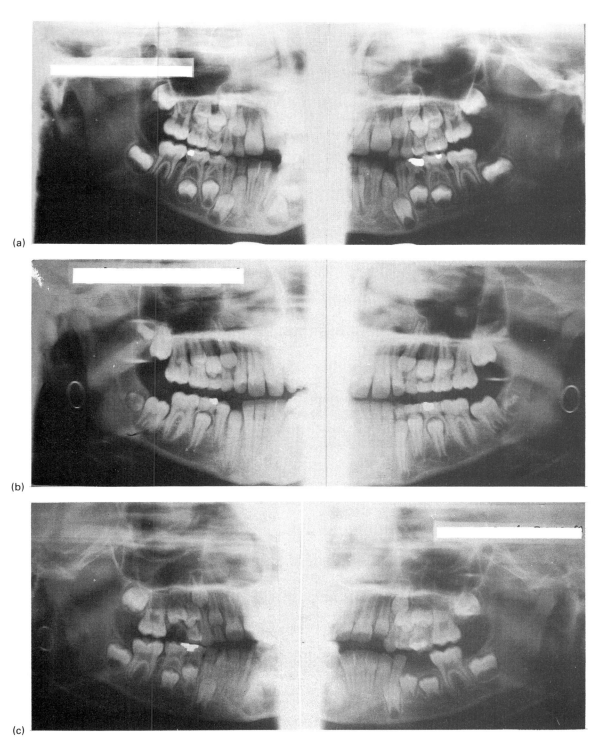

Fig. 7.2 The panoral radiograph provides one of the most convenient methods for dental ageing. Three specimens are illustrated: (a) boy aged 7 4/12 years; (b) girl aged 8 1/12 years; (c) girl aged 11 5/12 years (all × ½).

been determined by an analysis of the microscopic cross striations on the rod or prism structure of the enamel tissue which have been generally accepted as representing the daily growth pattern. This incremental pattern is also present on the microscopic tubules of dentine but is less discernible there; in some circumstances, the dentine pattern has been used as a confirmatory procedure. The total number of cross striations on the enamel are counted from the neonatal line, which is formed at birth as an accentuated incremental line, until the forming front of enamel tissue is reached where it is assumed that enamel formation has ceased at death. This count of cross striations has to be made on a suitably prepared longitudinal ground section of a tooth which shows a well-defined neonatal line. The total count will represent the total number of days that the enamel has been forming and, therefore, represents the age of the individual in days. If enamel formation has ceased in the tooth chosen, it is possible to transfer the count to the tooth which is next in line of development. So long as enamel was still forming at the time of the individual's death, the transfer can take place in a number of teeth providing the forming front of the enamel tissue is reached in the last tooth in the succession. This transfer technique assumes that all the teeth developing at the time were affected by the same stimuli despite the fact that each tooth was at a different stage of development. Systemic stimuli produce accentuated lines across the enamel called striae of which the neonatal line is one itself and results from the transition from fetal life to a separate existence. The first 2–3 weeks of the neonatal period involve disturbances in cellular activity and alterations in calcium metabolism which produce this 'birth line' in a characteristic position in each of the deciduous teeth and in the first permanent molars. Other factors can cause marked disturbances which follow the contours of the incremental lines. These include severe illnesses and the ingestion of some drugs such as tetracycline; a number of chemical elements – such as lead, strontium and fluorine – can form characteristic lines by reason of their affinity to the forming fronts of the calcifying tissues of bones and teeth.

When using this technique, an experimental error has to be taken into account with regard to the forming front of the hard dental tissues. If enamel is still forming at the time of death, the forming front is in its precursor form; it is not yet calcified and has no incremental pattern. The number of days taken to produce the uncalcified forming front is, therefore, speculative; this experimental error is taken into account by giving the age in days as between 20 days either side of the total count [11]. The procedure requires the facilities of a well-equipped laboratory with apparatus that will section the hard un-decalcified tissues in thin section without disrupting the material. In addition, the use of a projection microscope is of prime import-ance in order that the tedious count of the cross striations can be completed with accuracy.

As to the forensic application of the method, the presence of a neonatal line in the first permanent molar of a child's remains would indicate that it had been born and had lived beyond the neonatal period; a count of the striations would give the child's age in days taking into account the experimental error. However, in practice it has been found that variations in the accepted $4\,\mu m$ periodicity of incremental growth ranged from $2\,\mu m$ to $8\,\mu m$ in enamel and from $4\,\mu m$ to $16\,\mu m$ in dentine. Dentine can appear to develop at different rates in different regions of the same tooth and some incremental lines appear to be more pronounced at irregular intervals.

The application of this method of age assessment has been used successfully on a number of occasions involving very young children and fetal material but was not so successful in the identification of a female child of 11.5 years old.

Case 7.1

The badly decomposed bodies of a male and a female child were found 3 months after being reported missing. Confirmation of their true ages was obtained from the birth certificates. The girl was aged 11.5 and the boy 12 years. In the absence of dental records, identification had to proceed through age assessment. The anatomic, radiographic and dental development of the boy matched the details expected. The age of the girl, however, was anatomically and radiographically estimated as 16 years while the dental estimation was of 14 years of age. There was obviously some concern that, perhaps, an

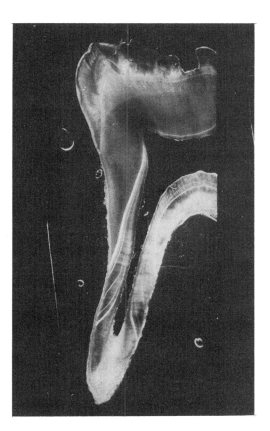

Fig. 7.3 Fluorescent tetracycline lines described in Case 7.1. (Undecalcified ground longitudinal section viewed under ultraviolet light).

older and entirely unexpected individual had been found rather than the missing schoolgirl [12].

The state of dental development of a 12-year-old female should be 6 months ahead of that of a male and, as the missing girl was 6 months younger than the missing male, their dentitions should have been at the same state; to be 2.5 years in advance dentally seemed to be well outside normal variation. It was found that the cross striations in the enamel were not sufficiently visible to carry out an incremental count. However, it became known that, when she was 9 months old, she suffered from a cervical abscess and that, subsequently, the sustained recurrent attacks of bronchitis and pneumonia which were treated with tetracycline on each occasion. As has been stated, tetracycline is one of the drugs which has an affinity for the forming fronts of calcifying tissues and will align itself along incremental lines in teeth; it also fluoresces under ultraviolet light. Re-examined under ultraviolet light illumination, a series of seven fluorescent incremental lines were seen in the dentine, the first being at the appropriate distance from the neonatal line to correspond with the treatment for her abscess at the age of 9 months (Fig. 7.3). Unfortunately, her medical documents indicated that there were only four tetracycline treatments recorded. The long interval from the first tetracycline line to those in closer pattern which came next fitted the medical history but not exactly; it was considered that the three extra lines were the result of treatment not recorded. It was at this time that it was observed that the assumption that hard dental tissue formation proceeded at a regular rate was not acceptable on all occasions and that variations, already referred to in the text, occurred. The dental evidence in this case was not conclusive in the positive identification of the missing girl but it did support the probability that it was her and not an unknown older girl. The matter was finally set to rest by the discovery of a print on a school book matching a portion of decomposed skin from the palm of her hand [12].

Not long after this criminal case, a number of age investigations were undertaken on behalf of appellants to the Immigration Appeal Tribunal. The first arose in 1978 as the result of the return to the United Kingdom of three children from Bangladesh. The question concerned the apparent discrepancy between the physical appearance and development of the children and the established records of their birth in the United Kingdom. They had been examined in Bangladesh in 1976 and the relevant reports and X-ray pictures had been submitted to the British High Commission in Dacca in 1977. The authority in Bangladesh considered that the children he had examined were much younger than was indicated by the documentary evidence and were not the same children.

In 1979, the results of the examination in the United Kingdom were reported to the tribunal in which the panoral radiographs of the teeth and the radiographs of the wrists of each child indicated that the dental age assessment was close to the recorded dates of birth for each child and that the osseous development was delayed within the limits set for development described by Modi [13]. The tribunal accepted the evidence that the children were entitled to reside in the United Kingdom. The doctor in Bangladesh would appear to have assumed that chronological and developmental age were synonymous.

It is now of prime concern to continue research into growth and development in worldwide populations as it would appear that the time is coming when dental restorations will be unnecessary in caries-free adults and children and the usual comparative methods of identification will be of little use; greater accuracy in age determination of unknown individuals will be needed.

7.5 PERSONAL IDENTIFICATION

As things stand at present, any investigation of identity, whether it be of a single victim of a homicide or of a number of victims in a mass disaster, depends upon a comparative study in which prospective ante-mortem details are submitted for comparison with the reconstructive data.

This phase of the procedure begins either at the site at which the human remains are found or, more conveniently, within the mortuary. The full oral examination should include details of the natural or artificial teeth; whether teeth are missing by reason of non-eruption, previous extraction treatment or have been lost port-mortem; the presence or absence of dental restorations and other conservative treatment and the materials or techniques used; the examination of skeletal pattern and Angle's classification together with description of abnormalities of tooth arrangement or tooth form; the presence or absence of orthodontic appliances either fixed or removable; and even the pattern of partial or full dentures. These details are recorded on an appropriate chart representing the five surfaces of the 20 deciduous teeth and of the 32 adult teeth.

If the details on both studies are comprehensive, it can be expected, at best, to achieve a positive result and, at worst, the elimination of a single or number of prospective identities.

The design of the standard grid form of the chart used in the United Kingdom and the European Economic Community has been accepted as the standard chart-form on the disaster-victim-identification forms of Interpol (Fig. 7.4). European and Interpol odontograms include a two-digit notation recommended by the Fédération Dentaire Internationale as a uniform dental recording method and one which is specifically designed for the recovery of data from computer records and for ease of transmission in radiocommunication. The standard chart used in the United Kingdom [14] is a modified

Zsigmondy's classification rather than the two-digit system. Other methods are in use and some are designed for specific purposes rather than for storage and retrieval; Haines' notation, for example, was introduced to ease transmission of information by telex (Fig. 7.5). Incidental findings such as staining of the teeth and localized trauma produced by occupation or leisure habits are recorded, although such conditions are seldom noted by dental practitioners on the records of their patients.

Ideally, it would be an advantage to have radiographs of the teeth and jaws and of the skull taken at the time of the autopsy. The obvious uses of radiographs would include enabling direct comparisons to be made between the ante-mortem radiographs of prospective identities with those taken post-mortem; to discover hidden details of unerupted teeth, root treatments, buried teeth and retained roots, etc. which may be recorded on ante-mortem chartings even if ante-mortem radiographs are not retrieved or available; finally, to allow comparison with ante-mortem radiographs when insufficient

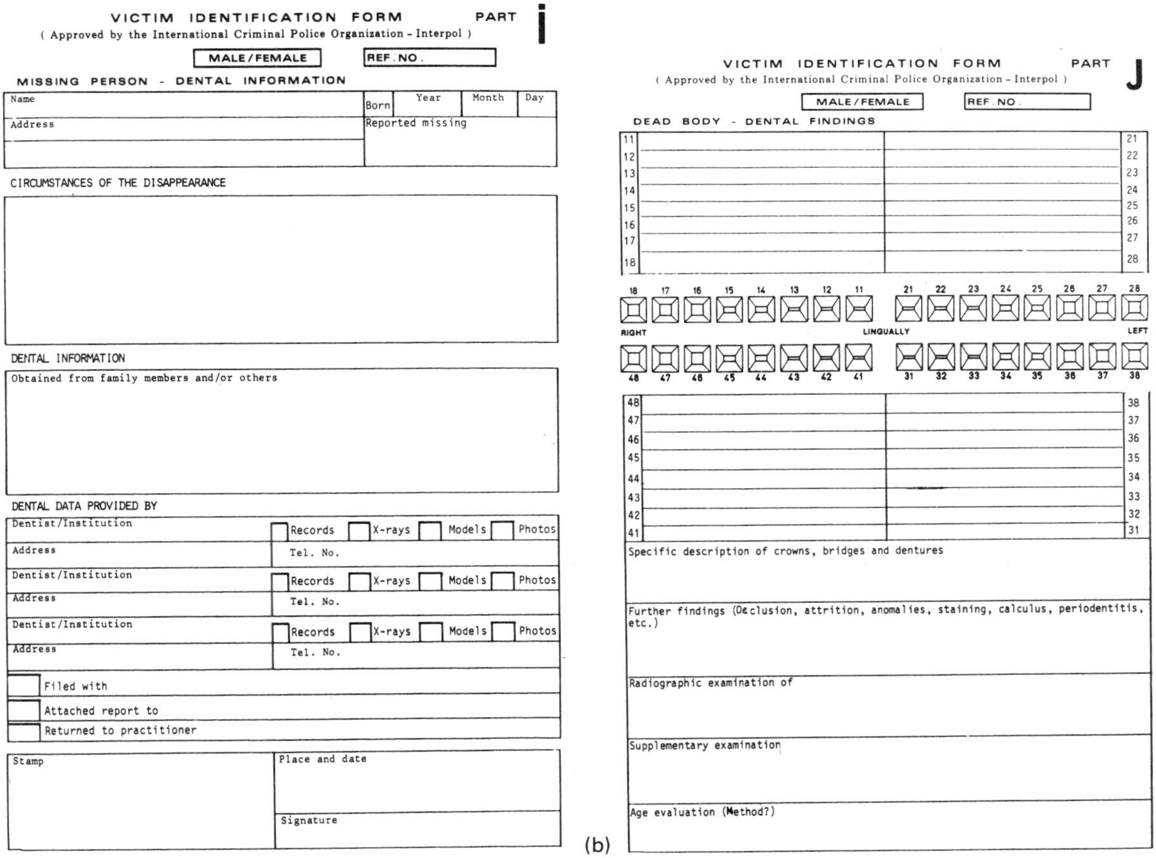

VICTIM IDENTIFICATION FORM PART i
(Approved by the International Criminal Police Organization - Interpol)
MALE/FEMALE REF. NO.
MISSING PERSON - DENTAL INFORMATION
Name | Born Year Month Day
Address | Reported missing
CIRCUMSTANCES OF THE DISAPPEARANCE
DENTAL INFORMATION
Obtained from family members and/or others
DENTAL DATA PROVIDED BY
Dentist/Institution | Records X-rays Models Photos
Address | Tel. No.
Dentist/Institution | Records X-rays Models Photos
Address | Tel. No.
Dentist/Institution | Records X-rays Models Photos
Address | Tel. No.
Filed with
Attached report to
Returned to practitioner
Stamp | Place and date | Signature

(a)

VICTIM IDENTIFICATION FORM PART J
(Approved by the International Criminal Police Organization - Interpol)
MALE/FEMALE REF. NO.
DEAD BODY - DENTAL FINDINGS
11 12 13 14 15 16 17 18 | 21 22 23 24 25 26 27 28
18 17 16 15 14 13 12 11 21 22 23 24 25 26 27 28
RIGHT LINGUALLY LEFT
48 47 46 45 44 43 42 41 31 32 33 34 35 36 37 38
48 47 46 45 44 43 42 41 | 38 37 36 35 34 33 32 31
Specific description of crowns, bridges and dentures
Further findings (Occlusion, attrition, anomalies, staining, calculus, periodentitis, etc.)
Radiographic examination of
Supplementary examination
Age evaluation (Method?)

(b)

Fig. 7.4 Interpol victim identification forms. (a) Obverse of missing person form; (b) Reverse of dead body form. The form originally recommended by ICAO for specific use in aircraft accidents is illustrated at (c).

Fatal Aircraft Accident Victim Identification & Autopsy Form

M2

Date of examination .... Body number

Examiner .... Sex Male

Clothing
Outer Garments

Garments

Jewellery

Other Effects
(Wallets, documents, etc.)

Dental Examination   M2

Date of examination   Examiner   Body number

Right   Left

18	17	16	15	14	13	12	11	21	22	23	24	25	26	27	28
55	54	53	52	51	61	62	63	64	65
85	84	83	82	81	71	72	73	74	75
48	47	46	45	44	43	42	41	31	32	33	34	35	36	37	38

Prostheses, Orthodontics, etc.

Malformations, Oral abnormalities, etc.

Dental estimates of age, sex, race, etc.

(c)

Fig. 7.4 *continued*

ante-mortem dental chartings are obtained – which is quite possible in the United Kingdom where the regulations oblige a dental practitioner to chart only standing teeth, missing teeth and those teeth intended for treatment [15].

Attention to detail and meticulous recording of all the dental data present is especially important with regard to the transient state of teeth of children and minors. Depending upon the precise age, there are three possible dentitions: the deciduous, the mixed dentition of deciduous teeth and permanent teeth (erupted or erupting), or 28 teeth of the adult dentition less the four wisdom teeth. The ante-mortem dental records may be out of date and refer to details of the dentition which no longer exist in the jaws of the unknown child. Teeth missing from a particular dentition may be the result of either the shedding of a deciduous tooth to make room for its permanent successor or of extraction as part of dental treatment. If the loss was recent, it may be possible to assess the presence of a blood clot within the socket and determine if the tooth was lost by extraction or post-mortem. In the living person, the blood clot becomes organized as the process of healing takes place and is replaced, first, by granulation tissue and is then invaded by woven bone; remodelling then occurs and adult lamellar bone of cancellous type obliterates the socket. The soft tissues heal normally within 2–3 weeks and bone formation continues for at least 6 months after extraction. Complete bony remodelling

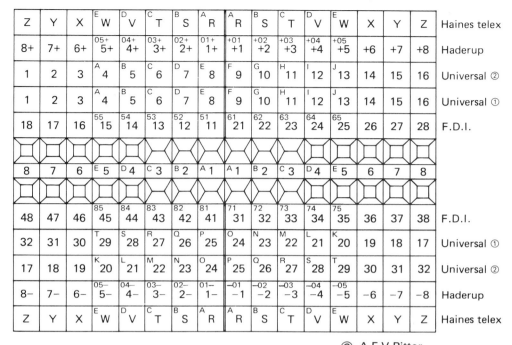

© A.F.V.Pitter

Fig. 7.5 Examples of various methods of charting in common use (by courtesy of Mr A.F.V. Pitter).

may take up to 5 years after the initial extraction and, due to the wide variations encountered, only a rough estimate can be made as to the time lapse.

Apart from the usual restorative techniques and materials used generally for patients of all ages, there are certain forms of conservation which are reserved for children and minors which will serve adequately until such time as it is appropriate to produce the adult permanent crown or bridge. Porcelain crowns are not usually fabricated until the patient is of a minimum age of 16 years. When a fracture of a central or lateral incisor occurs in a child the deficit of the crown shape may be repaired by the provision of a temporary gold 'basket' crown. Modern caries prevention techniques allow the fissures on the occlusal surfaces of posterior teeth to be sealed with plastic metals which are 'cured' by ultraviolet light.

It is not unusual to find either fixed or removable orthodontic appliances on the teeth of children and minors. A fixed appliance will suggest the possibility of an extensive description of the apparatus in the ante-mortem records, while misalignment of teeth or the recognition of an orthodontic problem in the teeth of an unknown child can sometimes be resolved by the finding of the appliance at the site or, in an air disaster, sometimes in the baggage; it can then be fitted to the teeth of the victim. There are occasions when the appliance is marked with the name of the patient or some other identifying code. Dentures are marked in a similar manner by various methods. Metal plates or strips can be processed into the dentures at some place which is the least likely to be destroyed by fire; absorbable materials which can be processed more easily than metal are the more common choice. One technique used in conservation and denture work involves the insertion of a personal dental identifier or information carrier composed of an alumina substrate, approximately 1.27 mm^2 in size with the data recorded in a micro-miniature mode. This ceramic tile can be placed inside the cavity preparation prior to filling or it may be cemented to the buccal side of a posterior tooth on a denture [16]. Many countries have a legal requirement for all dentures to carry an identification marker; marking a denture in the United Kingdom depends, at present, on the consent of the patient [15]. In any case formal markings of dentures are found less frequently than is the usual technician's mark of the first three initials of a patient's name; on other occasions, the laboratory may identify itself by incorporating a marked shape which will be identifiable if the laboratory, itself, can be located. The more general means of identifying dentures involves a full description of the shape and shade of the artificial teeth, the material from which the base is made, the shape of the relief chamber, the polished finish and, in the case of partial metal dentures, the design of the clasps and reciprocals and the position of the rests. This full description can then be matched with any ante-mortem information on the dentures known to have been made for particular persons.

It may be surprising to find that some children have to wear dentures at a very early age. There are those who suffer from the rare developmental condition of complete anodontia, in which no teeth develop at all, and there is the alternative condition in which the young patient has had all the deciduous teeth extracted by reason of rampant caries. It is necessary in both conditions to provide dentures in order to promote the necessary stimulus to the bone of the jaws to develop in a functional manner and to replace the dentures periodically as the jaws develop and grow. More common is the condition of partial anodontia in which individual teeth do not develop [17]. The usual tooth groups concerned are the lateral incisors, second premolars and the wisdom teeth in order of frequency. There are, of course, teeth which develop but, for some reason, are unable to erupt in the normal position and remain buried in the mouth. Radiographs will confirm the particular condition present which, in most instances, will have been observed and recorded ante-mortem.

Miscellaneous stigmata

Some identifying features described in textbooks refer to dental trauma produced by occupational habits. Most of this now relates to occupations which no longer exist. The origins of extrinsic, intrinsic and habitual stains of teeth are also well described [18] but have not been found to be of great value when applied to the examination of children's teeth. A black linear stain has been found on the teeth of non-smokers, females and children; orange and red stains can occur on children's teeth and are thought to be produced by chromogenic, or pigment producing bacteria. The colour of teeth may give an indication of the previous medical history. Amelogenesis imperfecta and dentinogenesis imperfecta, and the mottling due to high levels of fluoride, give characteristic colouring. Sometimes the haemolysis of blood cells and jaundice gives rise to a series of colours of the spectrum but these disappear when the underlying condition resolves. The forensic significance of 'pink' teeth originally described by Bell [19] has never been resolved.

7.6 RECOVERY OF DENTAL RECORDS

For nearly a decade, the Metropolitan Police

have had a system in operation by which the dental records of persons who have been reported missing for 1 month are submitted to the Missing Persons Bureau in anticipation of their being found dead – although many missing persons return home without any harm befalling them. Copies of dental chartings are obtained from the last known dental surgeon or information may be provided by relatives. All unknown bodies recovered in the London Metropolitan area, and especially from the River Thames, are dentally examined and the details are submitted to the Missing Persons Bureau for comparison with the index of dental charts of missing persons. If there are similarities with certain charts in the index then the original dental records together with any dental radiographs are requested from the dental surgeons and full comparisons are made. If a positive identification is not made, the records are returned and the chart pertaining to the unknown body goes into the unknown body index to await update information arriving from other police authorities in the United Kingdom, through Interpol or through any other country which requests information about its missing citizens. The success rate, therefore, depends on the existence and retrieval of ante-mortem dental records. In the United Kingdom, a dental surgeon is required to keep records of his patients for 4 years in Scotland and for 2 years in England and Wales. Other countries are more demanding; in Sweden, for example, the dental records are retained for 10 years. Dental records are held for long periods in private dental practice, in the dental schools of universities and in the armed forces but, because of the large numbers involved, the Dental Estimates Board of the National Health Service are only able to retain their records for under 18 months; the Board are, however, extremely helpful and willing to offer advice in any investigation.

7.7 ODONTO-LEGAL CONSIDERATIONS

The Scandinavian authorities have held for a number of years that, in order to achieve a positive identification by matching post-mortem with ante-mortem chartings, there should be a minimum of twelve points of correspondence or similarity [20]; recently, this recommendation has been brought down to six. It has always been the opinion in the United Kingdom that positive identifications could be made on fewer points if there were significant features present and that dental identifications could be made positively on non-dental skull radiographs if ante-mortem dental chartings were not available.

Case 7.2
V, aged 9 years, disappeared in 1981. His decomposed body was not found until 7 months later. The dental examination showed that he had a mixed dentition of deciduous and permanent teeth (Fig. 7.6). His first permanent molars had erupted as had his upper central incisors. The upper later incisor sockets were present as was the lower right lateral incisor socket indicating that the teeth had been lost post-mortem. There were sockets for the deciduous canine teeth and there were two amalgam fillings, one in the upper right second deciduous molar and one in the lower right deciduous first molar. His National Health Service dental records showed that he had attended for an examination some 3 months prior to his disappearance but no treatment was carried out and his dental surgeon stated that he would have charted fillings in his patient's teeth had he seen them. One radiograph was taken of the molars on the left upper jaw but this was found to be of no identifying value. The state of eruption of the teeth and the stage of development were consistent with the stated age. A recent photograph of V was obtained and a skull phototransparency was repro-

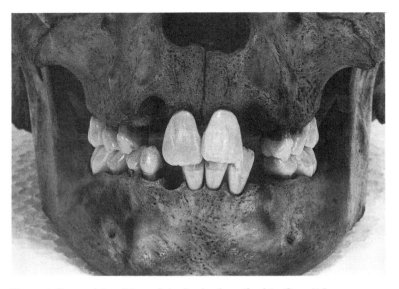

Fig. 7.6 State of dentition of the body described in Case 7.2.

duced to the same size and superimposed. The anatomical landmarks of the point of the chin, the angles of the jaw and cheek bones and the eye sockets matched with reasonable accuracy. The position and shape of the upper central incisors also matched with some accuracy. Though this could not be considered a positive identification by odontological means, there were other circumstantial features which aided the identification.

It may be pointed out that the presence or absence of other circumstantial evidence may be used to aid in an identification when the dental chartings are not adequate. Some dental charts which are submitted for comparison are in the attenuated form already referred to in the text; at other times, the records are not those including the latest treatment but are those of the last known dental surgeon that are some years out of date. There are occasions when the same dental charting appears to coincide with a number of individuals and, for reasons which have been discussed above, it may be very difficult to obtain a perfect match between ante-mortem and post-mortem charts when dealing with a completely unknown body. In circumstances such as an aircraft accident, however, one is dealing with a relatively well-known population; effectively, therefore, one can seek *best* matches rather than perfect matches and this accounts for the very considerable success of dental identification in such conditions.

In recent years, there has been some advance in techniques of facial reconstruction, originating in the work of Gerasimov, whereby modelling clay is applied in known thicknesses over the facial skeleton of an unknown skull [21]. This form of reconstruction has been found useful in a number of homicide cases in the United States by

Gatliff and Snow – especially in serial murders of juveniles [22]. Continuing research in this field is aimed at replacing the artist's intuitive portraiting of a face by precise cephalometric measurements derived from radiographic films taken by KLS Analytic Morphograph apparatus. This new method is known as Face Imaging Reconstructive Morphography [23]

and it is hoped that it will provide a useful adjunct to standard identifying procedures. This may be especially so in the case of juveniles in whom cephalometric and dental developmental features are present constantly but in whom dental pathology and associated features of treatment are often nonexistent.

(B) The dentist's role in non-accidental injury cases

D.K. Whittaker

7.8 INTRODUCTION

Since the first description of the battered child syndrome [24], it has been increasingly recognized that the dental surgeon may be the first health professional to see non-accidental injuries to a child [25]. In spite of the fact that 36 articles appeared in the dental literature between 1962 and 1986 which brought the attention of dentists to the syndrome [26], the problem is still not well appreciated by the profession. Dental surgeons are, however, in a good position to diagnose non-accidental injury provided that they are aware of the possibility of abuse and that they have some knowledge of the key factors in its diagnosis. These may be summarized [25] as a discrepancy between the history of injury as given by the adult accompanying the child and the type of injury presented to the clinician. The diagnosis of non-accidental injury is discussed in greater detail in Chapter 14. For the present, it need only be said that there should be physical signs of abuse, injury

inconsistent with the history given, delay in seeking medical attention, a history of previous injury and, perhaps, a history of violence within the family. The true extent of non-accidental injury in a population is difficult to determine but it was believed in 1967 that at least 300 cases occurred per year in London alone [27]. There were more than 72 000 suspected cases in California by 1977 and it was estimated that at least 2000 American children would die in any one year as a result of child abuse and neglect [28]. In 1974, 97 local authorities in the United Kingdom were approached by questionnaire, a survey covering 90% of the population. Some 5700 cases came to light in the last 9 months of that year with a mortality of 0.7% and a significant risk of re-injury [29]. By 1986, the reported incidence in the USA had risen to 1200 per million of the population [30] and it was anticipated that some 4000 children would die. Of all the patients seen in the Casualty Departments in this survey, 10%

had evidence of non-accidentally inflicted injuries. Whether or not the true occurrence is increasing, it is clear that increased awareness has resulted in many more cases being reported and, on the basis of current statistics, an individual dental surgeon may expect to encounter a case at least once every 3 years. In spite of this British dentists have not formally been requested to develop an awareness of non-accidental injuries to children and many Health Authority child abuse procedure documents make no mention of the possible role of the dentist [31].

Reporting of cases of child abuse is mandatory in the USA where ten sub-types of child abuse and neglect have been classified [30]. The most frequent of these is physical abuse with an incidence of nearly 32%, closely followed by educational neglect (28%) and by emotional abuse (26%). Suggestions as to how the dentist should examine a child thought to be suffering from child abuse or child neglect have been made [32]. Dentists are invited to note the relationships between the child and its parents, the cleanliness, stature and nutritional status of the child, the quality of its clothing and the presence of physical problems such as a limp or difficulty in climbing into the dental chair. It is recommended that the body be systematically examined for traumatic injury, bruises, previous scars, burn marks or injury caused by foreign bodies and, if the dentist's suspicions are aroused, the parents should be informed that an injury has been noticed; the dentist must then contact the appropriate child abuse or child neglect authority.

Accidentally acquired bruises or pseudo-bruises must be differentiated from inflicted injuries. Children who cannot crawl cannot cause a self-inflicted accident [30]; it follows that severe bruising or fractures in a child below the age of six to nine months are almost always inflicted non-accidentally by a second party.

The attention of the dental profession has also been drawn to the problem of child sexual abuse although the role of the paediatric dentist in these cases is not as clear as it is for other forms of child abuse [33]. Moreover, there is inadequate information in the dental literature to assist the paediatric dentist in examining these patients. Any physical examination should be confined to areas considered to be within the purview of the dentist; referral to a paediatrician for complete examination will be in the best interests of all concerned.

It is to be noted that non-fatal non-accidental injury to children is not compulsorily reportable in the United Kingdom nor have the General Dental Council given any ethical advice on the problem. The General Medical Council, however, in its annual report for 1987, regarded it not only permissible but an actual duty of the doctor to report cases of physical and sexual abuse.

7.9 FACIAL AND ORAL PATHOLOGY IN NON-ACCIDENTAL INJURY TO CHILDREN

Although there may be disagreement as to the role of the dentist in cases of physical abuse not involving the head and neck region and in those concerned with mental and sexual abuse, it is quite clear that he or she has an important role to play in the recognition, diagnosis and treatment of injuries to the face and oral cavity. The facial region is a common site of non-accidental injuries and it has been claimed that almost 50% of cases suffer injury to this part of the body [34]. In 260 cases of child abuse surveyed in Boston, 49% had sustained oro-facial trauma [35]; despite this, few of 537 dentists surveyed at that time knew of their legal responsibility to report these injuries. Others have reported an incidence of 60% of cases involving injury to the head and neck region [36] whilst the incidence in the United Kingdom has been cited as 43% [37].

(a) Extra-oral injuries

The head is a common area for child abuse injury; this may be because the face most clearly represents the persona of the individual. Bruises, lacerations, burns, cuts, scars and black eyes will suggest physical abuse. Extensive bruising of the face with a history of minimal trauma, especially if there are both old and new bruises, is almost diagnostic; bruising of the ear – which is often the result of a blow – and bruising of the cheeks produced by gripping the face are rarely accidental and may be typical [25]. Lesions to the jaw and neck are often well circumscribed and of a finger-tip character suggestive of gripping [24]. Burns to the face have been found to be the most frequent injury in some studies [37] although, in others, the most common type of injury was a facial contusion [35]. Burns from hot solid objects are the easiest to diagnose and are usually of second degree without blister formation. The shape of the burn often resembles the hot object producing it [30]. Cigarette burns, for example, result in circular, punched-out lesions of uniform size; these are, however, rarely seen on the face.

Non-accidentally produced fractures of the facial bones are uncommon in children and feature in about 2% of cases [35]. Of these, the most common fracture is of the nasal bones (45%), followed by the mandible (32%) and the zygomatic maxillary complex (20.5%). Specialized treatment is required for these and their definitive management has been comprehensively discussed in the oral surgery literature [38].

(b) Intra-oral injuries

The mouth is a frequent site of non-accidental injury in children, possibly because of its psychological significance; it is the organ of phonation and violence may be used against it in order to silence the child [28]. Contusions and bruises, which occurred in 43% of a series of 14 cases reviewed, are the commonest injuries to the mouth [35]; lacerations and trauma to the teeth each account for 28% of injuries.

Examination of the mouth should commence with the lips; the lips usually heal well following minor injuries and scarring should alert the dentist to previous severe trauma. Bruised and swollen lips or abrasions at the corners of the mouth are suggestive of blows from a fist; non-accidental injuries are especially likely if the bruises or injuries are at varying stages of healing.

The teeth themselves are vulnerable to blows to the mouth either from a fist, a hand slap or a weapon. It must, of course, be remembered that children frequently avulse or fracture teeth in the course of normal play activities, but an unsatisfactory history from the child or parent, or repeated attendance for treatment of injuries, will arouse the suspicion of the dentist. The roots of the anterior teeth may be incompletely formed in children and, as a result, blows to the face often result in complete avulsion and loss of the tooth rather than in fracture of the roots. When teeth are missing, full radiographs of the jaw should be taken to rule out some abnormality of development or conditions of partial anodontia; retained fractured roots should be sought as these will require surgical removal. Multiple healed micro-fractures of tooth roots may sometimes be visible in intra-oral radiographs – these are almost always indicative of trauma by repeated abuse.

Slight movements of the teeth may rupture delicate blood vessels passing through the apical foramina and, as a result, anterior teeth which survive trauma of this nature may become devitalized, especially if the root apices have completed their development. The crowns of the teeth are likely to become discoloured in the months following such trauma. A grey hue usually develops due to the presence of blood break-down products in the dentinal tubules and discoloured anterior teeth for which a satisfactory explanation is not forthcoming may suggest that non-accidental injury has occurred.

The report of the autopsy findings in 29 fatal cases seen during a two-year period at the London Hospital Medical College included one of the first assessments of soft tissue intra-oral injury following child abuse [34]. Of these, 50% had injuries to the head and neck and 45% of these had suffered damage to the upper lip region. This consisted of lacerations of the mucosa of the inner aspect of the upper lip close to the labial frenum, which were sometimes so severe that the reflected mucosa of the lip was completely torn away from that attached to the gingiva. Tearing of the labial frenum is not uncommon in very small children who fall accidentally onto the mouth whilst learning to walk, but this lesion should arouse suspicion as to a possible non-accidental cause when it is found in children less than about one year and more than about

2 years of age. These injuries can be produced by aggressive bottle feeding or by forcing a spoon into the mouth, as is sometimes done by a frustrated parent whose child is a slow eater. The labial frenum may also be damaged by blows to the mouth or by tearing the upper lip away from the gingival attachment (Fig. 7.7). Following this report, the torn labial frenum has been regarded as pathognomonic of child abuse but it must be noted that no later reports of intra-oral damage in cases of child abuse have indicated such a high incidence. Many paediatric dentists of considerable experience working in the United Kingdom have never seen a case of labial frenal damage which they could unequivocally relate to non-accidental injury. When it does occur, the condition is often associated with subluxation or fracture of the upper central incisors, damage to the teeth being caused by the same blow.

Penetrating injuries to the palate, the vestibule and the floor of the mouth resulting

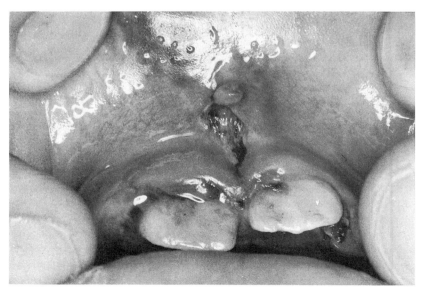

Fig. 7.7 Damage to the labial frenum may be caused by forcible feeding or, as in this case, by a blow to the mouth. Teeth may be displaced.

from forced feeding or forcible introduction of spoons and other implements into the mouth have been described. Burns of the oral mucosa following enforced ingestion of hot or caustic liquids are seen quite commonly [25] as are intra-oral cigarette burns and tearing of the oral mucosa by a parent's finger placed in the mouth. Dentists who are unfamiliar with the range of oral pathologies of a non-accidental nature that may occur in the mouth should refer patients to a specialist if they are in doubt as to the cause of a particular lesion.

7.10 THE DENTIST ACCUSED OF CHILD ABUSE

Child abuse or non-accidental injuries to children are frequently caused by adults in close relationship to the child. It has been pointed out [39] that this may include a child's professional adviser such as a dentist. Dental practitioners have, indeed, been accused of child abuse by using excessive restraint – for example, by placing the hand over the mouth in order to deal with a difficult patient. Questionnaires in the United States are currently being designed to discover how many dentists have been accused of battery or non-consensual 'touching'. The information is difficult to acquire and, up to 1987, only one report was available covering 3 cases [39]. All the incidents occurred during the course of normal treatment and all resulted in an arrest. Child abuse is a criminal offence and, accordingly, it is not covered by malpractice insurance in the United States.

7.11 BITE MARKS

The term bite mark has come to mean any mark produced in flesh, foodstuffs or a number of other materials by the teeth and the surrounding soft tissues. Whilst it is true to say that the mark is usually produced entirely by the teeth in foodstuffs and non-living materials, the mark in human flesh is often contributed to by pressure from the lips and the tongue as well as from the teeth themselves. Dental evidence has recently become increasingly important in the investigation of non-accidental injuries to children. Attention was first drawn to the incidence of bite marks in a report of 13 forensic dental cases, two of which involved teeth marks in battered babies; the child had died in both cases [40]. The incidence of bites in victims of all ages was given as 12 per 100 000 in the population of New York in 1977 [41] but there appears to be only one epidemiological study on the frequency of biting associated with child abuse [42]. In this study, nurses working in facilities which admitted child abuse patients were trained by forensic dentists to recognize bite marks on their patients. Bites were divided into incised bites without bruising, those incised with bruising or discoloration, marks with sucking bruises and marks where the teeth had been dragged over the tissue. Of 1100 children examined, 17 of these had evidence of bite mark abuse – an incidence of 1545 per 100 000 sheltered children. Most of the bites had been inflicted on children between the ages of 11 to 15 years but two were in children less than three years of age and four in children between 16 and 18 years. Most of the male victims were in the 4 to 10 year age group whilst females were most frequently in the 11 to 15 year old age group. The most common area to be bitten in children was the head and neck (43%); the limbs and trunk were also common sites of attack.

No studies have been carried out on the distribution of bite marks specifically in child abuse cases but the anatomical distribution has been investigated in a series of 67 cases of varying ages [43]. Of these cases 13 were aged below 15 years. Female victims were most commonly bitten on the breasts, arms and legs while the arms and shoulders were most often affected in males. These results differ somewhat from those reported in the United

Kingdom where bite marks on the breasts of females were found to be much more common than in the American sample, whereas bite marks on the arms were seen less frequently [44]. Other studies on the anatomical distribution of bites include those on 122 injuries observed in a New York hospital [45] and on 114 cases reported from Kansas [46]. In both of these studies, bites were most often seen on the hands and fingers; it appears that predilection for the different parts of the body has changed in more recent times. In non-accidental injuries in children, the entire surface of the child's body may be attacked resulting in bite marks on the cheeks, shoulders, chest, abdomen, arms, legs and buttocks [47]; multiple bites at the same site may be seen. Bites on the hands and fingers may be caused when the child attempts to protect him- or herself. Some forensic odontologists believe that bite marks found on infants tend to be in locations different from those found in older children or adolescents and are meant as punishments to the child in response to crying or soiling. These bites tend to be concentrated on the cheeks, arms, shoulders, buttocks or genitalia; bites intended as punishment for soiling are most commonly seen in the two latter locations. Quite frequently, there are other injuries such as pinch-marks, bruises or burns [48]. Bite marks in the older child may be less punitive in nature and are more likely to be related to physical or sexual abuse.

(a) Types of bite mark in children

There is general agreement that there are two main patterns of bite marks. The first of these is an aggressive or anger bite where, in the main, the teeth alone are used and the marks on the skin most nearly resemble the shape of the teeth making them. The mark results from an attack or defence bite and is the type most frequently seen in non-accidental injury to the child [48]. This kind of bite is a particularly aggressive one; no suction of lips and tongue is involved, the tissues being bitten directly between the teeth. On occasions, substantial abrasion marks may be associated with each tooth mark suggesting motion during the biting episode [49].

The second type of bite mark is one which is slowly, sadistically and deliberately inflicted, suction or, sometimes, presure being applied to the soft tissues via the lips and tongue. These types of mark are more often seen in abuse of older children with a sexual overlay. The injury demonstrates bruising in the central part of the bite and sometimes in the peripheral areas together with linear radiating abrasions caused by the incisal edges of the anterior teeth. The outlines of the teeth are usually quite clearly visible. The pressure exerted by teeth during biting can be considerable and may be as much as 11 kg (550 kPa) from the incisors and pressure from the tongue may reach at least 8 lb per square inch (55 kPa) during suckling activity [50]. Suction, as distinct from thrust from the tongue and lips, may reach a negative pressure of 20 mm Hg (2.75 kPa) in some bites [51].

Most children with bite mark injuries are brought to the casualty or paediatric department by the parents or adult guardians. The person who abused the child and produced the bites is likely to be among them [52]. This, however, is not always the case and the examiner should be aware of the fact that bites may be produced on small children by siblings or play-mates either aggressively as a means of punishment or occasionally in sexual play. The methods of distinguishing bites produced by children from those produced by adults will be described later.

(b) Self-inflicted bites

Cases have been reported in which bite marks found on the forearms of children have been caused by the victims themselves. It has been suggested that the arms may be pushed into the child's mouth by an assailant in order to stifle crying but, also, that young children may put their own arm or hand in their mouth because of the intense pain inflicted by other injuries and bite themselves through fear or as a counter irritant [53]. Self-biting may also be a type of self-destructive behaviour such as has been described in individuals who are mentally retarded or psychologically disturbed. Self-biting also occurs in adults, and a case has been described in which a 51-year-old man self-inflicted a bite mark on the left wrist during a fatal episode of myocardial ischaemia [54]. It is obvious that self-inflicted bite marks can only be made on parts of the body which may be placed in the mouth, but one suicide victim is reported as having managed to self-inflict a bite upon the left breast.

(c) Animal bites in children

Unsupervised infants, and even older children, may occasionally be attacked by domestic or wild animals. Animals may attack the face of a small child producing very serious injury. It is usually relatively easy for a dentist to distinguish between a human and an animal bite because of the size of the dental arch and, more particularly, the arrangement and size of the teeth – a carnivore such as a dog or a ferret, for example, has large canines and diminutive incisors in both the upper and lower jaws. The classical bite from these animals presents either as a four point puncture wound from the canines or as tearing of the tissue in more aggressive attacks (Fig. 7.8). Small animals such as rats have extremely sharp, razor-like incisors; these can inflict deep and extensive lacerations which may be mistaken for injuries using sharp implements (Fig. 7.9). It may be very important from a medico-legal point of view to determine which animal has made the bites since the parents or owners may be held responsible if it is a domestic animal, whereas

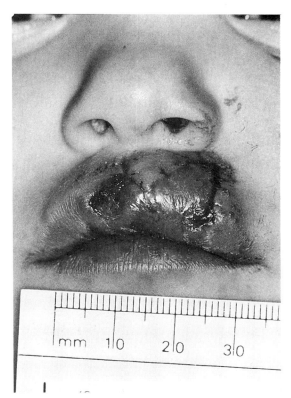

Fig. 7.8 Dog bites may result in four point puncture wounds or tearing of the tissues as in this case.

blame may be apportioned quite differently if, for example, the injuries have been produced by rats which have not been exterminated by the local authority as in the case shown in Fig. 7.9. Distinguishing between different animal bites requires not only a knowledge of comparative dental anatomy but also something of the habits of common animals. Watch dogs tend to bite and hold their victims whilst untrained wild dogs may move their heads as they bite, tearing the tissue and making the bite mark more difficult to evaluate [55]. A case has been described in which the body of a 13-month-old baby was discovered with more than 80 puncture wounds initially thought to have been caused

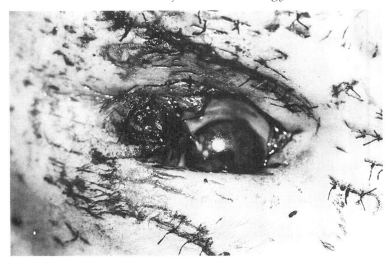

Fig. 7.9 Multiple bites from small animals may result in serious facial injury extending to loss of an eye. These injuries were caused by rats.

by a mechanical instrument. It was eventually shown that the child had been injured and finally killed by two German shepherd dogs [56]. Dogs are the commonest animal to bite children [57]; there have been a number of reports of serious infections following both dog and cat bites [58, 59].

Most injuries in children involve the extremities but, because of their small size, 33% of bites in children under 5 years of age are to the head and neck. There have been instances of damage to the central nervous system caused by an English bull terrier, a Doberman Pinscher – and a Bengal tiger [60]. The child has been less than two years of age – and usually less than one year old – in nearly all the reported cases of injury to the head from dog bites.

(d) The investigation of bite marks

The bite marks will be on the body of the victim in almost all cases of non-accidental injury to children although it must be remembered that, occasionally, they may be on an assailant – as when the victim has attempted to fight back or is attacking in self-defence. The same techniques of examination of the wound apply in both cases. Apart from the difficulty of examining the small child, the methods used to investigate bite marks on adults can be applied routinely in the child case. Bite marks, if present, are a particularly useful feature of non-accidental injury cases because not only do they demonstrate injury which is difficult to explain away as an accident but they are also one of the few injuries which relate directly to the assailant. The assessment of bite marks in human flesh requires considerable experience and knowledge on the part of the forensic dentist who should, therefore, be included in the team investigating a case of childhood abuse. This is still not the case in respect of many health authorities in the United Kingdom.

Even if a putative suspect is available, the bites on the victim should always be examined first and a full report of them should be made before the suspect is examined. This is because sight of a possible suspect's dentition inevitably injects an element of bias into the interpretation of the mark.

(e) The bite marks

Although the details of the method of examination of bite marks vary somewhat as a matter of personal preference, guidelines have been laid down by the American Board of Forensic Odontology and these form an extremely useful basis for the procedure. After recording the usual details of the victim, the location of the bite mark on the body, be it living or dead, is carefully described; at this stage, it is important to note whether the bite mark is on a flat or a curved surface and whether it overlies soft tissue, fat or bone. A human bite mark is usually identified readily because of the double arcade shape of the marks. If both upper and lower arches have left marks, the characteristics of the resulting bite include an elliptical or ovoid pattern containing tooth and arch marks [61] which are almost always produced by the canine to canine of the upper arch opposed to canine to canine of the lower arch. The incisor teeth tend to leave rectangular bruises or incisions whereas the canines at the periphery of the oval leave puncture or triangular marks. A decision as to whether an injury is, in fact, a human bite mark depends upon its shape, colour and size and on the impressions made by individual teeth. Bruising may be present not only in relation to the biting edges of the teeth but also in the central area of the bite because of the tongue thrust or suction against the palate of the assailant. If the marks of individual teeth in their correct alignment can be satisfactorily identified, then it is possible to say at this stage that the victim has suffered a human bite.

The next stage in examination of the bite is to obtain evidence from saliva traces which is best done using a teased out thread from well-washed cotton dipped into saline solution. This is used to swab the bite mark and is then sealed in a sterile test tube. One or more control swabs must be taken from skin in other parts of the body where no bite marks are suspected [62] – it is often convenient to use the contra-lateral area of the body; a saline 'control' swab should also be supplied. These specimens are needed to exclude any contamination by secretions of either the victim or the investigator; as a further precaution against the latter, gloves should be worn and, so far as is possible, there should be only instrumental contact with the swab. Subsequent grouping is usually limited to the ABO system only. A, B and/or H substances are secreted by some 75% of the population; a negative result may, thus, be due to the absence of saliva, to a non-secretor status of the biter or to poor sampling – the importance of a standard and satisfactory technique, is thereby, emphasized.

(f) The detail of the bite

Once a mark has been recognized as being due to a human bite its characteristics must be recorded. An arch mark is identified when 4 or 5 marks of adjacent teeth are present; if these include the maxillary canines, the distance between the two canine marks should be measured. In a human bite the inter-canine width will lie between 2.5 and 4.5 cm [52]; the bite has probably been caused by the deciduous dentition of a child if the inter-canine width of the maxillary teeth is less than 3 cm. Each bruise or laceration should be individually measured and described in an attempt to reconstruct the type of dentition which could have made the mark. Any missing teeth – or, at least, areas where no bruises have occured – must be noted. The alignment of the bruises and the possibility of their having been made by rotated teeth should also be examined. The mark caused by the maxillary arch is often more diffuse than that produced by the mandibular teeth. This results not only from the greater surface area of the incisal edges of the upper teeth but also because the maxilla is stable in relation to the skull; by contrast, the mandible is mobile and acts as a cutting instrument once the skin has been stabilized against the upper teeth (Fig. 7.10).

At this point in the investigation the forensic dentist should be prepared to explain the individual characteristics of the bite. A slowly produced bite results in stretching of

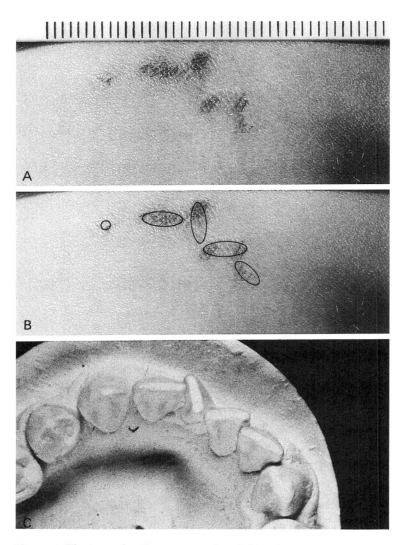

Fig. 7.10 The irregular abrasions on this child's shoulder were produced by lower incisor and canine teeth of an adult (A). Orientation and dimensions of the marks (B) can be compared with the unusual imbrication of the lower incisors of a suspect (C).

the skin over the cutting edges of the teeth and pressure or suction from the tongue and palate; this will be reflected in the extent of bruising both in the tooth marks and in the surrounding and central areas of the bite. A bite mark showing these characteristics was probably produced under amorous circumstances although even 'love bites' require considerable force to produce and can be painful to the recipient. A bite mark which consists of tooth marks only is of an aggressive nature and has probably been delivered rapidly and in anger – this is especially so if the teeth have penetrated the skin. It may also be possible to give an opinion as to the timing of the bite. In this respect, it is important to recognize differences between bites produced in victims who survive and in those who do not. The length of time for which a bite remains visible in living victims varies with the force applied and the amount of damage produced. Bites which do not penetrate through the skin may result in bruises which fade within a period of 24 hours [28]. It is therefore important that the forensic dentist be called in the early stages of the investigation of these cases. The marks may last for several days when the skin has been penetrated. Many investigators have recommended that bite marks be photographed at 24 hour intervals because their detail may improve in the first 2–3 days as swelling decreases and bruising increases [61]. In addition, the outline of the bite may change because of infection, oedema and discoloration of the skin.

Quite different appearances will result if the bite was inflicted immediately prior to or immediately after death. In the former case, provided that sufficient time has elapsed to allow extravasation of blood into the tissues, a very clear bite mark may be seen which changes very little until the onset of putrefaction. Bites inflicted after death rarely result in bruising; very considerable forces indeed are required to produce an appearance of bruising post-mortem.

(g) Recording the bite mark

In the majority of cases the most useful technique is to photograph the bite mark using both colour and black and white film. Some forensic dentists will argue that the photography should be carried out by a professional police photographer under the direction of the dentist so that questions in court regarding scale of reproduction, colour balance and other photographic questions may be answered with authority. However, in many cases such services are not available and photography must be carried out by the clinician.

A quality 35 mm camera with 100 mm lens, automatic extension tubes and available dedicated flash facilities will meet most requirements. In most cases of bite mark injury one or more standard flash guns and control of side lighting, will give better modelling than will a ring flash. The 100 mm lens will give satisfactory reproduction of the marks without distortion and will leave sufficient distance from camera to subject to allow of flexible lighting.

Whatever equipment is used, photographs should include low power distance shots of the bite and surrounding tissues which allow for orientation of the bite. A standard colour chart should be photographed along with the subject when colour film is used. In the case of black and white film, filters including ultraviolet may be used to enhance the contrast of the mark but the type of filter used must be recorded. Ultraviolet and infra-red illumination may bring out details that are not obvious when viewed by conventional lighting. The simplest method is to cover the flash-gun with the relevant filter. Increased exposures are needed to compensate for the reduced illumination. Each bite or suspected bite should be photographed with and without a millimetre scale. The scale, when used, should be placed in such a position that it does not cover any of the bite or the immediately surrounding tissues; it must be in the same focal plane as the bite mark. The use of an L-shape centimetre scale has been advocated; many of these devices have one or more circular designs imprinted on them so that any distortion at the time of photography will be obvious on the resultant prints. Some workers advocate the use of a flexible curve scale as well as a rigid scale if the bite is on a curved surface of the body. It is important that the camera be arranged in such a way that the film plane is as near parallel to the plane of the bite mark as is possible.

It is advisable to re-photograph marks on living victims every 24 hours for a number of days. One-to-one enlargements should be made of both colour and black and white photographs for measurement purposes and, in addition, larger prints should be prepared for demonstration in court.

Once the marks have been photographed they should be examined carefully through a hand lens to determine whether there are foreign bodies in the depth of the marks. These may include fragments of tooth fractured from the assailant at the time of the attack which should be removed carefully and stored as evidence. The depth of the bite mark and surface skin should be swabbed as described previously for saliva traces. Saliva samples are best used to eliminate suspects rather than to confirm identity.

(h) Impressions of the bite

Many bite marks in human tissue will not leave a three-dimensional imprint but will be visible only by way of the bruising in the underlying tissues; impressions are valueless in such cases. If the bite is deeper – and particularly when the skin has been penetrated – an impression may be useful and should be taken in a recommended silicone rubber base dental impression material. It is advisable to back the impression with a rigid material such as plaster of Paris to minimize distortion on removal, storage and casting. Subsequent models should be cast in quality dental stone; these may be useful for measurement purposes and study models prepared from possible suspects may be compared with the impression.

(i) Excision of skin samples

If the victim does not survive the attack, the bite marks and a large area of surrounding tissue may be excised and fixed; sections can then be prepared through the region of the injury. These may be stained for iron, other blood breakdown products and for changes in the elastic and collagen fibres (Fig. 7.11). The slides may demonstrate the classical features of bite mark injury which are: abrasion or penetration of the epithelium, compression and distortion or underlying collagen fibres, oedematous spaces and extravasation of erythrocytes from the blood vessels [63].

Various histochemical techniques may be useful to determine whether a wound is ante- or post-mortem. The most useful seem to be assays for serotonin (5-hydroxytryptamine) and histamine. A serotonin difference of a factor of 2 and a histamine difference of a factor of 1.5 between the wound and the control tissues are said to be indicative of ante-mortem injury [64].

(j) The suspect

Once a suspect has been apprehended steps should be taken to acquire records of his or her teeth which may be matched with the bite marks in question. It is normally essential that any suspect be asked for permission to be examined and the purpose of the examination must be explained to him. Written consent of the procedure should be acquired and witnessed, preferably in the presence of the suspect's solicitor. A dental history should be taken with particular emphasis on dental treatment both prior to and following the biting incident. Colour and black and white photographs should be taken or ordered of the extra- and intra-oral appearance of the suspect.

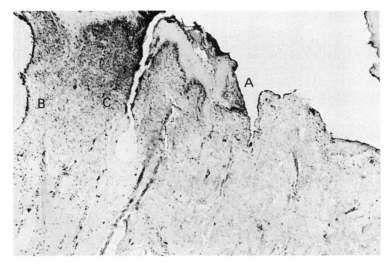

Fig. 7.11 Histological studies on a bite mark may demonstrate penetration of epithelium (A) oedema and disruption of underlying connective tissue (B) and the presence of extravasated erythrocytes demonstrated here by a positive benzidine reaction (C).

It may sometimes be useful to photograph a suspect with a scale in place showing the maximum opening between the incisor teeth. Suitable blood and saliva samples should be taken from each suspect when a saliva swab has been taken from the victim; the saliva sample must be boiled to prevent enzymatic destruction of the blood group substances. A comprehensive intra-oral examination must be undertaken charting teeth present, damaged, misaligned or fractured; teeth tender to biting forces and any abnormal chewing activity should also be noted.

Impressions in dental alginate should be taken of both upper and lower arches and the occlusal relationship between maxilla and mandible must also be recorded using a suitable technique. These impressions must be attested and labelled and cast in quality dental stone as quickly as possible. The technician making the castings must record the details of the procedure; the base of the study models must be marked with the individual's name and also signed and dated by the technician. Some dentists invite a suspect to produce a sample bite into a wax recording medium at the time of the examination. Dental impressions are classified as non-intimate samples for the purposes of the Police and Criminal Evidence Act 1984. A senior police officer can, therefore, authorize non-consensual investigations so long as the suspect is in detention in respect of a serious arrestable offence (s.63); in Scotland, an impression made by virtue of a Sheriff warrant would be admissible evidence.

(k) Comparison of evidence from the bite and from the suspect

Although it has been recommended that a fixed number of points of similarity should exist between the teeth of a suspect and the marks left by a bite, there is a danger in assuming that bite marks are equivalent to finger prints and that a reasonable number of matching points will prove the identity of the biter. Current opinion holds that a more important function is to note unusual features of both the mark and suspect's dentition which would tend either to eliminate him from or to indicate his involvement in the case. Thus, a single feature such as a missing, rotated or fractured tooth leaving a comparable mark in the bite may be a much more useful pointer than any number of matching features in an arch of normal size and arrangement (Fig. 7.12).

The methods of comparison of a dentition with a given bite will vary according to the circumstances. They include transparent overlays of the occlusion laid on scaled photographs of the injury, superimposition of colour slides, the use of dental articulators and the recording of bites in suitable media. They have involved sophisticated scientific analyses such as micro-contour mapping, scanning electron microscopic imaging and the use of the reflex microscope [65]. In practice, the simpler and more obvious is the method, the more likely are a jury to understand and appreciate its significance.

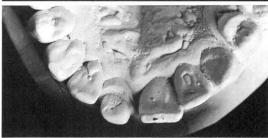

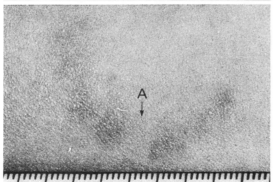

Fig. 7.12 Unusual features of a bite mark such as a gap left by a missing or fractured tooth (A) are important features in a comparison with the dentition of a possible suspect (B).

REFERENCES

1. Keiser-Nielsen, S. (1970), in *Legal Medicine Annual*, (ed. C.H. Wecht) Appleton-Century Crofts, New York.
2. Cameron, J.M. and Sims, B.G. (eds) (1973) *Forensic Dentistry*, Churchill Livingstone, Edinburgh.
3. Keiser-Nielsen, S. (1968) Forensic odontology. *Int. Dent. J.*, **18**, 668.
4. Langdon-Davies, J. (1966) *Shaftesbury and the Working Children*, Cape, London.
5. Schour, I. and Massler, M. (1941) The development of the human dentition. *J. Amer. Dent. Ass.*, **28**, 1153.
6. Moorrees, C.F.A., Fanning, E.A. and Hunt, E.E. (1963) Age variation of formation stages for ten permanent teeth. *J. Dent. Res.*, **42**, 1490.
7. Moorrees, C.F.A., Fanning, E.A. and Hunt, E.E. (1963) Formation and resorption of three deciduous teeth in children. *Amer. J. Phys. Anthr.* **21**, 205.
8. Johanson, G. (1975) Age determinations from human teeth. *Odontologisk Revy*, **22**, Supp. 21.
9. Ciapparelli, L. (1985) *An Assessment of Dental Age in Essex Schoolchildren Using Panoral Radiographs with Forensic Applications.* Dissertation, London Hospital Medical College.

10. Altini, M. (1983) Age determination from the teeth – a review. *J. Dent. Ass. Sth. Africa*, **38**, 275.

11. Sullivan, P.G. (1971) Observations on the rate of growth of human dentine. *Quarterly Dent. Rev.*, **5**, No. 2.

12. Sims, B.G. (1971) Disparity between real, skeletal, and dental age in a young female. *Quarterly Dent. Rev.*, **5**, No. 2.

13. Modi, N.J. (1972) *Medical Jurisprudence and Toxicology*, Tripathi, Bombay.

14. Sims, B.G. (1968) Identification by the teeth and jaws and other aspects of forensic odontology, in *Gradwohl's Legal Medicine* (ed. F.E. Camps), (2nd edn), Wright, Bristol, Chapter 12.

15. Sims, B.G. (1984) In *Taylor's Principles and Practice of Medical Jurisprudence* (ed. A.K. Mant) (13th edn), Churchill Livingstone, Edinburgh, Chapter 10.

16. Rawson, R.D. and Smith, E.S. (1986) *Current status of the oral ID disk*. Paper presented at 38th Annual Meeting of the American Academy of Forensic Sciences, New Orleans.

17. Stones, H.H. (1948) *Oral and Dental Diseases*, Livingstone, Edinburgh.

18. Stanley, H.R. (1976) The effect of systemic diseases on the human pulp. *Oral Surgery*, **33**, 606.

19. Bell, T. (1829) *Anatomy, Physiology, and Diseases of the Teeth*, Highley, London.

20. Keiser-Nielsen, S. (1980) *Personal Identification by Means of the Teeth*, Wright, Bristol.

21. Gerasimov, M.M. (1971) *The Face Finder*, Lippincott, Philadelphia.

22. Gatliff, B.P. and Snow, C.C. (1979) From skull to visage. *J. Biocom.*, **6**, 27.

23. Perper, J.A., Patterson, G.T. and Backner, J.S. (1988) Face imaging reconstructive morphography. *Amer. J. For. Med. Path.*, **9**, 126.

24. Kempe, C.H., Silverman, F.N., Steele, B.F., Droegemueller, W. and Silver, H.K. (1962) The battered child syndrome. *JAMA*, **181**, 105.

25. Macintyre, D.R., Jones, G.M. and Pinckney, R.C. (1986) The role of the dental practitioner in the management of non-accidental injury to children. *Br. Dent. J.*, **161**, 108.

26. Needleman, H.L. (1986) Orofacial trauma in child abuse: types, prevalence, management, and the dental profession's involvement. *Pediatr. Dent.* **8**, 71.

27. Simpson, K. (1967) *A Doctors Guide to Court*. Butterworth, London.

28. Sperber, N. (1981) The dual responsibility of dentistry in child abuse. *Int. J. Orthod.*, **19**, 21.

29. Fearn, J. (1987) Dental aspects of child abuse. (Letter). *Aust. Dent. J.*, **32**, 227.

30. Schmitt, B.D. (1986) Physical abuse: specifics of clinical diagnosis. *Paediatric Dent.*, **8**, 83.

31. Hobson, P. (1987) Child abuse: we can help (letter). *Br. Dent. J.*, **162**, 53.

32. Kittle, P.E., Richardson, D.S. and Parker, J.W. (1986) Examining for child abuse and child neglect. *Pediatr. Dent.*, **8**, 80.

33. Casamassimo, P.S. (1986) Child sexual abuse and the paediatric dentist. *Paediatric Dent.*, **8**, 102.

34. Cameron, J.M., Johnson, H.R. and Camps, F.E. (1966) The battered child syndrome. *Med. Sci. Law.*, **6**, 2.

35. Becker, D.B., Needleman, H.L. and Kotelchuck, M. (1978) Child abuse and dentistry: orofacial trauma and its recognition by dentists. *J. Am. Dent. Assoc.*, **97**, 24.

36. Fontana, V.J., Donovan, M.D., Wong, R.J. (1963) The maltreatment syndrome in children. *New Engl. J. Med.*, **269**, 1389.

37. Skinner, A.E., Castle, R.L. (1969) *A retrospective study*. Published by N.S.P.C.C. London W.1.

38. Sanders, B., Brady, F.A. and Johnson, R. (1979) *Injuries in pediatric oral and maxillofacial surgery*. (ed. B. Sanders). C.V. Mosby, St. Louis, p. 30.

39. Schuman, N.J. (1987) Child abuse and the dental practitioner: discussion and case reports. *Quintessence Int.* **18**, 619.

40. Hodson, J.J. (1971) Forensic odontology in cases of battered baby syndrome. *J. Dent. Res.*, **50**, 656.

41. Marr, J.S., Beck, A.M. and Lugo, J.A. (1979) An epidemiological study of the human bite. *Public Health Report*, **94**, 514.

42. Rawson, R.D., Koot, A., Martin, C., Jackson, J., Novosel, S., Richardson, A. and Bender, T. (1984) Incidence of bite marks in a selected juvenile population: a preliminary report. *J. Forensic Sci.*, **29**, 254.

43. Vale, G.L. and Noguchi, T.T. (1983)

Anatomical distribution of human bite marks in a series of 67 cases. *J. Forensic Sci.*, **28,** 61.

44. Harvey, W. (1976) *Dental identification and forensic odontology*, Henry Kimpton, London, page 91.

45. Lowry, T. McG. (1936) The surgical treatment of human bites. *Annals Surg.* **104,** 1103.

46. Speirs, R.F. (1941) Prevention of human bite infection. *Surg. Gynec. Obstet.*, **72,** 619.

47. Sims, A.P. (1985) Non-accidental injury in the child presenting as a suspected fracture of the zygomatic arch. *Br. Dent. J..*, **158,** 292.

48. Levine, L.J. (1977) Bite mark evidence. *Dent. Clin. North Amer.*, **21,** 145.

49. Wagner, G.N. (1986) Bite mark identification in child abuse cases. *Pediatr. Dent.* **8,** 96.

50. Kydd, W.L. (1956) Quantitative analysis of forces on the tongue. *J. Dent. Res.*, **35,** 171.

51. Harvey, W., Millington, P.F., Evans, J.H., *et al.* (1973) Bite marks – the clinical picture; physical features of skin and tongue. Standard and scanning electron microscopy. *Int. Microform J. Leg. Med.*, **8,** 3.

52. Levine, L.J. (1973) The solution of a battered child homicide by dental evidence: report of case. *J. Am. Dent. Assoc.* **87,** 1234.

53. Anderson, W.R., Hudson, R.P. (1976) Self-inflicted bite marks in battered child syndrome. *Forensic Sci.*, **7,** 71.

54. Warnick, A.J., Biedrzycki, L., Russanow, G. (1987) Not all bite marks are associated with abuse, sexual activities, or homicides: a case study of a self-inflicted bite mark. *J. Forensic. Sci.*, **32,** 788.

55. Triratana, T. (1970) Bite marks. *J. Dent. Assoc. Thailand*, **20,** 259.

56. Glass, R.T., Jordan, F.B. and Andrews, E.E. (1975) Multiple animal bite wounds: a case report. *J. Forensic. Sci.*, **20,** 305.

57. Belardi, F.G., Pascol, J.M. and Beegle, E.D. (1982) Pasteurella multocida meningitis in an infant following occipital dog bite. *J. Fam. Pract.*, **14,** 778.

58. Callaham, M.L. (1978) Treatment of common dog bites: infection risk factors. *J. Am. Coll. Emerg. Phys.*, **7,** 83.

59. Marcy, S.M. (1982) Infections due to dog and cat bites. *Pediat. Infect. Des.*, **1,** 351.

60. Steinbok, P., Flodmark, O., Scheifele, D.W. (1985) Animal bites causing central nervous system injury in children. A report of three cases. *Paediatr. Neurosci.*, **12,** 96.

61. MacDonald, D.G. (1974) Bite mark recognition and interpretation. *J. Forensic Sci. Soc.*, **14,** 229.

62. Pereira, M. (1971) Possibilities and limitations of saliva tests in forensic odontology. *Br. Dent. J.*, **130,** 161.

63. Millington, P.F. (1973) Histological studies of skin carrying bite marks. *J. Forensic Sci. Soc.*, **14,** 239.

64. Raekallio, J. (1966) Enzyme histochemistry of vital and postmortem skin wounds. *J. Forensic Sci.*, **13,** 85.

65. Ligthelm, A.J., Coetzee, W.J.C. and Van Niekerk, P.J. (1987) The identification of bite marks using the reflex microscope. *J. Forensic Odontostomatol.* **5,** 1.

CHAPTER 8

Withdrawing from invasive neonatal intensive care

Ian A. Laing

The author of this chapter is neither a lawyer nor an ethicist. The following discussion, therefore, touches only lightly on the evolution of neonatal care and on the legal and philosophical debates which have ensued. Too little attention has been paid in recent texts to the practical aspects of what is inaccurately termed 'non-treatment'. Only the practising neonatologist and other members of the team caring for a dying infant can know how demanding is this intensive work.

Neonatal special care units are a luxury limited to an affluent minority of the earth's population. The perinatal mortality is greater than 100 deaths per 1000 deliveries in parts of the Third World; by contrast, it has dropped to nearly 10 per 1000 in wealthy societies, including the UK, this being largely due to improved standards of nutrition and hygiene. About 700 000 infants are born every year in the UK; of these, more than 100 000 need some form of special care, while about 14 000 are offered a high level of neonatal intensive care. The commonest causes of neonatal death among live-born children in the Western World are extreme prematurity, severe congenital malformations and perinatal asphyxia. Neonatal intensive care units (NICUs) may provide life-support for such infants until recovery or inevitable death or, in a small number of instances, during a time when the outcome is uncertain.

8.1 HISTORY AND THE LAW

Intensive care of the sick newborn infant was first practised in the 1960s. Since then, an appreciation of the changes which prepare the fetus for an independent existence after birth has developed. Expanded knowledge of the physiological function of the infant's developing lung, brain and kidney has done much to advance the care of the newborn. The advent of ventilators and intravenous nutrition designed for the newborn child provided means of life-support, and development of these has continued in subsequent decades. Survival of infants weighing less than 600 g at birth is now possible and, occasionally, the child born at 23 weeks gestation (17 weeks premature) may also be managed successfully [1, 2]. Seventy-five per cent of infants weighing 751–1000 g at birth may survive to go home, and almost 90% of children with a birthweight of 1001–1500 g can leave the NICU [2]. A decreasing mortality associated with improvements in intensive care can be shown [3].

Infants with major handicaps which were previously considered to be fatal may also now survive. Unfortunately, some of these children – especially those with chromosomal abnormalities or those who have been profoundly asphyxiated at birth – are both severely mentally retarded and physically impaired. The stresses on society and, in particular on the child's family, have compelled paediatricians to review their policies as to who should receive intensive care, how much, and for how long. Society's attitudes to life-support for newborns have also altered in the past two decades. There was surprisingly little public debate in 1973 when Duff and Campbell reported that 14% of all deaths in the Yale NICU followed decisions to withdraw care [4]. In 1986, Whitelaw announced that 30% of deaths in the Unit in Hammersmith occurred after considered withdrawal of intensive therapy [2]. The public needs to be reassured that decision-making is open, thoughtful, legal and compassionate.

The three categories of illness which cause distress most frequently in the NICU are: (i) severe congenital abnormality; (ii) extreme prematurity; and (iii) perinatal asphyxia. In response to concerns about subjecting neurologically abnormal infants to recurrent surgical procedures, Lorber put forward criteria for the selective surgical treatment of newborns suffering from spina bifida and hydrocephalus [5]. An attempt to offer a practical approach to extreme prematurity prompted Campbell [6] to suggest a 'cut-off' birthweight of 750 g, below which full resuscitative measures would not be offered without first discussing the hazards with the parents. Guidelines for discontinuing resuscitation of severely asphyxiated babies have also been proposed [7]. These important papers have fuelled debate, but solutions are not universally applicable to each child; there

would rarely be agreement if the problems of an individual infant were put to outsiders of varying persuasions. A logical development in the 1980s has been the establishment of Ethics Research Institutes in several countries including the United Kingdom.

Paediatric technology is becoming increasingly sophisticated, and it is therefore not surprising that conflicts have arisen among the interested parties including the infants who will die, those who will survive with handicap, those who will survive intact, the families of all three groups of children and 'the society that seeks to give a chance to each sick child yet increasingly is eager to cut costs' [8]. One major difficulty arises from the lack of certainty as to the eventual outcome for an individual child. A study of predictions made in the first 24 hours of life regarding the survival of infants of birthweight less than 801 g described an error rate of approximately 20% in the opinions of the expert assessors [9]. Ultrasound scanning of a newborn's brain may become increasingly predictive of haemorrhage and brain destruction [10] but it cannot tell the clinician or parent precise details of the child's future handicaps and capabilities. Assessments of outcome are, therefore, based on probabilities and depend upon follow-up studies of graduates from the NICU who have had similar, but seldom identical, problems.

Can the law provide the ideal solution for difficult cases, when withdrawal of invasive support is being contemplated? Many of the problems which have been argued in the courts of law have centred on children with Down's syndrome; some of the decisions in both the United Kingdom and the United States have been of historic importance. In 1981, in London, the parents of a girl who had Down's syndrome associated with duodenal atresia decided against surgery to relieve the intestinal obstruction. The court of appeal, however, ordered that the infant have the operation which was duly carried out against the parents' wishes [11]. By contrast, and in the same year, a consultant paediatrician, who had prescribed repeated doses of di-hydrocodeine to a Down's infant rejected by his parents, was charged with murder at the instigation of an independent pressure group. The child died at the age of 3 days. The doctor was acquitted of both murder and attempted murder but the case continues to emphasize to paediatricians the potential conflict which lies between, on the one hand, the exigencies of the law and, on the other, of what may be perceived by a doctor as being in the best interests of the patient [12].

In the United States, 'Baby Doe' died in 1983, having been born with Down's syndrome complicated by tracheo-oeso-phageal fistula. His parents had withheld consent to surgery. Subsequent to this, a federal directive was issued to the effect that infants should not be discriminated against because of handicap [13] – it is unlawful under the Rehabilitation Act 1973, s.504 'to with-hold from a handicapped child nutritional sustenance or medical or surgical treatment required to correct a life-threatening condition if (1) the withholding is based upon the fact that the infant is handicapped; and (2) the handicap does not render treatment or nutritional sustenance medically contra-indicated'.

Apparently in response to a television programme featuring the film 'Who Should Survive?' (about a Down's syndrome infant who died at Johns Hopkins Hospital having not been fed by order of his parents), the federal administration caused NICUs to post notices reminding staff of the directive pro-hibiting discrimination against the handi-capped by institutions receiving federal funds. The above proposals were attacked by the American Academy of Pediatrics, how-ever, and the Department of Health and Human Services finally conceded in January 1984 that physicians had the right to make 'reasonable medical judgments' [14].

Extremely premature infants can also be the subject of legal controversy. A fatal accident enquiry was convened in Glasgow in 1987 to investigate the action of a paediatrician who was alleged to have withheld resuscitation from a preterm infant on the grounds that the child's birthweight was just below 800 g. The Sheriff found that the doctor was right to come to a decision based on the clinical evidence at the time [15]. Nevertheless, it may be that, today, paediatricians are obliged to resuscitate live-born neonates from as early as 22–24 weeks' gestation unless the individual infant is severely malformed at birth [16].

Retreating from an initial invasive step presents serious problems, whether the infant is malformed, premature or asphyxiated. The care-giving team should develop a sensitive approach which is structured to help the stressed families through these difficult decisions. Whether death is unavoidable or is chosen as the most compassionate outcome by the child's advocates, it is the responsibility of all to provide comfort, dignity and relief of distress to the infant and to his or her relatives. To consider this to be 'non-treatment' is to misunderstand its exacting nature and its potential contribution to the child, family and society.

8.2 BELIEFS

The law may provide boundaries within which the neonatal team should work and the care-givers may strive for what they consider to be the infant's best interests. But the spectrum of beliefs is wide and complex. Two extreme views of clinical care are attractive in their simplicity:

(1) All medical interferences in natural processes such as disease or death are intrusions into a pre-ordained course, and therefore such interferences should not be tolerated.

(2) Medical science has ever-increasing technology, and so all available resources should be directed towards sustaining sacred life, irrespective of the quality of that life in the future.

A great diversity of opinion lies between these two viewpoints.

It is apparent that a universal degree of intensive care is unrealistic and inappropriate if the reactions of individual patients and families are to be heeded. Christopher Nolan, a 22-year-old paralysed since a birth asphyxial episode, writes, 'Each day of my life is a bonus of comfortable blessings. My days of sadnesses are as of nothing compared with my serene days of sobbing fresh pleasure' [17]. By contrast, Robert Stinson reacted to the sufferings of his premature son by writing, 'As often as I wanted to gather him into my arms, I wanted him to be allowed to die' [18]. The intense emotional conflict which may affect the parents of defective children has recently been highlighted in the *Journal of Medical Ethics* [19]. Society may wish to be represented in decisions about the future of a gravely ill newborn child, but questions then arise as to how this representation can best be achieved. The larger the committee of representatives, the less likely it is that a consensus will be obtained; the smaller the team, the more it becomes probable that individual opinion will govern the outcome.

There are also philosophical difficulties involved in discussing critically ill neonates. Not all authors are agreed that a newborn infant is an independent human being with rights equal to those of older members of the human race. One argument is that, in order to be a person one must have awareness of oneself, and this may, therefore, not apply until later childhood. Gillon further points out: '"Viability", arbitrary dates of gestation, and passage through the birth canal and its associated physiological changes are, like

quickening, implausible criteria on which to base fundamental moral distinctions' [20]. The present author believes that the time of departure from the birth canal into the outside world is the first moment of a separate physical existence and, therefore, the first moment when the child's rights are independent of those of other members of the human race. This idea carries with it an important corollary. If it is wrong to withhold intensive care from an adult with a particular malformation or disability, then it may also be wrong to deny the opportunity of the same degree of intensive care to a newborn with a similar defect.

A child with severe mental retardation, limb paralysis, blindness and seizures may be thought to have a miserable existence, but at what degree of handicap is an infant to be considered better off dead? Decision-making becomes still harder when the uncertainty of outcome is acknowledged. Experience and advancing technology increase the accuracy of predicting the degree of handicap [10], but our expertise does not yet allow physicians to know exactly how a child with a neurological deficit would function in years to come. There is nevertheless a responsibility to provide a perspective for the care-giving team and the family, based on all available knowledge. It may, occasionally, be possible to be dogmatic. Referring to severely impaired children with trisomy 18, Smith recommends that, once the diagnosis has been established, there should be 'limitation of all medical means for prolongation of life' [21].

If the decision to withdraw from supporting the infant's life has been taken, is there any difference between an act of commission and one of omission? Is it 'wrong' to take an infant's life by administering a poison, but 'right' to allow the child to die slowly of malnutrition? Gillon states: 'while there may be some social benefits in distinguishing between actively "allowing to die" and painlessly killing such infants, there is, I believe, no other moral difference, and doctors who accept such "allowing to die" of severely handicapped newborn infants should not deceive themselves into believing that there is such a difference' [20]. Campbell replies: 'There may be no moral distinction between "killing" and "allowing to die" but there is a powerful psychological distinction which is important to the staff of intensive care units. To them there is a big difference between not using a respirator to keep an infant of 600 g alive and giving a lethal injection, although the end result is the same' [22].

It is certainly true that, if intensive care is withdrawn, the intention is that the infant should die. Bissenden points out that 'whether this is killing or allowing to die has no moral relevance – what is important is whether the decision is correct' [23]. Deliberately to stop an infant's heart beating with an injection of potassium chloride must nevertheless be unacceptable to us all; on the other hand, the relief from suffering achieved by administering opiates at the time of removal of the ventilator may provide a humane end to a painful existence. The parents also see this distinction.

It is also entirely appropriate that pressure groups should ask penetrating questions and should seek to influence others by developing their beliefs. There is, however, great danger to the child if critics who are ignorant both of a disease's course and prognosis seek to impose an outcome on a particular family, when the result would conflict with the considered view of a circle of experienced, compassionate and well-informed advisers who are fully aware of the facts of an individual case. Furthermore, Mason and Meyers rightly point out that the 'risk of prosecution, small though it may be, does not provide the best backdrop for informed and compassionate care of the defective neonate' [24].

8.3 THE APPROACH OF THE CLINICAL TEAM

In the author's opinion, there is little justification for the claim that one cannot *withdraw* from intensive care once a course of therapy has been started. The decision whether to *embark* on intensive care may first confront the junior resident at the moment of the infant's birth. Many senior paediatricians recommend that almost all live-born infants should be actively supported from labour ward to the NICU. The clear advantages of this approach are that senior staff can become involved, a mature decision can be taken in the light of a surer prognosis, and parents can begin to assimilate the reality of their child's situation. A decision on whether or not to withdraw from an established regimen of intensive care can then be taken. How this may be achieved in practice is the subject of the rest of this chapter.

The two primary responsibilities of a physician throughout an infant's terminal illness are to minimize the suffering of the child during those last minutes and to maximize family support. During the course of chronic, irreversible paediatric illness, there is every opportunity to become intimate with both the child and the family, and to adopt care strategies which are based on the detailed information available. It is unacceptable that a critical decision regarding the life of a newborn infant should be taken unilaterally by a fallible physician. Worse still is the idea that the parents should be presented with the bald facts and then be compelled to decide as to the next step. Their minds may be in a confused turmoil at the time and, whatever decision they take, they will be forced to live with their perceived guilt for decades to come. Outlined below is the process of guided consensus in which emphasis is laid on the practical responsibilities faced by the perinatal team and on the position of the infant's surrogate decision-makers.

When the question of withdrawal of invasive life-support is brought up, the consultant physician should lead the interested parties through an elaborate series of steps, the very complexity of which acts as a safety net for the infant. The child's parents should be involved during each stage. In addition, every aspect of the procedure should be documented in the child's case-notes and signed by the responsible doctors. Whenever the possibility of such a withdrawal is confronted, documentation should begin with why and how the initial question was raised. A summary should then be made which encompasses the child's past history and demonstrates clearly the course of events leading up to the serious problems under discussion. These facts should be presented in the full knowledge of up-to-date medical and scientific advances in the subject. One can describe what is known, what can still be discovered and what is currently un-knowable. Sometimes, the probabilities of brain damage and its anticipated severity contribute to the overall picture. An assessment is made of whether the child is suffering distress at the time. A conference, involving those members of staff who know the infant and parents well, should then meet to discuss all the details, including the family situation. Particular attention is paid to the parents' current knowledge, and their reactions to the severity of their child's illness, including any voiced or implied opinions they may have given about the infant's future. If the conference is unanimous that a course of 'comfort measures only' should be discussed with the child's family, then a small number (preferably not more than three) professionals are chosen to present the facts and options to the parents; two of the discussants will normally be a consultant physician and a senior nurse. This discussion *must* involve both father and mother if both parents are still involved in the child's welfare. The interview requires to be conducted with great sensitivity

and patience, so that a balance may be struck between giving the parents their rightful responsibility to participate in decision-making and, yet, providing recommendations which can help them. Freedom to reject such recommendations is essential and the staff should not be surprised if this occurs initially. For the sake of their future, the family must be confident that the management course was humane and that the experienced perinatal team concurred with the parents and, therefore, shared their moral and legal responsibility.

It is an essential principle that there is adequate time for discussion; this always involves several meetings. The parents may be encouraged to invite further advice from other members of their family, the clergy, the department of social work or from friends in whom they have confidence. The young, single, teenage mother may feel abandoned and will rely heavily on the tact of the care team to help her obtain counsel from her circle of relatives or friends.

If it is possible to consult with a subspecialty adviser then this should be arranged. For example, the child who is deteriorating on a ventilator because of a chronic lung disease may be seen by a paediatrician who has special expertise in respiratory disorders and who is not part of the neonatal team caring for the infant's needs. An independent opinion can be a source of great comfort to family and professionals alike. On the rare occasions when withdrawing or withholding invasive life-support becomes an ethical dilemma, advice may be obtained from many different sources including the British Medical Association or a corresponding body outwith the United Kingdom, medical defence organizations, senior colleagues in other regional institutions or from legal authorities. In the United States, Infant-Care Review Committees (including professional and lay members) have been set up in many hospitals which can arbitrate when parents and medical staff cannot agree [25,26]. If no consensus can be achieved, then it is reasonable to continue with invasive support until new clinical factors, or even the passage of time, alter the equation.

In the unusual circumstances of a continued, unresolved clinico/ethical dilemma, it may be necessary to seek the assistance of the courts of law. The most appropriate way to do this in England and Wales would be through an application for wardship; such a route was followed in the leading case of *Re B (a Minor)* [11]. The same result might be achieved in Scotland by referring the case to the Reporter to the Children's Panel (see Chapter 29a).

The above complex system of achieving a decision coincides with the best interests of the child and provides an environment in which outside interests are of secondary importance but are, nonetheless, necessary safeguards. It is possible that this intricate but overt structure might be strong enough to make court actions, such as that against Dr Leonard Arthur, less likely to occur.

8.4 DEATH

If death is inevitable or is regarded as being in the best interests of the child, the parents will be shown by words and actions that the chosen course is not one of 'selective non-treatment' [13] but, rather, a redirection of intensive care towards comfort measures. During preparation for death, the child can be offered warmth, freedom from pain and social comfort. Visits from relatives are to be encouraged, particularly from parents, grandparents and siblings. Small children are generally not frightened by the experience and can serve to enhance the feeling of a complete family supporting a dying member. Photographs are taken and the parents are encouraged to cuddle the infant even while he or she is still being ventilated. Clothes bought by the family can be used to emphasize the child's individuality. A religious service at this time is often a source of solace to both family and staff.

The senior physician will gradually become aware when the time for discontinuation of respirator therapy is at hand. Opiate relief for potential discomfort is given, the ventilator, monitors and all other impersonal equipment are removed, and the baby is placed in his or her parents' arms for what may be only minutes of remaining life. A small number of familiar staff should stay with the parents throughout this period, except at times when they feel the family wish to be alone; staff responsibilities to other patients should be taken on by colleagues during these critical hours. A warm, private room can be dedicated to this family for the time of bereavement, so that the infant's last minutes are spent away from the intrusive alarms of an intensive care unit. After death has been pronounced, the family should be encouraged to cradle their child for as long as they wish – this may be for several further hours. They often wish to groom the baby and may ask to have a lock of hair and the identification anklets as keepsakes. The staff may accompany the family to the local chapel on the following day to spend further moments in grieving.

8.5 AFTER DEATH

The bereaved family will usually require guidance through the administrative details and other anxieties which ensue, including procedures involving the provision of a birth certificate and a death certificate, the choice of burial or cremation, how to ensure that the infant wears the clothes of their choice at the funeral service, what to tell friends, and how and when their lives may become normal again. How soon will the weeping stop? How soon will regular sleeping return? How soon will appetites (including sexual) become normal? The commitment of the professional team must extend to these and many more aspects. Community support can begin only if the general practitioner, social worker and health visitor are kept in touch with the events in the NICU. The obstetrician looking after the mother must also know of the child's death so that the relationship can continue on a sensitive footing. The parents can be put in touch with self-help organizations such as (in the United Kingdom) 'Compassionate Friends' or the 'Stillbirth and Neonatal Death Society'. The family will realize that contact with the staff does not cease with the death of the child.

Two further aspects of after-care must be detailed. Usually within 24 hours of the infant's death, the senior paediatrician ought to interview both parents to request an autopsy examination. At first this may seem to be the final cruelty after the series of disasters which have befallen a child and its parents. However, there is one overriding factor which must be explained – without a post-mortem examination it is possible that information crucial to the parents may be lost and genetic advice regarding future pregnancies of the mother, and of members of her family, will be incomplete. There may be one surprising bonus for the couple who elect to have an autopsy performed on the remains of their baby. Weeks later, they often express relief and gladness to have the opportunity of seeing and possessing a copy of the report, which describes their infant's structure in detail. Staff who are experienced in follow-up interviews are in little doubt that this description contributes positively to the grieving process and allows parents to leave many doubts, and perhaps some guilt, behind. One follow-up interview should be dedicated to exploring in detail the genetic implications of the infant's death with reference to clinical and autopsy diagnoses. Further expert advice may be needed from a specialist in genetics.

The second aspect of after-care which needs further comment is the follow-up series of meetings. These may appropriately take place in an office outside the intensive care unit and away from the crying of babies. Ideally the nurse and doctor closest to the family should arrange for this. The meetings are often most successful when they are freely structured and offer the parents a chance to talk about their child. The conversation may range from medical details of therapy to humorous anecdotes of the infant's life. Friends and neighbours of the parents did not meet their baby and therefore find it difficult to be sources of strength through the early months of grief; it is understandable that both mother and father should wish to talk at length to the few people who remembered the nuances of their child's personality. A bereaved mother wrote: 'Most people did not know how to respond to us. They did not know what to say, but usually once we began to talk they would follow our lead. However, some people deliberately avoided the whole subject as if we hadn't had a baby, yet we knew they knew. It was both hurtful to us and hard since it was the subject uppermost in our minds and we both found relief in talking about it.' [27] The parents should be left in no doubt that the clinical team will maintain an interest in the family's future and that, if a further pregnancy occurs, the next child will be awaited with considerable excitement.

8.6 COST

Can even affluent Western societies afford to invest large sums to care for critically ill infants who may subsequently die despite the best efforts of the perinatal team? The cost of setting up equipment for an intensively cared-for baby, including the purchase of an incubator, ventilator, monitors and feeding pumps is £25 000–£30 000 [28]. Daily costings in 1984 on Merseyside were £297 for intensive care, £138 for special care and £71 for nursery care [29]. The same group showed that, when the costs of the total care of an infant born weighing less than 1500 g were calculated, survivors cost £4490 while non-survivors cost £3446. Another study has put the costs of non-survivors closer to £1000 [30]. Sandhu [29] observed that cost differences between survivors and non-survivors are very variable and may be due to 'differences in the duration of effort put into the management of an extremely sick infant with a poor prognosis. Such efforts are determined by professional and parental attitudes, which may vary between centres.' It has also been pointed out that there is relatively low viability and high cost when intensive care is offered to infants weighing less than 1000 g at birth [31]. Boyle [32] even went so far as to take expected future earnings into consideration and concluded that, if resources are scarce, money is best concentrated on infants of 1000–1499 g rather than on a group of lower birthweight.

It is not the intention here to prolong the debate on how much money should be devoted to intensive care and to which groups this care should be devoted. Clearly there must be some limit. Already in the United Kingdom such care is sometimes denied to infants, with fatal consequences, because of shortages of nurses or equipment [33]. Most infants who die in an intensive care unit do so in the first week of life. The cost to society of a child who undergoes a short course of critical care before death is not large. The value to the family of a few days spent with their dying infant is not measurable in any currency.

8.7 SUMMARY

To lay observers the discontinuation of life-support for a baby may seem callous 'selective non-treatment'. To the professional staff caring for the infant it is a task which is extremely demanding in time and in intellectual and emotional energy. All aspects of the infant's life must be considered before the most compassionate decision about its future can be taken. The autonomy of the parents as surrogate decision-makers must be respected, but they will require confident guidance and reassurance from the staff they have come to trust. The infant's dignity as a complete human being is of paramount importance at all times and it is the responsibility of the staff to provide this human being with freedom from distress and also with physical and social comfort.

Society will continue to debate the principle of the sanctity of human life and of the rights of human beings or their advocates to determine their future. Cognizant of these arguments, and remaining within the law, the neonatal physician and the small team of perinatal staff cannot avoid their moral and legal responsibility to provide the best care for their patient, including, if necessary, the withdrawal of invasive life-support. Redirection of care to comfort measures is, however, appropriate only after detailed exploration of the alternatives and after a guided consensus has been reached openly with the child's family. There should be no conflict with the law when these principles are followed.

REFERENCES

1. Yu, V.Y.H., Loke, H.L., Bajuk, B. *et al.* (1986) Prognosis for infants born at 23 to 28 weeks' gestation. *Br. Med. J.*, **293**, 1200.
2. Whitelaw, A. (1986) Death as an option in neonatal intensive care. *Lancet*, **ii**, 328.
3. Stewart, A.L., Reynolds, E.O.R. and Lipscombe, A.P. (1981) Outcome for infants of very low birthweight: survey of world literature. *Lancet*, **i**, 1038.
4. Duff, R.S. and Campbell, A.G.M. (1973) Moral and ethical dilemmas in the special care nursery. *New Engl. J. Med.*, **289**, 890.
5. Lorber, J. (1972) Spina bifida cystica. Results of treatment of 270 consecutive cases with criteria for selection for the future. *Arch. Dis. Child.*, **47**, 854.
6. Campbell, A.G.M. (1982) Which infants should not receive intensive care? *Arch. Dis. Child.*, **57**, 569.

7. Steiner, H. and Neligan, G. (1975) Perinatal cardiac arrest. Quality of survivors. *Arch. Dis. Child.*, **50**, 696.

8. Siegel, L.S. (1982) Low birth weight infants. *Semin. Perinatol.*, **6**, 265.

9. Zarfin, J., Aerde, J.V., Perlman, M. *et al.* (1986) Predicting survival of infants less than 801 grams. *Crit. Care Med.*, **14**, 768.

10. De Vries, L.S., Dubowitz, L.M.S., Dubowitz, V. *et al.* (1985) Predictive value of cranial ultrasound in the newborn baby: a reappraisal. *Lancet*, **ii**, 137.

11. *Re B (a Minor)* [1981] 1 WLR 1421.

12. Editorial Comment (1981) Paediatricians and the law. *Br. Med. J.*, **283**, 1280; Editorial Comment (1981) After the trial at Leicester. *Lancet*, **ii**, 1085; Brahams, D. and Brahams, M. (1983) The Arthur case – a proposal for legislation. *J. Med. Ethics*, **9**, 12.

13. Weir, R. (1985) *Selective Non-Treatment of Handicapped Newborns*, Oxford University Press, New York, pp. 131–4.

14. Gostin, L. (1985) A moment in human development: legal protection, ethical standards and social policy in the selective non-treatment of handicapped neonates. *Am. J. Law Med.*, **11**, 31.

15. Brahams, D. (1988) No obligation to resuscitate a non-viable infant. *Lancet*, **i**, 1176.

16. Walker, C.H.M. (1988) ... officiously to keep alive. *Arch. Dis. Child.*, **63**, 560.

17. Nolan, C. (1987) *Under the Eye of the Clock*, Weidenfeld and Nicholson, Letchworth.

18. Stinson, R. and Stinson, P. (1983) *The Long Dying of Baby Andrew*, Little Brown & Co, Boston.

19. Simms, M. (1986) Informed dissent: the views of some mothers of severely mentally handicapped young adults. *J. Med. Ethics*, **12**, 72.

20. Gillon, R. (1986) Conclusion: the Arthur case revisited. *Br. Med. J.*, **292**, 543.

21. Smith, D.W. (1982) *Recognizable Patterns of Human Malformation. Genetic, Embryologic and Clinical Aspects*, 3rd edn, W.B. Saunders, Philadelphia, pp. 14–15.

22. Campbell, A.G.M. (1988) Ethical issues in child health and disease, in *Child Health in a Changing Society* (ed. J.O. Forfar), Oxford University Press, Oxford.

23. Bissenden, G. (1986) Ethical aspects of neonatal care. *Arch. Dis. Child.*, **61**, 639.

24. Mason, J.K. and Meyers, D.W. (1986) Parental choice and selective non-treatment of deformed newborns: a view from mid-Atlantic. *J. Med. Ethics*, **12**, 67.

25. Gillespie, C. (1983) Letting die severely handicapped children. *J. Med. Ethics*, **9**, 231.

26. Berseth, C.L. (1987) Ethical dilemmas in the neonatal intensive care unit. *Mayo Clin. Proc.*, **62**, 67.

27. Boston, S. (1981) *Will My Son. The Life and Death of a Mongol Child*, Pluto Press, London.

28. Robertson, N.R.C. (1988) *Action for the Newborn*, Action for the Newborn, London.

29. Sandhu, B., Stevenson, R.C., Cooke, R.W.I. and Pharoah, P.O.D. (1986) Cost of neonatal intensive care for very-low-birthweight infants. *Lancet*, **i**, 600.

30. Newns, B., Drummond, F., Durbin, G.M. and Culley, P. (1984) Costs and outcomes in a regional neonatal intensive care unit. *Arch. Dis. Child.*, **59**, 1064.

31. Walker, J.B., Feldman, A., Vohr, B.R. and Oh, W. (1984) Cost-benefit analysis of neonatal intensive care for infants weighing less than 1000 g at birth. *Pediatrics*, **74**, 20.

32. Boyle, M.H., Torrance, G.W., Sinclair, J.C. and Horwood, S.P. (1983) Economic evaluation of neonatal intensive case of very low birth-weight infants. *New Engl. J. Med.*, **308**, 1330.

33. Sims, D.G., Wynn, J. and Chiswick, M.L. (1982) Outcome for newborn babies declined admission to a regional neonatal intensive care unit. *Arch. Dis. Child.*, **57**, 334.

CHAPTER 9

The epidemiology and sociology of the sudden infant death syndrome

Jean Golding

As infant mortality has dropped over the decades, attention has become focused on one cause of death for which little change appears to have taken place – the sudden infant death syndrome (SIDS). The diagnosis is derived by exclusion. It was defined by Beckwith [1] as, 'the sudden death of any infant or young child which is unexpected by history and in whom a thorough necropsy examination fails to demonstrate an adequate cause of death'. It is said that there are currently 1500 such deaths in the UK each year and about 8000 in the USA [2].

A newly created statistic YPLL (years of potential life lost before age 65) has highlighted the impact of SIDS on the community. Using the statistic, SIDS becomes the seventh most important cause of death in the USA; deaths in 1985 alone accounted for 313 386 years of potential life lost [3]. Thus, although using few health resources other than pathological services, the condition has wide-reaching implications for the community.

9.1 EPIDEMIOLOGICAL METHODS

The field of SIDS research is expanding rapidly; studies and theories are often being propounded by chemists, biochemists, physicists, physiologists, teratologists, geneticists and the lay-public. Hypotheses, however, need valid bases on which to build. In many instances in the past, they have been produced on the basis of one or two case reports or on poor uncontrolled studies or, even, on no evidence at all.

Balanced epidemiological studies can be used to put case reports into perspective. For example, a dramatic newspaper report of a pair of twins found dead 3 hours after a DTP injection tends to produce an immediate assumption of cause and effect. However, such injections are most likely to be given at the age when SIDS normally occurs. Population studies can be used to determine how often such a sequence could be expected by chance, and this can then be compared with the numbers that actually occur. The observed numbers are then found to be similar to those expected by chance [4–6] and one can conclude that immunization is not likely to be a cause of sudden infant death.

An epidemiological study, in order to be reliable, has to have the following data: (i) accurate information concerning which persons do or do not have the disorder; (ii) similar information on the social, biological and environmental backgrounds of those with and without the disorder; and (iii) if samples of cases with and without the disorder are chosen, there should be no difference in bias between their selection.

Where the condition is relatively rare, as in sudden infant death, it is often impossible to obtain the type of information which one wishes to analyse without bias creeping in. For example, if one wants an assessment by the local health visitor of the mothering ability or social problems of parents whose child has just died, one is likely to get a different response from that given when she is asked about parents of a child who is alive and well. Even though she may intend to view the two objectively, she is bound to be influenced by knowledge of the particular death. As we shall discuss later, it is unusual to get prospectively recorded information concerning such features, yet there is a body of opinion which considers that mothering ability and social factors may be very important in the aetiology of the syndrome.

9.2 INCIDENCE

Unfortunately, it is very difficult to obtain reliable incidence figures for SIDS. The term 'SIDS' has only been allowed to be written on British death certificates since 1971 and, since then, its use has become common. Nevertheless, there is still a number of pathologists who prefer to record conditions that are either not present at all, in the probably mistaken belief that parents would prefer something tangible rather than the intangible, or that may well have been part of an agonal event (e.g. aspiration of vomit) or minor changes which were unlikely to have caused the death (e.g. bronchiolitis) or even terms that can be totally misleading (e.g. asphyxia) [7].

Thus, in order to obtain reliable estimates of incidence, one has to consider all infant deaths in a defined population and to go

through the available clinical and post-mortem evidence case by case to determine which could possibly be considered as cases of SIDS using the Beckwith classification. In populations where autopsies are rare – and where there is no statutory *obligation* to carry out a post-mortem in an infant who has died suddenly – accurate incidence figures are impossible to obtain unless specific studies are undertaken.

Nevertheless, there has been a number of studies published which have been sufficiently carefully carried out to ensure reasonably reliable incidence figures. These show a remarkable picture. The reported incidences (per 1000 live births) from various areas in the British Isles are as follows: Northern Ireland 2.5 [8]; Edinburgh 2.1 [9]; Hartlepool 3.0 [10]; Scunthorpe 2.5 [11]; Grimsby and Cleethorpes 4.0 [12]; Newcastle upon Tyne 3.8 [12]; Oxfordshire and West Berkshire 2.8 for the years 1966 to 1970 [13] and 2.6 for the years 1971 to 1975 [2]; Gosport 7.8 [14]. Thus the incidence appears to be well over 2 per 1000 for all centres in the British Isles.

In North America the range has been less wide, with the following incidence patterns: King County, Seattle 2.3 [15]; Nebraska 2.5 [16]; Philadelphia 2.5 [17]; Chicago 3.4 [18]; Charleston, South Carolina 2.9 [19]; Cleveland 3.1 [20]; North Carolina 2.1 [21]; California 2.3 [22], 2.7 [23], 1.8 [24]; Oklahoma 2.0 [25]; Ontario 3.0 [26]. Thus for the British Isles the incidence appears to be between 2.5 and 3.0 whereas in North America it is perhaps slightly less.

Substantial variation has been found in the Antipodes, with rates of 2.9 in Tasmania [27], 2.2 in Western Australia [28], 2.1 in South Australia [29], while the most recent figures from New Zealand give an incidence of 4.9 for the whole country [30].

Within the rest of Europe the incidence varies markedly. A study from France found an incidence of 2.7 [31], one from Norway of

1.3 [32], one from Copenhagen of 0.9 [33], from Sweden of 0.5 [34] and from Finland of 0.5 [35]. Reported rates in West Germany have varied from 5.2 in Trier [36], to 1.9 in Stuttgart [37] and 1.6 in Hamburg [38].

Few studies have been mounted elsewhere in the world. Nevertheless, what information there is is interesting. For example, in an urban area of Southern Brazil [39], where there was a generally high infant mortality rate, the incidence of SIDS was only 1.5. In Israel, two studies of births to Jewish families have reported incidences of between 0.3 [40] and 0.7 [41] per 1000. An incidence of only 0.04 was reported in Hong Kong [42] but the study criteria were not appropriate. Nevertheless, since the total postneonatal mortality rate was only 3.1, the incidence of SIDS must, perforce, be relatively low in Hong Kong.

Thus, world-wide variation in incidence is large. Some of this variation may well be due to differential post-mortem rates and the assiduity with which the definition was applied but, nevertheless, one can conclude that the rates in the Scandinavian countries, especially in Sweden and Finland, differ substantially from those of the British Isles. For example, the total postneonatal mortality in Sweden was only 2.1 per 1000; one would have to assume that all these infants were dying of SIDS in order for the rate to approach even remotely that found in the British Isles. This would clearly be a nonsense – the postneonatal deaths in Sweden are, as expected, weighted with congenital malformations and with those infants with perinatal problems who survived the neonatal period [34].

(a) Ethnic group

Consistent differences have been reported between the incidences in black and white infants within the USA – the incidence among blacks being greater than that among whites. Thus, the contrasts were between rates of 1.9 among white and 3.0 among non-white in the longitudinal US Collaborative Study [43], 1.2 and 3.9 in Upper New York State [44], 1.2 and 3.8 in North Carolina [21], 1.9 and 5.9 in Nebraska [16] and 1.3 and 5.1 in Cook County, Illinois [45]. An interesting study from Oklahoma has shown recently that the American Indians resident in that state have an incidence rate that is intermediate between the two groups [25], even though their demographic and social conditions are close to those of the black population. In Illinois [45], the Hispanic population have an identical rate to the whites despite the fact that their socioeconomic status is much lower.

It has not been shown that West Indian or Asian immigrants in Britain have particularly high incidences when compared with that expected from their other characteristics; it has, however, been demonstrated that any immigrant group – whether from the West Indies, Australia or even Northern Ireland – has a higher rate than the indigenous population [46].

(b) Sex

All studies, whether they be in low-incidence areas such as Sweden [34] or in high-incidence subgroups such as the black population of the USA, show a similar sex ratio of 14 boys to every 10 girls [2].

(c) Age at death

There is a typical age pattern wherever the deaths arise [2], the peak incidence occurring at around 12–13 weeks of age and then tailing off (Fig. 9.1). Although the risk of SIDS decreases rapidly after 5 months of age, an occasional case occurs up to the age of 5 years [47].

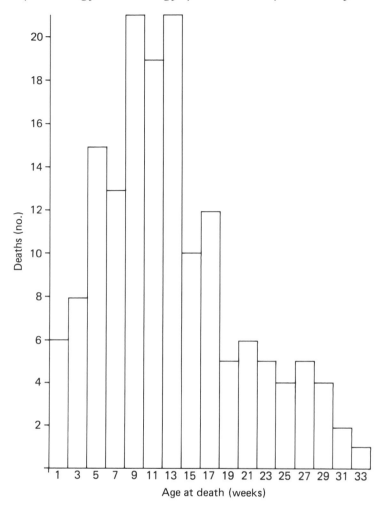

Fig. 9.1 Age at death (adapted from [13]).

(d) Month of death and month of birth

Although it is well known that sudden infant deaths occur at a much greater rate during the winter months (Table 9.1), it is less well appreciated that infants born at certain times of the year have a much decreased later risk of SIDS. Thus, although there is a marked increase of deaths in the winter months as compared with the summer in all areas in both the northern and southern hemispheres, infants born in the northern hemisphere in April or May have a much reduced risk of subsequent sudden infant death. Whether this is because the child born at that time is less likely to go through the winter during its vulnerable period of life, or whether there is an inherent advantage in being born in these 2 months, has yet to be assessed. It is, however, interesting that in Sweden, where the winter excess was only moderate (Table 9.1), there

Table 9.1 Examples of seasonal variation of deaths from SIDS

Place	Deaths (no.)			
	Winter	*Spring*	*Summer*	*Autumn*
UK				
Oxfordshire and West Berkshire [2]	129	77	57	111
North America				
Ontario, Canada [26]	152	79	72	130
San Diego, California [24]	56	47	33	65
Europe				
Sweden [34]	397	390	333	383
Antipodes				
Tasmania [27]	63	43	35	57

were still significantly fewer births of infants developing SIDS in April and May [34].

The relationship between the month of death and the weather pertaining at the time has been investigated by a number of people. Although, on the whole, the months in which the death is most likely to occur are those in which the temperature is lowest [2], there have been conflicting reports of a relationship between fall in temperature in the days prior to death once account has been taken of the ambient temperature of that particular month [2, 48]. Nevertheless, the suspicion that hypothermia may be a possible candidate for increasing the risk of SIDS is still viable. Only 37 of the 334 SIDS cases in the Swedish study [34] died while out of doors, but 31 (84%) of these deaths occurred in the winter as compared with 56% of all SIDS deaths. In 10 of the 31 winter deaths, the ambient temperature was between −6 °C and −14 °C. Thus, there was a highly significant relationship between season and dying out of doors.

The converse of the hypothermia relationship is that of hyperthermia. In this hypothesis, it is the infant who is overheated – possibly as a consequence of trying to keep the infant warm by either putting him near a radiator or fire or by putting too many clothes on – who is at risk [49]. Analyses by temperature of the day have failed to reveal an increased incidence on days when there is a heat wave or other objective criteria which might support such a hypothesis [2].

9.3 MATERNAL FACTORS

(a) Mother's age

It can be seen from Fig. 9.2 that the incidence of SIDS varies markedly with maternal age. This phenomenon is found in Europe [2,34], North America [2], Chile [50] and in every centre that has looked. It is found universally that infants of teenage mothers have the highest rate; mothers in the age-range 20–24 years have a somewhat lower rate but, thereafter, the incidence plateaus.

Peterson and his colleagues in the United States showed that the strong maternal age relationship was identical whatever maternal birth cohort was taken [51]. In addition, the trend was the same with each parity. The authors suggested that this is a fundamental clue to the aetiology of SIDS. The pattern is different from that associated with other

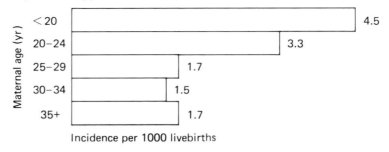

Fig. 9.2 Incidence of SIDS by maternal age (adapted from [2]).

causes of infant death and they suggested that nutrition in pregnancy may be of crucial importance.

(b) Parity and past obstetric history

The association with maternal youth might lead to the expectation that these are women who have had few previous pregnancies; yet, almost whatever population data one examine [2, 34], there is an increasing incidence of SIDS with rising parity – and this relationship obtains within each maternal age-group (Fig. 9.3).

Studies looking at the past obstetric history of these women have shown that they are less likely than expected to have had a previous miscarriage, stillbirth or neonatal death, and that the interval between the index pregnancy and the preceding delivery tended to be shorter than expected even after controlling for maternal age, parity and social factors [2].

It is possible that the relationship of SIDS with the maternal youth, high parity and short interpregnancy interval criteria indicates a biological problem – perhaps one of an immature or overworked system which cannot supply adequately the nutrients that the fetus needs.

9.4 SOCIOECONOMIC FACTORS

In Britain, we are well used to using an estimate of social class which is based on the occupation of the father of the baby. This classification groups those in the higher professions, e.g. doctors, solicitors, chartered accountants, university teachers, as social class I, those in the other professions, e.g. school teachers, nurses, managers, company directors, as social class II, and the other non-

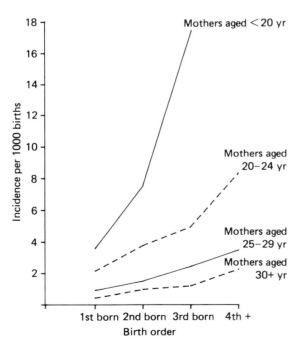

Fig. 9.3 Incidence of SIDS by parity within maternal age-groups (adapted from [2]).

manual occupations, such as clerks and secretaries, policemen and salesmen, as social class IIINM. These three groups together comprise the non-manual classes. The manual classes are divided into three. Social class IIIM are the skilled craftsmen, i.e. those that would have required training in order to be able to ply their trade or craft; these include carpenters, plumbers, car mechanics and lorry drivers. Social class IV are the semi-skilled manual workers and would include machine minders, caretakers and postmen. Social class V involve the unskilled labourers and mostly consists of labourers and cleaners. It should be noted that the classification is based on the occupation of the father. Women who are living on their own are classified to a remainder group. Those in the armed forces are usually unclassified.

It is possible to show that there are strong trends associating mortality with social class whether one looks at perinatal mortality, infant mortality or adult mortality (Fig. 9.4). In general, the trend is such that social class I has the lowest rate and social class V the highest. SIDS is no exception in that social class I tends to have the lowest rate and social class V the highest, but there is not a linear trend from I to V. As shown in Fig. 9.4, social classes I, II

and III tend to have very similar rates and an excess mortality for SIDS is found only in social classes IV and V; this relationship appears to be independent of maternal age and parity [2]. Social class classification is, however, only a marker of possible adverse associations. It has been shown that many different things vary with social class, including attitudes towards health care, diet, smoking habit, consumption of alcohol, housing circumstances, child care and exposure to pollutants [2]. No one has yet disentangled the various specific factors that might be influencing the incidence of SIDS.

There is also some evidence of socio-economic variation in incidence outside Britain. In California, a prospective study of data from the Kaiser Health Plan [22] showed that the incidence was higher in families of blue collar as opposed to white collar workers. In Cleveland, Ohio [20], the incidence in areas with low mean income was twice that found for census tracts with high mean income. In Denmark [52], the incidence among those paid a weekly wage was higher than among those paid a monthly salary. However, most studies have found no association between the incidence of SIDS and the educational level of the parents [2].

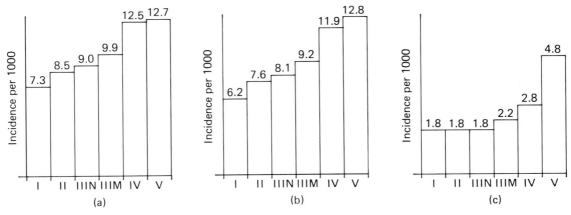

Fig. 9.4 Social class variation in mortality rates. (a) Perinatal mortality 1983. (b) Infant mortality 1983. (c) SIDS [2].

(a) Unemployment

There is no evidence available as yet from which to assess whether infants whose fathers are unemployed are at higher risk. It must be remembered that, at least in Britain, men in social classes IV and V are most likely to become unemployed at any time. It is, therefore, important to distinguish any unemployment effect from a social class effect. So far this has not been attempted.

(b) Marital status

Studies from California, Upper New York State, Northern Ireland, Canada, Copenhagen, Sweden and Britain have all shown an excess incidence of SIDS when the mother was unmarried (Table 9.2). This relationship

Table 9.2 Risk of SIDS among infants born to unmarried mothers relative to the risk of infants born to married mothers

Area	Relative risk	Overall proportion of unmarried mothers in the population (%)
UK		
Oxfordshire and West Berkshire [2]	2.5[a]	6
Southern England [53]	2.5[b]	8
Great Britain, 1970 [54]	2.2[a]	5
Rest of Europe		
Denmark [52]	3.4[a]	7
Sweden [34]	1.4[a]	33
Northern America		
Upper New York State [44]	2.2[a]	Not known
California [55]	1.9[a]	Not known

a, Risk based on incidence figures; b, risk based on case-control comparison.

has stayed constant even when controlled for factors such as maternal age.

It has been argued that, in the era of common law marriages, with no formal ceremony taking place, the incidence of SIDS among the unmarried should be the same as that among the married population. Evidence of cohabitation has not been collected in many studies but, in Sweden [34], where extra-marital deliveries are common (a third of all births), almost all of the unmarried mothers of the cases of SIDS were cohabiting with the father of the child. Nevertheless, this group had a 50% increase in risk. The authors of this study noted that the excess risk was mainly among the teenage mothers. It would seem possible, therefore, that the risks consequent upon being born to an unmarried mother are lower where the condition is common.

(c) Smoking in pregnancy

The maternal smoking habit is one of the factors that varies markedly with social class in the United Kingdom; women in the lowest social class are more likely to smoke, and to smoke heavily, than are those in the upper social classes. Various authors have now examined the risk to infants born to mothers who smoke compared with the risk to mothers who do not after allowing for maternal age, parity and social class. Invariably the same results are obtained – the infant of the mother who smokes has a markedly increased risk of SIDS compared with the risk to one of the mother who does not. This has been found in Britain, Canada and the United States (Fig. 9.5).

Very little information has been collected on postnatal smoking, although this is obviously a candidate in the aetiology of SIDS. It is well established that infants whose parents smoke have a higher risk of bronchitis in infancy and childhood. Information on parental smoking collected retrospectively after the infant has died is certainly very biased. What evidence there is suggests that smoking in pregnancy

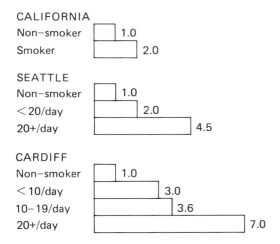

CALIFORNIA
Non–smoker 1.0
Smoker 2.0

SEATTLE
Non–smoker 1.0
<20/day 2.0
20+/day 4.5

CARDIFF
Non–smoker 1.0
<10/day 3.0
10–19/day 3.6
20+/day 7.0

Fig. 9.5 Risk of SIDS in infants of smoking mothers relative to non-smokers. (a) California [22]. (b) Seattle [58]. (c) Cardiff [59].

may be at least as important as postnatal smoking. This may well tie in with other published evidence on smoking in pregnancy. Recently, Taylor and Wadsworth [56] have shown that smoking in pregnancy is at least as important as is postnatal smoking in the genesis of infant bronchitis. In addition, smoking in pregnancy, rather than postnatal smoking, has been shown to be strongly associated with central apnoea in the infant [57].

(d) Other ingestions during pregnancy

No comprehensive study on the effect of diet during pregnancy has ever been carried out. There has been one which assessed the tea, coffee and cola consumption of mothers and controls and found no association, thus implying that caffeine in pregnancy was not associated with the condition [58]. Drug addiction, however, has been noted to be a strong association (see Chapter 3). Prospective studies of addicted women have shown the incidence of SIDS to be about 20 per 1000 among this group. Nevertheless, all

published studies to date have been concerned with the North American rather than the British or European scene. No study has been done on alcoholic women and their infants but one in California demonstrated no relationship between SIDS and mild to moderate alcohol consumption by the mother [22] (see also Chapter 3). Other studies have related to prescribed drug ingestions during pregnancy; two showed a consistent relationship with barbiturate-containing prescriptions [2].

(e) Housing

In view of the other social factors which are associated with SIDS, it is hardly surprising that there should be reports of an increased incidence where there is disadvantaged housing. Nevertheless, to date, none of the studies have controlled for those other factors that have been discussed above as being important in the aetiology of this syndrome. There were higher incidences in areas with houses of poor quality in both Copenhagen [52] and Cardiff [59], but no investigator has looked at whether the homes of the infants who died were actually of poorer quality than were other homes in the area.

There is no evidence that overcrowding is associated with SIDS [2]. The only other study to look at facets of housing was that by Eckert [38]. Taking information from West Germany and from Pennsylvania, he found that infants living in basement or ground floor areas had a higher incidence of SIDS than did those who lived at higher levels. He related this finding to electromagnetic fields, stating that the increased SIDS rate in the low-lying housing was due to increased magnetic fields and 'stray electric currents'. The validity of this argument has not been tested but electromagnetic fields induced by the electricity supply are of minimal strength in countries, such as Britain, where AC current is used.

One housing factor which may be of more relevance concerns the heating system. This has not been assessed in relation to SIDS in Britain. In Canada, however, where central heating is available universally, the crucial factor may be the temperature at which the thermostat is set. One study has shown that the homes of SIDS infants were more likely to have a high setting (70$^+$ °F). It was also shown that these children were far less likely to have the windows open at night in their bedrooms [60]. No other study has considered such information.

(f) Health behaviour

One of the most striking features of the pregnancies which subsequently resulted in a sudden infant death concerned the question of whether or not the mother knew the date of her last menstrual period. Mothers who confessed that they were not sure of such dates had a far higher subsequent incidence of SIDS than did mothers who were sure when it was [2]. Not surprisingly, in association with the finding of very short interpregnancy intervals, mothers of SIDS were also much less likely to have used the contraceptive pill in the period prior to conception.

A number of studies have attempted to determine whether mothers of SIDS were less likely to book early for antenatal care, or to have made fewer visits for antenatal care than expected. In four of these, such mothers were found to be more likely to book late and, in two, they had made fewer antenatal visits [2]. Interpretation of such visits is very difficult; delay in booking for antenatal care is associated with various risk factors that we have shown to be associated with SIDS – unmarried status, high parity, short interpregnancy interval, youthful mothers. No study has yet looked at antenatal care in order to assess whether socioeconomic status and gestation at delivery, as well as maternal age and parity, totally explain the associations found with late booking.

Several authors have also collected information on attendance by the mothers at 'well-baby' clinics. SIDS cases are less likely to have been immunized and mothers are more likely to have failed to keep appointments with health visitors [52]. These mothers were also less likely to keep their appointments for postnatal follow-up. Nevertheless, such findings have not taken account of whether the mother had defaulted because the infant was ill or for other reasons.

One of the most important facets of health behaviour concerns whether or not the mother attempts to breast-feed and whether she continues to breast-feed. Some years ago it was common to assume that breast-feeding protected against SIDS, this being on the basis that pathologists never came across deaths of infants who were wholly breast-fed. This was occurring at a time when breast-feeding was comparatively rare. In Northern Ireland, for example, only 27 of 162 mothers of SIDS (17%) had even attempted to breast-feed their babies, but this must be compared with the data for the matched controls (18%) [8]. Similar findings of a lack of association between breast-feeding and later SIDS have been reported from Britain, America and Canada [2]. Other studies, however, such as that in Copenhagen, have found that there were fewer deaths when the mothers were breast-feeding [33]. Nevertheless, the analysis did not fully take into account the social factors pertaining to the cases of SIDS. In Britain, for example, the breast-feeding rate was far higher in the upper than in the lower social classes (59% in social class I, 24% in social class V in 1970). There was also a much reduced chance of an attempt to breast-feed among mothers who were smoking; 41% of non-smokers attempted to breast-feed whereas only 23% of mothers who smoked 20 cigarettes or more per day did so. Thus, in analysing data on breast-feeding, it is essential to take both maternal smoking and social class into account. Where this has been attempted, it has been found that breast-feeding appears to have no protective effect against SIDS [2].

(g) Mothering

There have been several retrospective case-control studies where the quality of mothering was assessed by visiting health workers or by the mother's own health visitor. Each time, it was found that the mothers of cases of SIDS had poorer mothering qualities than did the mothers of controls [52,53]. It is not possible to proceed further with these results. Not only were they based on retrospective assessment after the death had occurred but, also, little account was taken of the social and other factors which are known to be important in the aetiology of SIDS. Thus, the question of whether mothering care has an independent association with SIDS must await a well-designed study with prospectively collected data.

9.5 THE CHILD

Infants destined to become cases of SIDS are not only more likely to be male, they are more likely to be slightly growth retarded and/or born at lower gestation. These two effects appear to be separate and are probably independent of other social factors – including a history of smoking during pregnancy.

Much research effort has been devoted to trying to assess whether particular signs and symptoms in the infant are predictive of SIDS. These studies have again been biased, details of symptoms being obtained from parents after the death had occurred. Fashion has swung from predicting that 'snuffles' in the infant were a strong predictor of SIDS, through apnoeic attacks in the neonatal period, to periods of sweating. There is no good prospective concrete evidence to

support any of these. Nevertheless, the children who do die of this syndrome are more likely to show objective indicators of illness during their life; not only are they more likely to have been kept in a special care baby unit after delivery but they are also more likely to have had subsequent hospital admissions. In addition, these children had more minor congenital malformations of various types, although, by definition, these abnormalities were not sufficiently major to be the cause of the child's death [2, 33].

9.6 OTHER EPIDEMIOLOGICAL CLUES

In spite of the fact that mothers of cases of SIDS are more likely to belong to a social group that is generally considered to be at risk of various types of morbidity, their pregnancies have appeared remarkably uneventful. The only conditions which appear to be associated with increased risk of later SIDS relate to infections during pregnancy. Such associations apply to both urinary tract and to respiratory infections. They are independent of age, parity and social class effects. It has not yet been assessed whether it is the infection or the medication taken for it that is primarily involved.

In contrast, there is no association between SIDS and maternal pre-eclampsia, bleeding in pregnancy, caesarean section or delivery by forceps, induction of labour or any other obstetric abnormality occurring during labour and delivery.

9.7 DISCUSSION

Many characteristics of the infant and his or her maternal background have been shown to be very strongly associated with SIDS. The first aim of the epidemologist is to search for such statistical patterns but, once these patterns are determined, and are shown not to be due to the various biases that could occur, the second important aim is to assign possible meanings to the results [61]. In this respect, sudden infant death research is currently largely failing to pick up the strong clues that are available.

At the moment, the bulk of research concerns either the respiratory physiology of the infant or a search for metabolic defects. As yet, few proponents of these projects have been able to indicate satisfactorily how, if at all, such research, with its built-in assumptions as to causes, can explain the strong associations that have been reported by epidemiological studies.

There are a variety of different hypotheses propounded in the literature. These include chronic mild carbon monoxide poisoning [62], poisoning from ammonia fumes from wet nappies [63], deficiencies of trace elements, excess of sodium, deficiencies of vitamins, immaturity of lung surfactant, abnormalities of sleep pattern, abnormalities of heart rate, immunological mechanisms or a disastrous sudden reaction to an infection [2]. In addition to these, Alice Stewart [64] has suggested that cases of SIDS may die suddenly from acute infections because they are in the process of developing a chronic myeloid leukaemia. Apart from that of Dr Stewart, very few of the hypotheses cited have adduced epidemiological findings in their support.

Consider once again what those epidemiological features are. First, the mother is much more likely to be young, and/or of high parity, at the time of the index conception. Infants of women in the very low social classes are at increased risk, as are those of unmarried mothers. Over and above these, however, the smoking of cigarettes during pregnancy, the ingestion of barbiturates and the infections which the mother may have during pregnancy all lead to an increased risk. Whether or not as a consequence of these features, the infant is more likely to be born at short gestation and/or to be somewhat growth retarded. He or she is more likely to have minor congenital abnormalities.

Features existing only after delivery and which affect the incidence of SIDS have not been found with reliability. The children themselves, however, indicate their susceptibility to various problems by being admitted to special care baby units and/or undergoing subsequent hospital admissions. The impression that one gets is of a child made susceptible, whether this be by virtue of his poor intrauterine environment (with possible malnourishment), the insidious effect of being a passive smoker *in utero* or suffering the infections of his mother and her remedies for them. All of these may be reflected in an increased incidence of minor congenital abnormalities. Thus, the major epidemiological findings may be doing no more than pinpointing an extremely vulnerable infant.

Most research is concentrated in the search for the final insult pathway. This may be foolish. Primary prevention should relate to eradicating the development of such vulnerable fetuses. One may, for example, be able to reduce the incidence of SIDS by persuading women to plan their families so that they are more mature when they first give birth, they then space their births well, their nutrition is good and they avoid smoking during pregnancy.

One of the crucial epidemiological questions that remains to be answered concerns whether smoking during pregnancy, rather than postnatal smoking, is the primary association with tobacco. No study has yet collected sufficient information to be able to tease out the two separate effects. Yet such a teasing out is crucial to the understanding of when the possible insults that result in SIDS occur.

It is tedious to end with a statement saying that more research is needed, yet in this instance it is emminently true. Before more effort is expended on chasing physiological findings, major research effort is needed to identify more closely the epidemiological factors that are associated with SIDS so that one can identify the point in time at which the major problems which are prodromal of SIDS occur.

REFERENCES

1. Beckwith, J.B. (1970) Observations on the pathological anatomy of the sudden infant death syndrome, in *Sudden Infant Death Syndrome: Proceedings of the Second International Conference on Causes of Sudden Death in Infants* (eds A.B. Bergman, J.B. Beckwith and C.G. Ray), University of Washington Press, Seattle.
2. Golding, J., Limerick, S. and Macfarlane, A. (1985) *Sudden Infant Death: Patterns, Puzzles and Problems*, Open Books, Shepton Mallet.
3. Editorial (1987) Premature mortality due to sudden infant death syndrome – United States, 1980–1986. *Morbid. Mortal. Week. Rep.*, **36**, 236.
4. Knowelden, J., Keeling, J. and Nicholl, J.P. (1985) *Postneonatal Mortality.* (A multicentre study undertaken by the Medical Care Research Unit, University of Sheffield), HMSO, London.
5. Pollock, T.M., Miller, E., Mortimer, J.U. and Smith, G. (1984) Symptoms after primary immunisation with DTP and DT vaccine. *Lancet*, **ii**, 146.
6. Roberts, S.C. (1987) Vaccination and cot deaths in perspective. *Arch. Dis. Child.*, **62**, 754.
7. Keeling, J.W., Golding, J. and Sutton, B. (1985) Identification of cases of sudden infant death syndrome from death certificates. *J. Epidemiol. Community Med.*, **39**, 148.
8. Froggat, P., Lynas, M.A. and MacKenzie, G. (1971) Epidemiology of sudden unexpected death in infants ('cot death') in Northern Ireland. *Br. J. Prevent. Soc. Med.*, **25**, 119.
9. Mason, J.K., Harkness, R.A., Elton, R.A. *et al.* (1980) Cot deaths in Edinburgh: infant feeding and socioeconomic factors. *J. Epidemiol. Community Health*, **34**, 35.
10. Milligan, H.C. (1974) The sudden infant death syndrome and its contribution to post neonatal mortality in Hartlepool, 1960–1969. *Public Health*, **88**, 49.
11. Robertson, J.S. and Parker, V. (1978) Cot deaths and water-sodium. *Lancet*, **ii**, 1012.
12. Clarke, J., Davidson, M.M., Downham, M.A.P.S. *et al.* (1977) Newcastle survey of deaths in early childhood 1974/76, with special reference to sudden unexpected deaths. *Arch. Dis. Child.*, **52**, 828.
13. Fedrick, J. (1973) Sudden unexpected deaths in infants in the Oxford Record Linkage area. An analysis in regard to time and space. *Br. J. Prevent. Soc. Med.*, **27**, 217.
14. Powell, J., Machin, D. and Kershaw, C.R. (1983) Unexpected sudden infant deaths in Gosport – some comparisons between service and civilian families. *J. R. Nav. Med. Serv.*, **69**, 141.
15. Bergman, A.B., Ray, C.G., Pomeroy, M.A. *et al.* (1972) Studies of the sudden infant death syndrome in King County, Washington – III Epidemiology. *Pediatrics*, **49**, 860.
16. Armitage, J. and Roffman, B.Y. (1972) Sudden unexplained death in infancy. *Nebr. Med. J.* **57**, 213.
17. Valdes-Dapena, M., Birle, L.J. and McGovern, J.A. (1968) Sudden unexpected death in infancy: a statistical analysis of certain socioeconomic factors. *J. Pediatr.*, **73**, 387.
18. Greenberg, M.A., Nelson, K.E. and Carnow, B.W. (1973) A study of the relationship between sudden infant death syndrome and environmental factors. *Am. J. Epidemiol.*, **98**, 412.
19. Bell, T.J., Sexton, J.S. and Conradi, S.E. (1975) The status of sudden infant death syndrome (1974), and SIDS in Charleston County, South Carolina. *J. SC Med. Assoc.*, **71**, 312.
20. Strimer, R., Adelson, L. and Oseasohn, R. (1969) Epidemiologic features of 1134 sudden, unexpected infant deaths. *JAMA*, **209**, 1493.
21. Bloke, J.H. (1978) The incidence of sudden infant death syndrome in North Carolina's cities and counties: 1972–1974. *Am. J. Public Health*, **68**, 367.
22. Lewak, N., van den Berg, G.J. and Beckwith, J.B. (1979) Sudden infant death syndrome risk factors. *Clin. Pediatr.*, **18**, 404.
23. Peterson, D.R. (1972) Sudden unexpected deaths in infants. Incidence in two climatically dissimilar metropolitan communities. *Am. J. Epidemiol.*, **95**, 95.
24. Borhani, N.O., Rooney, P.A. and Kraus, J.F. (1973) Post-neonatal sudden unexplained death in a California community. *Calif. Med.*, **118**, 12.

25. Kaplan, D.W., Bauman, A.E. and Krous, H.F. (1984) Epidemiology of sudden infant death syndrome in American Indians. *Pediatrics.*, **74**, 1041.

26. Steele, R., Kraus, A.S. and Langworth, J.T. (1967) Sudden, unexpected death in infancy in Ontario Part I: Methodology and findings related to the host. *Can. J. Public Health*, **58**, 359.

27. Grice, A.C. and McGlashan, N.D. (1978) Sudden death in infancy in Tasmania, 1970–1976. *Med. J. Aust.*, **2**, 177.

28. Hilton, J.M.N. and Turner, K.J. (1976) Sudden death in infancy syndrome in Western Australia. *Med. J. Aust.*, **1**, 427.

29. Beal, S. (1983) Some epidemiological factors about sudden infant death syndrome (SIDS) in South Australia, in *Sudden Infant Death Syndrome* (eds J.T. Tildon, L.M. Roeder and A. Steinschneider), Academic, New York.

30. Hassall, I.B. (1986) Sudden infant death syndrome – a serious New Zealand health problem. *NZ Med. J.*, **99**, 233.

31. Wagner, M., Samson-Dolfus, D. and Menard, J. (1984) Sudden unexpected infant death in a French county. *Arch. Dis. Child.*, **59**, 1082.

32. Irgens, L.M., Skjaerven, R. and Peterson, D.R. (1984) Prospective assessment of recurrence risk in sudden infant death syndrome siblings. *J. Paediatr.*, **104**, 349.

33. Biering-Sorensen, F., Jorgensen, T. and Hilden, J. (1978) Sudden infant death in Copenhagen 1956–1971. I. Infant feeding. *Acta Paediatr. Scand.*, **67**, 129.

34. Norvenius, S.G. (1979) Sudden infant death syndrome in Sweden in 1973–1977 and 1979. *Acta Paediatr. Scand.*, [*Suppl.*], **333**, 1.

35. Rintahaki, P. (1985) Sudden infant death syndrome in Finland in 1969–1980. *Publications of the National Board of Health, Finland, series original reports 3/1985*, Helsinki.

36. Schneider, H. (1977) Chacen either Weiteren Senkung der Sauglinssterblichkeit. *Oessentliche Gesundh-Wesen*, **39**, 642.

37. Canby, J.P. and Jaffurs, W.J. (1963) Sudden and unexpected death in childhood. A four year study in the United States Army Station Hospital in Germany. *Milit. Med.*, July, 613.

38. Eckert, E.E. (1976) Plötzlicher und Unerwarteter Tod im Kleinkindesalter und elektromagnistische Felder. *Med. Klin.*, **71**, 1500.

39. Barros, F.C., Victoria, C.G., Vaughan, J.P. *et al.* (1987) Infant mortality in Southern Brazil: a population based study of causes of death. *Arch. Dis. Child.*, **62**, 487.

40. Bloch, A. (1973) Sudden infant death syndrome in the Ashkelon district. *Isr. J. Med. Sci.*, **9**, 452.

41. Winter, S.T. and Emetarom, N.B. (1973) Sudden infant death. A pilot enquiry into its frequency in Israel. *Isr. J. Med. Sci.*, **9**, 447.

42. Davies, D.P. (1985) Cot death in Hong Kong: a rare problem. *Lancet*, **ii**, 1346.

43. Naeye, R.L., Ladis, B. and Drage, J.S. (1976) Sudden infant death syndrome. *Am. J. Dis. Child.*, **130**, 1207.

44. Standfast, S.J., Jereb, S., Aliferis, D. *et al.* (1983) Epidemiology of SIDS in Upstate New York, in *Sudden Infant Death Syndrome* (eds J.T. Tildon, L.M. Roeder and A. Steinschneider), Academic, New York.

45. Black, L., David, R.J., Brouillette, R.T. and Hunt, C.E. (1986) Effects of birthweight and ethnicity on incidence of sudden infant death syndrome. *J. Paediatr.*, **108**, 209.

46. Fedrick, J. (1974) Sudden unexpected deaths in infants in the Oxford Record Linkage area. The mother. *Br. J. Prevent. Soc. Med.*, **28**, 93.

47. Southall, D.P., Stebbens, V. and Shinebourne, E.A. (1987) Sudden and unexpected death between 1 and 5 years. *Arch. Dis. Child.*, **62**, 700.

48. Murphy, M.F.G. and Campbell, M.J. (1987) Sudden infant death syndrome and environmental temperature: an analysis using vital statistics. *J. Epidemiol. Community Health*, **41**, 63.

49. Stanton, A.N., Scott, D.J. and Downham, M.A.P.S. (1980) Is overheating a factor in some unexpected infant deaths? *Lancet*, **i**, 1054.

50. Puffer, R.R. and Serano, C.V. (1973) *Sudden Death. Patterns of Mortality in Childhood*, Pan American Health Organisation, ch. 11.

51. Peterson, D.R., Van Belle, G. and Chinn, N.M. (1982) Sudden infant death syndrome and maternal age. *JAMA*, **247**, 2250.

52. Biering-Sorensen, F., Jorgensen, T. and Hilden, J. (1979) Sudden infant death in Copenhagen 1956–1971. II Social factors and morbidity. *Acta Paediatr. Scand.*, **68**, 1.

53. Watson, E., Gardner, A. and Carpenter, R.G.

(1981) An epidemiological study of unexpected death in infancy in nine areas of Southern England, I. Epidemiology. *Med. Sci. Law*, **21**, 78.

54. Chamberlain, R.N. and Simpson, R.N. (1979) *The Prevalence of Illness in Childhood*, Pitman Medical, Tunbridge Wells.

55. Kraus, J.F. and Borhani, N.O. (1972) Post-neonatal sudden unexplained death in California: a cohort study. *Am. J. Epidemiol.*, **95**, 497.

56. Taylor, B. and Wadsworth, J. (1984) Breast-feeding and child development at five years. *Dev. Med. Child Neurol.*, **26**, 73.

57. Toubas, P.L., Duke, J.C., McCaffree, M.A. *et al.* (1986) Effects of maternal smoking and caffeine habits on infantile apnea: a retrospective study. *Pediatrics*, **78**, 159.

58. Bergman, A.B. and Wiesner, L.A. (1976) Relationship of passive cigarette smoking to sudden infant death syndrome. *Pediatrics*, **58**, 665.

59. Murphy, J.F., Newcombe, R.G. and Sibert, J.R. (1982) The epidemiology of sudden infant death syndrome. *J. Epidemiol. Community Health*, **36**, 17.

60. Kraus, A.S., Steele, R., Thompson, M.G. and de Grosbois, P. (1971) Further epidemiologic observations on sudden unexpected death in infancy in Ontario. *Can. J. Public Health*, **62**, 210.

61. Editorial (1987) Paediatric and perinatal epidemiology. *Paediatr. Perinat. Epidemiol.*, **1**, 1.

62. Cleary, J. (1984) Carbon monoxide and cot death. *Lancet*, **i**, 1403.

63. Tyler, J.W. (1983) *Cot-death – The Ammonia Factor*, J.W. Tyler, New Zealand, pp. 1–54.

64. Stewart, A.M. (1975) Infant leukaemias and cot deaths. *Br. Med. J.*, **2**, 605.

CHAPTER 10

The pathology of the sudden infant death syndrome

J.M.N. Hilton

As has been already remarked in Chapter 9, Beckwith defined SIDS, now the most common cause of death in the immediate postneonatal period, as follows: 'The sudden death of any infant or young child which is unexpected by history and in which a thorough post-mortem examination fails to reveal a cause' [1]. This definition has gained wide, if not universal, acceptance since its introduction in 1969. It implies that the morphological features of the disease must be subtle and not readily identified by the usual techniques; taken literally, it might inhibit any discussion of the pathology of the syndrome. However, if we add 'other than those manifestations usually observed in such disease', we may proceed without offending logic [2]. Alternatively, we can use Adelson's definition – which preceded that of Beckwith – 'the death of a child who was thought to have been in good health or whose terminal illness appeared to be so mild that the possibility of a fatal outcome was not anticipated' [3]; the implications of a negative necropsy are thereby avoided. In any event, should the consequent post-mortem examination reveal the unsuspected presence of pathology which might reasonably be expected to be of a life-threatening nature, then SIDS becomes an untenable diagnosis. A clear distinction must be made between SIDS and other conditions causing death in an infant no matter how sudden or unexpected is the presentation. The present author is as guilty as any in having failed to make this distinction abundantly clear in published work [4].

The detection of any 'characteristic' or pathognomonic lesion will require careful comparison with cases derived from a controlled group of children not dying of SIDS. The criteria for a control series in any study of the pathology of SIDS should include:

  (i) adequate numbers;
 (ii) the study must be of dead children – biopsies taken from living children will not bear the stigmata of death nor of post-mortem changes;
(iii) there must be a gestational age and sex match and, ideally, a racial match;
 (iv) the mode of death must be sudden and unheralded by prior illness or major congenital anomaly;
  (v) methods of investigation and recording must be comparable.

Sudden and unexpected death in children which satisfies these criteria is relatively rare in this age-group. Occasional deaths result from accidental or non-accidental immersion; even more rarely, accidental death occurs as a result of self-suspension between cot bars or of strangulation from clothing which is caught in crib structures and the like. However, each of these conditions has its own pathology which may or may not overlap with that of SIDS. Homicidal deaths do occur in this age-group (see Chapter 12) but, again, it is seldom that there is no pathology associated intrinsically with the method used. Even accidental deaths due to motor vehicle trauma, which are so often available as controls in adult life, are rare in this age-group – acute alcoholism and taking the baby out are seldom mutually compatible. Such a scarcity of control material is fortunate for society but is an almost insurmountable impediment to SIDS investigation. Accordingly, pathologists must be aware of the limitations which are imposed on the interpretation of pathological features seen in SIDS and should restrain themselves from a too-ready or uncritical acceptance of published studies which lack adequate control data.

As something of a corollary, appropriate steps must be taken to exclude violence in every case of sudden and unexpected infant death. Such exclusion may be difficult or, on occasion, impossible. However, no matter how innocent may be the external appearance, rigorous internal examination, coupled with appropriate ancillary investigations such as a full body X-ray, will disclose most instances of skeletal and soft-tissue trauma. Good lighting, effective magnification, a comprehensive history and a high index of suspicion should assist in the detection of subtle manifestations of 'gentle battering' [5] where the child may, for example, have been suffocated by having a hand or other object placed over the nose and mouth. Such sutble manifestations include superficial abrasions of the epithelium around the mouth and lips, bruising of the inner

aspect of the lips and of the gums with perhaps damage to the frenula of the lips. Repeated examination of the body may be necessary as initially concealed bruising may become obvious following the exsanguination caused by the original post-mortem. Care should be taken not to confuse post-mortem drying of the lips with the 'parchmenting' of ante-mortem pressure or abrasion. An additional complication is that many of these children will have been subjected to resuscitative efforts at some time after death; these efforts may have been applied with desperate vigour and may have produced post-mortem injury which is difficult to distinguish from that inflicted during life. Microscopic evidence of vital reaction, when present, will be helpful in this respect. The pathologist must maintain a high level of suspicion but equally avoid its premature articulation.

The typical presentation in the SIDS autopsy is the body of a baby of about 3 months of age, more often male than female, usually apparently well nourished and cared for, and without outward manifestations of injury or illness apart from an inconstant finding of froth, sometimes bloody, issuing from the nose and/or mouth (Fig. 10.1); there may, indeed, be sufficient blood present to mimic frank haemorrhage.

If the child has been dead for some time prior to presentation, gravitational lividity may indicate the position in which the body lay after death (Fig. 10.2). When present, the ease and extent to which such lividity may shift should be noted. This, together with the distribution of any rigor mortis and serial recordings of the body core temperature, may make it possible to estimate the time of death. The bereaved parents frequently seek to know this and the lack of precision inherent in the estimation must be emphasized. If the child is clothed, the napkin or equivalent is usually soaked with urine and frequently shows faecal soiling – but this is not an unusual

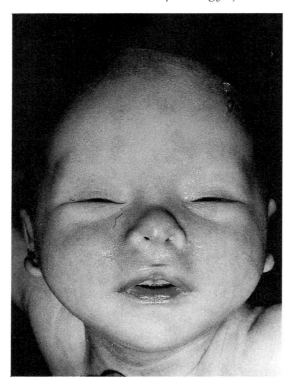

Fig. 10.1 SIDS: facial appearance.

'markers' for increased risk for SIDS, a proposition which merits further investigation.

Beckwith's definition indicates that the diagnosis can only be made on completion of a comprehensive necropsy. As in adult medicine, this entails the opening of all body cavities, the macroscopic examination and dissection of all organ systems and microscopic examination of what may be judged adequate representative tissue samples. Microbiological, biochemical, radiological, cytogenetic and toxicological studies of an appropriate nature should be undertaken [6].

On reflecting the scalp, evidence of bruising should be carefully sought; there can be extensive bleeding into the deeper zones

finding in any baby. Other garments may be soaked with sweat, thus indicating a vigorous diaphoresis before death. Fibres or other debris may be found entwined in the fingers indicating unusually active movement at some time prior to death. Marked cyanosis of the lips and nail-beds is common both to SIDS and to other causes of sudden infant death which are more readily demonstrable.

Minor departures from normal external morphology may indicate a chromosomal abnormality which may be, of itself, sufficient to cause death. Careful measurement of weight, head circumference and relevant lengths will detect any departure from expected stages of growth or development. Dysmorphisms, dysplasias, anomalies and growth retardation have been suggested as

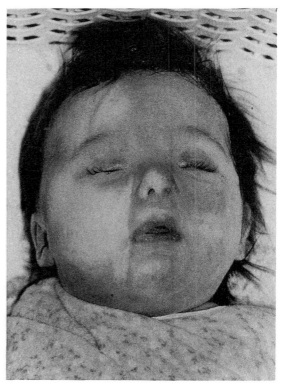

Fig. 10.2 SIDS: dependent lividity.

of the scalp or beneath the epicranium without any correlative external hint. The interpretation of any such appearance must be tempered by caution, expecially in the younger infant, for modest birth trauma can produce such bruising which may persist for several weeks and show remarkably little change either to the naked eye or on microscopic examination. In contrast, less florid bruises may indicate more recent, more subtle and more significant application of force. Bruising of this type should be sought assiduously around the lips and gums, and elsewhere on the face and neck.

The leptomeninges may show some congestion but the gyral and sulcal pattern of the brain in SIDS is in keeping with the developmental age of the child. Gross dissection reveals no further abnormality. As with much else that constitutes SIDS, the reported results of microscopic examination of the brain and its component parts are controversial, inconstant and subject to a range of interpretations. Focal glial proliferation at various sites in the cerebrum, cerebellum and brainstem [7–9], periventricular leukomalacia [10] and increased numbers of fat-bearing macrophages [11] have been reported and variously interpreted as being manifestations of prior hypoxia or impaired local perfusion or as being the cause or effect of apnoea. More peripherally, differences in the numbers of myelinated vagal fibres between SIDS babies and controls have been described but not confirmed.

Inspection of the middle ears, paranasal air sinuses and the nasal passages may reveal stigmata of acute or chronic inflammation. Minor microscopic manifestations of inflammation in the respiratory tract [12] are seen more commonly in the more crowded industrial societies of the Northern Hemisphere than in Australia [13]. Observation is easier than interpretation and the significance of this finding, like so many reported SIDS-related phenomena, remains obscure. The presence of acute inflammation anywhere in the body must raise the question of death having occurred during or in consequence of an unobserved febrile convulsion. Again, the problem arises of comparison with a 'control' group which is both appropriate in character and adequate in number.

The anatomical relationships between the tongue, the palate and uvula, the oropharynx, the epiglottis and laryngeal introitus in the infant differ somewhat from those in the adult. These structures are more crowded and the epiglottis is relatively larger. However, this is true of all infants in the age-group under discussion. Nevertheless, should another factor – such as a change in posture [14], reflex response to local irritation or a failure of neuromuscular control – be added to the equation, then life-threatening obstructive apnoea might ensue. While there would be little or no local physical evidence for such a sequence demonstrable at post-mortem examination, focal fibrinoid necrosis of the cords has been described in SIDS babies [15]. Chemical irritants, such as regurgitated gastric contents, might induce spasm and death could then ensue too rapidly for a local tissue response to be detectable histologically. The finding of gastric content even within the peripheral air passages must be interpreted with great caution for postural change associated with moving the body may cause 'passive' – and resuscitation 'active' – regurgitation and aspiration.

Elsewhere in the neck, careful dissection will disclose parathyroid glands which are normal in number and structure. Serial section of the thyroid may reveal a nub of parathyroid or thymic tissue beneath the capsule or within the substance of the gland; there is no departure from 'normal'. Altered cellular granularity in the carotid bodies has been proposed as a manifestation of deficient respiratory chemoreception – and, thus, a component of suboptimal control and regulation of breathing – but, again, no consistent difference between SIDS and non SIDS babies has been confirmed.

The major stigmata associated with SIDS may be seen within the chest cavity. The lungs (Fig. 10.3) show varying degrees of congestion, oedema and focal collapse with some acute hyperinflation lying between collapsed lobules or groups of lobules. Increased rib markings are common.

Petechiae (Fig. 10.4) are almost always present on the visceral pleurae but are seldom found on the parietal pleurae. They are also frequently seen on the epicardium, particularly adjacent to the atrioventriular sulcus, in the line of the septum anteriorly and on the posterior aspect of both ventricles, although they may be found in any cardiac area and occasionally extend subadventitially along the ascending aorta [16]. They are never present on the conjunctivae, eye-lids or on or in other soft tissues of the head and neck in SIDS. The thymus is usually a large fleshy structure in SIDS as it is in children dying instantly from trauma. Thymic petechiae may be seen most frequently on the surface of the gland but, when prolific, may extend

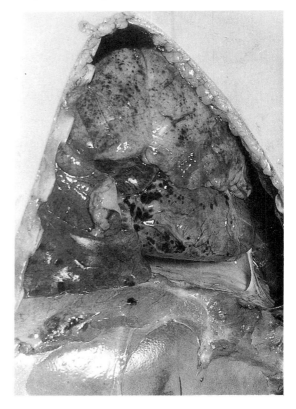

Fig. 10.4 SIDS: intrathoracic petechiae.

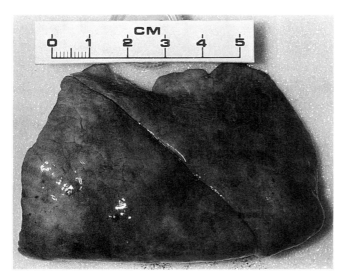

Fig. 10.3 SIDS: macroscopic appearance of lungs.

throughout the substance. Although their presence can no longer be regarded as pathognomonic of an asphyxial mode of death, they are seen to best advantage where an obstructive or compressive factor has prevented effective respiration, that factor having operated either intermittently or continuously.

Structurally, the heart appears normal although some authors have described microscopic narrowing of the nodal arteries [17], disorders of the conducting system [18], right ventricular hypertrophy and a variety of ostensibly minor abnormalities. The diagnosis of SIDS must be abandoned should areas of frank inflammation or necrosis be present. Controversy still surrounds the proposition that there is increased muscle mass in the right ventricular myocardium and in the pulmonary arteries [19]. Such findings might suggest pulmonary hypertension, perhaps in response to recurrent hypoxia, but a counter-claim has been made that they represent a normal part of the anatomical spectrum in this age-group.

Recently reported work from Sheffield [20] has caused renewed interest in both the structural and functional pathology of the liver in infants dying suddenly and unexpectedly. The liver in SIDS is usually macroscopically normal. Should it appear enlarged, yellow or fatty, then other causes of the infant's demise are likely, including fulminant Reye's syndrome [21], or inborn errors of metabolism. There may be no detectable abnormalities whatsoever on microscopic examination of the liver. Residual extramedullary haemopoiesis may be seen, especially in the younger victims. Glycogen depletion may be demonstrated by appropriate staining. Marked glycogenolysis and gluconeogenesis with consequent elevation of the blood sugar – at least in that obtained from the inferior vena cava or right heart chamber – is a common agonal phenomenon and is seen in a proportion of

sudden deaths from many other causes, hence the necropsy surgeon's preference for some other body fluids such as vitreous humour or cerebrospinal fluid for estimation of glucose levels in the fresh cadaver (see Chapter 13). Some hepatocytic cytoplasmic vacuolation is occasionally seen; although this may be hydropic and possibly hypoxic in aetiology, it is usually due to a fine steatosis and is not unique to SIDS [22].

The proposition that asphyxia is the most common mode of death in SIDS is supported by finding low oxygen levels in blood [23] which are similar when specimens are taken from both the left and right sides of the heart, provided always that samples are taken within 6 hours of death, with the same type of syringe and with the same attention to technique as is taken in intravital sampling. Post-mortem levels are always low in absolute terms and a single result from one chamber is of little value other than to exclude asphyxia when the pO_2 is above $25\,mmHg$ ($3.4\,kPa$) [24].

Recently published studies have tended to confirm a catastrophic failure of respiration – possibly of an obstructive nature – as being the most likely mechanism of death. The roles of central and mixed apnoea are still being investigated. The ethnic background, including a low incidence of smoking in mothers and the close physical supervisory environment of babies in non-Caucasian families, may afford linked protective factors for SIDS [25]. A possible association between the prone sleeping position and the sudden infant death syndrome has been postulated from the Netherlands and Australia [26, 27].

Infection, allergy and other immunological phemonena or aberrations have been proposed as aetiological factors. The role of bacteria was discounted early, perhaps too early, in the saga of SIDS. Infantile botulism and *Clostridium difficile* infection have recently emerged as contenders in at least some of these deaths. None were found in the cases in the present author's series which were examined for these organisms or their toxins in the microbiology laboratory. Likewise, the demonstration of viral infection either by culture or by serological methods (while accepting the limitations imposed on the latter in that the death of the subject precludes serial sampling) is seldom successful. If microbial or viral agents do play a role, it must be one of some subtlety without the production of the usual stigmata of major infection [28] – if such stigmata *are* present, then the diagnosis may not be SIDS.

The term infant is at greatest risk of dying by the way of SIDS at 3 months of age. The level of maternal IgG has by then declined in all infants; cell-mediated immunity and complement levels do not differentiate the SIDS from the 'control' baby. Anaphylaxis might manifest itself *de novo* as sudden death in a previously well person and the appearance of the body could be identical with that of a SIDS victim at necropsy. Sensitivities to cow's milk, house-dust mite and aspergillus have been proposed and, although early work showed an increase in IgE specific to these antigens, subsequent investigation has proved negative [29]. There is no evidence that prophylactic immunization of itself is a causative factor. In fact, evidence of major immune system disease should, again, cause the pathologist to question the validity of a diagnosis of SIDS.

The now voluminous literature pertaining to SIDS describes many other alleged deviations from normal [30–35]. These, by way of example, range from increased or persistent periadrenal brown fat, through subluxation of the cervical spine to epidural haemorrhage. Other reported aberrations include hyper- and hypoglycaemia, disturbances of calcium amd magnesium metabolism, thyroid and other endocrine problems and excesses or deficiencies of vitamins. Some phenomena would appear to have existed only in the eye of the original

beholder, others may be inconstant or infrequent findings or have no value in discriminating between SIDS victims and babies dying suddenly from other more easily demonstrable 'causes' – but, once proposed, each must be pursued if only to be excluded. The presence of major departures from normal should prompt the question, 'is the diagnosis still SIDS?'.

The pathologist's role in the diagnosis of sudden infant death and the management of the problems arising consequent to the child's demise are crucial. Early, precise and comprehensive investigation of all likely diagnostic possibilities and their confirmation or exclusion will assist materially in lifting the cloud of uncertainty which such a death evokes in the minds of both officials and families. The parents should be promptly appraised of a diagnosis of SIDS in the hope of lessening the burden of guilt and self-doubt which they inevitably experience consequent upon the death of their child. To this end, the pathologist should be experienced in, and alert to, the pitfalls implicit in the diagnoses associated with sudden death in an infant – pitfalls which may be social, emotional or legal rather than confined to the more familiar and comfortable discipline of pathology. Pathologists should give a high priority to the early completion of the necropsy without undue regard to personal, departmental or constabulary convenience. As far as it is possible, given the constraints of the medicolegal system within which they practise, they should ensure that any logistical problems or other causes of delay are overcome so that the interests of the parents, surviving siblings, children not as yet conceived and society as a whole are best served. Although a diagnosis of SIDS can only be provisional on the basis of the macroscopic examination – and to pretend otherwise would be quite improper – it can be offered with sufficient confidence to relieve parental and community doubt and to save the police from the onerous responsibility of further investigation.

The parents will often wish to discuss the post-mortem findings with the pathologist within a few hours or days of death, or at some later time. Because of their unqiue involvement in the diagnostic process, pathologists are well placed to speak of the findings in the baby, about the possible mechanisms and causes of the death and, if the diagnosis is SIDS, to refute some of the mythology which has accrued to that diagnostic label in times both ancient and modern.

Frequently asked questions include:

— Of what did our baby really die?
— Did we do anything to cause our baby's death?
— Did we neglect to do anything which could have prevented our baby's death?
— Was there any inherited abnormality which may affect later children?
— How can we avoid losing another baby in this manner?
— Did our baby suffer?
— What did you see when you looked at our baby and what was the significance of what you saw?

In answering these questions, pathologists must be attuned to the parents and their needs. A sensitive explanation that a post-mortem examination is like any other surgical operation and was as necessary as say, the removal of an inflamed appendix and that, as with any other surgical operation, incisions were made and stitched up afterwards, should help to put the necropsy in its proper context. It should be stated that tissue and body fluid samples were obtained for testing and the need for this, and the results of the investigations, should be explained. The legal requirements for a post-mortem examination should be outlined. Pathologists who sincerely believe that a competent and comprehensive post-mortem examination of each victim of SIDS contributes meaningfully

to the elucidation of the nature of the problem and its future elimination should not hesitate to say so; those who do not so believe should not practise in this field. There should be frank discussion of any theories of which the parents may have read or heard concerning SIDS. Expression of the pathologist's own views can be productive provided that the personal nature of these views is emphasized. Raising of false hopes and expectations, such as the utility of monitoring devices and screening tests in the prevention of SIDS, must be avoided. The temptation to fudge issues because they are painful to either party should be eschewed. The most valuable attribute of a pathologist undertaking this duty is an ability to listen with patience and understanding to the overt or covert expression of anguish and self-doubt which underlies even the most composed parental exterior.

REFERENCES

1. Beckwith, J.B. (1970) Observations on the pathological anatomy of the sudden infant death syndrome, in *Sudden Infant Death Syndrome: Proceedings of the Second International Conference on Causes of Sudden Death in Infants* (ed. A.B. Bergman), University of Washington Press, Seattle, p. 83.
2. Krous, H.F. (1984) Sudden infant death syndrome: pathology and pathophysiology. *Pathol. Annu.*, **19**, 1.
3. Adelson, L. and Roberts Kinney, E. (1956) Sudden and unexpected death in infancy and childhood. *Pediatrics*, **17**, 663.
4. Dunne, J.W., Harper, C.G. and Hilton, J.M.N. (1984) Sudden infant death syndrome caused by poliomyelitis. *Arch. Neurol.*, **41**, 775.
5. Taylor, E.M. and Emery, J.L. (1982) Two year study of the causes of postperinatal deaths classified in terms of preventability. *Arch. Dis. Child.*, **57**, 668.
6. Knoweldon, J. Keeling, J. and Nicholl, J.P. (1985) *Post-neonatal Mortality*, HMSO, London.
7. Summers, C.G. and Parker, J.C. (1981) The brain stem in sudden infant death syndrome:

a postmortem survey. *Am. J. Forensic Med. Pathol.*, **2**, 121.

8. Kinney, H.C., Burger, P.C., Harrell, F.E. and Hudson, R.P. (1983) Reactive gliosis in the medulla oblongata of victims of the sudden infant death syndrome. *Pediatrics*, **72**, 181.

9. Ambler, M.W., Neave, C. and Sturner, W.Q. (1981) Sudden and unexpected death in infancy and childhood: neurological findings. *Am. J. Forensic Med. Pathol.*, **2**, 23.

10. Allen, T.B. (1985) Sudden infant death with periventricular leukomalacia. *J. Forensic Sci.*, **30**, 1260.

11. Gadsdon, D.R. and Emery, J.L. (1976) Fatty change in the brain in perinatal and unexpected death. *Arch. Dis. Child.*, **51**, 42.

12. Williams, A.L. (1980) Tracheobronchitis and sudden infant death syndrome. *Pathology*, **12**, 73.

13. Emery, J.L. (1986) Cot deaths in Australia, 1985. *Med. J. Aust.*, **144**, 469.

14. Simson, L.R. and Brantley, R.E. (1977) Postural asphyxia as a cause of death in sudden infant death syndrome. *J. Forensic Sci.*, **22**, 178.

15. Cullity, G.J. and Emery, J.L. (1975) Ulceration and necrosis of vocal cords in hospital and unexpected child deaths. *J. Pathol.*, **115**, 27.

16. Krous, H.F. (1984) The microscopic distribution of intrathoracic petechiae in sudden infant death syndrome. *Arch. Pathol. Lab. Med.*, **108**, 77.

17. Anderson, K.R. and Hill, R.W. (1982) Occlusive lesions of cardiac conducting tissue arteries in sudden infant death syndrome. *Pediatrics*, **69**, 50.

18. Anderson, R.H., Ho, S.Y., Smith, A. *et al.* (1981) Study of the cardiac conducting tissue in the pediatric age group. *Diagnostic Histopathol.*, **4**, 3.

19. Weiler, G. and de Haardt, J. (1983) Morphometrical investigations into alterations of the wall thickness of small pulmonary arteries after birth and in cases of sudden infant death syndrome (SIDS). *Forensic Sci. Int.*, **21**, 33.

20. Howat, A.J., Bennett, M.J., Variend, S. *et al.* (1985) Defects of metabolism of fatty acids in the sudden infant death syndrome. *Br. Med. J.*, **290**, 1771.

21. Mason, J.K. and Bain, A.D. (1982) Reye's syndrome presenting as atypical sudden infant death syndrome? *Forensic Sci. Int.*, **20**, 39.

22. Mason, J.K. (1984) Fatty vacuolation of the liver in the sudden infant death syndrome, in *Proceedings of the Oxford Conference*, Oxford University Press, Oxford.

23. Hilton, J.M.N. and Turner, K.J. (1976) Sudden death in infancy syndrome in Western Australia. *Med. J. Aust.*, **1**, 427.

24. Mithoefer, J.C., Mead, G., Hughes, J.M. *et al.* (1967) A method of distinguishing death due to cardiac arrest from asphyxia. *Lancet*, **ii**, 654.

25. Milner, A.D. and Ruggins, N. (1989 Sudden infant death syndrome. *Br. Med. J.*, **298**, 689.

26. de Jonge, G.A., Engelberts, A.C., Koomen-Liefting, A.J.M. and Kostense, P.J. (1989) Cot death and prone sleeping position in The Netherlands. *Br. Med. J.*, **298**, 722.

27. Beale, S. (1988) Sleeping position and sudden infant death syndrome. *Med. J. Austral.*, **149**, 562; (1988) *Lancet*, **ii**, 512.

28. Zink, P., Drescher, J., Verhagen, W. *et al.* (1987) Serological evidence of recent influenza vira A (H3N2) infections in forensic cases of the sudden infant death syndrome (SIDS). *Arch. Virol.*, **93**, 223.

29. Turner, K.J., Baldo, B.A. and Hilton, J.M.N. (1975) IgE antibodies to *Dermatophagoides pteronyssinus* (housedust mite), *Aspergillus fumigatus* and beta-lactoglobulin in sudden infant death syndrome. *Br. Med. J.*, **1**, 357.

30. Robinson, R.R. (ed.) (1974) *SIDS 1974*, Foundation for the Study of Infant Deaths, Toronto.

31. Camps, F.E. and Carpenter, R.G. (eds) (1980) *Sudden and Unexpected Deaths in Infancy (Cot Deaths)*, Wright, Guildford.

32. Guntheroth, W.G. (1982) *Crib Death: The Sudden Infant Death Syndrome*, Futura, New York.

33. Tildon, J.T., Roeder, L.M. and Steinschneider, A. (eds.) (1983) *Sudden Infant Death Syndrome*, Academic, New York.

34. Golding, J., Limerick, S. and McFarlane, A. (1985) *Sudden Infant Death: Patterns, Puzzles and Problems*, Open Books, Shepton Mallet, Somerset.

35. Australian Rotary Health Research Fund Conference on Cot Death (1986) *Aust. Paediatr. J.*, **22**, Suppl. 1, 1.

CHAPTER 11

Causes of sudden natural death in infancy and childhood

C.L. Berry

It is, of course, true to say that a child may die suddenly from a number of conditions that affect adults – such as diabetes mellitus and bronchial asthma; indeed, these are significant causes of death in this age-group. This review will not deal with these types of condition but will concentrate on unusual or unexpected deaths, the latter sometimes occurring in an unpredictable way in otherwise well-defined illnesses. The entities discussed in the section on infections are those which may manifest themselves in ways which may not be familiar to those who normally deal with adults. Genetically determined conditions which run a predictable course – such as cystic fibrosis or Leigh's disease – are not discussed here, and other major sections of this book are devoted to the sudden infant death syndrome as a separate entity.

11.1 CONGENITAL MALFORMATIONS

Cases of undiagnosed malformation are becoming increasingly rare as a result of the great awareness and intensity of specialist investigation that are now the norm in neonatal care. However, it is clear that some clinically unascertainable defects, such as single kidney, Meckel's diverticulum or a bicuspid aortic valve, may well delay their presentation until late in adult life or may be detected at autopsy only after an uneventful existence. Between the group of conditions that are diagnosed and successfully treated by surgery and these incidental anomalies, are a number of defects which may not be amenable to treatment and which may cause death in childhood. Malformations remain a common cause of death in the first year of life.

This section deals only with those conditions which may cause *sudden* death – for a fuller account of such deaths in general, see Berry [1]. It is important to note that, in 1984, 1638 out of 3017 deaths resulting from malformations occurred in the first year of life. These consisted mainly of cardiovascular (972) and central nervous system (278) defects. The deaths in these two groups between 1 and 4 years of age totalled 236 (CVS) and 59 (CNS); between 5 and 19 years, the figures were 204 (CVS) and 41 (CNS). The importance of undiagnosed defects is real at all ages; the author has recently autopsied a 30-year-old male who died while taking part in an athletics programme and who had cardiomegaly

(540 g) due to an unsuspected ventricular septal defect.

(a) Cardiac anomalies

Left-sided hypoplasia of the heart, severe forms of Fallot's tetralogy, right heart hypoplasia and double-outlet right ventricle are those defects which may lead to sudden death despite therapy, as may some forms of transposition of the great arteries. Anomalies of venous drainage also have a poor prognosis if they are associated with severe obstruction to flow. Examples include those forms in which pulmonary venous blood drains into the portal vein and, thus, passes through two capillary networks.

Such deaths will be truly unexpected in only a minority of cases but major, and less predictable, contributors to the deaths in this group of patients are the cerebral complications of infarction and of brain abscess, both being related to polycythaemia; these complications may occur at any time.

Endocarditis on abnormal valves or prostheses, or in shunts used as palliative or facilitating procedures, is also commoner in cyanotic disease and has a mortality of between 30% and 40%.

(b) Central nervous system

The major structural anomalies generally cause death in early neonatal life. However, in a number of conditions a defect may not have been diagnosed and death may occur unexpectedly – for example, in tuberose sclerosis following convulsions or in cerebral angiomatosis as a result of haemorrhage.

(c) Gastrointestinal system

Atresias and stenoses are usually managed successfully in early life and are not an important cause of death. However, duplications may cause obstruction which may perforate, volvulus may occur in infants with abnormal mesenteric rotation and inguinal hernias may be missed both clinically and at autopsy.

The very rare smooth muscle defects in the bowel wall may perforate; the author has seen one case involving the stomach in a 10-month-old male infant and another in a 5-year-old boy, each of which presented as an acute abdomen. It is possible that this finding is under reported; it should be considered in all cases of unexpected perforation in infancy.

Heterotopic gastric mucosa may cause ulceration and perforation, usually at the site of a Meckel's diverticulum, but it should be remembered that perforation of peptic ulcers at classical sites is not rare in either infants or children [2].

(d) Respiratory system

Congenital anomalies of the lung with survival into postnatal life may cause death following infection. Accessory lung with bronchial connections, adenomatoid malformations and pulmonary lymphangiectasia are examples. Sequestration may be associated with heart failure due to shunting of the type in which the aortic blood supply drains into the pulmonary veins.

Respiratory distress and failure may be caused by lobar emphysema when the abnormal lung acts as a space-occupying lesion as air accumulates within it due to a valvular mechanism.

(e) Urogenital system

A number of undiagnosed anomalies may exist (e.g. horseshoe or doughnut kidney, ectopia), but these are unlikely to cause death in childhood either directly or indirectly. Medullary cystic disease (juvenile nephronophthisis) may cause death from renal failure in childhood and is associated with growth retardation and salt craving.

(f) Immunoreactive tissues

Infants and small children may present with failure to thrive, weight loss and diarrhoea in several of the conditions in which cellular immunity is deficient. Unusual infections, often involving persistent ulceration of the skin, are common. It is evident that this combination of signs and symptoms may indicate potential maltreatment and this had been suspected clinically in some instances included in one of the early studies of the morphological findings in this group of conditions [3]. However, the histopathological findings are well characterized and a diagnosis can be made post-mortem even if little or no immunological testing has been performed in life. The changes are described in detail in Berry and Revell [4], but it is worth reconsidering some basic points here.

In cases of this type, the thymus is small (less than 2 g), it is situated mainly above the innominate vein and, histologically, it has a distinctive glandular appearance without development of the cortex or of Hassall's corpuscles. The appearances are readily

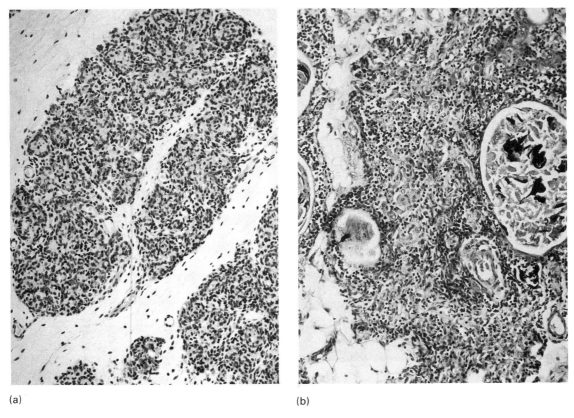

(a)   (b)

Fig. 11.1 (a) Thymus in the combined immunity deficiency syndrome from an 8-month-old male presenting with failure to thrive. There is a lobular, glandular appearance and no cortical development (haematoxylin and eosin, × 120). (b) Thymus in so-called stress involution from a case of congenital heart disease. Hassall's corpuscles are present and calcified. The cortex is present although lymphocyte depleted (haematoxylin and eosin × 140).

distinguished from those that are often attributed to stress (Fig. 11.1). Lymph nodes may be absent – a roll preparation of the mesentery is the simplest way of checking if in doubt – or they may consist of simple reticular networks (Fig. 11.2). Splenic histology is seldom very helpful since, although paucity of lymphocytes may be obvious, the normal range of appearances is wide. It is important to take blocks for histological examination from the tonsillar area and from the appendix in order to check the gut-associated lymphoid tissue which is often grossly deficient (Figs 11.3 and 11.4).

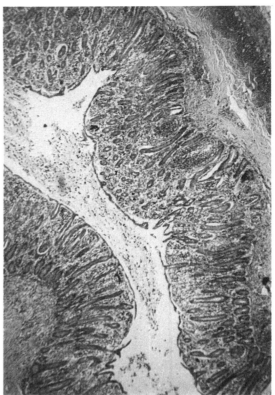

Fig. 11.3 Appendix showing paucity of lymphoid development (11-month-old female) (haemotoxylin and eosin, × 40).

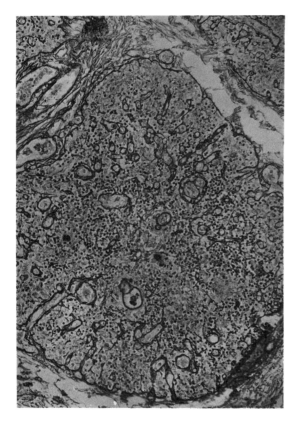

Fig. 11.2 Lymph node from the mesentery in the combined immunity deficiency syndrome. The node shows a reticular structure only (reticulin, × 80).

11.2 INFECTIONS

The role of infections in causing deaths in children is probably underestimated, often because of the speed of onset and the rapid course of the process. Infections which are mainly confined to the neonatal period, such as listeriosis, will not be considered here, nor will those conditions which have well-described features, such as tuberculosis or measles; a full account is given in Kaschula [5]. Infection should be considered in any unexpected death in childhood and the newer techniques which permit the histopathologist

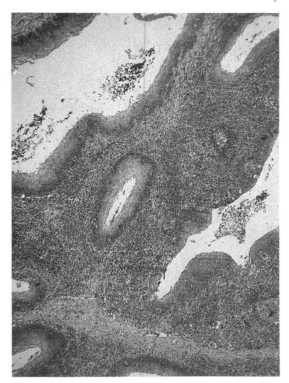

Fig. 11.4 Tonsil from a 15-month-old male. Little follicular development is seen (× 30).

to identify organisms in tissues help to resolve the many difficulties of post-mortem microbiology.

(a) β-haemolytic streptococci (βHS)

In the neonate and in the young, Lancefield group B βHS cause pneumonia and meningitis with a high mortality (20–30%) and significant neurological defect in survivors from infections of the central nervous system. A respiratory illness often precedes neurological involvement in older children. This organism has replaced *E. coli* as the most common cause of infections in the first 2 months of life [6]. Death may occur within 24 hours and fever may not be marked.

(b) Staphylococcal infection

Pneumonia in infants which is accompanied by haemorrhagic pneumonia (Fig. 11.5), abscess formation and by pneumothorax, frequently of tension type, is often due to infection by staphylococci which may follow a viral pneumonia or a skin lesion. Intrapulmonary haemorrhage may be so severe as to mimic the effects of trauma.

The scalded skin syndrome (Ritter's disease) resembles Lyell's syndrome and, like it, is a form of toxic epidermal necrolysis. In infants, it is due exclusively to an exotoxin

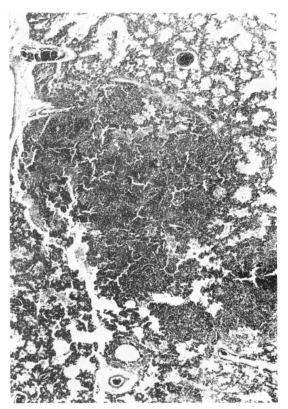

Fig. 11.5 Haemorrhagic pneumonia in an infant. Courtesy of Dr R.O.C. Kaschula, Cape Town, South Africa (haematoxylin and eosin, × 40).

isolated from phage group II, coagulase-positive staphylococci which can be cultured from the skin surface in some patients; this is in contrast to the multiple aetiologies described in adults [7]. The appearances of skin separation closely resemble those of scalding but will differ in distribution. They are due entirely to the toxin. It is important to remember that infection may also occur in operation wounds, for example, at the circumcision site [8].

The toxic shock syndrome has been reported in prepubertal girls and there is an account of its occurrence in a 3-week-old infant with staphylococcal infection at the site of a heel-prick [9].

(c) Pneumococcal disease

Pneumonia and meningitis, which is sometimes preceded by otitis media, are life-threatening conditions. A primary pneumococcal peritonitis may occur in young girls without a history of sexual activity.

The Waterhouse–Friderichsen syndrome may occur as a result of infection with this organism. Splenectomized children are particularly vulnerable to major pneumococcal illness, as are those with sickle cell disease.

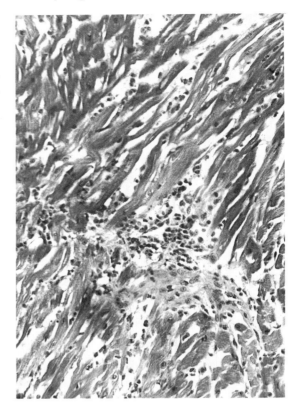

Fig. 11.6 Scanty infiltration of the myocardium is seen in myocarditis associated with *Neisseria meningitidis*. The lesion is often not marked but the change is widespread (haematoxylin and eosin, × 120).

(d) Infection with *Neisseria meningitidis*

Around 20% of children harbour *N. meningitidis* in the nasopharynx but the strains are mainly non-pathogenic. Disseminated infection is commoner in boys and respiratory symptoms often form the prodrome. In severe infection, there is petechial haemorrhage in the skin, ecchymosis and purpura. Some 70% of fatalities have meningococcaemia and 40% have meningitis. Most fatal cases die within 72 hours of onset; adrenal haemorrhages occur in less than 50%. Myocarditis is not uncommon and is a cause of sudden death (Fig. 11.6).

(e) Infection with *Haemophilus influenzae*

A large proportion of infants and children carry this organism in the upper respiratory tract, but only around 5% have the virulent form. The organism is a major cause of meningitis, with a peak incidence at 7–12 months; 66% of cases occur before the age of 18 months. Pneumonia with a high mortality rate (30%) may rapidly follow upon epiglottitis which occurs in older children (2–4 years) [10]. Septicaemia is not rare and septic arthritis is relatively common.

(f) Pertussis

The author has recently seen a fatal case of pertussis in a child of 11 months who had not been immunized. Patchy collapse with areas of overdistension of the lungs were the predominant findings.

(g) Respiratory syncytial virus (RSV) infection

This virus is an important cause of disease in childhood and a role for it in sudden infant death has often been proposed. It is the main cause of bronchiolitis in those under 6 months of age and has an incubation period of 2–6 days. Respiratory obstruction is a clinical feature. In fatal cases, there is epithelial necrosis with plugging of the bronchi by epithelial cells; air trapping may be prominent. Bronchiolar muscular hypertrophy may develop and permanent damage, which predisposes to bronchiectasis, may arise. Multinucleate epithelial cells are often seen in healing lesions.

In pneumonia, there are bronchial changes together with thickening of the alveolar walls and lymphocytic infiltration. Secondary infection is common in fatal cases.

(h) Herpes virus infections

The group of herpes DNA viruses includes cytomegalovirus, varicella, Epstein–Barr virus (EBV) and Herpes hominis 1 and 2. Although EBV may cause death from splenic rupture in the young, the syndromes associated with these infections seldom cause diagnostic difficulty and they will not be considered further.

Herpes virus type 2 produces necrotizing lesions in the liver, adrenals, oesophagus and skin. Where liver involvement is extensive, a disseminated intravascular coagulopathy (DIC) may develop and cause rapid death [11].

(i) Coxsackie and enterovirus infections

Coxsackie virus B4 and 5 may cause myocarditis and sudden death. The myocardium is usually pale and dilated and shows petechial haemorrhages and necrosis; mononuclear cell infiltration is seen and fibrosis occurs after about 10 days. Inflammation of the Islets of Langerhans is sometimes found at autopsy. Associated DIC is usually fatal.

Focal myocardial necrosis may also result from infection with enteroviruses.

Echovirus infections can cause massive hepatic and renal necrosis [12] and rapid death.

(j) Rickettsial infections

The group of spotted fevers are an important, but avoidable, cause of death in those countries where tick-borne infections are common. Two-thirds of cases of Rocky Mountain spotted fever occur in those under 15 years of age and there is a 5–7% mortality rate. Diffuse mononuclear cell infiltration of the myocardium occurs and microinfarcts are seen in the brain following widespread vascular involvement [13].

(k) Fungal infections

These infections occur mainly in the immunosuppressed – often in patients under treatment for leukaemia or other malignant disease. Infections by candida, aspergillus, cryptococcus and zygomyces are seen. The main sites of infection appear to be the gut for candida, the lung for aspergillus, the lung and central nervous system for cryptococcus and the sinuses and blood vessels for zygomyces. However, wide dissemination of candida and aspergillus may be found in severe illness.

(l) Protozoal infections

Malaria is a common cause of death in childhood worldwide and may occur in

Europe in travellers, particularly in immigrant children who are returning from family visits to Africa and Asia.

Amoebic infections may also cause death rarely and the various complications of amoebiasis due to *Entamoeba histolytica* may all occur in children. Other amoebae, such as those in the *Limax* group – in particular, *Naegleria fowleri* – have caused meningo-encephalitis, with death in 5–16 days, following swimming in contaminated pools or rivers [14].

(m) Gastroenteritis

Deaths from gastroenteritis still occur in the United Kingdom. The author has recently seen a case associated with superior sagittal sinus thrombosis. They are common in many countries in the developing world. Important causative organisms include salmonella, shigella, enteropathic *E. coli*, campylobacter, rotarviruses and *Giardia lamblia*.

11.3 MISCELLANEOUS CONDITIONS

Not unexpectedly, the majority of these affect the cardiovascular system.

Polyarteritis nodosa is not uncommon in childhood and is a frequent cause of that rare event in this age-group – myocardial infarction. The relationship of polyarteritis to Kawasaki disease has been discussed extensively; in the author's view, it is likely that they are related [15].

Coagulation defects are a rare cause of myocardial infarction in the young with normal coronary arteries [16] and, in the

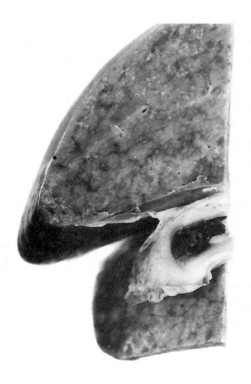

(a)

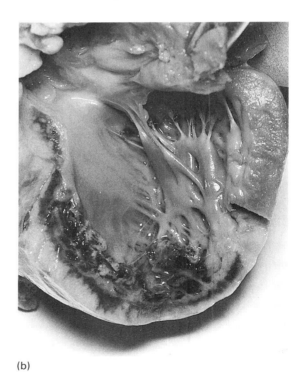

(b)

Fig. 11.7 (a) Thrombus is seen in the ductus venosus. (b) Recent myocardial infarction caused by thromboembolism to the coronary vessels.

neonate, coronary embolism from the ductus venosus with subsequent infarction has been documented [17] (Fig. 11.7).

Schönlein–Henoch purpura may cause sudden death from haemorrhage into specific sites, including the lung [18]. Other defects of the coagulation mechanism seldom cause death in the young but pulmonary bleeding has been fatal in at least one reported case of thrombocytopenic purpura [19].

11.4 REYE'S SYNDROME

Reye's syndrome was first described by an Australian pathologist [20] as a severe neurological disorder complicated by hepatic dysfunction. It is extremely rare, probably occurring in around five per million infants and children per year.

Typically, a prodromal, viral-like illness in a previously healthy child is followed by the onset of effortless vomiting and, later, by altered consciousness and encephalopathy. Liver involvement is indicated by grossly elevated serum levels of aspartate and alanine transaminases and the blood ammonia is usually also raised. Blood glucose is low and the prothrombin time may be prolonged. There are histological and ultrastructural changes in the liver, the cells of which show swollen and ultimately disrupted mitochondria and fatty change which often appears in the form of microvesicular droplets. This form of storage is identifiable in frozen sections if rapid diagnosis is necessary, and squash preparations have been used for cytological diagnosis by Wigger [21].

The pathogenesis of Reye's syndrome depends on acute mitochondrial dysfunction which is probably produced by the uncoupling of oxidative phosphorylation with effects on the mitochondrial dehydrogenases.

(a) Epidemiology

A major problem in the study of this entity is that of specificity of diagnosis. The Centers for Disease Control in Atlanta have maintained a national surveillance of Reye's syndrome in the United States since 1974 and have used the following diagnostic criteria:

(1) There should be encephalopathy but no signs in the cerebrospinal fluid or in brain histopathology to indicate infection or inflammation.
(2) There should be typical fatty change *or* raised transaminases *or* raised blood ammonia.
(3) There should be no other more reasonable explanation for the condition [22].

This is a good working definition but, of course, there are many reasons for children to present with encephalopathy and abnormal liver function tests – including inherited metabolic disease which may mimic Reye's syndrome histologically (see below). The third criterion described above requires diagnostic awareness and also laboratory facilities which are not always available.

A British Reye's Syndrome Surveillance Scheme was set up jointly by the British Paediatric Association and the Public Health Laboratory Service Communicable Diseases Surveillance Centre in 1981. In 4 years (August 1981 to July 1985), 229 cases were reported in the British Isles, giving an annual incidence in 1983–84 of 0.7/100 000 children [23].

The epidemiological features may be summarized:

In the United States, there is an equal sex distribution, a median age of 8–9 years, an excess of cases living in rural areas and a constant time/place association with influenza B and, to a lesser extent, with influenza A. There is also a prodromal association with varicella. Mortality is around 20%.

Some important differences are found in Britain. The median age is younger at 14 months and there is an association with a wide variety of viruses rather than a specific relationship with influenza. The mortality is higher at 50%. An equal sex distribution and an excess of cases in rural areas are also seen in Britain.

(b) Reye's syndrome and aspirin

It was noticed in the 1960s that the symptomatology of Reye's syndrome was similar to that of salicylism and that a significant proportion of cases had a history of aspirin ingestion [24]. In a case-control study carried out in 1980, a dose–response relationship between the stage of coma and the total dose of aspirin was noted [25]. Close similarities between the histopathological changes in the two conditions were pointed out by Starko and Mullick [26].

The evidence from four case-control studies published between 1980 and 1982 (from Arizona, Michigan (two studies) and Ohio) was said to demonstrate a positive association between the use of aspirin and Reye's syndrome. However, these studies were seriously flawed in important respects; a further investigation, designed to eliminate errors, was started in 1983 and was reported in 1985 [27]. Thirty patients with Reye's syndrome and 145 controls, matched for age, race and antecedent illness, were compared; the controls were chosen from different groups based on the hospital emergency room or school or were identified by random digit dialling. It was found that significantly more cases had received salicylates than had members of the four control groups or of all controls combined. In the same year, Rennebohm *et al.* [28] reported an increase of Reye's syndrome in children who were treated with acetyl salicylic acid for connective-tissue disease.

These data collectively, together with an apparent reduction in the incidence of the syndrome where aspirin use has been restricted, have led to a recommendation that acetyl salicylic acid-containing medicines should not be used in childhood.

It is not entirely clear that this recommendation is justified since a number of important areas of bias remain. Selection bias probably existed in the early work, recall bias has occurred, the data may be flawed by the awareness of questioners of the hypothesis to be examined and a case is now more likely to be diagnosed as Reye's syndrome if salicylate has been ingested. Currently, with less aspirin being used, alternative diagnostic labels may be being attached to this type of case.

(c) Reye's syndrome and the sudden infant death syndrome

Consideration of the criteria described above makes it clear that Reye's Syndrome cannot properly be confused with SIDS because of the history of prodromal viral infections. Sinclair-Smith *et al.* [29] reported a high incidence of fatty liver in SIDS but, as is so often found in the literature on this difficult topic, the diagnostic criteria were unclear and no attention was paid to the *systematic* study of fatty change in other modes of death. In general, fatty liver, defined by the presence of visible fat in more than 20% of liver cells, is seen in about 40% of sudden deaths in the community [30]. Cystic fibrosis and alpha-1-antitrypsin deficiency are the commonest causes of steatosis in children but the change may be acquired after prolonged intravenous alimentation, in malnutrition, after drug ingestion and in severe infections.

11.5 METABOLIC DISEASE

If a macroscopically fatty liver is found at autopsy, it is prudent to freeze a portion of this and other organs. The material can be discarded if histological findings indicate simple steatosis; if not, this precaution may help to clarify many issues which are otherwise difficult to resolve.

(a) Glycogen storage diseases

Sudden death is not infrequent in some lysosomal storage diseases, in particular, in glycogenosis type 2a (infantile type of Pompe's disease). In addition to the presence of cardiomegaly, storage is widespread in the central nervous system and the liver, kidney and skeletal muscle are also involved. This autosomal recessive condition is seldom missed providing adequate histological examination is carried out. Moderately distended hepatocytes, with multivacuolated cytoplasm, are seen in the liver; glycogen is also stored in the cell nucleus. Deposition in the cardiac muscle is evident from a yellowish-brown discoloration seen macroscopically and from the distinctive histological appearances (Fig. 11.8).

(b) Disorders of fat oxidation

In conditions in which inadequate glycogen is present in the liver to provide the metabolic source of energy production, long-chain fatty

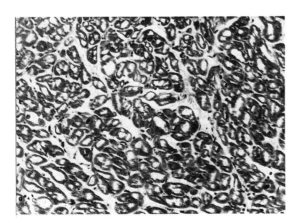

Fig. 11.8 Myocardium in glycogen storage disease. Vacuolation is seen, here exaggerated by post-mortem change (haematoxylin and eosin, × 120).

acids are mobilized from adipose tissue and are β-oxidized in mitochondria. The first step in this metabolic path is a dehydrogenation, and three distinct dehydrogenases deal with long-, medium- and short-chain acyl CoA esters. Genetically determined abnormalities of all these three dehydrogenases have now been described, with medium-chain acyl CoA deficiency (MCAD) being the commonest [31].

This disease usually presents with episodic encephalopathy and hepatomegaly and the illness is often wrongly diagnosed as Reye's syndrome. SIDS may occur but some of those affected by these diseases have never been acutely ill.

(c) Disorders of carnitine metabolism

Long-chain fatty acids enter the mitochondria via a carnitine-dependent step and disorders of fat metabolism may occur if this substrate is deficient. Carnitine deficiency and carnitine palmitoyl transferase deficiency may present with an encephalopathy resembling Reye's syndrome. Sudden death may occur in these conditions.

(d) Urea cycle enzyme deficiencies

This is an important group because a presentation as a sudden death in a family with a history of previous sudden death is not infrequent. Hepatomegaly and hyper-ammonaemia may suggest Reye's syndrome but the hepatic architecture is undisturbed. The biochemical types include ornithine transcarbamylase deficiency, carbamyl phosphate synthetase-1 deficiency, ornithinaemia, citrullinaemia and argino-succinic aciduria [32].

(e) Hypoglycaemia

Hypoglycaemia is an undoubted, if rare, cause of death in children. Hyperinsulinaemic hypoglycaemia occurring in infancy is associated with what has been called the islet cell dysmaturational syndrome – an ugly and inaccurate term; the criteria for diagnosis are discussed by Ansley-Green [33]. It is important to distinguish between hyperplasia of the islets seen in the infants of diabetic mothers, the cases associated with multiple endocrine adenomatosis and true nesidio-blastosis. Judging from cases which are referred, nesidioblastosis appears to be over-diagnosed. For the diagnosis to be made,

small islets and single islet cells should be found scattered around the pancreas; normal islets may either be present or, much less commonly, absent (Fig. 11.9). The total number of insulin-producing cells may not be increased in the pancreas [34] and the paracrine relationship of insulin-producing cells to somatostatin producers in the abnormal glands may be critical [35].

11.6 POISONING

Aspects of this problem are dealt with in Chapter 17. For present purposes, it is only remarked that the pathologist should remember that lead poisoning and poisoning by organic mercurial compounds may cause death without there being a history suggestive of a distinct incident of ingestion of a toxic substance.

(a)
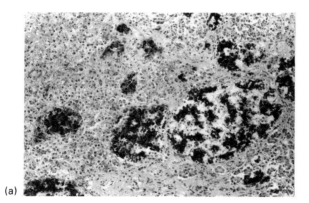

(b)
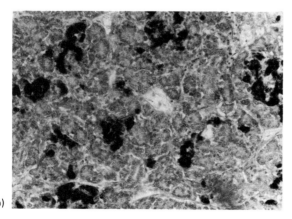

Fig. 11.9 (a) Pancreas in nesidioblastosis. Insulin-producing cells are present in small clumps in the parenchyma as well as in islets (immuno-peroxidase, × 120). (b) Isolated groups of insulin-containing cells are seen throughout the gland.

REFERENCES

1. Berry, C.L. (1989) Congenital malformations, in *Paediatric Pathology*, 2nd edn (ed. C.L. Berry), Springer, Berlin, pp. 41–61.
2. Seagram, C.G.F., Stevens, C.A. and Cumming, W.A. (1977) Peptic ulceration at the Hospital for Sick Children Toronto, during the twenty year period, 1949–1969. *J. Pediatr. Surg.*, **8**, 407.
3. Berry, C.L. (1968) The neonatal thymus and immune paresis. *Proc. R. Soc. Med.*, **61**, 867.
4. Berry, C.L. and Revell, P.A. (1989) Spleen, lymph nodes and immunoreactive tissues, in *Paediatric Pathology*, 2nd edn (ed. C.L. Berry), Springer, Berlin, pp. 565–605.
5. Kaschula, R.O.C. (1989) Infectious diseases, in *Paediatric Pathology*, 2nd edn (ed. C.L. Berry), Springer, Berlin, pp. 653–735.
6. Baker, C.J. and Edwards, M.S. (1983) Group B streptococcal infections, in *Infectious Disease of the Fetus and Newborn Infant* (eds J.S. Remington and J.O. Klein), W.B. Saunders, Washington.
7. Lyell, A. (1967) A review of toxic epidermal necrolysis in Britain. *Br. J. Dermatol.*, **79**, 662.
8. Shinefield, H.R. (1983) Staphylococcal

infections, *Infectious Disease of the Fetus and Newborn Infant* (eds J.S. Remington and J.O. Klein), W.B. Saunders, Washington.

9. Whitley, C.B., Thompson, L.R., Osterholm, M.T. *et al.* (1982) Toxic shock syndrome in a newborn infant. *Pediatr. Res.*, **16**, 254A.

10. Smith, A.L. (1981) Haemophilus influenzae, in *Textbook of Pediatric Infectious Diseases* (eds R.D. Feign and J.D. Cherry), W.B. Saunders, Philadelphia.

11. Whitaker, J.A. and Hardison, J.E. (1978) Severe thrombocytopenia after generalised herpes simplex virus (HSV-2) infection. *South. Med. J.*, **71**, 864.

12. Berry, P.J. and Nagington, J. (1982) Fatal infections with Echovirus 11. *Arch. Dis. Child.*, **57**, 22.

13. Walker, D.H. and Bradford, W.D. (1981) Rocky Mountain spotted fever in childhood. *Perspect. Pediatr. Pathol.*, **6**, 35.

14. Culverton, C.G. (1981) Nageleria and acanthaemoeba (Hartmannella) infections, in *Textbook of Pediatric Infectious Diseases* (eds R.D. Feign and J.D. Cherry), W.B. Saunders, Philadelphia.

15. Berry, C.L. (1983) Kawasaki's disease. *Pediatr. Cardiol.*, **4**, 233.

16. Penny, W.J., Colvin, B.T. and Brooks, N. (1983) Myocardial infarction with normal coronary arteries and factor XII deficiency. *Br. Heart J.*, **53**, 230.

17. Berry, C.L. (1970) Myocardial infarction in a neonate. *Br. Heart J.*, **32**, 412.

18. Leatherman, J.W. Sibley, R.W. and Davies, S.F. (1982) Diffuse intrapulmonary haemorrhage and glomerulonephritis unrelated to anti-glomerular basement membrane antibody. *Am. J. Med.*, **72**, 401.

19. Heiner, D.C. (1977) Pulmonary haemosiderosis, in *Disorders of the Respiratory Tract in Children* (eds E.L. Kendig and V. Chernick), W.B. Saunders, Philadelphia.

20. Reye, R.D.K., Morgan, G. and Baral, J. (1963) Encephalopathy and fatty degeneration of the viscera, a disease entity in childhood. *Lancet*, **ii**, 749.

21. Wigger, H.J. (1977) Frozen section of the liver in the diagnosis of Reye syndrome. *Am. J. Surg. Pathol.*, **1**, 271.

22. Center for Disease Control (1986) Reye syndrome – United State, 1985. *CDC Mortal. Morbid. Week. Rep.*, **35**, 66.

23. Public Health Laboratory Service Communicable Disease Surveillance Centre and British Paediatric Association (1985) Reye's syndrome surveillance scheme. Third annual summary report. *Br. Med. J.*, **291**, 329.

24. Rodgers, G.C. (1985) Analgesics and Reye's syndrome: fact or fiction?, in *Reye's Syndrome IV* (ed. J.D. Pollack), National Reye's Syndrome Foundation, Bryan.

25. Starko, K.M., Ray, C.G., Dominguez, L.B. *et al.* (1980) Reye's syndrome and salicylate use. *Pediatrics*, **66**, 859.

26. Starko, K.M. and Mullick, F.G. (1983) Hepatic and cerebral pathology findings in children with fatal salicylate intoxication: further evidence for a causal relationship between salicylate and Reye's syndrome. *Lancet*, **i**, 326.

27. Hurwitz, E.S., Barrett, M.J., Bregman, D. *et al.* (1985) Public Health Service study on Reye's syndrome and medications. Report of the pilot phase. *New Engl. J. Med.*, **313**, 849.

28. Rennebohm, R.M., Heubi, J.E., Dougherty, C.C. and Daniels, S.R. (1985) Reye syndrome in children receiving salicylate therapy for connective tissue disease. *J. Pediatr.*, **107**, 202.

29. Sinclair-Smith, C., Dinsdale, F. and Emery, J. (1976) Evidence of duration and type of illness in children found unexpectedly dead. *Arch. Dis. Child.*, **51**, 424.

30. Berry, C.L. (1987) Liver lesions in an autopsy population. *Hum. Toxicol.*, **6**, 209.

31. Stanley, C.A., Hale, D.E. and Coates, P.M. (1983) Medium chain acyl CoA dehydrogenase deficiency in children with non-ketonic hypoglycemia and low carnitine levels. *Pediatr. Res.*, **68**, 284.

32. Syderman, S.E. (1981) Clinical aspects of disorders of the urea cycle. *Pediatrics*, **68**, 284.

33. Ansley-Green, A. (1982) Hypoglycemia in infants and children. *Clin. Endocrinol. Metab.*, **11**, 159.

34. Grotting, J.C., Kassel, S. and Dehner, L.P. (1979) Nesidioblastosis and congenital neuroblastoma. *Arch. Pathol. Lab. Med.*, **103**, 642.

35. Hirach, H.J., Loo, S., Evans, N. *et al.* (1977) Hypoglycaemia of infancy and nesidioblastosis. Studies with somatostatin. *New Engl. J. Med.*, **296**, 1323.

CHAPTER 12

Concealment of birth, child destruction and infanticide

D.A.Ll. Bowen

While the subjects of concealment of birth, infanticide and child destruction form a compact group for forensic or medicolegal consideration and although, historically, there are similarities in their legal development, they are not necessarily alternative charges in a court of law. It might be thought that these matters are now much less important than was formerly the case. But, quite recently, considerable interest in the Infant Life (Preservation) Act 1929 surrounded a case involving a father's petition to prevent an abortion on the grounds that it would constitute the offence of child destruction [1]. The statute has also been invoked recently when a child's death occurred *in utero* following an assault on its mother [2]. A thorough knowledge of the subject is, therefore, essential.

12.1 CONCEALMENT OF BIRTH

This offence was first outlined in a statute of 1623 [3] as concerning a live-born illegitimate child whose body is disposed of by its mother in order to conceal its death. Its concept was to allow prosecution of those women who would otherwise escape a charge of murder or infanticide due to the difficulty of proving live

birth; it was provided that the woman, if found guilty, should suffer death as in the case of murder.

This savage Act was repealed in 1803 [4], after which conviction for the offence was possible only after acquittal on an initial indictment for murder. Until 1922, it was the only alternative to a conviction for murder when, following a birth in poor conditions, a woman had caused the death of her newly born child. The possibility of conviction for concealment of birth following an acquittal of murder, manslaughter or child destruction was, however, abolished by the Criminal Law Act 1967, Sch. 2. The offence of concealment of birth was included in the Offences Against the Person Act 1861, s.60 and is still a competent charge irrespective of a live or stillbirth or how the death occurred; it is not necessary to produce the child's body if it can be shown otherwise that the mother has been delivered of a child recently. The charge can, therefore, be used as an alternative to that of infanticide and it does not involve serious punishment – the maximum sentence on conviction is imprisonment for 2 years; the Offences Against the Person Act has, thus, served to dilute the importance of the offence. In past years, much effort was expended in showing some secret disposition of the body, and, thus, providing a case for concealment of birth, so that the matter could be dealt with under s.60 of the 1861 Act; if this failed, the woman had to be sentenced to death on a conviction of murder – although a reprieve was highly likely. It was not until 1922 that the Infanticide Act provided for an alternative to murder or manslaughter in such cases.

The essence of the offence relating to secret disposition of the body of the baby is of some importance. It depends, basically, on whether the body will be found easily; it does not, necessarily, involve burial or partial destruction of the body – indeed, actual physical concealment is not necessary. A dead baby left in an unfrequented field in winter would fulfil all the requirements of secret disposition; it might not be so if it was left on a pathway in the summer, the likelihood being that the baby would be found. Secret disposition, therefore, depends not so much on the place where the body is discovered, i.e. whether it be a mountain peak, the cliff or the seashore, but, rather, on the likelihood of the place being secluded, i.e. not visited by a number of people. This would certainly exclude such simple areas of disposition as the top of a bedroom wardrobe or, for instance, on a lavatory cistern. It must be remembered that the disposal of the child's body must occur after death; the conditions of murder or manslaughter are fulfilled if a living child is concealed and later dies in that concealment. The child must be mature – presumably of legal viability (see below); no offence is committed if a fetus of 2–3 months' gestation is concealed.

From a purely practical viewpoint, the pathologist will seldom have difficulty in dealing with the case. The finding of a decomposed or mummified baby in the absence of a mother or other responsible person is a matter which the coroner will investigate initially, although it is not usually a matter which benefits from detailed forensic investigation. In the absence of serious injuries, the examination of the body will, as likely as not, shed no light as to a separate existence and this leads, almost invariably, to a conclusion of stillbirth. Following a police inquiry, and if no charges are forthcoming, the coroner will transmit to the registrar a certificate setting out the facts so far as they are known.

The legal history of the comparable offence in Scotland is remarkably similar; it is now defined in the Concealment of Birth (Scotland) Act 1809. This provides that the offence is committed:

> if . . . any woman in Scotland shall conceal her being with child during the whole period of her pregnancy, and shall not call for and make use of help or assistance in the birth, and if the child be found dead or be amissing . . .

Thus, the offence is really that of concealment of pregnancy and is, in practice, even more difficult to prove. The rationale of the Act is that, but for the concealment of the child, it would have been born alive; it is thus probable that no offence is committed if the fetus is not viable or if it is stillborn [5].

12.2 CHILD DESTRUCTION

This offence, which exists in the lacuna between unlawful abortion and infanticide, is defined in the Infant Life (Preservation) Act 1929. Child destruction is committed when any person, with intent to destroy the life of a child capable of being born alive, by any wilful act causes it to die before it has an existence independent of its mother; this is subject to the provision that no person shall be found guilty of the offence unless it be proved that the act which caused the death of the child was not done in good faith for the purpose of preserving the life of the mother. The immediate purpose of this exception was to ensure that the operation of cranioclasis – or crushing of the fetal head – was not a criminal act when it was performed so as to relieve an obstructed labour. Caesarian section is now commonplace in such circumstances and the main medical interest of the Act now lies in the management of the living abortus (see Chapter 25).

Child destruction is an offence alternative to murder or manslaughter of a child or to infanticide or to unlawfully procuring the miscarriage of a woman – a person who is charged initially with murder or manslaughter or under the Offences Against the Person Act 1861, ss. 58 or 59 and who is found not guilty may, nevertheless, be found guilty of child destruction. Thus, the distinction between illegal abortion and child destruction is not clear cut and was rendered even less so through the well-known case of R v. Bourne [6]. In this instance, the distinguished gynaecologist, Mr Alec Bourne, terminated the 6 weeks' pregnancy of a 14-year-old girl on the grounds that continuation of the pregnancy would endanger her life; he was subsequently charged under the Offences Against the Person Act 1861 as having unlawfully procured her miscarriage. Mr Bourne's defence was that he had acted with the highest motives owing to the patient's health having been endangered by pregnancy and that, in such circumstances, it was lawful to cause abortion. At the trial, McNaghten J drew heavily on the Infant Life (Preservation) Act 1929, his view being, first, that it referred explicitly to the law on abortion in that a person should not be convicted unless the operation was not done in good faith in order to preserve the life of the mother and, secondly, that any distinction between danger to life and danger to health was artificial insofar as impairment of health might reach the stage at which there was a danger to life and that, in the instant case, continuation of the pregnancy might make the mother a physical or mental wreck. Mr Bourne was acquitted.

Other circumstances in which criminal charges may be brought under the Infant Life (Preservation) Act include assault. A young man was so charged in 1986 following an incident involving an assault on a pregnant woman which resulted in stillbirth [7]; he was later found guilty of child destruction and was sentenced to 16 years' imprisonment [2].

The importance of the 1929 Act in abortion legislation was highlighted in February 1987 when an Oxford University student sought a High Court injunction to prevent his former girl friend, who was 18 weeks' pregnant by him, from obtaining an abortion [1]. The father's case depended upon the interpretation of the words' capable of being born alive' in the 1929 Act. In defining the offence of child destruction, the Act simultaneously introduces the legal presumption that a fetus which has reached 28 weeks' gestation is capable of being born alive; but it does not state – or even imply – that an infant of lesser gestational age is incapable of live birth. The father contended that a fetus of 18–21 weeks' gestation would show discernible signs of life including that of a beating heart; it would, therefore, be born alive and would fall to be registered as a live birth under the Births and Deaths Registration Act 1953. Expert evidence was, however, that the fetus, if delivered by hysterotomy, would be unable to breath either naturally or with the assistance of a ventilator. Judgement was to the effect that a fetus which was incapable of breathing was incapable of being born alive within the meaning of the Act and, accordingly, termination of pregnancy would not constitute an offence under the 1929 Act. This was sufficient to justify – indeed, to compel – the court to dismiss the application irrespective of all questions as to the right of a father to apply for an injunction of this nature or of the fetus to be regarded as a legal person with a right to representation. (See Chapter 25 for further discussion.)

It is noted that the Infant Life (Preservation)

Act 1929 does not run to Scotland where the comparable offence would be dealt with at common law [8]. Similar statutory provisions are in force in Northern Ireland by virtue of the Criminal Justice Act (Northern Ireland) 1945, s.25.

12.3 CHILD MURDER AND INFANTICIDE

(a) Historical aspects

Child murder may be defined as murder of a person less than 18 years of age and as such forms a large and important group of deaths in young persons. It is important to differentiate between various forms of child homicide. 'Neonaticide' is a somewhat contrived and inexact term which has been used by some to mean the killing of an infant in the first 24 hours of its life [9]; others have attempted to apply the word to the passive 'letting-die' of the deformed newborn [10] (see Chapter 28) – in any event, the word has no special legal connotation. In many jurisdictions, infanticide means the killing of a child below the age of 1 year; it has a particular statutory meaning in England and Wales where it is confined to killing by a mother – the term must, therefore, be used with caution unless it is qualified. Filicide involves the killing of a person below the age of 18 years by a parent or step-parent; but such a term, including others, such as matricide or uxoricide, is again purely descriptive. The numerous accounts throughout the world literature of child murder have adopted varying attitudes from century to century and from culture to culture. Infanticide, in the broad sense, was common in Biblical times, the worst recorded example being Herod's slaughter of the infants. Many tribal societies have practised infanticide. There are references in Greek mythology to ritual sacrifice (after killing their two sons, Medea told the unfaithful Jason: 'Thy sons are dead and gone, that will stab

thy heart') [11]. Bedouins buried unwanted daughters in desert sand and Eskimos exposed their children on the ice. Violent disposal of children has been prevalent in the past in the United Kingdom; 25% of all deaths recorded in the nineteenth century were of infants less than 1 year, and this is probably an underestimate. Records made between 1843 and 1858 show that from 46% to over 80% of all illegitimate infants died under 12 months of age; those babies born to single women in poverty were particularly susceptible. The practice of wet nursing allowed a mother to provide milk for another child – something which provided a powerful financial incentive – while, at the same time, her baby might have been taken away and placed 'in the care of' another family or 'farmed out'. The scandal of baby farming was exposed when it was discovered that many such infants died from starvation [12].

The crime of child murder has been considered over the centuries as being less serious than that of adult homicide; the distinction rested on the questionable concept of personhood (q.v.) and on the view that infants were replaceable. In the Middle Ages, unmarried mothers were often driven to destroy their babies rather than be ostracized by society and, in particular, castigated by the forces of Church and State. Martin Luther advocated the drowning of mentally defective children as he thought they were instruments of evil [13]. Hunter [14], addressing the British Medical Society in 1783, referred to special circumstances surrounding the events of killing babies which required that the crime be differentiated from adult homicide.

The Infanticide Act 1938 also has an interesting historical background. Prior to 1922 any act carried out by the mother of a child which resulted in its death was the subject of a charge of murder or manslaughter but there was a considerable body of both medical and legal opinion which argued on humanitarian and social grounds that infanticide is less reprehensible than are other forms of murder. Consequently, a conviction was seldom obtained and, even when it happened, the sentence of death pronounced by the judge was not confirmed.

The basic considerations were that an injury causing the death of an infant causes less suffering than does one inflicted on an adult; the evil in the crime was less, in that the motive on the mother's part depended on the wish to conceal the birth from society; moreover, it was often promoted or precipitated by disturbance of the mother's mind following the birth. The 1938 Act provides that where a woman, by any wilful act or omission, causes the death of her child being less than 12 month of age and where, at the time, the balance of her mind is disturbed by reason of her not having fully recovered from the effects of giving birth, or, further, by reason of the effect of lactation consequent upon the birth, the offence which would normally be regarded as murder, may be considered as the offence of infanticide – which, in practice, amounts to manslaughter. The original Act of 1922 restricted infanticide to a newly born child but it soon became clear that such an imprecise status required clarification; the precipitating case was one in which a mother was found guilty of murder of her baby because the alternative of infanticide was thought to be inapplicable to a child aged as much as 35 days [15].

The concept of mental illness being a cause of infanticide is no longer acceptable as, in many cases, the relationship between incomplete recovery from the effects of childbirth and infanticide is not clear cut. The Butler Report [16] considered that a defence to a charge of a mother murdering her baby would fall into the category of diminished responsibility; the Criminal Law Appeal Committee, however, thought that a charge of infanticide was preferable in such circumstances as it clearly excluded the possibility of the mother being charged with murder.

There are other good social reasons why the charge of infanticide should depend on whether or not the mother's mind was disturbed by reason of giving birth to the child or, more significantly, on circumstances consequent upon the birth; the environmental stress associated with childbirth, the psychological demands on the mother, her inability to care for the child, and the lack of accommodation and physical poverty may all cause great mental stress. Such mitigating factors are widely recognized irrespective of statute; there is no Infanticide Act in Scotland but, nevertheless, a mother killing her infant will always be charged with culpable homicide rather than with murder.

(b) Medical aspects and autopsy studies

It is here that the pathologist plays a vital part and whether or not a charge is brought will depend upon his findings; this is particularly applicable if the child is found dead shortly after birth. It is essential in such circumstances to ascertain whether the child has had a separate existence and whether legal viability has been established although, in theory, the proof or not of this does not necessarily prejudice a prosecution or committal proceeding. It must also be remembered that the death of a newly born infant may be due to natural causes or that it may be associated with a lack of care or facilities at birth which do not necessarily involve foul play.

The circumstances of infanticide can include those involving frank or obvious harm to a baby where, even to lay eyes, the child had a separate existence. On the other hand, it may be the circumstances surrounding the finding of the dead body themselves which are inherently suspicious, such as when a dead baby is found abandoned on waste ground or concealed in a cupboard.

External examination

The pathologist must first consider how his findings relate to the legal viability of the baby he is examining at autopsy. In law a child of 28 weeks' gestation is presumed to be capable of being born alive; nowadays, however, survival of babies well below 28 weeks of development is not uncommon in neonatal units. The relevant examination must include measurement of both height and weight. The child's length must be measured using a paediatric measuring rule from crown to heel and crown to rump. Taking the former, a well-known formula is that the measurement in centimetre length is divided by 5, e.g. a 7-month fetus is 35 cm in length. A baby weighing less than 2500 g is considered to be premature and, in general, an assessment of viability depends upon the infant being at least 5.5 lbs or 2500 g regardless of the presumed gestation period (Fig. 12.1).

The development of the centres of ossification is also important: at 28 weeks, the talus and calcaneum will contain centres; the cuboid bone, the lower end of the femur and the upper end of the humerus are ossified at 40 weeks. A quick rule of thumb is that there should be six centres of ossification in a mature baby – the proximal head of the humerus, the distal condyle of the femur, the proximal condyle of the tibia, the talus, calcaneus and cuboid.

Ossification centres may also be estimated by X-ray serial sectioning, a highly specialized procedure. Examination of the teeth is the province of a forensic odontologist. The deciduous dentition begins to calcify at 2–4 months before birth, i.e. after 20–28 weeks in utero; the jaw should be X-rayed and the state of the whole dentition compared with standard charts. Stack [17] used a method based on the increasing weight of developing teeth, calculated after dissecting them out, and compared this against a weight/age regression line. This method is said to be valuable from 5 months before birth to 7 months afterwards but it obviously requires skill and considerable experience.

There may be clear findings which indicate live birth, including separation of the umbilical cord, which usually dries in about 24 hours after birth and detaches after 4 days. Microscopical studies on the umbilical cord

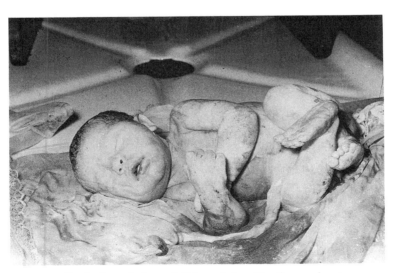

Fig. 12.1 Typical newly born full-term fetus. Death was due to drowning.

indicate that an inflammatory reaction begins between the cord and navel skin after 3 hours of the mature infant's life, but more slowly in premature infants, disappearing after seven hours. Thrombotic changes in the umbilical vessels indicate survival for several days after birth [18]. Conversely, maceration of the fetus is clear evidence of a stillbirth (Fig. 12.2). There is little distinctive change in the appearance of the fetus or baby if death occurs *in utero* 12–24 hours prior to delivery; there will be no evidence of post-mortem change in the tissues and, externally, there will be no blistering or discoloration. Early signs of maceration, consisting of a few blistered areas chiefly over the pressure points on the limbs, with general discoloration of the skin, are seen

if death occurs 24–48 hours before delivery. Maceration will be quite obvious if 3–5 days have elapsed between death and delivery.

Internal examination

The examination of a newborn child must include provision of evidence as to the state of aeration of the lungs; the presence of air in the stomach, intestines and the middle ear; whether there is milk in the stomach; and the state of the umbilical cord.

Examination of the lungs must be carried out after ligation of the trachea; the results have long been considered as being invaluable in distinguishing live from stillbirth but this is not necessarily correct. The lungs may be obviously expanded and aerated and this is presumptive evidence of a live birth so long as decomposition changes are excluded. Microscopical demonstration of the presence of hyaline membrane provides additional evidence [19]; contrariwise, the finding of

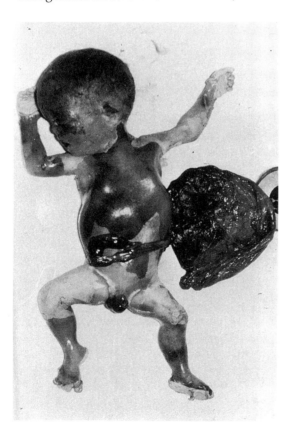

Fig. 12.2 Maceration of the fetus.

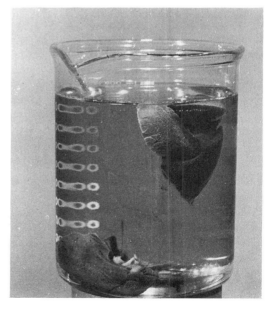

Fig. 12.3 Lung flotation test. There is a clear distinction between the aerated lungs which have floated and those from a stillbirth which have sunk.

squames and/or meconium in the alveoli is indicative of a stillbirth. Recent immuno-histochemical work suggests that, where pulmonary surfactant is not produced, the lung parenchyma is unable to open the alveoli by respiration; a diagnosis of respiratory distress syndrome rather than infanticide may, then, be presumed [20]. Not infrequently, the lungs may appear solid, congested and collapsed when a live birth has followed resuscitative measures and artificial respiration has failed to expand the lungs. The flotation or hydrostatic test is that which is traditionally described and performed in order to distinguish living lung tissue from that derived from a stillbirth (Fig. 12.3), but it must be remembered that lung tissue from an infant with pneumonia, atelectasis or decomposition may give a false result [21]. The lungs from a live-born baby should float in water. If they do so, cut portions of the lung are similarly treated and, should these float, a compression test is performed – the lung tissues are enclosed in a piece of material and are firmly compressed. If the original flotation was due to post-mortem decomposition and gas formation, the firm pressure should be sufficient to expel the gas from the tissue – the compressed lung will sink. Initial failure of the lung tissue to float may indicate stillbirth. One should bear in mind the possibility that breathing may have taken place during the process of birth and that, therefore, a positive test would not necessarily indicate a separate existence [22]. Microscopical examination may also reveal particles of foreign bodies in fluid obtained from the air passages in suspected cases of drowning, but it is important to differentiate these from the normal amniotic fluid debris which may be present. The stomach should be tied off at both ends, floated in water and opened under water to ascertain whether air is present. Similarly, the middle ear cavities should be examined under water as air may reach the middle ear cavities while swallowing during

life. Again, decomposition must be excluded. In practice, proof of live birth is difficult, and probably impossible, in the face of severe decomposition of the body .

A further difficulty facing the pathologist is that, even though there may be signs of lung aeration, the fact of a separate existence cannot be confirmed unless it can also be shown that the child has been completely separated from its mother. It is certainly possible for a baby to have breathed during the process of delivery but the fact that it has breathed would not prove that a separate existence was established in a child who was found dead following delivery. The difficulty in assessing whether a newborn child has had a separate existence is such that, in the majority of cases, a dogmatic statement on the point can now be made; interpretations of the results of examinations designed to assess a separate existence should be treated with great caution. Nevertheless, the pathologist cannot conclude that the infant was stillborn simply because the fact of a separate existence is in doubt; the possibility of a charge of child destruction still remains and this was, indeed, a major reason behind the Infant Life (Preservation) Act 1929. The distinction between stillbirth and child destruction – as between natural death and infanticide – depends, ultimately on whether or not a cause of unnatural death is discovered.

(c) **Cause of death**

It will be appreciated, therefore, that it falls to the pathologist to ascertain the cause of any perinatal death in which there are grounds for suspicion. The supportive role of a paediatric pathologist is particularly important in this field as there is a number of pathological conditions, particularly those demonstrable only on microscopic examination, of which specialized knowledge is essential. The cause of death will be either natural or unnatural,

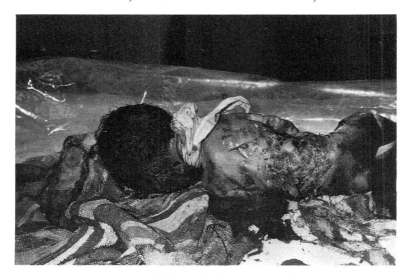

Fig. 12.4 A ligature around the neck of a neonate who was, in fact, considered to have been stillborn.

the former including the respiratory distress syndrome, cranial birth trauma, infection and septicaemia. Unnatural causes of death may result from acts of omission such as inattention at birth, airway obstruction, hypothermia, precipitate delivery followed by drowning in the lavatory pan – or from acts of commission which may be due to obstruction of the airway, stabbing, strangulation, cut throat or poisoning.

The two most common methods of infanticide are strangulation and suffocation. There may be obvious signs of suffocation due to imprint of the hand across the mouth or neck, with or without asphyxial changes, the development of the latter depending on the speed with which interruption of the airway has occurred. The presence of a cord or ligature around the throat (Fig. 12.4) or obstruction of the mouth by a gag may or may not be prima facie evidence of infanticide or, since others than the mother may be involved, murder. On the one hand, it is not known for distraught mothers at the time of delivery to thrust a wad of material into the baby's mouth or secure the neck by a piece of string in the hope and belief that it will not breath – a successful effort would amount to child destruction. On the other, a distinction must be made from efforts by the mother to release the child during the process of birth which can result in abrasions around the neck and on the face; their pattern is usually different from that produced by other forms of malicious external violence. Much will depend on the background history and the precise findings. Cerebral injury, with or without skull fractures, will require careful evaluation, particularly because innocent birth trauma is likely to arise in just that situation where · infanticide might be suspected – the single, young girl undergoing an unassisted labour. Blunt injuries to the skull or crushing blows will give a different pattern from those produced by a birth injury, in which the examination usually reveals torn dura particularly in the sharp edge of the tentorium or falx. Less common causes of violent death include stabbing and infanticidal throat wounds – as was alleged on the basis of the examination of the clothing in the celebrated Australian case involving Mrs Chamberlain and the dingo [23]. Drowning in a lavatory pan (Fig. 12.5) may be responsible for death

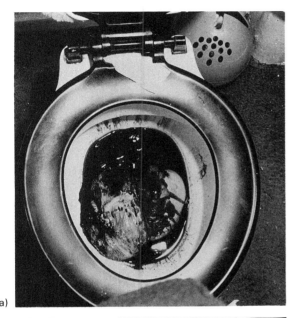

(a)

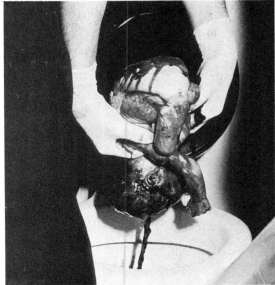

(b)

Fig. 12.5 (a),(b) Precipitate delivery in a lavatory pan.

immediately after birth [24]. Although the lung changes may be characteristic of inhalation of water and the diagnosis of death by drowning not in dispute, the history must be carefully assessed as it is not unknown for the mother to be unaware that she was about to give birth to a child and, even, for her not to have known about or understood her pregnancy. In such circumstances, the short time elapsing between intra- and extra-uterine environments may prevent the development of pulmonary expansion and inhalation of water. In cases involving older childen – late infanticide or murder – poisoning may be most difficult to detect owing to the lack of history and the absence of abnormalities at initial examination. It is therefore important to collect samples of the stomach contents, blood and liver for toxicological analysis in any suspicious infant death – and it has to be appreciated that there is an overlap between sudden natural and unnatural death in this age group.

In general, it is important, both from the medical and investigative legal points of view, to be aware of the need to differentiate between infanticide and cot death. Some years ago, Asch [25] suggested that many apparent cot deaths occurring during the period of potential post-partum depression were, in fact, instances of hidden infanticide. In the face of the difficult pathology of the sudden infant death syndrome (see Chapter 10) it is difficult to deny or prove this thesis objectively; indeed, the whole concept and its investigation causes considerable reaction in the individuals, groups and societies dealing with supportive care of cot death parents. The proposition was studied by Kukull and Peterson [26] after SIDS became a certifiable cause of death in 1963. Their premise was that, if homicides had been misclassified as SIDS after that time, the trend in figures for criminal deaths would have changed; instead, the death rates remained unaltered. The possibility of infanticide, *vis-a-vis* cot deaths, has also been investigated in Sheffield where there is a closely knit organization relating the autopsy to the psychosocial investigation of cot deaths. The results give some credence to the view that up to 1 in 10 cot deaths could be cases of filicide [27].

Resnick [28, 29] made a major study of infanticide and considered that there are two distinct types which he designated as neonaticide and filicide; the former refers to the death of an infant on the day of its birth and the latter to the murder of a son or daughter over 24 hours old. Most neonaticides, as thus defined, are perpetrated by mothers, a small percentage of whom are psychiatrically disturbed; mothers are again responsible for the majority of filicides, although here fathers contribute significantly (Table 12.1). Resnick further divided filicides into five categories according to causation (Table 12.2). The 'unwanted' group is self-explanatory as are the 'acutely psychotics'. 'Altruistic' murders are intended to relieve the victim of real or imaginary suffering; 'accidental' deaths essentially comprise the category of baby battering; and 'spouse revenge' filicide is regarded as a reactive

Table 12.1 Age of murderers [28]

Age (years)	Maternal filicide		Paternal filicide	
	No.	(%)	No.	(%)
20–24	11	(18)	0	
25–29	16	(26)	8	(50)
30–34	15	(25)	5	(31)
35–39	9	(15)	1	(6)
40–44	6	(10)	2	(13)
45–50	4	(6)	0	
Subtotal	61	(100)	16	(100)
Unknown	27		27	
Total	88		43	

Table 12.2 Classification of child murder by apparent motive [29]

Category	Maternal neonaticide		Maternal filicide	
	No.	%	No.	%
'Unwanted child' murder	29	83	10	11
'Acutely psychotic' murder	4	11	21	24
'Altruistic' murder	1	3	49	56
'Accidental' murder	1	3	6	7
'Spouse revenge' murder	0		2	2
Total	35	100	88	100

mechanism designed to cause suffering to the spouse. The main distinction between neonaticide and filicide is to be found in their different motivating circumstances. Children who are the victims of neonaticide are not wanted, the mothers rarely seek abortion, they fail to seek advice on the pregnancy, they sometimes deny pregnancy and, in general, assume that the child will be stillborn. Neonaticides are also associated in some cases with cool premeditation; mothers do not harm themselves and seldom use guile to escape detection. In practice, the law does not differentiate between neonaticide and filicide; both are legally infanticide when maternal in origin and they are treated similarly – but it is clear that, from the medical point of view, not every case of maternal child murder is the result of a post-partum psychosis.

D'Orban [30] emphasized this differentiation in a study of 89 women charged with killing or attempting to murder their children in a female remand prison. Fifty per cent of these maternal filicides resulted in a verdict of infanticide, the courts, thus, recognizing that psychiatric disorder was probably responsible for the offence; d'Orban's clinical opinion, however, was that 9 of the 23 women convicted of infanticide could not be regarded as suffering from mental disorder as defined in the Mental Health Act 1969, s.4 [31]. A parallel study from Japan [32] reported on 71 cases involving 18 filicides and 53 neonaticides. The authors divided these into the anomie type – that is those involving disregard of the law – which were associated with single unmarried mothers having a first child, and 'Mabiki' involving married mothers with several children who were living in poverty.

There is some difficulty in English law as to whether there is such an entity as attempted infanticide; in so far as infanticide itself is a partial defence to murder, it would seem that only charges of attempted murder or concealment of birth would be appropriate following an unsuccessful attempt by a mother to kill her infant. This interpretation has, however, been overtaken judicially. In the relevant case, a child was wrapped in towelling and placed in a cupboard – it was rescued alive by neighbours; McCOWAN J ruled that a charge of attempted infanticide was proper and an appropriate indictment was formulated under the Criminal Attempts Act 1981, s.1 [33]. This seems only right and the probability is that this precedent will be followed in the future.

In fact, legal attitudes to maternal filicide have demonstrated a remarkable swing of the pendulum in the last century. Infanticide once carried savage penalties; it is now doubtful if any woman convicted of the offence would be sentenced to anything more than a period of probation.

12.4 OTHER FORMS OF CHILD HOMICIDE.

Murder or manslaughter of older children differs little from such homicide of adults. Frequently, the death of a child is the culmination of the period of prolonged physical abuse which is discussed in Chapter 14; motivation for killing is, however, seldom overt and convictions for manslaughter, rather than for murder, are the rule.

Finally, a word must be said of the new product of high-technology civilization – the allowing to die or selective non-treatment of the defective newborn [34], a concept which is discussed in detail in Chapter 8. While the great majority of instances are solved on the basis of good professional practice, a particularly interesting situation arises when parents refuse to consent to treatment of their neonate in opposition to medical advice. It is only in these circumstances that the deaths are likely to be subject to medicolegal inquiry and, here, the forensic pathologist would do particularly well to obtain the advice and assistance of his paediatric colleague; more commonly, the problems are those of an ethical nature which are discussed in Chapter 28.

REFERENCES

1. *C* v. *S* [1988] QB 135.
2. *R* v. *Virgo* (1987) *The Times*, 26 September, p. 3.
3. 21 Jac 1 (1623), c. 27.
4. 43 Geo 3 (1803), c.58.
5. Gordon, G.H. (1978) *The Criminal Law of Scotland*, 2nd edn, W. Green, Edinburgh, p. 810.
6. [1939] 1 KB 687.
7. [1987] *The Times*, 19 January, p.3.
8. Gordon, G.H. (1978) *The Criminal Law of Scotland*, 2nd edn, W. Green, Edinburgh, p. 727.
9. Wilkey, I., Pearn, J., Peters, G. and Nixon, J. (1982) Neonaticide, infanticide and child homicide. *Med. Sci. Law*, **22**, 31.
10. Mason, J.K. and McCall Smith, R.A. (1987) *Law and Medical Ethics*, 2nd edn, Butterworths, London, p. 102.
11. Oates, W. and O'Neill, E. (eds) (1938) Euripides *Medea*, in *The Complete Greek Drama*, Random House, New York.
12. Cohen, D. (1969) To live or let die. *Aust. N.Z. J. Surg.*, **56**, 429.
13. Haffter, C. (1968) The Changeling. History and psychodynamics of attitudes to handicapped

children in European folk lore. *J. Behav. Sci.*, **4**, 55.

14. Parry, L.A. (1931) Dissertation by William Hunter on uncertainty of signs of murder in the case of bastard children. *Br. Med. J.*, **2**, 1143.
15. *O'Donoghue* (1927) *Cr. App. R.*, **20**, 132.
16. Report of the Committee on Mentally Abnormal Offenders (1975) Cmnd 6244, paras 19.23 – 19.24.
17. Stack, M.V. (1960) Forensic estimation of age in infancy by gravimetric observations on the developing dentition. *J. Forensic Sci. Soc.*, **1**, 49.
18. Janssen, W. (1984) *Forensic Histopathology*, Springer, Berlin.
19. Kuoda, S., Namon, H., Ebe, M. and Sasarki, M. (1965) Medico-legal studies on the foetus and the infant. Histological characteristics of the lungs of liveborn and stillborn infants. *Jpn J. Legal Med.*, **19**, 7.
20. Morita, M., Fujiwara, H., Shionoh, H. and Ohtani, O. (1987) Studies on the pulmonary surfactant – with special reference to using monoclonal antibodies against human pulmonary surfactant and its application, in *Proceedings of the 11th Meeting of the International Association of Forensic Science*, Vancouver.
21. Knight, B. (1987) *Legal Aspects of Medical Practice*, 4th edn, Churchill Livingstone, Edinburgh, p. 249.
22. Rentoul, E. and Smith, H. (eds) (1973) *Glaister's Medical Jurisprudence and Toxicology*, 13th edn, Churchill Livingstone, Edinburgh, p. 406.
23. Cameron, J.M. (1984) The dingo murder in retrospect. *Medicolegal J.* **52**, 173; Gerber, P.

(1987) Playing dice with expert evidence: the lessons to emerge from *Regina* v. *Chamberlain*. *Med. J. Aust.*, **147**, 243.
24. Mitchell, E.K. and Davis, J.H. (1984) Spontaneous births into toilets. *J. Forensic Sci.*, **29**, 591.
25. Asch, S.W. (1968) Crib deaths; their possible relation to post-partum depression and infanticide. *Mt. Sinai J. Med.*, **35**, 214.
26. Kukull, W.A. and Peterson, D.R. (1977) Sudden infant death and infanticide. *Am. J. Epidemiol.* **100**, 485.
27. Emery, J.C. (1985) Infanticide, filicide and cot deaths. *Arch. Dis. Child.*, **60**, 505.
28. Resnick, P.J. (1969) Child murder by parents. A psychiatric review of filicide. *Am. J. Psychiatry.*, **126**, 325.
29. Resnick, P.J. (1970) Murder of the newborn. A psychiatric review of neonaticide. *Am. J. Psychiatry*, **126**, 1414.
30. d'Orban, P.T. (1979) Women who kill their children. *Br. J. Psychiatry*, **14**, 560.
31. See now Mental Health Act 1983, s.1; Mental Health (Scotland) Act 1984, s.1.
32. Sakuta, T. and Saito, S. (1981) A socio-medical study on 71 cases of infanticide in Japan. *Keio J. Med.*, **30**, 155.
33. *R.* v. *K A Smith* [1983] *Crim. L. R.*, 739. See Wilkins, A.J. (1985) Attempted infanticide. *Br. J. Psychiatry*, **146**, 206.
34. Lund, N. (1985) Infanticide, physicians and the law. The 'Baby Doe' amendments to the Child Abuse Prevention and Treatment Act. *Am. J. Law Med.*, **11**, 1.

CHAPTER 13

Post-mortem biochemistry of blood and vitreous humour in paediatric practice

John I. Coe

The utility of post-mortem chemistry is receiving increasing recognition in forensic laboratories; this parallels a steady expansion of the body of literature addressing the topic. Biochemical studies may identify the cause of death, they may help in assessing the physiological effects of the anatomic findings at autopsy or they may aid in determining the time of death.

A significant proportion of the published reports concerns infants and children. It is the purpose of this chapter to review those articles that deal with natural deaths in the paediatric population, including the sudden infant death syndrome (SIDS), and with certain forms of child abuse. To this end, discussion will be directed primarily towards articles concerned with blood and vitreous humour. For the most part, material on cerebrospinal fluid, joint fluid, bile, urine, pericardial fluid and tissue will not be included.

13.1 FACTORS FOR EVALUATION OF POST-MORTEM BIOCHEMISTRY

There are four major factors to be considered in the proper evaluation of post-mortem studies of blood or vitreous humour:

(a) Time of sampling

Samples must be obtained during the early post-mortem period. This is defined as the time between death and the onset of putrefaction; it may vary from a few hours to several days. In blood specimens, it represents the period prior to the onset of significant haemolysis. The vitreous humour specimens during this interval consist of crystal-clear, colourless fluid; they become cloudy and brownish in colour with the onset of decomposition.

(b) Sample source and acquisition

Studies on blood glucose [1], insulin [2], pH [3], oxygen tension [4], lactate dehydrogenase [5], alkaline phosphatase [6] and certain drugs [7–9] all demonstrate significant differences between specimens which are taken from the two sides of the heart or between specimens of cardiac blood and those obtained from peripheral vessels. It is, therefore, critical to know the source of blood that is submitted for examination. Blind cardiac puncture is never acceptable; in general, peripheral venous specimens – either femoral or subclavian – are the most satisfactory in providing post-mortem values that best approximate to those found in the living individual.

Vitreous humour should be obtained by means of a needle and small syringe with *gradual* application of suction. The use of Vacutainer, or similar, tubes, which have a strong initial suction, often causes fragments of retina or other tissue to contaminate the specimen; such particulate matter will distort the biochemical values. With care, over 1 ml of vitreous can usually be aspirated from each eye, even in newborn infants. Centrifugation, with eventual use of the supernate, prevents clogging of the fine tubing that is used in most current analytical instruments. All the vitreous that can be extracted should be withdrawn, as the concentration of many solutes varies between the humour next to the retina and that obtained from the centre of the globe.

(c) Analytical methodology and normal values

Studies on serum and vitreous samples show that the values obtained for many components vary according to the particular analytical methods used [10, 11]. Such variations may not cause any problems of interpretation for some substances but they may be critical to the proper evaluation of other chemicals. The forensic scientist must, therefore, determine reference ranges for his or her own laboratory. Only then can useful attempts be made to compare the data obtained with those provided in the literature.

(d) Variations in the individual vitreous humours

A number of different investigators have compared the chemical values obtained from the vitreous of each eye [12–15]. Most of these studies demonstrated no significant difference between the two eyes when the specimens were withdrawn simultaneously, but they were all small series. Recently, Balasooriya *et al.* [16] found that, in 60 individuals from whom vitreous specimens were drawn from both eyes at the same time, there were variations in the concentrations of potassium, sodium and/or urate between the eyes. The values for potassium alone varied by more than 10% from the mean values from both eyes in 18.6% of the group studied. It must be concluded that comparison of the values in specimens drawn from the two eyes at different times after death may not always give a true indication of what the post-mortem change has been.

13.2 CARBOHYDRATES

Several articles concerned with glucose and lactic acid concentrations have paediatric forensic implications.

(a) Glucose

Experimental and autopsy studies [1, 17] have demonstrated the importance of proper specimen selection in the evaluation of post-mortem glucose values. This is due to several factors. Samples from the right side of the heart or from the inferior vena cava will usually have a very high glucose content as a result of glycogenolysis in the liver with diffusion of the resultant glucose into adjacent vessels. Thus, blind cardiac puncture or the use of pooled blood from the pericardial sac may give high serum values indicative of a diabetic condition when none exists. Parenthetically, the demonstration of a low glucose concentration in blood from the right atrium, particularly if in conjuction with a positive test for ketones, is evidence of starvation and may support other findings of abuse or neglect.

Very high glucose values may be found in

non-diabetics even when blood is obtained from an extremital vessel [1, 17, 18]. This may be due, in part, to the secretion of catecholamines in terminal stress but, as documented by the author [18], it is more commonly the result of cardiopulmonary resuscitation. I found that the peripheral serum glucose values exceeded 500 mg/dl (27.8 mmol l^{-1}) in over 10% of 1000 consecutive deaths and this can cause problems in diagnosing diabetic hyperglycaemia. Gormsen [19] substantiated that cardiopulmonary resuscitation could increase post-mortem peripheral vascular glucose but concluded that uncontrolled diabetes could still be diagnosed from properly performed blood studies.

Because of the difficulty of interpreting post-mortem blood glucose values, an increasing number of investigators are turning to the vitreous glucose content for evidence of ante-mortem hyperglycaemia [18, 20–23]. Glycolysis routinely causes a marked fall in the blood glucose of non-diabetics within a short time after death but it has little effect on the elevated vitreous glucose of the uncontrolled diabetic. The author, in analysing over 6000 vitreous humour specimens using glucose-specific laboratory procedures, has never found values exceeding 200 mg/dl (11.1 mmol l^{-1}) in the non-diabetic population, even in individuals dying under acute stress or receiving cardiopulmonary resuscitation. The diagnosis of diabetic ketoacidosis is, thus, easily made by showing a high glucose value and the presence of ketones in the vitreous humour. These findings remain valid even after embalming [24].

The following published cases from the author's experience [23, 24] reveal the significance of vitreous glucose analyses in the paediatric population:

Case 13.1
A 10-year-old female in apparent good health developed a fever and acute pharyngitis with an elevated leucocyte count. A throat-swab culture revealed β-haemolytic streptococci. She was treated with penicillin and improved initially but continued to suffer from a sore throat and fever. A second physical examination showed the pharynx to be still mildly inflamed and revealed evidence of dehydration. Following this, the patient became listless and was found dead in bed 7 days after the onset of her symptoms. No urinalysis had ever been performed. The autopsy revealed no significant gross or microscopic findings. The glucose content of the vitreous humour was 924 mg/dl (51.3 mmol l^{-1}) and there was a 4+ qualitative test for ketones. Vitreous sodium concentration was 176 mEq/l (176 mmol l^{-1}), chloride 134 mEq/l (134 mmol l^{-1}) and urea nitrogen 64 mg/dl (22.8 mmol l^{-1}). These studies established a diagnosis of diabetic ketoacidosis with a severe terminal dehydration.

Case 13.2
A 17-year-old insulin-dependent girl entered a religious group who persuaded her to discontinue her medications. She deteriorated rapidly and died in coma. Autopsy showed no cause of death and no biochemical studies were made. Vitreous humour obtained after exhumation – 11 days after death – revealed a glucose content of 772 mg/dl (42.8 mmol l^{-1}) and an acetone of 17 mg/dl ($2900 \mu\text{mol l}^{-1}$). The embalming fluid contained a significant amount of isopropanol but no glucose or acetone.

Mildly elevated vitreous glucose values (60–180 mg/dl) ($3.3–10.0 \text{ mmol l}^{-1}$) have also helped to support a diagnosis of hypothermia in paediatric deaths [21].

The normal vitreous glucose levels which are found in many cases of SIDS exclude hypoglycaemia as being a significant factor in this syndrome.

(b) Lactic acid

Attempts to diagnose ante-mortem hypoglycaemia from post-mortem glucose studies alone have proved unsuccessful because of the glycolysis which occurs in blood, vitreous humour and cerebrospinal fluid. Traube [25] proposed that hypoglycaemia might be diagnosed by combining the values for glucose and lactic acid in the cerebrospinal fluid but he did not substantiate the concept. Working on Traube's hypothesis, Sippel and Mottonen [26] examined the combined values for glucose and lactic acid in the vitreous humour of both diabetics and non-diabetics. When expressed in milligrams per decilitre, combined values above 375 mg/dl excluded hypoglycaemia and over 410 mg/dl represented decompensated fatal diabetes mellitus; they suggested that combined values below 160 mg/dl might indicate hypoglcaemia but had no cases with which to support their hypothesis. By contrast, Sturner *et al.* [27] presented several examples of children without ante-mortem hypoglycaemia whose combined values of vitreous glucose and lactic acid were less than 100 mg/dl. Thus, it seems that there is still no reliable way in which hypoglycaemia can be diagnosed by post-mortem studies at the present time.

The study of lactic acid by Sturner's group [27] concerned 102 infants dying from a variety of causes including SIDS, respiratory disease and mechanical asphyxia. There was variation in the average value for each group, with the lowest average value (137 ± 51 mg/dl) (15.4 ± 5.7 mmol l^{-1}) being found in the cases of mechanical asphyxia. Sturner felt that such low values are an additional diagnostic marker which, in combination with the circumstances and autopsy findings – especially the presence or absence of petechiae – might be useful in distinguishing mechanical asphyxia from SIDS.

13.3 NITROGEN RETENTION

(a) Urea and creatinine

Many studies have demonstrated the stability of urea and creatinine in the body after death so that nitrogen retention may be evaluated by analysis of post-mortem blood, vitreous humour or cerebrospinal fluid [12, 20, 28, 29, 30, 31, 32, 33, 85]. The author [24] has also shown that there is only mild dilution of urea nitrogen in the vitreous after embalming so that cases of uraemia are easily identified in such cadavers. The stability of creatinine and urea nitrogen has been helpful in evaluating equivocal renal autopsy findings in paediatric cases in which the kidneys were damaged either through natural disease or through toxic processes. In addition, discovery of mild nitrogen retention, in association with evidence of electrolyte imbalance, can be used to verify ante-mortem dehydration.

(b) Other nitrogenous compounds

Other nitrogenous compounds, such as amino acids, ammonia, etc., all increase in value in the serum with an increasing post-mortem interval. This precludes their use as a measure of ante-mortem renal function but did encourage Schleyer to include them among a group of substances that he analysed in an attempt to evaluate the early post-mortem interval [50].

13.4 ELECTROLYTES

(a) Sodium and chloride

Both sodium and chloride, the values for which fall erratically in the serum after death [37], tend to remain quite stable in the vitreous humour during the early post-mortem period [12, 15, 30, 34]. It has been shown that elevated or depressed sodium and chloride values in the vitreous humour indicate an ante-mortem serum abnormality of comparable direction and degree; this is true not only in adults but also in the paediatric population including infants [15, 20, 35, 36]. As a consequence, it is possible through vitreous studies to determine the pre-existence of an ante-mortem hyperosmolar electrolyte imbalance with or without apparent physical evidence of dehydration. Clinical dehydration is commonly accompanied by evidence of moderate urea nitrogen retention (40–100 mg/dl) (14.3–35.7 mmol l^{-1}).

Likewise, the pre-existence of conditions resulting from an excessive salt loss will be apparent from the finding of significantly depressed vitreous sodium and chloride concentrations. Whereas sodium in the vitreous mirrors that in the serum, chloride values in the former tend to be around 120 mEq/l (120 mmol l^{-1}). Thus, vitreous humour values of 100 mEq/l (100 mmol l^{-1}), which would be within the normal range for serum, actually indicate ante-mortem hypochloraemia.

A problem connected with the interpretation of vitreous sodium and chloride results lies in the variation in the normal values for these two substances which results from the use of different analytical methods. For example, values indicative of hypernatraemia obtained by flame photometry fall within the normal range when the sodium is measured by ion-specific electrode in the Ektachem system. Similar variations are found in the normal range for chlorides, depending upon the laboratory methodology in use. The author [10] determined the range of values for these two ions using four different laboratory instruments; the results are shown in Table 13.1.

Concurrent determination of the vitreous potassium is important when evaluating the possibility of an ante-mortem hyponatraemia or hypochloraemia in order to separate the true ante-mortem salt-deficiency conditions from the effects of post-mortem decomposition; the latter is also accompanied by a fall in vitreous sodium and chloride values. The concentration of potassium in the vitreous rises with increasing time since death; a low potassium value can, therefore, be used as evidence that low sodium and/or chloride values really do represent an ante-mortem abnormality.

Table 13.1 Range values of sodium and chloride by different tested methods

Ante-mortem abnormality	Vitreous humour values		
	Flame photometry or SMA 6/60	Ektachem 400	Beckman Astra
Dehydration			
Sodium mEq/l or mmol l^{-1}	>155	>165	>155
Chloride mEq/l or mmol l^{-1}	>135	>125	>140
Urea nitrogen (mEq/l)	40–100	40–100	40–100
Urea nitrogen (mmol l^{-1})	14.3–35.7	14.3–35.7	14.3–35.7
Low salt condition			
Sodium mEq/l or mmol l^{-1}	<130	<135	<130
Chloride mEq/l or mmol l^{-1}	<105	<95	<110
Potassium mEq/l or mmol l^{-1}	<15	<15	<15

Emery *et al.* [38] and Huser and Smialek [35] have each reported evidence of dehydration manifested by hypernatraemia and uraemia in infants with symptoms of gastrointestinal infection. Other cases of dehydration, probably associated with the use of hyper-osmolar feeding formulae, were manifested by a marked hypernatraemia alone. Conversely, Blumenfeld *et al.* [36] have reported evidence of hypochloraemia in two infants. The author has noted hypochloraemia in several children who suffered from prolonged vomiting before death.

Several surveys have been made of the vitreous electrolytes in the sudden infant death syndrome. Sturner and Dempsey [39] and Blumenfeld *et al.* [36] showed only minimal variations in infants dying from SIDS as compared to control series. By contrast, Emery *et al.* [38] and Huser and Smialek [35] found cases with hypernatraemia indicating dehydration. Andrew [40] found high urea values in most of his cases of sudden infant death; he attributed these to dehydration but undertook no electrolyte studies to support this view. Mason *et al.* [85] also found elevated urea levels in many cases of sudden death in bottle-fed infants but no evidence of hypernatraemia.

Whether dehydration does, or is thought to, contribute to SIDS will depend upon how this group is defined. If it is strictly limited to those cases for which no cause of death can be found by autopsy including such ancillary studies as post-mortem microbiology, toxicology and chemistry, then many of the dehydration cases of Emery, Huser and Andrew would be excluded. If, on the other hand, the SIDS group is delineated only by there being a sudden death in which there are no significant gross or microscopic morphological findings, then it incorporates a much larger group of infants of which fatalities due to electrolyte imbalance may form a fair proportion.

The use of vitreous electrolytes has also proved invaluable in some cases of child abuse, as is shown in the following two examples. The first case, previously reported by the author [20], provides an instance of a fairly common form of neglect:

Case 13.3
Two children, aged 1 and 2 years, were found unattended after their parents had been absent for several days. The 2-year-old was moribund from dehydration and the infant was dead in his crib. An autopsy on the infant revealed no anatomic abnormalities other than sunken eyes and poor skin turgor. Vitreous studies revealed a sodium concentration of 170 mg/dl $(170 \, \text{mmol} \, l^{-1})$ and a urea nitrogen of 58 mg/dl $(20.7 \, \text{mmol} \, l^{-1})$. The post-mortem chemical analyses provided the most convincing pathological evidence of dehydration when the parents were later brought to trial for neglect.

The forced feeding of salt as a form of punishment is far less common but has been reported by Zumwalt and Hirsch [49]. Another example of such brutality was presented at a forensic seminar by Dr James Benz, Medical Examiner for Palm Beach, Florida:

Case 13.4
A 3-year-old girl was brought by her parents to hospital where she was found to be dead on arrival. An autopsy revealed numerous skin bruises but no internal injuries or natural disease. There was no anatomic evidence of dehydration. Routine vitreous humour studies showed a sodium value of 210 mEq/l $(210 \, \text{mmol} \, l^{-1})$, chlorides 167 mEq/l $(167 \, \text{mmol} \, l^{-1})$, urea nitrogen 31 mg/dl $(11.1 \, \text{mmol} \, l^{-1})$ and osmolarity 442 mOsm/kg. Subsequent investigation established that the child had accidentally spilled a large amount of table salt on her spaghetti dinner. She was forced to eat this

as well as drink a strong solution of salt water which the mother had prepared for 'dessert'. The child shortly became too ill to stand, vomited on the way to the hospital, had a seizure and expired.

Other unpublished examples of child abuse have involved lethal water intoxication due to forced water ingestion. These have been established from the marked hyponatraemia and hypochloraemia which developed.

(b) Calcium and magnesium

Post-mortem studies of serum calcium initially mirror the ante-mortem values. There is then a slow rise with increasing post-mortem time [37, 41]. In contrast, the vitreous calcium, running between 6 and 8 mg/dl (1.5 and 2.0 mmol l^{-1}), maintains a constant value until decomposition sets in and seems to be independent of the serum calcium [12, 13, 42]. No studies to date have implicated calcium in SIDS [36, 38, 39], nor have calcium levels been proved to be of value in elucidating ante-mortem pathology in either infant or adult cases of unexpected death.

Magnesium deficiency has been proposed as a possible cause of SIDS [43] but numerous studies have disproved this hypothesis [36, 38, 83]. Vitreous magnesium values decrease with increasing age. Immature infants average 6.06 ± 0.85 mg/dl (2.05 ± 0.35 mmol l^{-1}; this falls to 2.3 ± 0.3 mg/dl (0.95 ± 0.12 mmol l^{-1}) by adulthood. No post-mortem studies with paediatric forensic applications beyond the investigation of SIDS have been published to date.

(c) Potassium

Vitreous post-mortem values have been found to increase in a linear fashion with increasing post-mortem time. Initially, this was thought to be independent of environmental factors and to give an accurate estimate of the post-mortem interval [44, 45]. However, many more recent studies have indicated that the margin of error is greater than was originally recognized and that the rate of increase is very dependent on the ambient temperature [12, 13, 46, 47]. The author has found vitreous potassium to be of help in estimating the post-mortem interval in adults or older children when the environmental temperature is taken into account [48, 86] but he, along with Mason *et al.* [85], has found it useless in infants, whose vitreous potassium tends to rise much more rapidly than it does in the mature individual. Thus, its use as an indicator of the post-mortem interval in paediatric cases is very limited and is not to be recommended. Because of this rapidly increasing level after death, the post-mortem determination of potassium in either the serum or the vitreous humour cannot be used to determine ante-mortem hyperkalaemia or hypokalaemia.

13.5 PROTEINS AND IMMUNOLOGICAL STUDIES

Several investigators [52, 53] have shown that the ante-mortem and post-mortem total serum proteins and their electrophoretic patterns are essentially the same. This has enabled the author to identify agammaglobulinaemia in one infant in whom it had not been suspected prior to death. Other investigators [54, 55] have studied immunoglobulins and have found good general correlation between ante-mortem and post-mortem specimens. Immunoglobulin studies in cases of SIDS have been reported by three groups whose findings vary [56–58]. Two reported high IgM levels compared with normal infants, while the third reported no difference between IgM or IgE levels found in SIDS victims and healthy infants.

Recently, Guilian *et al.* [59], using electrophoretic separation of the haemoglobin from cases of SIDS, found significantly higher levels of haemoglobin F than was present in age-matched controls. They felt that infants with SIDS are characterized by a marked delay in the switch from haemoglobin F to haemoglobin A, a phenomenon which may reflect an underlying chronic abnormality.

Routine serological studies of post-mortem specimens are being increasingly undertaken and a number of these involve paediatric cases. McCormick [55] studied viral antibodies in a case of Reye's syndrome and the author has used such techniques to identify the aetiological agents in cases of infantile viral myocarditis.

Studies using the Radioallergosorbent test (RAST) to identify bee-sting venoms as the agents of anaphylactic shock and death in adults have been reported by Schwartz *et al.* [60]. Use of the same technique has been reported by two groups of investigators [61] to substantiate the diagnoses of fatal penicillin reactions and of fatal anaphylactic reactions to food, including some cases in the paediatric age-range.

Despite the essential absence from the vitreous humour of proteins which are found in the plasma, certain antibodies have recently been demonstrated in the former when their levels have been high in the post-mortem serum [65, 66].

13.6 ENZYMES

Most enzymes which have been studied to date in blood, vitreous humour or tissue have shown such erratic post-mortem variation as to make interpretation impossible. These include acid phosphatase, alkaline phosphatase, amylase, lactic dehydrogenase, total serum esterase, creatinine kinase, aspartate aminotransferase, alanine aminotransferase, gamma-glutamyl transferase and phosphophenylpyruvate carboxykinase. The one exception is cholinesterase which is discussed below.

While individual values cannot be used in specific cases, it is interesting to note that, as a group, infants dying of SIDS show a significant variation from paediatric control cases in values for transferases, creatinine kinase, lactic dehydrogenase [62] and phosphophenylpyruvate carboxykinase [63].

(a) Cholinesterase

In contrast to the other enzymes studied to date, cholinesterase is stable and shows no significant decrease in activity in non-refrigerated samples up to 3 weeks after death [64]. This is of great significance to the forensic scientist who may be able to establish the presence of organic phosphorus poisoning by noting low cholinesterase values.

13.7 HORMONES

(a) General

Post-mortem studies of 17 hydroxycorticosteroids, cortisol, catecholamines, thyroxin, T_3, TSH, insulin, parathormone, growth hormone, testosterone, luteinizing hormone, chorionic gonadotrophin and melatonin have been reported in the literature. Reference to the early relevant articles may be found in Coe's review [50]. Certain of these have present paediatric interest.

(b) Cortisol

Finlayson [67] established that post-mortem cortisol levels were the same as those during life in both infants and adults and that they remained stable for at least 18 hours. Use of this information has helped to resolve several cases in which congenital hypoplasia or chronic inflammation of the adrenal glands has indicated the possibility of Addison's disease.

(c) Catecholamines

Lund [68] has shown that levels of epinephrine and norepinephrine in the blood rise rapidly after death but that the levels found tend to depend on the acuteness of the lethal process preceding death. The longer the period of terminal stress, the higher the catecholamine level tends to be. On this basis, Hirvonen and his associates [69, 70] have used the discovery of high levels of catecholamines in the urine or vitreous humour as supporting evidence of death from hypothermia.

(d) Thyroid function

The author [71] has demonstrated that thyroxin (T_4) tends to fall slightly with increasing post-mortem time, while thyroid-stimulating hormone (TSH) remains quite stable. Use of these two parameters has enabled investigators to detect true cases of abnormal thyroid function in children although, as Bonnell has pointed out [72], care must be exercised in the interpretation of low thyroxin levels.

Rachut *et al.* [73] found that T_3 values in post-mortem blood taken from normal individuals showed a wide variation from ante-mortem values, ranging both high and low, so that they could not be used for the evaluation of thyroid function. In 1981, Chacon and Tildon [74] made the interesting observation that there was an apparent mean increase in T_3 values in SIDS victims as compared with control groups. This was verified by others [75, 76] but was later shown to be most likely a post-mortem effect [77, 78].

(e) Melatonin

Sturner *et al.* [84] have studied the melatonin levels in the body fluids of infants who died during the night. They found that the levels were markedly lower among children dying from SIDS (blood 11 ± 2 pg/ml, CSF 15 ± 3 pg/ml) than children dying from other causes (blood 35 ± 9 pg/ml, CSF 51 ± 17 pg/ml); they feel that the lower melatonin levels correlate with the diagnosis of SIDS and could represent an impairment of the normal physiological circadian rhythm.

13.8 BLOOD GASES

(a) Oxygen tension

Mithoefer *et al.* [4] performed blood gas analyses on animals in which fatal cardiac or respiratory arrest was induced under controlled conditions; they found that the pO_2 of systemic arterial blood was quite different for these two mechanisms of death. If the pO_2 was greater than 25 mmHg (3.4 kPa), it was indicative that the heart had stopped before the breathing. This was substantiated in humans by Osterberg [50]. While this has not been used as a routine test in paediatric forensic reports, it was studied in association with SIDS by Patrick [51]. He found the mean pO_2 in cases of SIDS to be 13.7 mmHg (1.9 kPa) compared to values of 21.0 and 24.8 mmHg (2.8 and 3.4 kPa) for sudden 'explained' deaths and a random autopsy series respectively. This finding may tie in with the fetal haemoglobin study discussed above.

13.9 VITAMINS

While Rhead *et al.* [79] found values for vitamin E to be low in deaths from SIDS, there is no indication that hypovitaminosis E is either a cause or a good marker of SIDS. In 1982, Davis *et al.* [80] reported that infants dying of SIDS had much higher serum thiamine levels that did their control series. However, Wyatt *et al.* [81] showed these to be simply a port-mortem artefact similar to the high T_3 levels described above.

13.10 HEAVY METALS

Abnormal selenium levels have been postulated as a possible aetiological factor in SIDS but Rhead *et al.* [79] found no difference between the selenium levels of victims of SIDS and controls.

It is not truly germane to this chapter to discuss poisoning by heavy metals such as lead, mercury or arsenic. However, an article by Mittleman *et al.* [82], describing the vitreous findings in a case of acute iron poisoning involving a 21-month-old child, provides an opportunity to stress that vitreous analysis can frequently aid in the evaluation of a variety of toxic substances such as alcohol and the tricyclic drugs.

13.11 SUMMARY

In a significant proportion of cases involving both natural deaths and child abuse, routine chemical analyses of vitreous humour for glucose, urea nitrogen and electrolytes will provide very valuable, and often unexpected, information concerning diabetes mellitus, uraemia and electrolyte imbalances associated with regular dehydration, hyperosmolar dehydration or low salt conditions. The judicious use of a wide variety of other biochemical tests such as protein analysis, immunology, hormone studies and the like may greatly aid in elucidating the cause of death in unusual cases. The forensic pathologist must know what procedures he can expect to provide interpretable post-mortem results.

A large number of biochemical studies have been performed on cases of SIDS with few positive results. Hypoglycaemia, hypocalcaemia, magnesium deficiency, hypogammaglobulinaemia, immunoglobulin anomalies, hormone deficiencies, vitamin abnormalities and selenium poisoning have all been eliminated as aetiological factors. Considering all the cases of sudden unexpected infant deaths, a significant minority have demonstrated hyperosmolar dehydration. Whether these should be included in the true SIDS group is open to definition. Other reported abnormalities in SIDS include low post-mortem pO_2 values, persistence of fetal haemoglobin, lower melatonin levels and an enzyme profile which differs from that of other babies. However, each of these last observations have been made only by single groups of investigators and, so far, they have not been verified by other independent studies. Insofar as SIDS probably represents a physiological death, it remains possible that the key to its aetiology may lie in the biochemical laboratory.

REFERENCES

1. Hill, E. (1941) Significance of dextrose and nondextrose reducing substances in post-mortem blood. *Arch. Pathol.*, **32**, 452.
2. Lindquist, O. (1973) Determination of insulin and glucose postmortem. *Forensic Sci.*, **2**, 55.
3. Straumfjord, J.V. and Butler, J.J. (1957) Evaluation of antemortem acid-base status by means of determining the pH of postmortem blood. *Am. J. Clin. Pathol.*, **28**, 165.
4. Mithoefer, J.C., Mead, G., Hughes, J.M.B. *et al.* (1967) A method of distinguishing death due to cardiac arrest from asphyxia. *Lancet* **ii**, 654.
5. Lythgoe, A.S. (1980) The activity of lactate dehydrogenase in cadaver sera: A comparison of different sampling sites. *Med. Sci. Law*, **20**, 48.
6. Lythgoe, A.S. (1981) Postmortem activity of alkaline phosphatase in serum from different sites of the cadaver cardiovascular system. *J. Forensic Sci. Soc.*, **21**, 337.
7. Gee, D.J. (1974) The poisoned patient: the role of the laboratory. In *Ciba Foundation Symposium 26 (new series)*, Associated Scientific Publishers, New York.
8. Aderjan, R., Buhr, H. and Schmidt, G. (1979) Investigation of cardiac glycoside levels in human post mortem blood and tissues

determined by a special radioimmunoassay procedure. *Arch. Toxicol.*, **42**, 107.

9. Vorpahl, T.E. and Coe, J.I. (1978) Correlation of antemortem and postmortem digoxin levels. *J. Forensic Sci.*, **23**, 329.

10. Coe, J.I. and Apple, F.S. (1985) Variations in vitreous humour chemical values as a result of instrumentation. *J. Forensic Sci.*, **30**, 828.

11. Daae, L.N.W., Teige, B. and Svaar, H. (1978) Determination of glucose in human vitreous humour. *Z. Rechtsmed.*, **80**, 287.

12. Coe, J.I. (1969) Postmortem chemistries on human vitreous humor. *Am. J. Clin. Pathol.*, **51**, 741.

13. Farmer, J.G., Benomran, F., Watson, A.A. and Harland, W.A. (1985) Magnesium, potassium, sodium and calcium in postmortem vitreous humour from humans. *For. Sci. Int.*, **27**, 1.

14. Foerch, J.S., Forman, D.T. and Vye, M.V. (1979) Measurement of potassium in vitreous humor as an indication of the postmortem interval. *Am. J. Clin. Pathol.*, **72**, 651.

15. Swift, P.G.F., Worthy, E. and Emery, J.L. (1974) Biochemical state of the vitreous humour of infants at necropsy. *Arch. Dis. Child.*, **49**, 680.

16. Balasooriya, B.A.W., St. Hill, C.A. and Williams, A.R. (1984) The biochemistry of vitreous humor. A comparative study of the potassium, sodium and urate concentrations in the eye at identical time intervals after death. *Forensic Sci. Int.*, **26**, 85.

17. Hamilton-Paterson, J.L. and Johnson, E.W.M. (1940) Postmortem glycolysis. *J. Pathol. Bacteriol.*, **50**, 473.

18. Coe, J.I. (1975) Postmortem peripheral blood glucose and cardiopulmonary resuscitation. *Forensic Sci. Gaz.*, **6**, (4), 1.

19. Gormsen, H. and Lund, A. (1985) The diagnostic value of postmortem blood glucose determinations in cases of diabetes mellitus. *Forensic Sci. Int.*, **28**, 103.

20. Coe, J.I. (1972) Use of chemical determinations on vitreous humor in forensic pathology. *J. Forensic Sci.*, **17**, 541.

21. Coe, J.I. (1984) Hypothermia: autopsy findings and vitreous glucose. *J. Forensic Sci.*, **29**, 389.

22. Sturner, W.Q. and Gantner, G.E. (1964) Postmortem vitreous glucose determination. *J. Forensic Sci.*, **9**, 485.

23. DiMaio, V.J.M., Sturner, W.Q. and Coe, J.I. (1977) Sudden unexpected deaths after the acute onset of diabetes mellitus. *J. Forensic Sci.*, **22**, 147.

24. Coe, J.I. (1976) Comparative postmortem chemistries of vitreous humor before and after embalming. *J. Forensic Sci.*, **21**, 583.

25. Traube, F. (1969) Methode zur Erkennung von tödlichen Zuckerstoffwechselstorungen an der Leiche (diabetes mellitus und hypoglykamie). *Zentralbl. Allg. Pathol.*, **112**, 390.

26. Sippel, H. and Möttönen, M. (1982) Combined glucose and lactate values in vitreous humour for postmortem diagnosis of diabetes mellitus. *Forensic Sci. Int.*, **19**, 217.

27. Sturner, W.Q., Sullivan, A. and Suzuki, K. (1983) Lactic acid concentrations in vitreous humour: their use in asphyxial deaths in children. *J. Forensic Sci.*, **28**, 222.

28. Hamilton, R.C. (1938) Postmortem blood chemical determinations: a comparison of chemical analyses of blood obtained postmortem with degrees of renal damage. *Arch. Pathol.*, **26**, 1135.

29. Jensen, O.M. (1969) Diagnosis of uraemia postmortem. *Dan. Med. Bull.*, Suppl. VIII, 1.

30. Leahy, M.S. and Farber, E.R. (1967) Postmortem chemistry of human vitreous humor. *J. Forensic Sci.*, **12**, 214.

31. Levonen, E., Raekallio, J. and Saikkonen, J. (1963) Postmortem determination of blood creatinine and urea. *J. Forensic Med.*, **10**, 22.

32. Naumann, H.N. (1949) Diabetes and uremia diagnosed at autopsy by testing cerebrospinal fluid and urine. *Arch. Pathol.*, **47**, 70.

33. Paul, J.R. (1925) Postmortem blood chemical determinations. *Bulletin Ayer Clin. Lab. Pennsylvania Hosp.*, **9**, 51.

34. Jaffe, F. (1962) Chemical postmortem changes in the intra-ocular fluid. *J. Forensic Sci.*, **7**, 231.

35. Huser, C.J. and Smialek, J.E. (1986) Diagnosis of sudden death in infants due to acute dehydration. *Am. J. Forensic Med. Pathol.*, **7**, 278.

36. Blumenfeld, T.A., Mantell, C.H., Catherman, R.L. and Blanc, W.A. (1979) Postmortem vitreous humor chemistry in sudden infant death syndrome and in other causes of death in childhood. *Am. J. Clin. Pathol.*, **71**, 219.

37. Coe, J.I. (1974) Postmortem chemistries on blood: particular reference to urea nitrogen, electrolytes and bilirubin. *J. Forensic Sci.*, **19**, 33.

38. Emery, J.L., Swift, P.G.F. and Worthy, E. (1974) Hypernatraemia and uraemia in unexpected death in infancy. *Arch. Dis. Child.*, **49**, 686.

39. Sturner, W.Q. and Dempsey, J.L. (1973) Sudden infant death: chemical analysis of vitreous humor. *J. Forensic Sci.*, **18**, 12.

40. Andrews, P.S. (1975) Cot deaths and malnutrition: the role of dehydration. *Med. Sci. Law*, **15**, 47.

41. Hodgkinson, A. and Hambleton, J. (1969) Elevation of serum calcium concentration and changes in other blood parameters after death. *J. Surg. Res.*, **9**, 567.

42. Dufour, D.R. (1982) Lack of correlation of postmortem vitreous humor calcium concentration with antemortem serum calcium concentration. *J. Forensic Sci.*, **27**, 889.

43. Caddell, J.L. (1972) Magnesium deprivation in sudden unexpected infant death. *Lancet* **ii**, 258.

44. Sturner, W.Q. and Gantner, G.E. (1964) The postmortem interval: a study of potassium in the vitreous humor. *Am. J. Clin. Pathol.*, **42**, 137.

45. Lie, J.T. (1967) Changes of potassium concentration in the vitreous humor after death. *Am. J. Med. Sci.*, **254**, 136.

46. Hanson, L., Votila, V., Lindfors, R. and Laiho, K. (1966) Potassium content of the vitreous body as an aid to determining the time of death. *J. Forensic Sci.*, **11**, 390.

47. Coe, J.I. (1973) Further thoughts and observations on postmortem chemistry. *Forensic Sci. Gaz.*, **5**(5), 2.

48. Coe, J.I. and Curran, W.J. (1980) Definition and time of death, in *Modern Legal Medicine, Psychiatry, and Forensic Science* (eds W.J. Curran, A.L. McGarry and C.S. Petty), Davis, Philadelphia, ch. 7.

49. Zumwalt, R.E. and Hirsch, C.S. (1980) Subtle fatal child abuse. *Hum. Pathol.*, **11**, 167.

50. Coe, J.I. (1976) Postmortem chemistry of blood, cerebrospinal fluid and vitreous humor, in *Legal Medicine Annual 1976* (ed. C.H. Wecht), ACC, New York, pp. 55–92.

51. Patrick, J.R. (1970) Cardiac or respiratory death, in *Sudden Infant Death Syndrome.*

Proceedings of the Second International Conference on Causes of Sudden Death in Infants (eds A.B. Bergman, J.B. Beckwith and C. Ray), University Press, Washington, p. 131.

52. Coe, J.I. (1973) Comparison of antemortem and postmortem serum proteins. *Bull. Bell Museum Pathobiol.*, **2**(1), 40.

53. Robinson, D.M. and Kellenberger, R.E. (1962) Comparison of electrophoretic analysis of antemortem and postmortem serum. *Am. J. Clin. Pathol.*, **38**, 371.

54. Brazinsky, J.H. and Kellenberger, R.E. (1970) Comparison of immunoglobulin analyses of antemortem and postmortem sera. *Am. J. Clin. Pathol.*, **54**, 622.

55. McCormick, G.M. (1972) Nonanatomic postmortem techniques: postmortem serology. *J. Forensic Sci.*, **17**, 57.

56. Khan, W.N., Ali, R.V., Werthmann, M. and Ross, S. (1969) Immunoglobulin M determination in neonates and infants as an adjunct to the diagnosis of infection. *J. Pediatr.*, **75**, 1282.

57. Urquhart, G.E.D., Logan, R.W. and Izatt, M.M. (1971) Sudden unexplained death in infancy. *J. Clin. Pathol.*, **24**, 736.

58. Clausen, C.R., Ray, C.G., Habestreit, N. and Eggleston, P. (1973) Studies of the sudden infant death syndrome in King County, Washington: IV. Immunologic studies. *Pediatrics*, **52**, 45.

59. Giulian, G.G., Gilbert, E.F. and Moss, R.L. (1987) Elevated fetal hemoglobin levels in sudden infant death syndrome. *New Engl. J. Med.*, **316**, 1122.

60. Schwartz, H.J., Squillace, D.L., Sher, T.H. *et al.* (1986) Studies in stinging insect hypersensitivity: Postmortem demonstration of antivenom IgE antibody in possible sting-related sudden death. *Am. J. Clin. Pathol.*, **85**, 607.

61. Abstracts of papers by Sweeney, K.C. *et al.* and Menchel, S.M. *et al.* presented at the meeting of the American Academy of Forensic Science, San Diego, California, February 1987.

62. Richards, R.G., Fukumoto, R.I. and Clardy, D.O. (1983) Sudden infant death syndrome: a biochemical profile of postmortem vitreous humor. *J. Forensic Sci.*, **28**, 404.

63. Sturner, W.Q. and Susa, J.B. (1980) Sudden infant death and liver phosphophenylpyruvate carboxykinase analysis. *Forensic Sci. Int.*, **16**, 19.

64. Petty, C.S., Lovel, M.P. and Moore, E.J. (1958) Organic phosphorus insecticides and post-mortem blood cholinesterase levels. *J. Forensic Sci.*, **3**, 226.

65. Gregora, Z. and Bruckova, M. (1986) Attempts to demonstrate specific antibody responses in the vitreous body of the eye. *J. Hyg. Epidemiol. Microbiol. Immunol.*, **30**, 195.

66. Pepose, J.S., Pardo, F.S. and Quinn, T.C. (1986) HTLV-III ELISA testing of cadaveric sera to screen potential organ transplant donors. *JAMA*, **256**, 864.

67. Finlayson, N.B. (1965) Blood cortisol in infants and adults: a postmortem study. *J. Pediatr.*, **67**, 284.

68. Lund, A. (1963) Adrenaline and noradrenaline in blood from cases of sudden, natural or violent death, in *Proceedings of the Third International Meeting in Forensic Immunology, Medicine, Pathology and Toxicology*, London, England, April.

69. Hirvonen, J. and Huttunen, P. (1982) Increased urinary concentrations of catecholamines in hypothermia deaths. *J. Forensic Sci.*, **27**, 264.

70. Lapinlampi, T.D. and Hirvonen, J.I. (1986) Catecholamines in the vitreous fluid and urine of guinea pigs dying of cold and the effect of postmortem freezing and autolysis. *J. Forensic Sci.*, **31**, 1357.

71. Coe, J.I. (1978) Postmortem values of thyroxine and thyroid stimulating hormone. *J. Forensic Sci.*, **18**, 20.

72. Bonnell, H.J. (1983) Antemortem chemical hypothyroxinemia. *J. Forensic Sci.*, **28**, 242.

73. Rachut, E., Rynbrandt, D.J. and Doutt, T.W. (1980) Postmortem behaviour of serum thyroxine, triiodothyronine, and para-thormone. *J. Forensic Sci.*, **25**, 67.

74. Chacon, M.A. and Tildon, J.T. (1981) Elevated values of tri-iodothyronine in victims of sudden infant death syndrome. *J. Pediatr.*, **99**, 758.

75. Ross, I.S., Moffat, M.A. and Reid, I.W. (1983) Thyroid hormones in the sudden infant death syndrome (SIDS) *Clin. Chim. Acta*, **129**, 151.

76. Peterson, D.R., Green, W.L. and van Belle, G. (1983) Sudden infant death syndrome and hypertriiodothyroninemia: comparison of neonatal and postmortem measurements. *J. Pediatr.*, **102**, 206.

77. Lee, W.K., Strzelecki, V. and Root, A.W. (1982) Serum T$_3$ values and SIDS. *J. Pediatr.*, **101**, 161.

78. Schwartz, E.H., Chasalow, F.I., Erickson, M.M. *et al.* (1983) Elevation of postmortem triiodothyronine in sudden infant death syndrome and in infants who died of other causes: a marker of previous health. *J. Pediatr.*, **10**, 200.

79. Rhead, W.J., Cary, E.E. Allaway, W.H. *et al.* (1972) The vitamin E and selenium status of infants and the sudden infant death syndrome. *Bioinorganic Chem.*, **1**, 289.

80. Davis, R.E., Icke, G.C. and Hilton, J.M. (1981) High serum thiamine and the sudden infant death syndrome. *Clin. Chim. Acta*, **123**, 321.

81. Wyatt, D.T., Erickson, M.M., Hillman, R.E. and Hillman, L. (1984) Elevated thiamine levels in SIDS, non-SIDS and adults: postmortem artifact. *J. Pediatr.*, **104**, 585.

82. Mittleman, R.E., Steele, B. and Moskowitz, L. (1982) Postmortem vitreous humor in fatal acute iron poisoning. *J. Forensic Sci.*, **27**, 955.

83. Sturner, W.Q. (1972) Magnesium deprivation and sudden unexpected infant death. *Lancet* **ii**, 1150.

84. Sturner, W.Q., Lynch, H.J., Deng, M.H. and Wurtman, R.J. (1987) Melatonin levels in body fluids of SIDS infants. Abstract of paper presented at the XI International Association of Forensic Science, Vancouver, British Columbia, Canada.

85. Mason, J.K., Harkness, R.A., Elton, R.A. and Bartholomew, S. (1980) Cot deaths in Edinburgh: Infant feeding and socioeconomic factors. *J. Epid. Comm. Health.*, **34**, 35.

86. Coe, J.I. (1989) Vitreous potassium as a measure of the postmortem interval: an historical review and critical evaluation. *Forensic Sci. Int.* In press.

CHAPTER 14

Physical abuse of children

John Pearn

The important subject of non-accidental injury involving children has overtones for all involved with the professional care of children and their families. Timely diagnosis of the syndrome of child abuse and neglect almost always prevents a fatal outcome; correct autopsy diagnosis may prevent sibling injury or deaths in the future; in few areas of medicine are there greater responsibilities for pathologists and clinicians, nurses, teachers and neighbours of abused children. It is now realized that the most important preventive stratagem is the development of a high index of suspicion of possible non-accidental injury when suspicious signs become evident.

Health professionals may be called upon to help in a clinical emergency related to a battered child or in securing custody orders to keep children 'at risk' in a place of safety, in giving evidence in court and in performing tests which range in scope from clinical photography to the forensic autopsy. The results of such tests will have to be interpreted in cases in which there is a suspicion of child abuse. Two different types of expertise commonly become intermingled in this area – clinical skills on the one hand and forensic ability and experience on the other [1]. The whole approach to the living child who may have been battered, or the investigation of a fatality, requires the most scrupulous

attention to both these aspects. This chapter is a consideration of the different types of child abuse and the clinicopathological and forensic themes which are inherent in the subject.

14.1 TERMINOLOGY

The phenomenon of physical abuse of children is given different names in different countries. 'Non-accidental injury' (NAI), the 'syndrome of child abuse and neglect' (SCAN) and 'child battering' or 'the battered child' are terms which are used frequently. It was this last term which the late C. Henry Kempe used in 1962, to bring to the notice of a complacent medical profession that this hitherto unthinkable syndrome truly existed [2]. In 1946, the radiologist, Caffey, had first drawn attention to a puzzling association of long bone fractures and subdural haematomata in a series of infants and very young children, a constellation of signs which was difficult to interpret in that era [3]. This was followed in the 1950s by further papers in the radiological literature, calling attention to the occasional occurrence during childhood of fractures without known pathogenic cause [4,5]. Since that time some clinicians have used the term 'Caffey's syndrome' as a form of veiled speech to describe this condition; 'Kempe's syndrome' has been used in like form, usually in a euphemistic sense and often in the context of a low-level code jargon. The two terms which are in majority use currently are non-accidental injury (NAI) and the syndrome of child abuse and neglect (SCAN); this latter term will be used in this review. The whole subject, which is one with a history of less than three decades, is one which is still evolving [6].

14.2 CLASSIFICATION

Debate continues as to whether or not cases of unlawful physical abuse of children are variants of one spectrum or whether distinct and separate conditions exist [7]. Studies of unselected consecutive fatal cases indicate that the latter is correct. Eight such distinct syndromes can be recognized (Table 14.1), each with its specific predispositions, acute precipitating triggers, clinical features and preventive approaches. A summary of these separate SCAN syndromes is shown in Table 14.2, which excludes the subjects of sexual interference with children (see Chapter 15) and emotional abuse (Chapter 16).

14.3 PREDISPOSING FACTORS – HIGH-RISK GROUPS

It is truly said that children of all social classes, from all types of family, and of all subcultures within the broader society may be physically

Table 14.1 Eight syndromes of child abuse

Neonaticide
Infanticide
Euthanasia
Syndrome of repetitive physical child abuse
Child neglect
Murder – suicide
Murder (homicide)
Sexual abuse (non-violent)

abused [8]. However, SCAN is disproportionately more common in families of lower socioeconomic status [9]. It is well recognized that certain predictive factors can be used: (i) to identify individual children 'at risk' prospectively and (ii) to heighten awareness of the possibility of SCAN in the differential diagnosis of specific cases [10].

Syndrome profiles of abusing parents and custodians are now well established. High risk factors include young parents – usually teenagers in the 15–20-year age-bracket, the fact that a parent himself or herself was abused as a child, a mother who was, herself, subjected to incestuous approaches as a child, a family already known to welfare agencies in an unfavourable context, one in which the partners are living in a *de facto* relationship and the presence within the family of handicapped children. Families in which there is manifest ignorance of age-appropriate behaviour of children are also at high risk.

Male consorts of foster mothers, single mothers and baby-sitters are overrepresented in all unselected case series [11]. Studies of children who survived confinement in the concentration camps of World War II, and anecdotal evidence from numerous child abuse treatment centres, have shown that children who live and grow formatively within a violent microenvironment come to accept this as the norm and are more likely, themselves, to indulge in violent and aggressive behaviour in their postchildhood years. This quasigenetic clustering of child abuse [12] is universally accepted but, in fact, has never yet been subjected to prospective confirmatory studies.

Personality testing has revealed that abusive parents relate poorly to their children and to other people and that they have immature and impetuous personalities [13]. Low self-esteem in the child's mother and increased rates of sickness in immediate family members also raise the potential for SCAN.

Table 14.2 Features of the syndrome of physical child abuse

Syndrome	Relative frequency (%)	Victim's age	Predisposition	Time-course	Notes
Neonaticide	20–25	Premature and full-term infants, at or soon after birth	Usually single young mother, often living with parents	Single act, and one of either commission, or an omission of care	Pregnancy often concealed. Antenatal care very uncommon. About half the cases are accompanied by attempted concealment of the body
Infanticide	5	0–6 months	Mother almost always the perpetrator. *Two groups are recognized – maternal psychopathy and maternal psychosis (especially puerperal depression)	Single act	Differential diagnosis includes sudden infant death syndrome; the distinction often impossible
Euthanasia	1–3	Throughout childhood; usually under 3 years	Child almost always has significant physical or mental abnormalities (or both)	Single act	A parent almost always the perpetrator. Perceived to be a subjective altruistic act. Full revelation of facts usually made by the perpetrator. Some parents misguided
Syndrome of repetitive physical child abuse	30–40	6 weeks– 5 years. Rarely older	Often single parents often living in changing, *de facto* or other relationships. History of psychopathy common. Lower socioeconomic status families predominate in diagnosed cases	Multiple pleomorphic assults, often crescendo in severity and frequency	Injuries of all types. Almost always parental (or custodial) denial of the assault. Collusion between knowledgeable parties usually occurs

Child neglect	10	0–3 years	Gross parental psychosis, or mental retardation present. In affluent societies, children always from deprived socio-economic status subgroups	Chronic time-course	Usually in socially or geographically isolated families
Murder–suicide	5–15	0–10 years	Parents always depressed. Both reactive and endogenous depression occurs. An acute pre-disposition (trigger) usually identifiable in retrospect	Single constellation of acts	Psychodynamics include subjective *altruistic* motivation in some cases. Often a whole family is killed, usually in one incident. Sometimes a serious disappointment is the precipitant (trigger) which is superimposed on the background of a chronically depressed person
Murder (homicide)	5–10	0–15 years, usually 0–8 years	Great majority of victims are girls. Most such incidents occur in the context of a sexual assault (in both sexes)	Single act, or an event lasting over several hours	Perpetrators almost always have a history (in retrospect) of psychopathy or psychiatric illness. Sometimes perpetrators are male–female pairs with a dominant male and a *folie à deux* relationship

* The specific English crime of infanticide can *only* be committed by the mother, otherwise, it is murder—[Ed.].

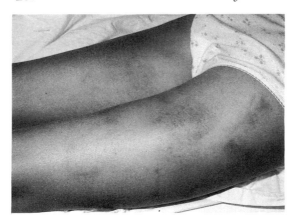

Fig. 14.1 Severe contusions on the thighs of a 12-year-old-girl, beaten with a broad belt by her father as an extreme form of discipline.

Some teenagers – almost exclusively teenage girls – who live in strict conservative family groups are also at risk from severe physical beatings. Such conditions occur particularly in families of central or southern European or Islamic backgrounds who have emigrated to liberal Western societies. Young growing children may be torn between two cultures in such circumstances; extreme physical chastisement may occur if traditional mores are flouted (Fig. 14.1).

Table 14.3 The syndrome of child abuse and neglect: baselines and superimposed acute precipitants (triggers)

Baseline predisposition	Acute triggers
Isolated parent(s)	Acute jealousy of a child
Parent(s) dependent on	in *de facto*
another person;	relationships
Immaturity	Demanding, crying
Personality defects	infant
(psychopathic,	Child faecal soiling
psychotic or antisocial	
backgrounds)	
Low socioeconomic	
status	

A disproportionate number of abusive adults are known to the police unfavourably in respect of matters which are unconnected with a specific suspicious SCAN case. Psychopathic personalities, psychotic parents and parents with low impulse control are all overrepresented in 'at risk' families. SCAN victims sustain their injuries as the result of violent acts which are precipitated by acute situational triggers set against a background of a heightened predisposing baseline. Examples are shown in Table 14.3.

14.4 HISTORY

Presenting symptoms are very important in arriving at a diagnosis of child abuse which, from the forensic point of view, is almost always difficult to prove. Physical evidence of abuse may be totally lacking and is often equivocal. History-taking in such circumstances assumes an even greater significance than it has in clinical medicine or forensic pathology generally. The child victim is usually the only eye-witness to the abuse and the physician's role in eliciting and documenting statements from that source is crucial from the forensic point of view – history-taking must be undertaken in such a way that the statements will be admissible in evidence in any subsequent legal proceedings [14].

Children's initial statements to a parent, neighbour or school teacher are usually considered to be hearsay. Some children under the age of 4 years are able to testify in certain circumstances and many who are older have the psychological competence to give evidence [15]. However, because of their tender years, children are, as a rule, naturally intimidated into silence. They may recant, or deny, earlier descriptions of abuse or of the abuser. For these reasons, history-taking from the child is now often undertaken in association with unobtrusive videotape recording. This subject is, however, also an evolving one and the techniques require special skills and training in legal and forensic approaches. Several exceptions to the normal inadmissibility of hearsay evidence can be made in the case of suspected child abuse in the United States [14].

In taking a history from a child suspected to be a victim of SCAN, the questioning should always be non-leading and the nature of the questions – as well as the answers – should be formally recorded in a hospital chart or on videotape. Questioning should take the form of such approaches as 'What happened?', 'Tell me more', 'Did anything else happen?' etc. [14] and it is essential to have a second adult present as an independent witness. Some important points in interpreting the responses of young children to questioning include:

(1) The duration of the time elapsed between any suspected abuse and the child's statement.
(2) Whether the statement is made spontaneously or in response to questioning by an adult.
(3) Whether the child's statement was a product of reflective thought or was proffered spontaneously.
(4) If in response to questioning, whether the questioning was leading or non-leading. Open-ended questions are less subject to legal challenge.
(5) The state of the child – excited, distressed, what signs of distress.
(6) The child's physical condition when the statement was made.
(7) The exact words used by the child.
(8) Whether the statement was made at the first opportunity when the child felt safe to talk [14, 15].

The history of the presenting injuries is usually taken from parents or care-takers of the child. In the great majority of cases, parents or custodians collude in the history in order to protect each other. For this reason, the parents or custodians will often present together with the child – and often at unsocial

hours. A discrepancy in the history of what has happened can be an important factor in the interpretation of an otherwise puzzling history if the parents present separately [16]. Concerned relatives, such as grandparents or aunts, will sometimes find an excuse to bring the child to the doctor or to medical attention; veiled speech is often used in such circumstances. This, when recognized by the doctor, should heighten suspicions that all is not as it seems. Features in the presenting history which suggest the likelihood of SCAN are shown in Table 14.4.

The commonest history in true SCAN cases is that of a fall or minor accident. Usually, only a single event is acknowledged and a claim that a major traumatic incident, albeit accidental, was the cause is made in very few cases. A common history is 'fell from a couch or settee' or 'fell from the cot'. This history is often extended after it is pointed out by the doctor that multiple asynchronous injuries are present. Abusive parents sometimes state that a child has been injured by a sibling.

Important as the details of presenting symptoms – and their proper documentation – are, it has been found that one of the most significant features is the reaction to the history by the doctor taking it. 'An indefinable feeling of disquiet' or 'a feeling that all is not as it seems' on the doctor's part has been shown in retrospect to be a most valuable point in

Table 14.4 History-taking in cases of suspected child abuse: some characteristic points

---

Unexplained delay in seeking treatment
Submitted history (presenting symptoms) are changed after initial presentation
Discrepancy in the stories given by each parent or care-giver separately
A history incompatible with (or very unlikely at) the age and development of the child
Ambivalence or hostility in the parent or care-giver
Injuries blamed upon a sibling or another child

---

itself. Although it is not, of course, in any way admissible as evidence, the knowledge that such suspicion exists should bring confidence to the health professional who is, thus, encouraged to trust his or her instincts; this will often lead to a more meticulous forensic approach to history-taking, to better documentation and to a more complete investigation of cases that might otherwise have occurred. From the forensic point of view, 'a problem for the pathologist who is not a forensic pathologist may be disbelief leading to denial that a child can be beaten to death' [17]. All who are confronted with social, clinical or autopsy evidence that a child has been abused feel affronted. Some are reluctant to accuse the abuser; others feel guilty themselves, a phenomenon which may be expressed as hostility or self-righteous criticism [18]. It is important to recognize these feelings and to use them as a self-acknowledged cue to adhere to meticulous clinical and pathological techniques on which accurate diagnosis and, in many cases, prevention of further abuse ultimately depend.

14.5 PHYSICAL SIGNS

A wide range of physical signs – protean in form, extent and severity – has been recorded in the physically abused child. At one extreme, no physical, radiological or ophthalmological signs may be present [18]; this is the case in some children who are deliberately partly drowned [19,20] or suffocated. Some children who are killed by the use of pillows and the like may show the usual signs of petechial haemorrhages on the pericardium and pleura and on the meningeal surfaces of the brain; non-fatal cases, however, may not manifest any clinical signs.

At the other extreme, children may present with the most severe injuries. Such tragic cases present either to the clinician in the emergency room or to the forensic pathologist in the mortuary. Burns, contusions, lacerations and fractures may all be present in extreme cases [17]. Features which raise the index of suspicion of SCAN are shown in Table 14.5. Some representative lesions are shown in Figs 14.2–14.10; details of some lesions which are characteristic of SCAN are summarized in Table 14.6.

Ocular damage is a particularly significant sign of child abuse. Typically, periocular signs of trauma are absent; the eye changes that are so frequently encountered in abused infants suggest a cause other than direct contusion of the globe itself. Subretinal, retinal, preretinal, subhyaloid and vitreous haemorrhages have all been described; they are typically bilateral [21]. Vitreous haemorrhages may not develop until after a delay of several days and later scarring of the macula shows a cystic or crater-like configuration [11]. It is believed that the retinal haemorrhages and damage result from splitting of the retina which is due to the direct mechanical effects of violent shaking. Retinal scarring and subsequent loss of visual acuity is less likely to occur if no blood enters the

Table 14.5 Physical signs in the syndrome of child abuse and neglect: principles of interpretation

Child is excessively alert, apathetic or submissive; child manifests a stoic response to painful procedures

Injuries that appear older than the alleged history would suggest

Presence (concurrently) of different types of injury (e.g. fractures together with burns)

Presentation of multiple lesions of different ages (e.g. both acute and chronic fractures or separate burns at different stages of healing)

Multiple lesions from a single cause (e.g. two separate cigarette burns)

Unusual soft-tissue injuries (e.g. avulsion of the frenulum of the tongue or lips; tears of the preputial frenulum)

Suspected lesions covered by sticking plaster, by hair or by clothes

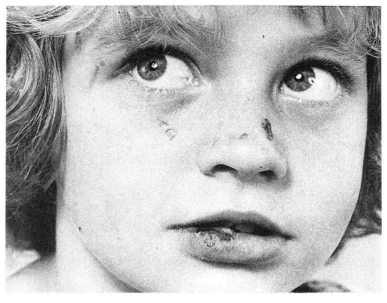

(a)

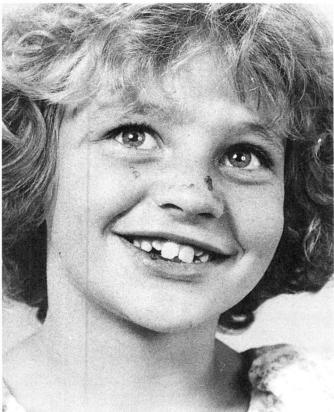

(b)

Fig. 14.2 (a) Facial brusing and lacerations. Syndrome of child abuse and neglect in an 11-year-old-girl. (b) The same girl showing dental trauma from blows to the teeth and mouth.

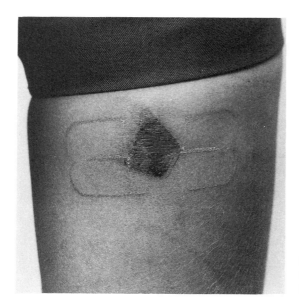

Fig. 14.3 Burn on the thigh of a boy subject to repeated abuse. Note the unusual site, and its typical concealment by adhesive plaster.

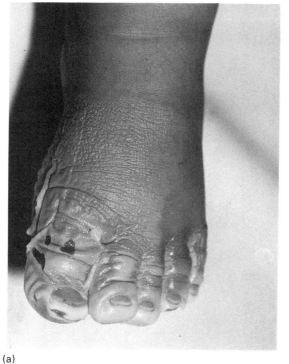

(a)

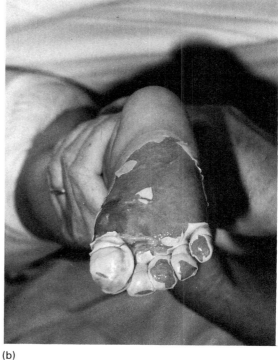

(b)

Fig. 14.4 (a) Foot of a 7-month-old infant deliberately immersed in hot water. Dorsal aspect; note clear-cut upper 'immersion line'. (b) Case in (a). Plantar aspect showing third-degree burns.

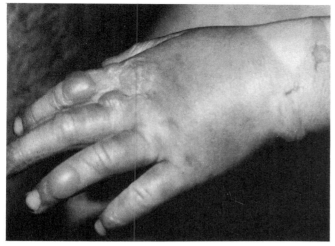

Fig. 14.5 Scalded hand of a 1-year-old infant, deliberately immersed in hot water by an abusing parent. Note depth of immersion, and 'immersion line' implying abuse.

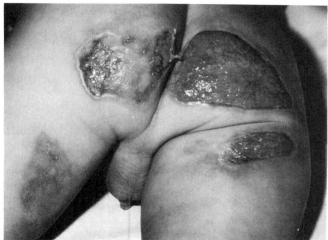

Fig. 14.6 Buttocks of a 10-month-old male infant sat on a stove hotplate by an abusing custodian. Note spanning of intergluteal folds.

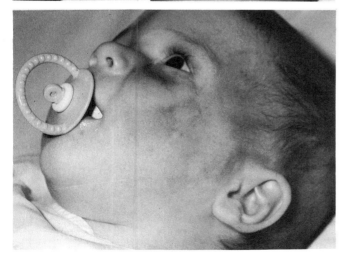

Fig. 14.7 Facial contusions on the left cheek and forehead of a 6-month-old female infant caused by battering by a psychopathic mother.

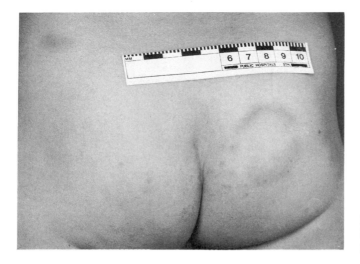

Fig. 14.8 Bite-mark contusion on the buttocks of a 15-month-old infant. Note pattern of adult dentition.

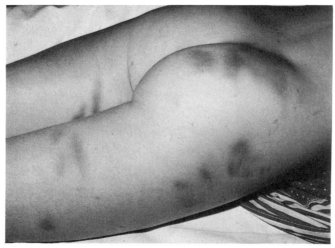

Fig. 14.9 Contusions on the buttocks and thighs of an abused child. Note imprint of finger marks and of a flexible cord-rope-like object.

vitreous humour within a week after the production of retinal haemorrhages [22].

Whiplash injuries and intracranial haemorrhages also result from the 'shaken baby syndrome' [23, 24]. Acute hemiplegia – which is often permanent – and mental retardation are not infrequent sequelae of intracranial haemorrhages due to direct and indirect trauma.

It is essential to examine the hidden parts of the body in both fatal and non-fatal cases of

SCAN. In living children, full fundoscopic examination with an ophthalmoscope, and the use of the fundus camera, are mandatory. Both the vitreous and aqueous humours opacify quickly after death; the fundi cannot be visualized accurately after 6 hours at a standard mortuary temperature of 5 °C (42 °F) – a whitish-ground glass appearance is all that can be discerned and no details are visible. In fatal cases of suspected child abuse, it is essential to remove the eyes – optimally by

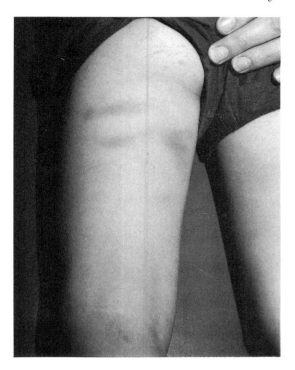

approaching these through the supraorbital plate for aesthetic and cosmetic reasons – for formal histological examination.

Abused children almost always attempt to hide the stigma of abuse; parents often attempt to do so also. Lacerations and contusions about the neck, ears and forehead may be concealed by the arrangement of hair (Fig. 14.2(b)), or by clothes (Figs 14.3 and 14.10). Telltale bruising, imprints from buckles or straps used to thrash children, or burns from branding with cigarettes or hot metal objects may be hidden by adhesive plaster (Fig. 14.3). It it important to preserve a high degree of suspicion when examining a child in which SCAN forms one of the possible differential diagnoses.

Fig. 14.10 Contusions on the posterior aspect of the thighs of a boy, beaten with a strap. Note normal covering by clothing.

Table 14.6 Specific clinical findings which raise the probability that an injury is part of the SCAN syndrome

Lesion	SCAN features
Burns	Burns in unlikely sites (e.g. buttocks). Children may be sat on hot plates, branded with irons or hot metal. Cigarette burns on areas normally covered by clothing, multiple burns
Scalds	Scalds show a clear-cut 'line of immersion' or 'Plimsoll line'. A child reacts to a deliberate scalding incident by reflex flexion resulting in relative protection of the body creases. This often results in a striped pattern [7]. The location or extent of a scald may not be as important as its skin pattern [35]
Bite-marks	Site is important – e.g. buttock lesions are more significant than arm bites. Size of the dental impression (adult vs. child) is important (see Fig. 14.8)
Strap-marks	Clear-cut lesions. Outline of abuse objects (such as electric flex) may be present. Lesions from pieces of wood, straps or whips are seen more commonly in children who are over the age of 3 years
Retinal haemorrhages	Highly suggestive – if not pathgnomonic [36] – of physical abuse in children older than 2 months. Result from shaking, from raised intracranial pressure due to intracranial contusion and haemorrhage [37] or from strangulation
Fractures	Often multiple. May involve ribs as well as long bones and/or skull. Spiral fractures of long bones imply twisting injury. Skull fractures not often parietal as in accidents [33]. Stellate fractures indicate abuse

14.6 DIFFERENTIAL DIAGNOSIS

A differential diagnosis should be constructed in the usual way after the clinical or coronial history has been taken and the child examined externally – or the body in fatal cases. In cases of suspected SCAN, the problem is often not so much that a differential diagnosis is difficult but, rather, that there is a surfeit of potential possibilities. Some of the confounding possibilities of forensic significance are listed in Table 14.7.

In the case of contusions, two points require special attention. The first is that children's bruises heal more quickly than do those of adults. Therefore, the normal time-course of colour changes has to be interpreted with great care. Secondly, most children over the age of 12–15 months have bruises on their arms and legs for most of the time. Bruises on the shins are particularly common, but these ubiquitous innocent lesions virtually never bear any specific imprint or diagnostic feature.

One particularly confusing diagnosis is that of 'pseudobattering', which results from the application of oriental or folk medicine

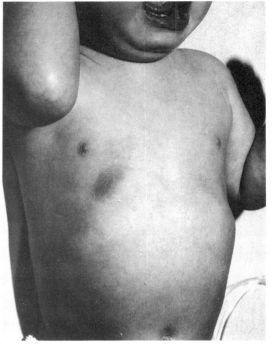

Fig. 14.11 Contusion on the chest of a 7-month-old Vietnamese infant. Lesion caused by coin-rubbing, a form of oriental folk medicine. No abusive intent.

Table 14.7 Differential diagnosis of some clinical signs in the abused child

Sign	Confounding diseases
Fractures	Osteogenesis imperfecta [38]
	Menkes' syndrome [30]
	Atypical skull suture lines
Limb tenderness	Congenital syphilis with periostitis and osteochondritis [39]
Scars	Chickenpox lesions resembling cigarette burns
Bruising	Haemophilia [40]
	Hypersensitivity vasculitis [41]
	Bacteraemia with DIC [28]
	Folk medicine ('Pseudobattering syndrome'); Oriental folk medicine
	Phytophotodermatitis [42, 43]
	Mongolian spot
	Erythema multiforme [44]
Retinal haemorrhages	Resuscitation retinopathy (Purtscher's retinopathy) [45]
Burns	Car-seat burns [46]
	Self-inflicted skin lesions due to sucking (dermatitis artefacta) [1]
Diarrhoea	Administration of magnesium sulphate (one form of Polle syndrome) [47]

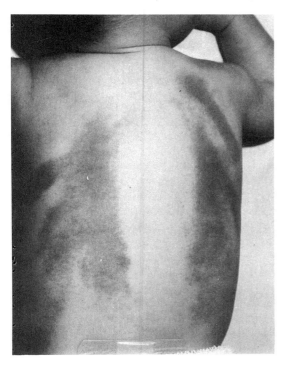

Fig. 14.12 Back of an infant subjected to coin-rubbing and cupping as a form of oriental folk-medicine. No abusive intent.

parents who were the victims of error also tended to be from poorer families, and that mistaken attitudes of suspicion, or hostility, on the part of doctors contributed to the misdiagnosis. Purpura fulminans and disseminated intravascular coagulation (in acute meningitis), Purtscher's retinopathy following resuscitation, the presence of a simple Mongolian spot and normal relaxation of the anal sphincter after death have all been causes of such disasters [30]. Most parents whom the stress of losing an infant is compounded by the severe emotional upset of false accusations of SCAN suffer long-term traumatic psychiatric scars.

Child abuse should, nevertheless, always be considered when a child dies unexpectedly. One recent study from Chicago has suggested that 20% of such unanticipated and unexpected deaths – particularly those occurring in children over the age of 1 year – may be due to child abuse [31].

treatments (Figs 14.11 and 14.12). The condition is particularly common in children of Vietnamese or Chinese extraction and may be due to coin-rubbing of the skin over parts of the body according to ancient medical practice, to 'cupping' or to the application of astringent herbs or chemicals [25, 26]. Such injuries have been noted quite extensively in the last decade [27, 28] and have been observed in most Western countries in which first-generation refugee oriental families are living [29].

A mistaken diagnosis of child abuse leads to some of the worst tragedies in all of clinical or forensic medicine. Physicians or pathologists may mistake life-threatening illness or post-mortem artefacts for intentional injury. A Chicago series of 10 such cases showed that

14.7 INVESTIGATIONS AND RECORDING

The normal meticulous approach to any forensic or coronial autopsy is required in the case of a child who has died suddenly and unexpectedly. In particular, a total radiological skeletal survey is needed and special thought must be given to the administration of drugs and to the possibility of immersion.

In the living child, skilled clinical photography with particular emphasis on the importance of colour matching, the use of videotaped interviews with individuals skilled in both the medical and legal aspects, haematological studies for blood clotting factors, bacteriological assessment of infections – especially those which are sexually transmitted, examination in some cases for spermatozoa and radiographic skeletal survey (see Chapter 19) are particularly needed.

Cranial X-rays have traditionally been regarded as key investigations in the investigations of children suspected of having been physically abused. Skull fractures resulting from accidental falls or impacts tend, as a group, to be single and of narrow linear type [32]; they are seen most commonly in the parietal bones [33]. Such accidental skull fractures are not commonly associated with extradural or subdural bleeding. Features of skull fractures which are the result of child abuse are shown in Table 4.8.

The use of computerized axial tomography (CAT scans) and, more recently, of nuclear magnetic resonance (NMR) has provided a quantum leap in the investigation of children suspected of child abuse. In the absence of frank skull fractures, the discovery of intracranial bleeding due to direct trauma, or resulting from the 'shaken baby' syndrome, or of intracerebral bleeding due to abusive transient anoxia, e.g. from partial drowning, will be of great significance.

Radiological studies are especially important in the case of young children (see Chapter 19). No unexpected lesions were encountered in verbal school-age children over the age of 5 years in a large New York study (involving over 300 skeletal surveys of children suspected of being abused) [34]. The positive diagnostic rate may be expected to be higher in some special groups such as those children who are intellectually disabled, or neurologically abnormal. The particular value

of CAT scans, NMR investigations and X-ray skeletal surveys is that children may manifest no overt clinical signs of quite dramatic underlying bony lesions. Cases are known where infants with recent fractures of the femur and similar severe injuries have crawled and played happily, apparently without pain.

14.8 PROGNOSIS

If a case of child abuse can be diagnosed before serious injury is sustained the chances of further injury or death are low. The likelihood of a crescendo of attacks of physical abuse going on to a fatal termination is somewhere between 2% and 10% [7, 10]; murder is an unwelcome concomitant of abuse to the abuser – it removes the object of his or her attentions and, at the same time, leads to almost certain discovery. In the last decade, most centres in the Western world have established detailed principles of management for cases of suspected SCAN. These have included the implementation of 'standing orders' for emergency rooms and casualty departments of hospitals and the development of skilled SCAN teams with interdisciplinary input from paediatricians, social workers, child welfare officers and specially trained police officers. These latter are, in the most part, plain-clothed skilled operatives, who enter police child protection teams after more general detective or constabulary work. Although the general approach is now everywhere very similar, there are so many national – and intranational – variations that there would be little point in giving a detailed description of any one system. Some aspects of the legal and social protection of children in the United Kingdom and the United States are provided in Chapter 29.

Table 14.8 Radiographic features of skull fractures due to SCAN [33]

Fractures presenting more than 1–2 hours after injury
Multiple complex fractures
Depressed fractures
Maximum fracture width >3 mm
More than one bone involved
Associated intracranial injury on CAT scan or NMR

REFERENCES

1. Reid, D.H.S. (1985) Pitfalls in determining child abuse. *Lancet*, **i**, 1316.

2. Kempe, C.H., Silverman, F.N., Steele, B.V. *et al.* (1962) The battered child syndrome. *JAMA*, **181**, 17.

3. Caffey, J. (1946) Multiple fractures in the long bones of infants suffering from chronic subdural hematoma. *Am. J. Roentgenol.*, **56**, 163.

4. Silverman, F.N. (1953) The roentgen manifestation of unrecognised skeletal trauma in infants. *Am. J. Roentgenol.*, **69**, 413.

5. Caffey, J. (1957) Some traumatic lesions in growing bones other than fractures and dislocations: clinical and radiological features. *Br. J. Radiol.*, **30**, 225.

6. Helfer, R.E. (1977) Where to now, Henry? A commentary on the Battered Child Syndrome. *Pediatrics*, **76**, 993.

7. Wilkey, I., Pearn, J., Petrie, G. and Nixon, J. (1982) Neonaticide, infanticide and child homicide. *Med. Sci. Law*, **22**, 31.

8. Heins, M. (1984) The 'Battered Child' revisited. *JAMA*, **251**, 3295.

9. Shepherd, J.R. (1987) Children as burn victims. *FBI Law Enforcement Bull.*, July, 9.

10. Pearn, J.H. (1982) Child abuse – an overview, with priorities for the future, in *Proceedings of the Second Australasian Conference on Child Abuse*, Government Printer (Qld), Brisbane.

11. Greenwald, M.J., Weiss, A., Desterle, C.S. and Friendly, D.S. (1986) Traumatic retinoschisis in battered babies. *Ophthalmology*, **93**, 618.

12. Argles, P. (1980) Attachment and child abuse. *Br. J. Soc. Work*, **10**, 33.

13. Oates, R.K. (1984) Parents who physically abuse their children. *Aust. NZ J. Med.*, **14**, 290.

14. Myers, J.E.B. (1988) Role of the physician in preserving verbal evidence of child abuse. *J. Pediatr.*, **109**, 409.

15. Summit, R.C. (1983) The child sexual abuse accommodation syndrome. *Child Abuse Neglect*, **7**, 177.

16. Schanberger, J.E. (1981) Inflicted burns in children. *Topics Emerg. Med.*, October, 86.

17. Norman, M.G., Newman, D.E., Smialek, J.E. and Horembala, E.J. (1984) The postmortem examination on the abused child. *Perspect. Pediatr. Pathol.*, **8**, 313.

18. Isaacs, S. (1968) Physical ill-treatment of children. *Lancet*, **i**, 37.

19. Nixon, J. and Pearn, J. (1977) Non-accidental immersion in the bath; another extension to the syndrome of child abuse and neglect. *Child Abuse Neglect*, **i**, 445.

20. Nixon, J. and Pearn, J.H. (1977) Non-accidental immersion in bath-water: another aspect of child abuse. *Br. Med. J.*, **1**, 271.

21. Tongue, A.C. (1986) Discussion of 'Traumatic retinoschisis in battered babies'. *Ophthalmology*, **93**, 618.

22. Mushin, A.S. (1971) Ocular damage in the battered-baby syndrome. *Br. Med. J.*, **3**, 402.

23. Caffey, J. (1974) The whiplash shaken infant syndrome: manual shaking by the extremities with whiplash-induced intracranial and intraocular bleedings, linked with residual permanent brain damage and mental retardation. *Pediatrics*, **54**, 396.

24. Ludwig, S. and Warman, M. (1984) Shaken baby syndrome: a review of 29 cases. *Am. J. Emerg. Med.*, **13**, 104.

25. Asnes, R.S. and Wisotsky, D.H. (1981) Cupping lesions simulating child abuse. *J. Pediatr.*, **99**, 267.

26. Feldman, K.W. (1984) Pseudoabusive burns in Asian refugees. *Am. J. Dis. Child.*, **138**, 768.

27. Yeatman, G.W., Shaw, C., Barlow, M.J. *et al.* (1976) Pseudobattering in Vietnamese children. *Pediatrics*, **58**, 616.

28. Kaplan, S.L. and Feigin, R.D. (1976) Pseudobattering in Vietnamese children. *Pediatrics*, **58**, 616.

29. Du, J.N.H. (1980) Pseudobattered child syndrome in Vietnamese immigrant children. *Can. Med. Assoc. J.*, **122**, 394.

30. Kirschner, R.H. and Stein, R.J. (1985) The mistaken diagnosis of child abuse. A form of medical abuse? *Am. J. Dis. Child.*, **139**, 873.

31. Christoffel, K.K., Zieserl, E.J. and Chiaramonte, J. (1985) Should child abuse and neglect be considered when a child dies unexpectedly? *Am. J. Dis. Child.*, **139**, 876.

32. Helfer, R.E, Slovis, T.L. and Black, M. (1977) Injuries resulting when small children fall out of bed. *Pediatrics*, **60**, 533.

33. Hobbs, C.J. (1984) Skull fracture and the diagnosis of abuse. *Arch. Dis. Child.*, **59**, 246.

34. Ellerstein, N.S. and Norris, K.J. (1984) Value of radiological skeletal survey in assessment of abused children. *Pediatrics*, **74**, 1075.

35. Jewett, T.C. and Ellerstein, N.S. (1981) Burns as a manifestation of child abuse, in *Child Abuse and Neglect: A Medical Reference* (ed. N.S. Ellerskein), Wiley, New York.

36. Eisenbrey, A.B. (1979) Retinal hemorrhage in the battered child. *Childs Brain*, **5**, 40.

37. Tomasi, L.G. and Rosman, P. (1975) Purtscher retinopathy in the battered child syndrome. *Am. J. Dis. Child.*, **129**, 1335.

38. Adams, P.C., Strand, R.D., Bresnan, M.J. *et al.* (1974) Kinky hair syndrome: serial study of radiological findings with emphasis on the similarity to the battered child syndrome. *Radiology*, **112**, 401.

39. Fisher, R.H., Kaplan, J. and Holder, J.C. (1972) Congenital syphilis mimicking battered child syndrome. *Clinical Pediatrics*, **11**, 305.

40. Schiver, W., Brueschke, E.E. and Dent, T. (1982) Family practice grand rounds: hemophilia. *J. Fam. Pract.*, **14**, 661.

41. Waskerwitz, S., Christoffel, K.K. and Hauger, S. (1981) Hypersensitivity vasculitis presenting as suspected child abuse: case report and literature review. *Pediatrics*, **61**, 283.

42. Coffman, K., Boyce, T. and Hansen, R.C. (1985) Phytophotodermatitis simulating child abuse. *Am. J. Dis. Child.*, **139**, 239.

43. Wickes, I.G. and Zaid, Z.H. (1972) Battered or pigmented? *Br. Med. J.*, **2**, 404.

44. Adler, R.A. and Kane-Nussen, B.K. (1983) Erythema multiforme: confusion with child battering syndrome. *Pediatrics*, **72**, 718.

45. Bacon, D.J., Sayer, G.C. and Howe, J.W. (1978) Extensive retinal haemorrhages in infancy. An innocent cause. *Br. Med. J.*, **1**, 281.

46. Schmitt, B.D., Gray, J.D. and Britton, H.L. (1978) Car seat burns in children: avoiding confusion with inflicted burns. *Pediatrics*, **62**, 607.

47. Clark, G.D., Key, J.D., Rutherford, P. and Bithoney, W.G. (1984) Munchausen's syndrome by proxy (child abuse) presenting as apparent autoerythrocyte sensitization syndrome: an unusual presentation of Polle syndrome. *Pediatrics*, **74**, 1100.

CHAPTER 15

Incest and other sexual abuse of children

W.D.S. McLay

To those reared in the Judaeo-Christian tradition, the proscription of incest is scriptural. The Incest Act 1567, which applied in Scotland until 1986, was based on the injunction: 'No man shall approach a blood relation' (Leviticus 18: 6) (Fig. 15.1). The Act, following the detailed words of the chapter, forebad intercourse between a man and his granddaughter, daughter, sister, mother, half-sister, stepmother, aunt, niece, aunt-in-law, daughter-in-law, mother-in-law, sister-in-law, greatgranddaughter and step-daughter; there were, of course, comparable proscriptions of a woman having intercourse with her male relations. The developing parity of authority and responsibility as between male and female has led Western society to soften its attitudes to these biblical rules – and certainly insofar as they would constrain adult behaviour. There are many differences between states and even within states in both law and practice regulating sexual relationships [1]. Thus, the relevant statute in force throughout the larger part of the United Kingdom is the Sexual Offences Act 1956 which declares the offence of incest to be committed when a man has intercourse with a woman he knows to be his granddaughter, daughter, sister or mother, the sister including half-sister and the relationships pertaining whether or not they can be traced through lawful wedlock; the offence may be committed, *mutatis mutandis*, by a woman over the age of 16 years.

The mediaeval Scottish statute is now repealed by the Incest and Related Offences (Scotland) Act 1986 but intercourse with near relatives is still forbidden according to the list shown in Table 15.1. It will be seen that the Act has removed relationship by affinity from those forbidden but, at the same time, introduces adoptive relationships into the list. A special offence of having intercourse with a stepdaughter is introduced (s.1 (2B)) and, most interestingly, an offence is created of having intercourse with a person in respect of whom one holds a position of trust and authority (s.1 (2C)). Certainly, the two last offences are limited by domicile and by the age of the dependant but the trend is, thereby, made even more clear – the current concentration in respect of protection against intrafamilial sexual abuse is on the concept of abuse of authority rather than on that of genetic proximity [2]. It is also to be noted that, while incest is circumscribed in the United Kingdom as involving vulval intercourse between man and woman, it is not

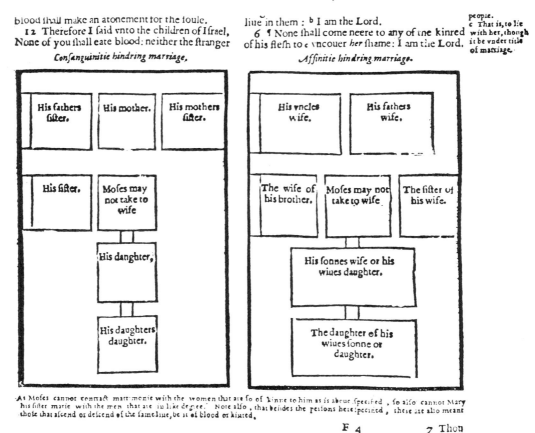

blood fhall make an atonement for the foule.

12 Therefore I faid vnto the children of Ifrael, None of you fhall eate blood: neither the ftranger

Confanguinitie hindring marriage,

liue in them : **b** I am the Lord.

6 ¶ None fhall come neere to any of the kinred of his flefh to c vncouer *her* fhame: I am the Lord.

Affinitie hindring marriage.

people.
c That is, to lie with her, though it be vnder title of marriage.

·As Mofes cannot contract matrimonie with the women that are fo of kinne to him as is aboue fpecified , fo alfo cannot Mary his fifter marie with the men that are in like degree.' Note alfo , that befides the perfons here fpecined , there are alfo meant thofe that afcend or defcend of the fame line, be it of blood or kinred.

F 4   7 Thou

Fig. 15.1 An early 'flow diagram' illustrating the law as laid down in Leviticus (from the 1599 London edition of the Bible – the rather poor quality reproduction is due to very justifiable library restrictions).

everywhere so limited. Thus, for example, in all the United States and in other countries which have a wider definition of sexual intercourse, incest includes penetration of any orifice and may be committed homosexually [3].

Why are sexual relationships within the family other than between husband and wife seen as reprehensible? The easy answer has always been that children born of a closely related union are more likely to suffer the genetic disadvantages of a mating between two persons carrying disadvantageous recessive genes. But intercourse or other

sexual activity can no longer be viewed as necessarily leading to reproduction – in practice, the genetic hazards of reproduction are catered for in the Marriage Act 1949 and as amended, the Marriage (Scotland) Act 1977. The title of this chapter takes the better and commonsense view that incest and sexual abuse, although separate, are closely related phenomena. The abuse is all the more heinous when it arises in a family context – however the particular legal system may define the family – for the important question is not: 'Are the participants in a particular legal or family relationship?', but rather: 'Has this

Table 15.1 Forbidden relationships set out in Incest and Related Offences (Scotland) Act 1986

Degrees of incestuous relationship

For male persons	*For female persons*
Relationships by consanguinity	
Mother	Father
Daughter	Son
Grandmother	Grandfather
Grand-daughter	Grandson
Sister	Brother
Aunt	Uncle
Niece	Nephew
Great grandmother	Great grandfather
Great grand-daughter	Great grandson
Relationships by adoption	
Adoptive mother or former adoptive mother	Adoptive father or former adoptive father
Adopted daughter or former adopted daughter	Adopted son or former adopted son

perpetrator a particular duty towards the victim?' There will be little argument that one of the marks of civilization is the care and concern shown by society to children and other dependants. Sexual behaviour that is wrong in exploiting a child for the gratification or profit of an adult attracts particular opprobrium when that adult has an especially influential or trusted position such as father or teacher. Incest is usually a prolonged course of conduct producing psychological and emotional consequences in the child which are all the greater when the appearance of an otherwise normal life is so often maintained, perhaps for years on end.

Case 15.1
The mother of a girl aged 13 had not lived with the family for 10 years. The child had intercourse twice a week with her father for 3 years. After a row at home she told an older sister, who reported the matter. On questioning, the complainer said that for about 2 months she had been subjected to anal intercourse also. The hymen was found to be thickened and torn at the 10–11 o'clock position. The introitus easily accepted two examining fingers. The anal sphincter had good tone, there was no radial splitting within the canal, but there was some circumferential abrasion. Both anal and vaginal intercourse had taken place.

The following themes must be kept in mind when thinking professionally about incest. Sexual abuse within a family does happen quite commonly, but what finally – or ever – brings it to light may be trivial; the doctor ought to be as ready to believe what a child recounts of sexual abuse as of other medical matters. Sexual abuse is not always synonymous with sexual intercourse or sodomy; therefore, signs are often not to be found despite careful clinical examination.

15.1 PRESENTATION

Those who commit these offences may well try to embroil their victims in a conspiracy of silence; this is maintained by a combination of threats and cajolery. In time, too, erotic pleasure experienced by the victim [4] – and perhaps the knowledge that she has displaced her mother as the object of her father's affection – add to the internal pressure for secrecy.

Case 15.2
A 30-year-old male was seen repeatedly by his doctor because of increasing weight. His depression and poor work record were at first attributed to his lack of success in dieting, but he finally revealed what he knew about his wife's medical history. She was agoraphobic, frightened to remain alone in her home when her husband

worked a night shift and had attempted suicide. Psychological enquiry into her symptoms later led to her recounting a history of incest during childhood. In spite of counselling, he never really understood the consequences to her nor the reasons for the extreme marital difficulties they experienced.

Case 15.3

A girl aged 9 twice visited the house of a man recently discharged from prison for sexual offences although she was aware of the history and had been involved with him before. The matter came to light when she became very difficult at home and then admitted that the accused had rubbed his penis against her and put a finger in her anus and vagina. On examination the hymen fell back on each side leaving a rectangular introitus. Any attempt at inserting a fingertip met substantial resistance; it was concluded that there had been no penetration, the configuration of the hymen being a natural variation.

Thus, early disclosure cannot always be expected. In some cases psychological enquiry in later life into sexual or marital difficulties or into apparently unrelated symptoms inculpates abuse during childhood. Recognition of this possible nexus on the part of both patients and practitioners allows the latter to put direct questions without seeming offensive or prurient.

A wife's reaction to the discovery of an incestuous relationship between father and daughter will vary with her own experience and with the family circumstances as she sees them. Some wives are tempted to tacit acceptance, such collusive behaviour having the object of relieving her of unwanted sexual duties and, by failing to expose the abuse, preserving the seeming integrity of the family. Police and social work involvement is likely to cause disruption leaving a, perhaps, already inadequate wife to try to cope on her own without the security of her husband's income; the family may prefer to close ranks.

Case 15.4

A boy aged 9 who attended a special school was reported as having complained of repeated sodomy by his father. He described getting wet when his father did this. He had seen his father do similar things to a brother and sister, the latter always lying on her back. When no clinical evidence was found, he said that the intercourse had been between the buttocks. His brother, a year older, denied the first's story and said that the father had never done anything to him; no evidence of injury was seen. The sister, aged 12, also denied any physical or sexual abuse; again, no abnormality was found. Clinical examination in this family was inconclusive.

The older siblings may have been protecting the father, although there seemed to be no reason for this. It is possible that abuse was directed solely towards the youngest, most vulnerable, child.

Many of the families involved are already under social work supervision or the children are attending clinics of one kind or another. Members of such families may hint to the professionals that there has been sexual abuse without putting the allegation into so many words, but will quickly withdraw these suggestions in the face of professional obtuseness or embarrassment [5].

Following the recent, often sensational, publicity given to this subject, inhibitions on disclosure are lessening and the third option, a straightforward statement to some authoritative figure, must now be expected more often. Direct complaint is now quite commonly made by the child victim herself for whom various telephone services have been established for just such use – a development which may indicate how unresponsive doctors and others have been in the past.

Case 15.5

Blind and of low IQ, this female, aged 16, was in the care of the local authority. She asked her house-mother to telephone the 'Childline' alleging intercourse with her brother over a period of years. The brother, also of low IQ, admitted this. The vulva showed prominent candidal infection. The hymen was defective at the 8 o'clock position, the defect not quite extending to the periphery. The picture was thought to support her allegation.

Recognition that child sexual abuse may have occurred and still be occurring can follow investigation of behaviour, infection or injury. Symptoms and signs are protean and may come to the attention of many of those who work with children, including playgroup leaders, school teachers, social workers, nurses, psychologists, paediatricians, general practitioners and police officers. Pressure to sniff out sexual abuse should not blind anyone to the need for caution before pronouncing this as a cause of some abnormality. Some of the pitfalls are discussed below.

Case 15.6

A boy aged 10 with a long history of seriously disturbed behaviour had spent many months in a residential school and had been out of his father's care for a year. When first admitted he had frequently described nightmares in which a boy was attacked by a man. He and the other children had been subjected to repeated violence by the father, usually when he was drunk. Examination of the boy's anus showed its sphincter to have good tone but, anteriorly, there was a small pit lined with a thinned epithelium just within the margin which could well have represented old injury.

Case 15.7

This girl, aged 10, had a mental age of 3. On admission to hospital because of behavioural problems, some bruising of the limbs was found and examination of the vulva suggested to staff that there had been sexual interference although the girl herself made no such complaint. Her father had struck her frequently. She had a history of masturbation and of severe constipation requiring the use of enemata. On examination 3 days later, a few bruises were seen on all four limbs but with no particular pattern. The vulva showed evidence of developing secondary sexual characteristics but an intact fourchette. The hymen was thicker than average. While she was being examined the child was completely relaxed; the introitus fell open but showed no sign of dilatation on digital examination. There was certainly no tear of the hymen extending towards its periphery. There was a degree of chronic inflammation. These findings could not support an allegation of sexual interference.

The ethical response to disclosure or suspicion is not simple. As has been discussed in Chapter 1, physicians have a clear statutory requirement to report suspected abuse in many of the United States but the incidence is still thought to be greater than the figures suggest [6]. Failure to report may be passive in the sense that an individual practitioner's experience is likely to be small thus causing underdiagnosis, or active because, for example, the doctor feels capable of managing the problem himself. In most cases this is a delusion. Moreover, no doctor can be certain that he is the sole repository of a patient's confidence. Some signs suggestive of sexual abuse are described in the following paragraphs.

Behaviour

Virtually any change in behaviour pattern from that normally accepted for chronological age may be a pointer. Totally non-specific examples include depression [7], mood swings, secondary enuresis, attention seeking and aggressive disobedience. Although deteriorating schoolwork is to be expected, some children will welcome the opportunity to spend unusually long hours at school [8] or in pastimes which keep them away from home. While it is true that alienation from peers – the 'loner' reaction – is often seen, some children revel in their sexual sophistication and use it to command respect from a group of contemporaries.

Case 15.8

A woman whose daughter was aged 15 had remarried 9 months earlier. The girl had been having regular weekly intercourse with her stepfather in the past 3 months. Contraceptive precautions were taken only just before and after (*sic*) her period. She experienced pain and bleeding on the first occasion and was quite happy to recount the whole history, saying that they were very much in love. Smegma was present within the vulva and its lining reddened. The hymen was defective to the left of the midline posteriorly and the introitus easily accepted two examining fingers.

Children often play out their future roles as parents with siblings, friends or alone, but an overtly sexual theme to this play or a precocious acquaintance with the intimacy expected between parents are highly suspicious of personal involvement. Although the expectation is not always borne out, most adults retain a prudery which shields children from the mechanics of intercourse even when living in overcrowded conditions. Preoccupation with sex may also be revealed in drawing or in writing and by the suggestive manner in which girls approach male visitors. The opposite reaction, that of avoiding male company, is often

found. Yates [4] makes it clear that male children are also corrupted by their mothers.

Infection

Vulvovaginitis is a common cause of pruritis or vaginal discharge. The aetiology is multiple. If it is found to be venereal then, by definition, there has been sexual abuse, but innocent sources of infection must also be considered. These include parasites, notably threadworms, yeasts such as *Candida albicans* and bacteria such as coliforms, all of which may come from the alimentary canal (Fig. 15.2). These and the undoubtedly venereal infections – most commonly gonorrhoea and trichomoniasis – must be identified positively if transfer of infection is to play any part in confirming the diagnosis of abuse or, even, in implicating a suspect. The bacteriology of many cases of genital infection will remain

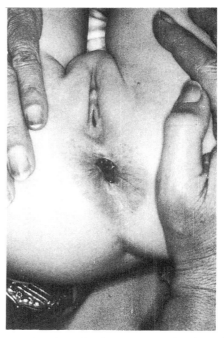

Fig. 15.2 A girl aged 4 showing examination of the anus without traction on the buttocks. There is anal thrush due to the use of antibiotics.

unclear. The advice of a venereologist should be sought, particularly when faced with the rarer infections.

Recurrent urinary infection is another possible presenting sign. The relapsing pattern is common and must lead to adequate urological investigation, whatever the underlying cause.

Case 15.9

Ten days earlier, a friend had thought that an 8-year-old girl had passed blood while urinating. A social worker was consulted and the child was later examined by her own doctor and then at two hospitals. The last of these examinations reported confirmation of finger penetration with scarring of the hymen. The medical history included epilepsy which was treated inadequately because her often drunken mother did not make sure she took her anticonvulsants. She had repeated urinary tract infections. The parents were separated and she was in the habit of spending one night a week with her father, sleeping in his bed. The regular social worker reported that the girl was frequently incontinent of urine, especially when at home. On examination, the vestibule showed reddening and there was some apparent thickening of the hymen on both sides. Small vesicles were seen on the superficial surface of the hymen but it was not possible to say that these had been caused by attempted penetration rather than by infection. The anus was unremarkable.

Injury

Sexual abuse may coexist with physical abuse or be found alone. Within the family, a father may be particularly ready at times to chastise the same sexually abused victim; in other cases, all the children may suffer, which suggests that physical abuse is not designed simply to secure compliance. The pattern of injuries, therefore, is that to be found in other cases of non-accidental injury (see Chapter 14).

Genital injury

Pain may be a symptom of both infection and injury. The most common presenting sign of injury to the vulva is bleeding but it, too, may be due to infection. A tempting explanation of bleeding from the vulva is a fall astride some object; this, however, produces a typical blunt force injury, any laceration of the skin being associated with bruising. Genital penetration stretches and bursts the skin, usually with little more than local bruising. Appropriate cutting lesions will be produced when the penetrating object is some instrument or fingers with sharp nails. It is usually assumed that the hymen will be broken by penetration but this must depend on the distensibility of the introitus, the force used, the diameter of the object inserted and the depth of any thrusting. Accident has been found to be an uncommon cause (Table 15.2) [9]. Bleeding with or without vaginal discharge may indicate a retained foreign body [10]. A deeper lesion is not necessarily excluded when bleeding apparently arises from the perineum, the labia or the readily inspected parts of the genitalia. In general, however, perforation of the vaginal wall causes surgical

Table 15.2 Respondents' recollection of how the hymen came to be broken (abstracted from Table 101 of The Kinsey Data)

Cause of hymen breakage	%
Coitus	79.7
Petting	2.1
Homosexual activity	0.2
Accident	5.9
Deliberate dilatation	0.4
Surgery	8.5
Tampon use	2.1
Other	1.0

shock and the child will be obviously ill. It is surprising that the child described below as having quite serious vulval injury was capable of normal activity over several days.

Case 15.10

A girl aged 8, abducted and raped, was examined cursorily and no injury was found. Seventy-two hours later she was re-examined and found to have a full thickness perineal tear extending for 2 cm from the fourchette towards the anal margin. Her only complaint was of minor discomfort but her mother noticed a little blood spotting on her pants. Interview and initial examination were woefully inadequate.

15.2 INVESTIGATION

(a) History

Although the clinical history is unquestionably of major importance, this is one of the rare instances in medicine when examination may have to be conducted before a knowledge of a coherent sequence of events is available. The urgent need to take action either to protect the child or to mount a prosecution clashes with the equally necessary slow deliberate teasing out of the story. Those with therapeutic responsibility often find themselves in opposition to those who are anxious to gather evidence for legal purposes. Wherever possible, these different

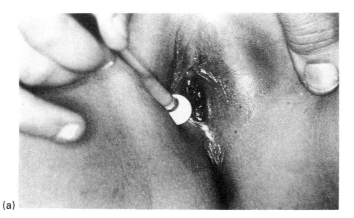

(a)

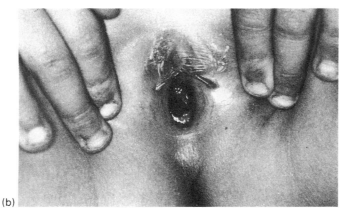

(b)

Fig. 15.3 (a) A girl aged 10 demonstrating with an illuminated rod what had been done to her. (b) Shows her displaying the introitus where a tear is seen at 3 o'clock.

stances should be reconciled beforehand, so allowing the various agencies to act in concert. It is too easy to say that the interests of the child are paramount and that, therefore, she should be handled only by, say, paediatricians. On the other hand, although the public interest demands that wrongdoers be brought to justice, this must surely not be at the expense of increasing the harm which has already been done to the victim.

The doctor's sources of information will depend on how the case presents. When this is in a purely clinical context, make careful note of the initial complaint and the names and addresses of witnesses. Accept that the child, even if nearing her teens, may wish to disclose little. The gathering of detailed information about family background, the identity of the alleged perpetrator and the previous history are all the responsibility of the relevant statutory and voluntary agencies – the social service departments, societies for the prevention of cruelty to children and the police.

It may take many sessions by a skilled psychologist to draw from a child the details of what has been done to her. A trusting relationship can only be developed over time and is certainly not achieved in the atmosphere of an accident and emergency department, no matter how concerned is the house officer. Do not, therefore, attempt to press the child for more information as this will often increase her distress; this, in turn, makes clinical examination impossible or, at least, unsatisfactory. Among the techniques available to the psychologist is the use of play and drawing. Dolls, especially those equipped with genitalia, are now commonly given to victims to let them demonstrate what has been done to them; their use should be limited to those who have developed appropriate skills lest there be a suggestion of leading or even coaching a potential witness (Fig. 15.3).

(b) Clinical examination

Careful thought must be given beforehand to where the examination is to be conducted and by whom. Social workers who are under instruction to have abused children examined immediately often take them to general practitioners or to casualty officers who are unfamiliar with the normal anatomy and, thus, with departures from the normal and how to assess their significance (Fig. 15.4). Local procedures should be developed to obviate this problem.

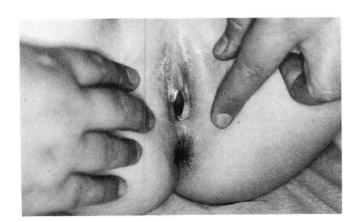

Fig. 15.4 An 11-year-old girl with an intact hymen but whose vagina appears more open than normal. Tissue around the vaginal orifice seemed to the naked eye to be flattened. An anal skin tag added to suspicion. These findings supported the child's story well enough to secure conviction on a charge of rape.

Case 15.11

The aunt of a 6-year-old girl found her to be bleeding from the vulva. Her father took her to hospital where the casualty officer immediately referred her to the social work department. The child maintained that she had fallen on a brick while attempting the splits. On examination 3 days later there was a 2 mm bruise to the right of the vulva and a 1 mm bruise on the inner side of the left labium majus. There was a deep 1 cm tear along the right labium majus. No bruising was found within the vulva or vestibule. The findings supported the child's explanation.

Case 15.12

A mother took her 3-year-old son to her general practitioner saying that he fell from furniture in the house. When bruising was found behind both ears, on the legs and in the groin he was immediately referred to a paediatric unit and a place of safety order was obtained. On examination 5 days later there was no evidence to support an allegation of sexual abuse. There was a fading scar on the right side of the base of the penis and fading bruising above the right groin and on the right side of the scrotum. Family circumstances did not justify the action taken.

A report giving merely a conclusion does not help the court to reach a proper conclusion. Statements such as 'there were signs of sexual abuse' or 'in my opinion, there has been penetration' are useless without a clear description of the findings giving rise to such inferences. Better by far to refuse involvement in these cases unless you are determined to build up experience and ready to give credible evidence. Although recruitment of medical students in the United Kingdom is now shared equally between the sexes it remains true that most senior clinical positions are held by men. There are occasions when the sex of

the examiner is important to the child, and every effort should be made to accommodate his/her wishes. Gynaecologists, paediatricians and police surgeons are those most likely to provide a satisfactory service.

The essential features of the examination facilities are a clinical atmosphere which, at the same time, provides comfort for children and parents. There is much to be said for examining abused children where they first report, be it a general practitioner's surgery, hospital or police station – but convenience and available, suitable accommodation must match. A good level of general illumination and directional lighting are equally important.

General physical

It has already been pointed out that non-accidental injury and sexual abuse often coexist. A full clinical inspection, if necessary including a skeletal radiological survey, must be undertaken. Note the appearance of clothing, the state of nutrition, hygiene, development and demeanour. When lesions are described, record their size and position and try to assess their age and cause.

Perigenital

Most acts of sexual abuse to children are accomplished without significant physical violence. Bruising to the inner thighs or the lower abdomen, perhaps on the wrists or ankles indicating restraint, are all unusual but their rarity makes them all the more significant. Small round bruises arranged in a crescent are characteristic of fingertip pressure.

Female genitalia

The anatomy of the pudenda changes gradually as the child grows until pubescence when the adult form is attained quite rapidly. The young girl's labia majora show much less contour and the labia minora are often not visible until a little lateral traction is applied. The labia majora become more prominent with the onset of puberty and hair appears well in advance of the menarche. The labia minora elongate, often protruding noticeably, and lose the sharp free margin seen in childhood. The frenulum of the labia minora, which is thrown into prominence as the labia are parted, is a frequent site of injury following even partial penetration. It must be inspected with care, for stretching is often accompanied by superficial splitting at the midline – perhaps accompanied by a little fresh bleeding which recurs when an examination is made within a few hours of defloration.

Tissue heaped up in a line from the fourchette towards the introitus along the posterior wall of the vestibule indicates a deeper tearing which has left a scar. It is unsafe to put an age on such an injury. The vulva is a very vascular structure and the lining of its vestibule very thin, especially in childhood. This imparts a perhaps unexpected redness, but a brighter colour still is seen with fungal infection in which patches of white exudate are not always present; a persistent infection is at times responsible for splitting of the mucous membrane and bleeding.

Penetration of a child's vulva by an adult penis causes distraction between the greater and lesser labia and may produce antero-posterior laceration of the sulcus (Fig. 15.5). Such an injury will seldom be associated with much bleeding or bruising. Violent penetration can cause laceration with perforation of the vagina and tearing of the anal sphincter, even to the extent of rectovaginal fistula, but florid damage of that kind is very much the exception in child sexual abuse.

Close to the surface in infancy, the introitus recedes with age but, in most examinees, it is easily seen when the thighs are abducted. For closer inspection, parting the labia with the fingers has the added benefit of putting the hymen on the stretch (Fig. 15.6). A solid plastic nasal speculum, designed to fit in a pen torch, helps to provide light and may be used to transilluminate the hymen from the vagina. Gentle pressure allows the whole free edge to be inspected for, even in prepubertal girls, folds and notches will mislead the unwary. It has been postulated [11] that measurement of the transverse diameter of the introitus is an infallible guide to whether or not penetration has occurred, the critical figure being 4 mm; however, the hymen varies so substantially in extent and shape that doubt must be cast on the general use of such a criterion.

Parts of the vaginal wall proper are seen through the introitus without further instrumentation; in most cases, a satisfactory view

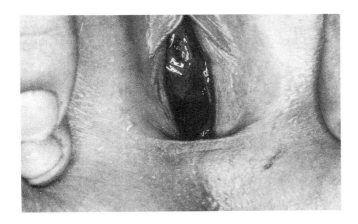

Fig. 15.5 An 11-year-old girl whose vagina has an open appearance and whose hymen is torn at 6 o'clock.

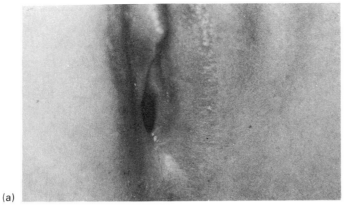

(a)

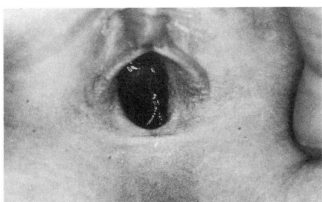

(b)

Fig. 15.6 A 5-year-old girl who complained of vulval soreness and who behaved in a sexual way. At first sight, the appearance is normal (a) but, with time to let the child settle and a little traction, the vagina opened readily and a tear of the hymen could be identified (b).

is obtained by placing the child in the left lateral position, one which often causes less distress to a child than having her lie supine. Full theatre facilities and general anaesthesia may be employed in cases of severe injury which indicate a possible need for repair.

Male genitalia

Adhesions prevent full retraction of the prepuce in childhood. Forcible retraction, poor hygiene and infection may all cause splitting and ulceration. Note the condition of the prepuce and meatus, together with the presence of smegma or discharge. Erection during examination is not significant. Having inspected the penis and scrotum, palpate the testes. Suction during fellatio may cause petechial haemorrhages but masturbation, even when repeated, will leave no trace unless it is accompanied by violence. Masturbation is often a mutual act, so that ejaculate or pubic hair should be looked for even within the preputial sac.

The anus

Clinical examination of the anus is often disappointing in the sense, first, that little is to be found and, secondly, that the correct interpretation of abnormalities remains a matter of serious doubt. Indeed, what constitutes abnormality is uncertain. There is gross disproportion between the child's

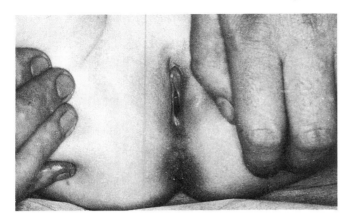

Fig. 15.7 The child is aged 2.5 years. Attempted sodomy caused perineal brusing, seen here at an examination soon after the offence was committed.

anus and an erect adult penis, although the sphincter permits substantial dilatation, especially if lubrication is used. Children will often not be able to distinguish in their minds and statements between intercrural, intergluteal or perineal intercourse and buggery. Both buggery and anal penetration using a finger will usually cause pain until such time as sphincter relaxation becomes a learned response.

Most young children should be placed in the conventional left lateral position for examination of the anus, although the knee/elbow posture is easily adopted by older boys; some may prefer simply to bend over a couch. Instrumentation and digital examination are seldom required unless there are indications suggesting the need for an operating theatre. Good lighting which can be easily directed is essential in all cases (Fig. 15.7).

Even careful gentle parting of the buttocks may provoke some tightening of the sphincter but this passes as traction is maintained [12]. Inspect the perianal area for reddening, inflammation, bruising or other lesions such as warts. Traction applied nearer the anus allows part of the anal canal to be seen. Skin tags, fissures and radial scars are all evidence of previous dilatation to the point of rupturing or tearing the lining but these findings will not necessarily indicate the aetiology.

(c) Trace evidence [13]

The exchange principle of Locard (Fig. 15.8) is a basic tenet of forensic science. Persons in contact with others or with a place leave traces behind and some traces will adhere to them; the identification of these traces is an essential task of the forensic scientist. To assist in this, the clinician who is cast in an investigative role must preserve the clothing and take possession of any material adhering to the skin such as fibres and vegetation. Most of the contact identification is irrelevant in the context of sexual abuse within a family, but forensic science techniques provide corroborative evidence when, for example, pubic hair is found between the buttocks of a prepubertal child. When relevant, swabbings of the mouth, anus or vagina are taken and should be allowed to dry in the atmosphere before being sealed. The swabs themselves should be made of plain cotton-wool; albumen-treated fibres interfere with serological investigations. Samples of seminal or salivary staining on the skin are taken by applying a lightly moistened swab and treating it in the same way. Forensic science laboratories vary somewhat in their particular requirements and prior consultation smooths the path. There is a preference in some laboratories for slides to be made from swabs

Principle of Locard

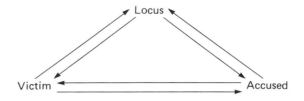

Specimens   1. Contact: debris, hairs, fibres, body fluids

                 2. Control: unstained clothing, vegetation etc.

                 3. Diagnostic: swabs for sperm and bacteriology

NB. Danger of third party contamination

Fig. 15.8 Locard's principle of exchange of evidence.

immediately, but others prefer to make their own.

Much sexual abuse leading to ejaculation does not entail intercourse. Traces of ejaculate are found on the child's skin, apparel or bedclothes. Towels, face flannels and handkerchiefs are all used to confine the ejaculate or to clean up afterwards and such material may provide important evidence.

(d) Pitfalls in examination

Clinical examination has a relatively minor part to play in the investigation of sexual abuse, the result often being inconclusive. This will certainly be the case if there has been no penetration and no violence. The lack of evidence of injury is, by itself, a source of comfort to concerned parents and, where possible, they should be reassured on that score.

Case 15.13
A girl aged 13 gave a history that she had been raped twice during an evening.

Questioning included attempts to ascertain whether or not ejaculation had occurred, but her understanding of 'wetness' was confined to urine. She had been using cream for a vaginal infection over a number of years, but no real medical investigation had ever been undertaken. There was a little vaginal discharge with chronic inflammation of the vestibule. It was possible to demonstrate that an apparent defect of the hymen at the 9 o'clock position was, in reality, a deep notch in a fimbriated hymen. No penetration could be substantiated, nor was it established why she made the allegation.

Hobbs, Wild and Wynne have written a valuable series of articles [14–16] concerning sexual abuse in the Leeds area and have drawn particular attention to anal injury and to the deductions to be made from anal appearances. These authors do not recommend routine examination of children's anuses [16], yet how else is one to gain the necessary experience? We must become much more familiar with the normal before any confidence can be placed in our evidence; the incidence of skin tags, for example, is unknown.

There is certainly a danger of overdiagnosis in this and other aspects of child abuse, partly because medical examiners are under pressure to confirm that legal proceedings are justified. The standard of evidence required to secure a conviction in the criminal courts is much higher than that on which care proceedings is based, but the objectivity of the examiner must not be allowed to falter in either instance. The importance of a particularly high 'probability' standard when a parent/child relationship is at issue has recently been emphasized in the family court [17]. Misinterpretation of the normal and lack of adequate investigation have founded mistaken support for sexual [18, 19] as for physical [20, 21] abuse (Fig. 15.9). There is no disgrace in saying, 'I don't know'.

Case 15.14
Over a period of 2 years, the stepfather of a girl aged 12 had made repeated attempts at intercourse, putting fingers into her vulva and making her masturbate him. Two weeks before examination she had some vaginal bleeding. Secondary sexual characteristics were appearing and the hymen showed a wide anteroposterior split. From this it was impossible to substantiate vaginal penetration, the appearance of the introitus being simply a natural variant. She herself was quite confident that her stepfather's finger had never gone within the introitus. The vaginal bleeding was menstrual.

Chronic pruritis or vaginal discharge is tolerated in many houses in which hygiene is poor. Reddening is certainly not to be taken as an indication of injury – especially in the vulva where the normal coloration is often quite unjustifiably mistaken for 'evidence of interference' in young children. On the other hand, venereal disease – and trichomoniasis should be included in this category [22] – cannot be acquired from fomites and its presence must give powerful support to the presumption of abuse.

15.3 INITIATIVES IN INVESTIGATION AND MANAGEMENT

Should doctors be compelled to notify cases of sexual abuse encountered in their practice? There is legislation requiring physicians to report suspected child abuse in many of

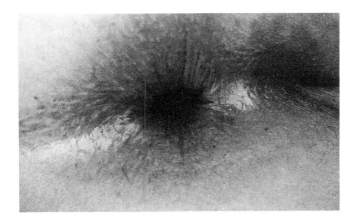

Fig. 15.9 'Reflex dilatation' of the anus in a 5-year-old suffering from constipation.

the United States of America but there are indications not only that doctors' case experience is low, but also that nearly 10% of recognized cases are not reported, despite the statutory compulsion [6] (see also Chapter 1, p. 15). A purely legal framework is not necessarily conducive to full co-operation but primary-care practitioners do sometimes need to be reminded of their obligations.

Disparaging comment on the ability of particular groups of doctors or the sex of examiners [23] should give way to the recognition that the outcome of intervention is improved when all the properly interested professionals are involved rather than when an individual attempts management [24]. In essence, therefore, there must be local discussion among the police and prosecuting authorities, the judiciary, the social service departments and doctors – who are concerned in investigation as well as in immediate and in long-term care – to establish a procedure which is, on the one hand, workable yet, on the other hand, eschews what is too elaborate.

Case 15.15

A general practitioner visited the parents of a 3-year-old boy, saying that their neighbour's wife thought that her husband was exposing himself to the child. The boy's father wanted to contact the police but the doctor said that this would be unwise as the boy could be further damaged by the tests to which he would be subjected. Next day the boy remarked that the neighbour could produce milk from his penis. His sister of 7 said to her mother that the brother was talking about dirty things. It transpired that the neighbour had threatened the child that the police would take him away if he told anyone; the boy did react hysterically when he later saw a uniformed officer in the police station. The general practitioner's action was inept and a co-ordinated approach might have saved much distress.

The social services department of the London

Borough of Bexley and the Metropolitan Police, working together, have established an eclectic procedure in which their personnel have looked beyond traditionally prescribed rules, yet without abrogating duties which are laid on them by law. The investigation of the incident becomes the joint responsibility of a police officer and a social worker. Interviews are conducted in a room within a hospital paediatric unit and are recorded on videotape. The striking feature of this still experimental project is its co-operative nature.

Such units are in existence in several parts of the world, their structure based on work done for victims of sexual assault in older age-groups [25]. For example, some 4 years ago, Strathclyde Police appointed four policewomen who had been given special training to each of its divisions. These officers have responsibility for a variety of offences involving children and women.

Perhaps the two elements giving rise to most concern in all investigations leading to a prosecution are, first, the taking of evidence from children in the initial stage and, second, how this is to be proved in court. Modern closed-circuit television allows the recording of interviews which should be available for later court use just as would be a signed statement or a photograph of injuries. Objections to this have centred on who should conduct the recorded interview and on fairness to the accused – who, it will be generally thought, is entitled to cross-examine a verbal witness.

As early as 1955 the Israeli parliament passed a law designed to protect children who had to give evidence in 'offences against morality' cases [26]. The law provided for the appointment of youth interrogators whose sole prerogative it is to examine witnesses who are under 14 years of age. The interrogator is under a duty to disclose to the police the particulars of the examination and to lay his or her conclusions before them. The child may appear in court only with the consent of the interrogator who also has the authority to ask the court to bring such evidence to an end on the ground that the child may be affected adversely. When the interrogator has interviewed the child in private, the record is admissible as evidence. Interrogators are appointed by the Minister of Justice after consulting a committee consisting of a judge dealing with juveniles, a mental hygienist, an educator, a child-care expert and a senior police officer. There seems no reason why a corps of such qualified individuals should not be appointed elsewhere.

The arguments in favour of video recordings rather than live evidence by a victim were put forcefully by Williams in 1987 [27]; the author also considered, albeit with reduced enthusiasm, the middle road of live-linked television between the witness in a separate room and the court itself – a proposal which is now statutorily discretionary as regards witnesses under the age of 14 years by virtue of the Criminal Justice Act 1988, s.32(1)(b). His counter arguments to the suggestion that video recording is unfair to the accused included the facts that any recording would be available in advance of trial and would indicate lines for further questioning of the witness; in the event of an accused being identified at the time of interview, the defence would be able to put their own questions through the interrogator; the defence would no longer be deterred from cross-examination for fear of antagonizing the jury; and, in any event, a right to cross-examine the witness could be preserved. Such proposals are not without critics [28] but, surely, the time is ripe for a much more radical approach by the courts. The technology is available and it seems inevitable that there will be a general increase in the use of modern techniques within our system of justice.

15.4 OTHER FORMS OF ABUSE

Several paedophile rings are known to operate by having young boys picked up in provincial cities and then solicited for clients in London, where they are traded. Examination of the often willing subjects of these rings frequently demonstrates a lack of physical damage despite an admission of repeated sodomy; this makes one sceptical of the significance of funnelling of the anus and other signs reported as being characteristic in the catamite. The greater physical danger to these children now is venereal disease and a compromised immune system.

Girls are also encouraged early into prostitution. Investigation of 11 child sex rings within one working class community showed no less than 175 children (171 of them girls) aged between 6 and 15 years to have been recruited by 14 adults [15]. The age of these adults ranged from 30 to 82 years.

Pornography is used by some adults to introduce children to inappropriate sexual behaviour, the children, themselves, being used as pornographic subjects. This is an offence struck at in England and Wales by the Protection of Children Act 1978 and, in Scotland, by the Civic Government (Scotland) Act 1982, s.52; the mere fact of the subject's age may be sufficient to invoke the provisions of the statute [29].

Although, thus far, this chapter has concentrated on the abuse of girls, mainly within the family, it must not be forgotten that boys, too, have sexual encounters; by contrast, these are commonly outwith the immediate family circle. Many of these events flow from a developing sexual awareness and do not necessarily indicate a homosexual orientation and, certainly, not when the participants are of similar ages – peer pressure and the desire to demonstrate pubertal prowess are involved; parents may need to be reassured that masturbation in these circumstances is no more harmful than is that practised in private. So benign a view cannot, of course, extend to incidents when adults are intent on molesting children, for this readily falls within the definition of exploitation [3]. Moreover, laboratory measurement of response to a variety of sexual stimuli applied to offenders suggests that their tastes are unlikely to be confined to one type of victim – much depends upon availability [30]. Adolescent males have been found to abuse boys twice as often as girls [31]. It is to be expected, also, that the type of abuse will not necessarily be constant for a single perpetrator or a single victim – the pattern develops over time.

15.5 INCIDENCE

How common are these problems? Certainly, there are no reliable statistics in the United Kingdom. In official terms, criminal convictions are recorded and cases reported to the police are tabulated in the annual Criminal Statistics for England and Wales and for Scotland; these data, however, can take no account of undisclosed crime.

The National Society for the Prevention of Cruelty to Children has been conducting research since 1973 on the children placed on those child abuse registers covering 9% of the children living in England and Wales. The figures, in general, show absolute increases for all forms of abuse over these years, but there was a rise of more than one and a quarter times in reported cases of sexual abuse between 1984 and 1985. The figures in Table 15.3 have been taken from the Child Abuse Register maintained by the Social Work Department of Strathclyde Region (total population 2 358 727) and show registrations at the end of 1986 in representative areas. These tiny percentages contrast strangely with many other estimates of prevalence.

A recent retrospective study in Great Britain [32] seems to confirm the now widely quoted rule of thumb that 10% of the population have experience of sexual abuse in childhood. It must, however, be emphasized that the abuse ranged from erotic talk, through exhibitionism and fondling, to full intercourse. Other analyses have shown the importance of definitions and semantics in this area; thus, in a major study of adults in the United Kingdom who claimed to have been sexually abused as children, it was found that physical contact was involved in only 49% and that 63% of the reports referred to single incidents [33]. Various studies in the USA and Canada [34] have assessed prevalence rates as varying from 6% to 62% in females and from 3% to 30% in males; it is evident that the information obtained in one study is not necessarily comparable with that in any other.

While this chapter was in preparation, a furore arose in Cleveland, England, over the greatly increased number of children who were taken into care on suspicion of sexual abuse. Many of these children were brought to hospital by their parents to be examined for quite unrelated complaints and several parents made successful applications to the courts for judicial review of place of safety orders; in at least one case, the judge in the family court went so far as to impute professional negligence to the diagnosing physicians [35]. Allegations of incompetence and bad faith resulted in the setting up of a Public Inquiry under a High Court Judge. The findings have now been reported [36] and, in the end, they add little to what has been said above in respect of awareness, caution and cooperation in the diagnosis and management of child sexual abuse. The point is firmly made, however, that diagnostic confusion will persist until a clear definition of both clinical and anatomical terms is agreed upon. It is clear that a serious lack of inter-professional trust has contributed to the loss of confidence the public must have in mechanisms which are designed ostensibly to protect a child's welfare yet which may, at the same time, be seriously disruptive of the family. The Cleveland affair will not have been an unmitigated disaster if the lessons have been learnt and it is salutary that a number of well-considered governmental guidelines have been issued subsequent to the publication of the report [37]. While much of

Table 15.3 From Strathclyde Region Child Abuse Register, with the addition of population figures

| District | Type | Population | | Registrations | | | | Sexual abuse |
		Total	Children	Families	Children	Injury	Sexual abuse	$\dfrac{\text{Sexual abuse}}{\text{Child population}} \times 100$
Argyll/Bute	Rural	65 586	14 029	9	11	3	2	0.014
Clydesdale	Rural	58 293	12 876	4	5	2	1	0.008
Motherwell	Urban	148 016	32 963	47	76	25	3	0.009
Glasgow SE	City	201 645	39 970	25	46	16	16	0.040
Glasgow SW	City	276 851	54 698	70	131	39	16	0.029

the advice is pitched at an administrative level, no individual doctor can fail to benefit from a careful look at their contents [38].

15.5 THE AIMS OF POLICIES

The incidence of child sexual abuse is no better known than is that of incest or of physical abuse but, by their very nature, these offences must be much under-recorded; it follows that increased awareness may simply be unearthing what has always been there. The aim in clinical practice is to be alert enough to recognize abuse and so to bring it to an end for the individual victim; in a patient's later life, no clinician need hesitate to explore such a possibility as the aetiology of a wide variety of neurotic and psychosomatic symptoms.

A doctor's first duty is to do no harm. Similarly, the agents of any civilized society must try to cause no unnecessary distress to those who are already victims either during the inquiry into an incident or during the subsequent judicial process. That can be achieved only by a properly co-ordinated system of investigation and by having evidence led in humane ways.

Although damage to the already abused individual may be thus, to some extent, mitigated, the wider incidence will only be lessened when both adults and children better understand the proper place of sexuality in life. Yet however much is done by way of education to improve the child's ability to protect itself from abuse, the responsibility lies always with the offending adult. This chapter opened with a consideration of the biblical foundation of the law of incest. It is appropriate to end with a quotation recounted in St Luke's Gospel: 'Causes of stumbling are bound to arise; but woe betide the man through whom they come. It would be better for him to be thrown into the sea with a millstone round his neck than to cause one of those little ones to stumble.'

REFERENCES

1. Noble, M. and Mason, J.K. (1978) Incest. *J. Med. Ethics*, **4**, 64.
2. Mason, J.K. (1981) 1567 and all that. *Scots Law Times*, 301.
3. For a general review, see Batten, D.A. (1983) Incest – a review of the literature. *Med. Sci. Law*, **23**, 245; American Medical Association (1985) Diagnostic and treatment guidelines concerning child abuse and neglect. *JAMA*, **254**, 796.
4. Yates, A. (1982) Children eroticized by incest. *Am. J. Psychiatry*, **139**, 482.
5. Porter, R. (ed.) (1984) *Child Sexual Abuse Within the Family*, Tavistock, London, p. 65.
6. Saulsbury, F.T. and Cupples, R.E. (1985) Evaluation of child abuse reporting by physicians. *Am. J. Dis. Child.*, **139**, 393.
7. Anonymous (1987) Childhood depression and sexual abuse. *Lancet*, **i**, 620.
8. Porter, R. (ed.) (1982) *Child Sexual Abuse Within the Family*, Tavistock, London, p. 8.
9. Gebhard, P.H. and Johnson, V.E. (1979) *The Kinsey Data*, W.B. Saunders, Philadelphia, p. 148.
10. Paradise, J.E. and Willis, E.D. (1985) Probability of vaginal foreign body in girls with genital complaints. *Am. J. Dis. Child.*, **139**, 472.
11. Cantwell, H.B. (1983) Vaginal inspection as it relates to child sexual abuse in girls under 13. *Child Abuse Neglect*, **7**, 173.
12. Clayden, G. (1987) Anal appearances and child sex abuse. *Lancet*, **i**, 620.
13. Davies, A. (1986) The sexual abuse of children: cases submitted to a police laboratory and the scientific evidence. *Med. Sci. Law*, **26**, 103.
14. Wild, N.J. (1986) Sexual abuse of children in Leeds. *Br. Med. J.*, **292**, 1113.
15. Wild, N.J. and Wynne, J.M. (1986) Child sex rings. *Br. Med. J.*, **293**, 183.
16. Hobbs, C.J. and Wynne, J.M. (1986) Buggery in childhood – a common syndrome of child abuse. *Lancet*, **ii**, 792.
17. *In re G (a minor)* [1987] *The Times*, 30 July per Sheldon J.
18. Handfield-Jones, S.E., Hinde, F.R.J. and Kennedy, C.T.C. (1987) Lichen sclerosus et atrophicus in children misdiagnosed as sexual abuse. *Br. Med. J.*, **294**, 1404.

19. Kean, H.B. and Clarke, M.D.B. (1988) Sexual assault or skin disease? *Police Surg.*, **33**, 6.

20. Davies, H. de la H. (1985) Adolescent lumbar striae mistaken for non-accidental injury. *Police Surg.*, **27**, 72.

21. Paterson, C.R. (1986) Unexplained fractures in childhood: differential diagnosis of osteogenesis imperfecta and other disorders from non-accidental injury. *J. Neurol. Orthoped. Med. Surg.*, **7**, 253.

22. Jones, J.G., Yamauchi, T. and Lambert, B. (1985) *Trichomonas vaginalis* infection in sexually abused girls. *Am. J. Dis. Child.*, **139**, 846.

23. Shepherd, R.C. (1985) Child abuse injuries. *Lancet*, **i**, 1511.

24. Anonymous (1985) Where you stand depends on where you sit. *Am. J. Dis. Child.*, **139**, 867.

25. Dellar, C. (1981) The development of a sexual assault referral centre. *Police Surg.*, **19**, 90.

26. Law of Evidence (Protection of Children) Law 5715-1955.

27. Williams, G. (1987) Videotaping children's evidence. *New Law J.*, **137**, 108; (1987) More about videotaping children. *New Law J.*, **137**, 351, 369.

28. The debate is continued by Morton, J. (1987) Videotaping children's evidence – a reply. *New Law J.*, **137**, 216.

29. *R v. Owen* [1987] *The Times*, 10 October per Stocker L.J.

30. Travin, S., Bluestone, H., Cullen, K. and Mellella, J. (1986) Pedophile types and treatment perspectives. *J. Forensic Sci.*, **31**, 614.

31. Reinhart, M.A. (1987) Sexually abused boys. *Child Abuse Neglect*, **11**, 229.

32. Baker, A.W. and Duncan, S.P. (1985) Child sexual abuse: a study of prevalence in Great Britain. *Child Abuse Neglect*, **9**, 457.

33. Quoted in Findlay, A. (ed.) (1987) *Practice Paper on Child Sexual Abuse*, Lothian Regional Council, Edinburgh, p. 6.

34. Finkelhor, D. (1986) *A Source Book on Child Sexual Abuse*, Sage, Beverley Hills, Table 1.2.

35. Davenport, P. (1987) Wrong diagnosis of sex abuse on sisters 'devastated family'. (1987) *The Times*, 23 October, 3; Dyer, C. (1987) First High Court judgment on sex abuse in Cleveland. *Br. Med. J.*, **295**, 382.

36. Lord Justice Butler-Sloss (Chairman) (1988) *Report of the Inquiry into Child Abuse in Cleveland 1987*, HMSO, London.

37. Department of Health and Social Security and the Welsh Office (1988) *Working Together*, HMSO, London; Department of Health and Social Security (1988) *Diagnosis of Child Sexual Abuse: Guidance for Doctors*, HMSO, London.

38. Valman, B. (1988) Implications of the Cleveland inquiry. *Br. Med. J.*, **297**, 151.

FURTHER READING

Finkelhor, D. (1986) *A Source Book on Child Sexual Abuse*, Sage, Beverly Hills.

MacFarlane, K. and Waterman, J. (1986) *Sexual Abuse of Young Children*, Holt, Rinehart and Winston, London.

McLay, W.D.S. (ed.) (1985) *The New Police Surgeon: Rape*, Association of Police Surgeons of Great Britain, Creaton.

Porter, R. (ed.) (1984) *Child Sexual Abuse Within the Family*, Tavistock, London.

Acknowledgement

Dr Raine Roberts of Manchester has very kindly allowed me to prepare Figs 15.2–15.7 and 15.9 from slides taken of her cases and to abstract relevant clinical information.

CHAPTER 16

The emotional abuse of children

Ann Gath

Different cultures, and even different strata of society within a culture, apply different standards as to the degree of violence towards a child that is tolerated or regarded as part of the parents' right, or even obligation, to chastisement. Behaviour to children which is manifested as an attack or series of attacks resulting in actual physical injury is, however, generally recognized as cruelty. Similarly, most observers would regard a child as being neglected if he or she was exposed to malnourishment, filthy living conditions or grossly inadequate clothing – although such conditions are common in those areas in the world where extreme poverty still exists. Contrasting with these still familiar forms of severe parenting failure is that more subtle form of ill-treatment of children which does not, in itself, involve any physical injury and which is usually referred to as emotional abuse. Examples of such treatment include active abuse – such as terrifying children by means of verbal threats or belittling them with sarcasm or constant criticism – and more passive maltreatment in refusing to speak to them or depriving them of any affection. Exposure to frightening or grossly indecent scenes can also be considered as ill-treatment without physical injury.

Emotional abuse of this sort frequently accompanies physical abuse and is almost invariably present in cases of prolonged or severe cruelty or neglect. Proof of cruelty can be established in court – and the protection of the child from further misuse is, consequently, a relatively simple matter – where there is physical abuse with objective evidence that can be systematically recorded using photographs of bruises or X-rays of broken bones. Such straightforward evidence can be produced in court and can be readily understood by the judiciary or lay magistrates. In addition, the parents, caretakers or others whose behaviour produced the damage can recognize the existence of a serious problem, even if they are unable to accept their own responsibility for it. By contrast, the injury sustained by a child who is emotionally abused rarely leaves visible marks. The purpose of this chapter is to define emotional abuse and to discuss the recognition and management of this intangible, but sometimes pernicious, form of cruelty to children.

16.1 THE LEGAL DEFINITION OF EMOTIONAL ABUSE

Emotional neglect, including deprivation of affection, has long been recognized as being associated with delinquency and this view has been confirmed in specific studies [1].

Parental rejection has also been recognized by some child psychiatrists as being a causative factor in behavioural and emotional disorders [2, 3]. The law, however, has hesitated to intervene between parents and children in the absence of a clearly defined offence [4]. There are major problems in the definition of abuse or neglect where the principal ill-effects are in the mental or emotional sphere. After the publication of Bowlby's work in 1951 [5], emotional neglect was seen in terms of 'maternal deprivation' but, more recently, it has been appreciated that it is the quality of contact with parents or parent-substitutes, rather than the undivided attention of the mother, that is important [6]. The definition of emotional abuse must be more specific than mere condemnation of any particular lifestyle or cultural background.

Emotional abuse as a variant of abuse to be included in the Child Care Central Register system has been recognized by the Department of Health and Social Security since 1980. It was then defined as applying to: 'Children under the age of 17 years whose behaviour and emotional development have been severely affected and where medical and social assessments find evidence of either persistent or severe neglect or rejection.'

The concept underlying the inclusion of this category in the 1980 circular [7] was not new since some of the more severe cases could already be brought before a juvenile court, and protected by varying degrees of supervision, under the Children and Young Persons Act 1969, s.1(2)(a) if it could be proved that: 'A child's proper development is being avoidably impaired or neglected or he is being ill-treated'. Under this Act, it was essential to demonstrate that the child's mental or emotional development had fallen significantly behind the norm. The proof required might include school reports which showed an increasing inability to learn with poor performance being indicated by written work or class tests. The report from school would need to be substantiated by standardized psychological tests which could also be used to repudiate any suggestion that the problems were inborn or due to a developmental disorder. In addition, psychiatric evidence concerning emotional development and present mental state might all be required to prove that a child's proper *mental or emotional* development was, indeed, impaired. It was also necessary to demonstrate that these effects could be ameliorated by ordinary good parental care so as to prove the point that such damage was, in fact, 'avoidable'. Such cases which could be dealt with in court under the 1969 Act would include the child who is fed and kept clean and warm but who is isolated and never given company, affection or opportunity to learn. Once discovered, the most serious cases can be recognized as neglect or maltreatment without much difficulty. Neighbours may not even know of the existence of the child who will be found apparently grossly retarded, particularly in verbal skills. Rapid improvement is noted when the child is removed to a foster home. These extreme examples of parental neglect are rare but they can occur in all strata of society. They are distinguished from other severe developmental disorders such as mental retardation and autism by their improvement after removal to a more congenial environment and, for that reason, they are sometimes referred to as 'pseudo-retardation' and 'pseudo-autism'. The Czechoslovakian twins, described and studied by Koluchova [8], who showed complete recovery from severe retardation when brought up in a stimulating environment, are a classic example of severe emotional abuse and neglect.

Under the 1969 Act, therefore, not only must damage to the child be established but there must also be evidence that damage could have been prevented. 'Avoidable' damage is caused either by neglect or by more deliberate cruelty and these two factors are taken into account in the DHSS circular of 1980 which established emotional abuse as a definite entity in its own right. In all cases, there are two major areas in which evidence is needed to establish the fact of abuse. First, there must be proof of cruelty or neglect. Second, there must be proof of damage to the emotional and/or mental development of the child.

16.2 THE STANDARDS AGAINST WHICH SEVERE DEFICITS IN PARENTING AND CHILD ABUSE MUST BE MEASURED

Before the welfare of a child or the capacity of an adult to act as a parent is called into question, there has to be some agreement as to what are acceptable standards as regards the rearing of children in any particular culture. The state of the child and also the behaviour and attitudes of the care-taker must be examined.

(a) Measures of well-being in children

Health – and, particularly, mental health – is not easy to define because of its enormous variability in growing children. Physical health and development depend in part on emotional well-being. Yardsticks measuring physical development are easier to comprehend and may be more objective than are those which attempt to measure cognitive growth or emotional development. These physical measures, which can give some indication of emotional health, are considered first.

Growth

Physical growth is a useful measure of emotional as well as physical well-being in childhood. The simplest reliable measure is a regular assessment of height and weight, preferably measured on the same scales, recorded meticulously on standardized growth charts; the child's rate of growth can thus be seen over time and can be compared with that of the normal population [9]. Healthy, happy children grow along a known curve on which the boundaries of normality are now well defined. Persistent poor growth – below the third percentile at each age – requires investigation, as does a falling off of the rate from a higher percentile to a much lower one.

Prolonged misery is one cause of inadequate growth. Inadequate food intake is the obvious primary cause of the growth problem but that may be due, either, to less than sufficient food becoming available, or to a deterioration in the quality of the food, or to a diminution in the child's appetite or ability to digest the food effectively.

Failure to thrive

Failure to thrive, despite allegedly adequate food intake and in the absence of any medical disorder such as malabsorption, can indicate an overlap between emotional abuse and neglect of basic needs. The child's weight gain is shown to be satisfactory while in hospital or in a foster home but weight is lost and growth is impeded on return to the care of the parents [10].

The continuation of this state may result in a markedly reduced stature which has been called deprivation or psychosocial dwarfism. The cause of this has been postulated as a direct effect of the emotional disturbance on the hypothalamus with inhibition of the production of growth hormone [11]. There is also some evidence that emotionally deprived children actually may not eat or may not absorb competently the food that is put before them. Widdowson [12] described a study in an institution in which the children under the care of one matron grew much more effectively than those under the care of another, despite improvement of both the quantity and the quality of the food available to those under the latter. The atmosphere at meal-times was very different and the children were more likely to eat and enjoy the food when under a kindly regimen than when under a more strict one. Poor appetite will contribute to poor growth as does emotionally induced intestinal hurry [13] since an anxious child will not absorb food efficiently. An accurate dietary history, with direct observation, is important because the parents may not give a true account of what the child eats [14]. The mechanism of deprivation of psychosocial dwarfism is, however, not clear and some would argue that the condition is nothing more than that of malnutrition [15].

Poor growth without any positive findings following medical investigation cannot be assumed to be deprivation dwarfism without the demonstration of 'catch-up' growth under other conditions. The behaviour of children subject to non-organic failure to thrive has been noticed to be unusual, with particular deficits in response to physical contact or affectionate overtures, in facial expression and in eye contact [16].

Case 16.1

Figs 16.1 and 16.2 show the height and weight charts for a child, R.S., between the ages of 4 and 10 years. He was first admitted to hospital (first weight estimate) when well below the third percentile in weight and was discharged home after gaining significant weight. The rate of growth was not continued at home and he was re-admitted (first arrow). The rapid gain in weight followed by a more normal growth period, coupled with negative investigations for any pathological explanation, finally led to a care order being made (second arrow). From then on, his growth proceeded along normal lines until he was

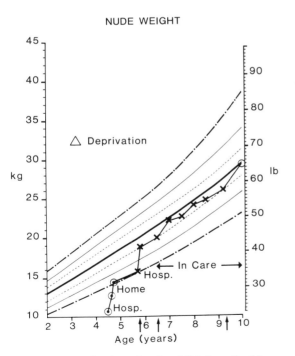

Fig. 16.1 Weight chart for the child described in Case 16.1.

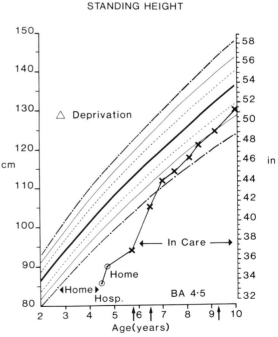

Fig. 16.2 Height chart for the child described in Case 16.1.

discharged from follow-up at the age of 9 years 3 months.

(b) Developmental milestones

Few children are followed meticulously throughout infancy and early childhood so that the ages at which particular skills are acquired are not often recorded with accuracy. Parental recall is notoriously unreliable and this is particularly so of the dates at which one of several offspring have achieved such milestones as smiling, sitting independently, speaking words singly or in phrases and the like. Walking alone, without support from furniture or adults, is the one milestone that can be remembered by most parents with some reliability. Retrospective data about development are, therefore, unsatisfactory. Children who have been seen regularly in a well-baby clinic or by a health visitor will have some records that will enable an opinion to be given as to whether development has been normal up to any given point in time. Unfortunately, many children who are at risk of poor parenting will not have been seen at clinics and statutory checks by health visitors may have been evaded by repeated changes of address or even of name. Indeed, it has been estimated that non-attendance at infant-welfare clinics and subsequent omission of the statutory developmental checks can be as high as 40% and that non-attenders have a higher incidence of abnormalities as well as many more social problems [17].

Even with accurate prospective records, deviation of developmental milestones from the normal is less easy to demonstrate than in the case of growth. There are a number of standardized tests that can be used to determine developmental quotients but their ability to predict later development has been disappointing – hence their multiplicity. Nonetheless, serial testing, using the same standardized test, which shows a clear fall-off of scores in relation to each age tested can

be very useful evidence that a child's development is impaired. However, other reasons for such fall-off must be explored and excluded before the damage can be established as being the result of abuse. It is, for example, common for children with Down's syndrome to show an apparent deterioration in terms of developmental quotient as they grow older [18]. Yet children with Down's syndrome are not exempt from emotional abuse; on the contrary, they may, like other retarded children, be particularly vulnerable [19].

(c) Progress in school

All children in the United Kingdom must, by law, attend school between the ages of 5 and 16 years. Records are kept by each class teacher and are passed on to the next at the start of each school year. These ordinary school records will, of course, vary very greatly in quality and many will consist of little more than subjective comments by the teachers. However, a stop or a marked decrease in the rate of progress should be apparent. There are some standardized tests of educational achievement in both reading and arithmetic, e.g. the Neale tests of reading comprehension and accuracy and of arithmetic [20]. More than one estimate is very helpful and serial testing at regular intervals is particularly valuable; but these are rarely available since deprived children have many changes of school.

However, the importance of school records as evidence of the well-being of children is recognized by those courts concerned with the future arrangements for the care of children in divorce or wardship proceedings.

(d) Increasing competence in childhood

There are few positive measures of well-being in childhood. Although some attempts have been made to measure competence for research purposes [21], there are no standardized questionnaires available which would monitor the progress of children in a less negative way than can the instruments that search for behavioural problems and symptoms of emotional distress. As they grow up, healthy children acquire more and more skills in day-to-day living, more confidence in dealing with their own problems and more independence, both in functioning and outlook, from their parents. The development of these skills may be referred to collectively as the acquisition of competence, a process which is geared towards the end of emotional childhood when the young adult can stand on his or her own feet and can make mature relationships. Emotional health is indicated by the acquisition of a range of skills, the enjoyment of hobbies and of outside interests and of pleasure and skill in social relationships – particularly with a peer group. It is clear, however, that there is a wide variation in competence in any age-group, even among children who have not been exposed to severe adversity. Inborn advantages – such as good looks, intelligence and athletic ability – influence a child's view of him or herself and the way in which they tackle the problems that face them [22].

16.3 MEASURES OF PARENTING

The ability to parent is a most important indication of emotional competence in an adult. Thus, two ends of the same process are seen in cases of abuse when one looks at the damage – as shown by the impairment in any child – and at the cause – which is the failure of the capacity to parent [23]. Since personality development is never perfect, most ordinary parents find that bringing up is a task which is seldom carried out to one's complete satisfaction. All parents are, at times, unjustifiably angry or too preoccupied with other matters to recognize every need of the child. Yet, the majority of parents, despite acknowledging many human failings, do manage to bring up children without causing serious damage or distress in childhood and without impeding their progress to independence. A useful concept here is that of Winnicott [24] who described 'good enough parents' – those who bring up their children with success and enjoyment despite the hard times which the family may meet on the way.

Behaviour of parents that is emotionally abusive to children is either neglect or rejection or a mixture of both. Neglect implies a failure to meet the child's needs. In the emotional field, these needs are for affection and approval, for stimulation and teaching, for discipline and control and, finally, for the opportunity and encouragement to acquire independence and self-confidence. The 'good enough' parent will also have provided physical care and protection.

Rejection is most commonly a failure to meet the needs for affection and approval and, instead, a demonstration of undisguised dislike, punishing words and creation of a punishing atmosphere around the child. Crude language is not always seen as abusive by a child; by contrast, hidden barbs that cause deep wounds may be masked by flowery language that is freely interspersed with endearments. In addition to distortions of communication, there may be abnormal attitudes to the child in which roles are reversed, so that the child, effectively, has to parent the mother or father, or where hateful and developmentally inappropriate motives are attributed to the child. Social workers, and even judges, may collude with the parents in this last form of abuse when a small child is accused of an evil plot against the parents – even though the concepts involved are way beyond his or her cognitive development at the time.

There is no typical parent who mistreats children emotionally, any more that there is a typical parent in other forms of child abuse [25, 26]. Many abusing parents have no psychiatric disorder. Psychotic parents may involve their children in their delusions and the abuse becomes part of the symptomatology. However, psychosis is not a common cause of emotional abuse although the severely depressed parent may fail to meet the child's emotional needs, particularly those for stimulation and the opportunity for independence [27]. More commonly, the parental diagnosis, if any, is that of personality disorder. Although uncontrolled, aggressive types of personality are more common in instances of physical abuse, subtler disorders are found associated with cases of emotional abuse. An example is the very shallow type of personality who is constantly craving attention and is oblivious of the needs of those who have to live around someone who is always acting as if he/she were centre stage.

16.4 THE SIGNS OF EMOTIONAL ABUSE

Children may show signs of emotional damage which is due to a number of different causes. Those that are reacting to rejection or neglect by the parents may show many signs that are very similar to those in children suffering from the chronic distress of an emotional disorder which may be due to a wide variety of alternative aetiologal factors. Although there are no signs that are pathognomonic of emotional abuse, there are some clinical features that are more characteristic of that particular form of maltreatment than of others. Nonetheless, there is a marked overlap between the symptoms in children who have been rejected or starved of affection and those in children suffering from psychiatric disorder related to other antecedents.

(a) Disorders of attachment

There are unusual features to be seen in the attachment behaviour towards the usual care-taker, and towards any substitute, of young children who have been treated in an abusive, cold or rejecting way. Some react angrily to the parents and clearly avoid contact but, more commonly, they cling excessively and fear separation – as if heeding the advice of Hilaire Belloc (1870–1953):

> And always keep a hold of Nurse
> For fear of finding something worse.

Others are ambivalent, showing both hostile and clinging behaviour. Those who show anxious attachment obviously demonstrate their fear that something worse may happen, while the child who has had some experience of good parenting is able to react with what can be recognized as understandable anger. Indifference to human contact has been seen in young children who have been severely deprived of both nourishment and affection over a long period. Attachment behaviour varies in ordinary children who have a normal experience of parenting since some are outgoing while others venture forth only slowly from the safe base of the parent. The variation is due as much to innate temperamental characteristics as to environmental factors. Most children are different in a clinic from what they are in their own homes and this, in turn, will produce another repertoire of behaviour which differs from that seen in a familiar playgroup. The observation and interpretation of attachment behaviour requires considerable experience of children from a wide variety of backgrounds in many different situations.

(b) Self-esteem

Older children who are never praised but who are frequently criticized or punished will have developed a low opinion of themselves. This low self-esteem shows itself by the emergence of problems in relationships with other children as well as with adults. Children so afflicted cannot believe that they are likeable, let alone loveable, and, accordingly, are slow to trust. All children have to learn about making friends and will suffer some set-backs in so doing. Most can return for comfort to parents whose love is experienced as dependable and can try again; but those who have suffered years of rebuff from parents will be very hesitant to risk further rejection and will tend to withdraw from interpersonal relationships – a pattern of behaviour which can last for a long time, often up to and including adult life. A few abused children with a different temperament, who have also been reared coldly or harshly, may face the world with an aggressive stance and oppose anyone coming near, attacking first each time.

(c) Signals of distress from emotionally abused children

Drug overdoses taken by adolescents and young adults are often interpreted as 'cries for help' and, indeed, a number of young adolescent girls who are seen following a para-suicide gesture are found to have been abused emotionally or sexually and have discovered no other effective way of communicating their distress [28].

The cries for help of younger children are at least as incoherent, and can be even more maladaptive, leading to the risk of further rejection and even more punishment. Unruly or aggressive behaviour in school is common in those children who have many problems to cope with at home. It occurs in, but is by no means confined to, children who have been emotionally abused. A more specific cry for help is the attention-seeking complaint where a child plays what seems to be an exaggerated role of victim – this is sometimes known as the 'Cinderella syndrome' [29]. In such cases, the original dramatic complaint may be found to lack foundation but the child is, nonetheless, in an unenviable position due to mistreatment of another type or from another quarter. Such a 'no smoke without fire' situation, where the

child is too terrified of the real perpetrator to lay the complaint in the proper quarter, is common in sexual as well as emotional abuse.

The sudden onset of soiling and wetting, without any attempt being made to get to the toilet, may represent another way of attracting attention in mid-childhood. This is an unusual symptom in general child psychiatric practice but it is found in children who have been emotionally abused, some of whom will have also suffered the added trauma of sexual abuse. The behaviour may continue for a time after the child is safe in a loving foster home.

16.5 EMOTIONAL ABUSE AS PART OF OTHER FORMS OF ABUSE

(a) Emotional abuse accompanying sexual abuse

Mention has already been made above of signs that are common in emotional abuse and that occur also in children who have been sexually abused. There is a wide range of abnormal sexual behaviour towards children; the boundaries are ill-defined and extend from that which is little more than unwise to frankly abusive acts – and even the latter will affect children emotionally in varying degree. Child sexual abuse within the family invariably involves *violation of trust* and misuse of power of one member over another. The power of parents of younger children is such that the wishes of the parents may not be questioned and the admonishment not to tell anyone else will be adhered to without the need for further threats. The parents' acts become more open to question as children grow older and are influenced by others outside the family, such as friends and teachers or by what they see on television; strict obedience to an order for secrecy cannot, then, be counted upon and threats may be used. The most common threats are that, if the child tells, he or she will be taken away and put into a home or that Daddy will go to prison and it will be his or her fault. Other threats that are heard include those of death or damage to a loved pet or to a younger sibling. These threats unquestionably constitute emotional abuse. Even in the least coercive forms of sexual abuse, where there is a very slow progression over the years from light touching to full sexual intercourse, the relationship has been distorted – not just with the perpetrator but also with other members of the family from whom the child gradually feels more estranged as the unusual nature of the secret behaviour with the abusing parent is realized and the feeling of guilt increases.

This experience of guilt is often long-lasting and is potentially very damaging. A frightening, indeed, very dangerous, attack from a stranger can produce less lasting ill-effects when the child is later comforted and supported by a loving family than will arise from a long-term illicit relationship with little physical damage but with the child left feeling blameworthy and stigmatized by the experience. Two cases seen in the same month will illustrate this point:

Case 16.2
A girl had been abducted near her home and been taken 30 miles away where she was raped and then stabbed, being left for dead. She recovered from serious wounds so as to be able to give evidence to the police which enabled them to arrest her attacker. She was surrounded by the love of her family and the concern, not only of them, but of strangers as well as of friends who had heard about the incident. The police even made a collection to buy her a dog for her future protection. She returned to school and made an excellent emotional as well as physical recovery.

By contrast:

Case 16.3
A boy had been seduced over a 2-year period by a trusted friend of the family who had high standing in the neighbourhood. He had been subjected to many threats to keep the secret and, when he finally broke down and told his parents, both he and they were subjected to vilification by the perpetrator – who loudly protested his innocence – and by others whom the boy and his family had previously held in esteem; all this despite the fact that the case was proved in court. Two years after the event, the boy still had severe emotional distress and experienced great difficulty in leaving his home.

The murderous attack upon the young girl appears to have absolved her from blame while the fact that the boy's abuser was a respected individual who used only emotional violence left the victim with a crippling burden of guilt which was greatly compounded by the misplaced virtuous indignation of the community. The comparison of these two cases supports the findings in a number of studies of children who have sustained appalling trauma [30]. The ill-effects were diminished if the parents shared the horrifying experience or were able to provide strong support for the child afterwards. The worst outcome for the child arose when the parent, him or herself, was the instigator of the horror.

The emotional trauma suffered by the sexually abused child or adolescent is often continued in court. There is often a lag of several months between the attack and the court hearing, during which time a victim may have begun to recover from the symptoms of 'post-traumatic stress syndrome' as it is called in the American psychiatric classification [31]. The main symptoms of such a disorder include recurrent and intrusive recollections of the event and recurrent dreams together with loss of interests, problems of sleep or concentration and the avoidance of anything that can remind the child of the attack. Where these symptoms have been severe, such as when there has been a serious attempt at suicide, the doctor in charge of the case may have considerable misgivings about exposing the child to the ordeal of cross-examination during which it is permitted to make a major onslaught on the victim's personality and past history, with neither redress nor correction.

Studies of sexually abused children indicate that a large proportion show signs of emotional disturbance [32]. Studies of adults suggest that these effects can be long lasting, although studies of healthy young women in university samples have indicated that, when minor abuse, such as a single exposure to exhibitionism, is included, few associations can be found between that widely defined sexual abuse – which includes what is a relatively common sort of childhood experience – and their later psychological adjustment [33].

(b) Emotional abuse and physical abuse

Emotional abuse is a common companion of prolonged physical abuse. It is not found as frequently in cases where the alleged abuse is either a punishment which is inappropriately harsh or is that which causes injury through accident or carelessness. Where punishment has been both frequent and random, the child remains fearful between attacks. In many cases, an ordinary parent is able to see that threats are as effective as is actual physical punishment. This can be seen as simple training and differs from the situation in which a child cannot distinguish between behaviour that deserves a reprimand and that which does not. Random punishment induces considerable anxiety similar to the condition of 'learned helplessness' which is demonstrable in rats which are given electric shocks at random and contrasts with the reaction of those that come to know that the shocks always accompany a perceived stimulus and, hence, learn to avoid punishment [34].

Physical neglect is almost inevitably accompanied by neglect of the emotional needs of the child. In the few cases where neglect can be attributed to a significant degree of mental retardation in the mother, the child may be treated affectionately despite its basic needs of adequate food, cleanliness and warmth being unmet. However, a mother who is intellectually incapacitated will have great difficulty in understanding the child's need for increased freedom to enable him or her to develop any sort of competence. When the small child can be treated as a doll, the mother treats it with affection, but she reacts with hostility to the emergence of an independent personality which is evinced by lack of compliance or tantrums of temper.

16.6 CHILDREN WHO ARE PARTICULARLY VULNERABLE

Much attention has been paid to the development of attachment in the first hours after birth. Prematurity and treatment in a special-care baby unit were, until recently, both regarded as being risk factors in the development of mother/child relationships. The recognition of this risk – and improvements in the atmosphere in the special-care baby units, with an emphasis on welcoming parents and promoting their relationship with their new babies – has led to these two factors no longer being significant in themselves. Emotional problems in connection with conception, pregnancy and, later, the labour and delivery may discolour the view that a vulnerable woman has of her child. For example:

Case 16.4
A woman, referring to her 5-year-old daughter, first said: 'I don't know why I dislike her.' She gave a history that the pregnancy resulted from a conception following intercourse with a drunken man, that the marriage precipitated by the pregnancy was over before the child was even born and that the subsequent months spent in moving from hostel to hostel, because none could tolerate the presence of

a crying baby, had started her drinking and had initiated a degrading cycle of drying-out and readmissions. She then gained some insight and was able to say spontaneously: 'I must be blaming her for all that'.

Illegitimacy was often cited as a reason why a child was neglected or abused emotionally. In modern times, it is not the matter of whether the child was or was not born within a legal marriage that appears to be important but, rather, it is the retrospective quality of the relationship between the child and its father that seems to matter. An increasingly common situation is that in which the child is held to blame for a previous unhappy marriage.

Children who lack competence or the attributes particularly prized by their parents may be at special risk. Glaser and Bentovim [35] found that chronically ill or handicapped children were more likely to suffer abuse 'by omission' than were potentially healthy children. The severity of the handicap itself was not associated with the degree of abuse but problems involving social and emotional disturbance in the handicapped children were.

Many cases of child emotional abuse can be seen as a problem in the parents' perception of the child rather than as being due to a factor which is more objectively recognizable. The child may remind the abusing parent of a cruel adult in that parent's childhood. A difficult, and potentially dangerous, situation is where the child serves as a constant reminder of the parent's hated self.

Unusual families may sometimes be regarded as being emotionally abusive because of the demands that are put upon the children. Those with a tradition of excellence in academic, musical or sporting fields often expect a degree of compliance in hard schedules of practice or study which would appal many other children. There is,

however, little evidence that the child is damaged provided that the main motivation comes from the child and is not entirely imposed by ambitious parents. The line between high standards and abuse can be far from clear in certain fields. Yet, excellence in any particular sporting, artistic or academic arena appears to protect the child from reacting adversely to emotional trauma from other directions. The childhood of Mozart or of the Brontë sisters was far from ideal and the desire to produce great art or to acquire an Olympic medal in the family does not justify ill-treatment. Unusual exposure of a young child to danger [36] could seem questionable with regard to parenting, yet growing up in conditions such as are described in Murphy's series of travel books can lead to exceptional competence [37].

16.7 MANAGEMENT

The treatment of all forms of abuse is difficult but that of severe emotional abuse is particularly fraught with problems. The fact that there is an element of abuse in many referrals to a child psychiatric clinic and that there is a huge overlap between several diagnoses as to the results of abuse mean that emotional abuse covers the whole field of child and adolescent psychiatry. There is no one treatment to be prescribed with confidence and the results of treatment vary widely. It is usually necessary to employ a combination such as individual therapy for the child conjoined with family therapy to involve all members. Frequently, marital therapy for the parents together or individual treatment for one parent alone, as in Case 16.4 above, may also have to be used. Several therapists will be needed. Certainly two will be required to work with a family group in which serious emotional abuse has been recognized and they, themselves, will benefit from regular and skilled supervision by a colleague who is not directly involved.

Parents who have to face up to the unpalatable fact that their behaviour has caused serious damage to their child are likely to be extremely hostile towards the person who has made the diagnosis. The invisibility of the ill-effects, in contrast to those of physical abuse, makes denial stronger. There is also a good argument to be made for a therapist not being involved in either any legal action or in the making of plans for future placement. A second therapist for the severely damaged child may also have to be someone who is not involved with the family as a whole.

It may be very difficult to establish a therapeutic alliance. Abusive parents put a price on their cooperation, thus placing the therapist in the position of the child-victim who has had to pay dearly for what a loved child has never had to question. The conditions imposed by parents may run counter to the needs or rights of the child.

The problems of working with a child who has for years – perhaps for all his or her life – been exposed to confusion, distortion of messages and emotions, random punishment and discouragement of achievement are great. The child may need years of skilled work and child psychotherapists are rarely to be found outside a few big cities. The time required to treat the parents or family successfully and the fast disappearing time in terms of childhood which is left to the child are often incompatible. The child's need for nurture cannot always wait for therapy to succeed.

actually possible in the case of a particular family or individual parent. It is necessary to work with the future foster parents if a substitute family has to be found and the child is to be placed away from home. Too often, children who have suffered years of subtle abuse have been labelled as destructive and 'unfosterable'. They have learnt ways of coping with the bizarre functioning of their family which are totally out of place in a normal family setting.

16.8 ABUSE IN CARE

As has been indicated above, children who have been emotionally abused remain extremely vulnerable. Those who fail to learn to adjust to the give and take of family life and who maintain maladoptive behaviour are at high risk of rejection by foster parents. They then repeat the sad pattern of appearing to goad adults who are meant to be caring into using behaviour that is, once more, abusive. Even given the best of intentions, the future of children who have a past history of emotional abuse from their parents can go badly wrong in care. Where there is a low standard of child care – characterized by poor training and support of foster parents or by badly run or demoralized children's homes – it is those children who have learnt to regard themselves as unloveable or even hateful who suffer most and who may proceed to more and more punitive, euphemistically called 'secure', placements until they end up as the youngest inmates in the hospital wing of a prison.

16.9 EMOTIONAL ABUSE AND THE DIVORCE COURT

Divorce is a painful process for all concerned. Very few parents caught up in the misery of terminating a marriage would hurt their children deliberately. Nonetheless, many are unintentionally hurt although their number could be much reduced by sufficient conciliatory services. A small minority of children are used cruelly as pawns in the bitter battle between the spouses. In some ways, these are the easiest cases of emotional abuse to deal with from the legal point of view because the welfare of the children must be brought before the court. Matrimonial care orders can be made or supervision orders, with a condition of attendance for treatment, can be arranged when successful treatment seems possible.

Unfortunately, children whose parents have never been married miss even this opportunity of being heard. No one knows, or appears to care, about arrangements for children of irregular unions.

16.10 THE INVOLVEMENT OF THE COURTS

Whenever possible, it is preferable to retain the cooperation of the parents within a programme of treatment which involves the abusers as well as the abused, often within the setting of the whole family. However, a policy of always putting the interests of 'the family' first can have tragic results. The extent of the damage done to an abused child can never be appreciated without a careful individual psychiatric assessment of the child – this being additional to whatever may be done to assess the family and the social background.

Protection must be obtained through the courts if a child is too seriously damaged to risk leaving with the family. Informal arrangements, such as sending the child to boarding school or allowing voluntary reception into care, can only be successful if remedial work continues within the family. Unfortunately, the family can successfully sabotage any therapeutic plan for the child which is made without any formality. The proponents of the boarding school option often forget that the child will return on holiday at those times when there is most stress for the family and least help from agencies, such as at Christmas and in the long summer holidays. The four-term school year, which is often favoured by boarding schools for children with special needs, can also mean that the child is at home when there are no others available in the neighbourhood for company. Only a few highly specialized, and highly expensive, schools can deal with the psychiatric repercussions of emotional abuse.

There is virtually no guidance available from previous court decisions to help those trying to take legal measures to protect a child from emotional abuse. As has been stressed, all the symptoms occur in other psychiatric disorders and the child psychiatrist is, therefore, in some difficulty when being cross-examined. In practice, it is very hard to make a case in the magistrates' court and these highly problematical cases are best dealt with in the more appropriate atmosphere which attends wardship proceedings in the High Court.

16.11 CONCLUSION

The successful rearing of children to independent adult life is one of the most exacting tasks demanded of the adult. The principal duty of each generation is to pass on hope, love and accumulated skills to the next. There is no sure recipe for success in any culture. Awareness of the existence of emotional abuse of children should not lead to a narrow perception of correct parenting but, rather, to an appreciation of the infinite variety of healthy living.

REFERENCES

1. West, D. (1985) Delinquency, in *Child and Adolescent Psychiatry – Modern Approaches*, 2nd edn, (ed. M. Rutter and L. Hersow), Blackwells, Oxford.
2. Lukianowicz, N. (1972) Rejected children. *Psychiatr. Clin.*, **5**, 174.
3. Pemberton, D.A. and Benady, D.R. (1973) Consciously rejected children. *Br. J. Psychiatry*, **123**, 575.
4. Gesmonde, J. (1972) Emotional neglect. *Conn. Law Rev.*, **123**, 575.
5. Bowlby, J. (1951) *Maternal Care and Mental Health*, World Health Organization, Geneva.
6. Rutter, M. (1972) *Maternal Deprivation Reassessed*, Penguin, Harmondsworth.
7. Local Authority Social Services Letter (1980) Hn (80)20–2.2e(ii), DHSS, London.
8. Koluchova, J. (1976) A report on the further development of twins after severe and prolonged deprivation, in *Early Experience; Myth and Evidence* (eds A.M. Clarke and A.D. Clarke), Open Books, London.
9. Tanner, J.M. Goldstein, H. and Whitehouse,

R.H. (1970) Standards for children's heights at ages 2–9 years based on parents' heights. *Arch. Dis. Child.*, **45**, 566.

10. Powell, G.F., Brasel, J.A. and Buzzard, R.M. (1967) Emotional deprivation and growth retardation simulating idiopathic hypopituitarism. I. Clinical evaluation of the syndrome. *New Engl. J. Med.*, **276**, 1279.

11. Gardner, L. (1972) Deprivation dwarfism. *Sci. Am.*, **227**, 76.

12. Widdowson, E.M. (1951) Mental contentment and physical growth. *Lancet*, **i**, 1316.

13. Patton, R.G. and Gardner, M.D. (1962) Influence of family environment on growth: the syndrome of 'maternal deprivation'. *Pediatrics*, **30**, 957.

14. Whitten, C.F., Pettit, M.G. and Fischoff, J. (1969) Evidence that growth failure from maternal deprivation is secondary to undereating. *JAMA*, **209**, 1675.

15. Green, W.H., Campbell, M. and David, R. (1984) Psychosocial dwarfism – a critical review of the evidence. *J. Am. Acad. Child Psychiatry*, **23**, 39.

16. Powell, G.F. and Low, J. (1983) Behaviour in non-organic failure to thrive. *Dev. Behav. Pediatr.*, **4**, 26.

17. Drillien, C. and Drummond, M. (1983) *Developmental Screening and the Child with Special Needs*, Heinemann, London.

18. Gibson, D. (1978) *Down's Syndrome – The Psychology of Mongolism*, Cambridge University Press, Cambridge.

19. Frodi, A.M. (1981) Contribution of infant characteristics to child abuse. *Am. J. Ment. Def.*, **85**, 341.

20. Williams, P. (1973) Slow learning children and educational problems, in *The Psychological Assessment of Mental and Physical Handicaps* (ed. P. Mittler), Tavistock, London.

21. Kokes, R.F., Harder, D.W., Fisher, L. and Strauss, J.S. (1980) Child competence and psychiatric risk. IV. Relationship of parent diagnostic classification and parent psychopathology severity to child functioning. *J. Nerv. Ment. Dis.*, **168**, 343.

22. Berger, M. (1985) Temperament and individual differences, in *Child and Adolescent Psychiatry – Modern Approaches*, 2nd edn (eds M. Butter and L. Hersov), Blackwell, Oxford.

23. Rohner, R.P. and Rohner, E.C. (1980) Antecedents and consequences of parental rejection: a theory of emotional abuse. *Child Abuse Neglect*, **4**, 189.

24. Winnicott, D.W. (1965) *The Maturational Processes and the Facilitative Environment*, International Universities Press, New York; see also Adcock, M. and White, R. (1985) *Goodenough Parenting – A Framework for Assessment* (Practice Series 12), British Agencies for Adoption and Fostering.

25. Oates, M.R. (1982) Different types of abusing parents, in *Understanding Child Abuse* (ed. D.N. Jones), Hodder and Stoughton, London.

26. Steinhauer, P.D. (1983) Assessing for parenting capacity. *Am. J. Orthopsychiatry*, **53**, 468.

27. Susman, E.J., Trickett, P.K., Iannotti, R.J. and Hollenbeck, B.E. (1985) Child rearing patterns in depressed, abusive and normal mothers. *Am. J. Orthopsychiatry*, **55**, 237.

28. Anderson, L.S. (1981) Notes on the linkage between the sexually abused child and the suicidal adolescent. *J. Adolescence*, **4**, 157.

29. Goodwin, J., Cauthorne, C.G. and Rada, R.T. (1980) Cinderella syndrome: children who simulate neglect. *Am. J. Psychiatry*, **137**, 1223.

30. Rutter, M. and Garmezy, N. (1985) Acute reactions to stress, in *Child and Adolescent Psychiatry*, 2nd edn (eds M. Rutter and L. Hersov), Blackwells, Oxford.

31. American Psychiatric Association (1980) DSM-III *Diagnostic and Statistical Manual of Mental Disorders*, American Psychiatric Association, Washington, DC.

32. Mannarino, A.P. and Cohen, J.A. (1988) A clinical-demographic study of sexually abused children. *Child Abuse Neglect*, **10**, 17.

33. Fromuth, M.E. (1988) The relationship of child sexual abuse with later psychological and sexual adjustment in a sample of college women. *Child Abuse Neglect*, **10**, 5.

34. Seligman, M.E.P. (1975) *Helplessness: On Depression, Development and Death*, Freeman, San Francisco.

35. Glaser, D. and Bentovim, A. (1979) Abuse and risk to handicapped and chronically ill children. *Child Abuse Neglect*, **3**, 565.

36. Murphy, D. (1977) *Where the Indus Is Young – A Winter in Baltistan*, John Murray, London.

37. Murphy, D. (1985) *Muddling Through in Madagascar*, John Murray, London.

CHAPTER 17

Poisoning in children

A.T. Proudfoot

Poisoning in childhood covers a much wider range of problems than arise in adults, simply because of the rate at which children change physically, psychologically and socially between conception and adulthood. Before birth and during the first months of life they are almost entirely at the mercy of the behaviour of those caring for them, while in the early preschool years they may suffer not only from their acquired mobility and innate curiosity but also from their environments. Later, in the often turbulent years of adolescence, they adopt the patterns of drug use and abuse of their elders all too rapidly.

17.1 THE AGE DISTRIBUTION OF CHILDHOOD POISONING

While children may be exposed to potential toxins *in utero* and in the first few months of infancy, there is no doubt that the major part of clinical childhood poisoning is encountered after the age of about 9 months simply because this is the time at which infants acquire independent mobility and, consequently, have greater opportunities for access to poisons. A bimodal distribution is constantly demonstrable beyond that age. The first peak occurs in the second and third years and is followed by a successive decline in the fourth and fifth; the great majority of these episodes result from accidental poisoning. Between the ages of 5 and 10 years the number of poison exposures in each year of life remains very low but starts to increase again towards a second peak at age 16. This peak, however, is not discrete but is merely the first part of the incline to that which occurs in adulthood. Not only have the two age-groups merged but the causes of poisoning have done so also. From the age of 12 years on, and in some cases even earlier, poisoning is almost always self-inflicted – either as a response to emotional distress or in the search for pleasure. The adult pattern has been attained.

(a) The need for a critical approach to the statistics

Before discussing poisoning at the different stages of childhood, it is appropriate to comment on the interpretation of statistics pertaining to the topic. Poisoning in childhood has attracted much attention over the past two or three decades. Indeed, its increasing prevalence in the 1940s and 1950s was a potent stimulus to the establishment of poisons information centres throughout the Western world; recent reports from the National Poisons Information Service in London and the American Association of Poisons Control Centers testify to the effort which has gone into collecting information which might aid in the understanding and prevention of the problem [1, 2]. Not surprisingly, the volume of other medical and lay literature on the subject has also become extensive.

However, as is not unusual with statistics of any type, interpretation is not always as straightforward as might appear at first sight. In the first place, the term 'poisoning' is widely misused in being applied not only to events in which there is uncertainty as to whether exposure to a potential toxin has acually occurred but also when, despite a known exposure, there are no symptoms or physical signs to confirm that actual intoxication has resulted. The main reason for this dilemma is simple. The common scenario of such events is that of a parent, having left a child alone, returning to find him or her surrounded by a split product and with the skin and clothes soiled with it. How much may have been swallowed or absorbed by other routes can never be known but the alarm is raised and the event is ultimately incorporated into the statistics. There is now an extensive body of evidence to show that 'non-toxic exposures' comprise as much as 70–80% of childhood 'poisonings' [1].

Such incidents commonly provoke telephone enquiries to poisons centres where a further impediment compromises the collection of adequate data and, subsequently, the interpretation of statistics. Poisoning is not a static phenomenon but one which evolves and resolves over a period of hours or days according to the rate of absorption, metabolism and elimination of the substance or substances involved; it may also be modified by the effects of the poison itself and by the therapeutic measures undertaken. Enquiries about childhood exposures, however, are frequently made within a few minutes of the event happening and before features of toxicity have developed. The collection of clinical data at this stage obviously does not give a true picture of the morbidity associated with exposure to the product in question – but the limitations of the data are seldom indicated in publications. Attempts have been made to overcome this particular deficiency by making repeated telephone calls from the poisons centre to the family so as to assess the evolution of possible poisoning, but this solution remains less than ideal. The most reliable data would be expected to come from observations on children admitted to hospital since they are under constant supervision until the episode has run its course. However, even this is unlikely to yield the information one might wish for because there are no specialist paediatric poisons units and details of an accident will probably not be published unless the paediatrician has a special interest in the subject or the case has been of particular interest. While the consequences of exposure of groups of children to individual poisons have been reported frequently, there are few data on overall morbidity. Death is the clearest and most easily measured result.

17.2 THE MORTALITY FROM ACUTE POISONING IN CHILDHOOD

The mortality from acute poisoning in childhood has been falling in recent years throughout the developed world and is now very low. Indeed, children aged up to 10 years accounted for only 6 out of 269 deaths from poisoning (excluding those from carbon monoxide) in a recent New Zealand series [3]. Ninety-nine children aged less than 5 years died from this cause in England and Wales between 1974 and 1980, but the yearly number fell from 21 in 1974 to 10 in 1980 [4]. In the USA the figures were 456 in 1959 falling to 57 in 1981 [5]. Similarly, only 13 children in the same age-group died from poisoning in Brisbane, Australia, during the 15 years 1968–82 [6].

The low mortality from accidental poisoning in children under the age of 5 is not surprising since it has been repeatedly shown that the proportion who develop features of toxicity after an exposure is no more than a quarter. Of just over 2000 episodes in this age-group reported in the recent London survey, 78% of the children had no symptoms or signs on admission. Seven of those with features of intoxication were admitted to intensive care units but only two were seriously affected and none died [1].

Poisoning deaths in children in this young age-group are more commonly due to drugs than to household products, gases or the many pesticides which are available to the general public. Thus, 69 of the 99 instances in England and Wales were caused by a relatively small number of medicines [4] which tend to feature regularly in mortality statistics regardless of their country of origin. However, the nature of the drugs involved depends, to a large extent, on the time at which the statistics are collected since drug availability reflects prescribing fashions. For some time now, tricyclic antidepressants have been the commonest cause of psychotropic drug deaths having long since superseded barbiturates; their prescription for enuresis has been blamed by some for increasing their availability to young children.

Iron preparations, which were once held to be a serious cause of poisoning deaths in childhood, are now seldom involved [7] and there was not a single pesticide death in this age-group in England and Wales between 1979 and 1983 [8]. The number of childhood deaths from aspirin has also fallen considerably but older drugs such as digoxin and quinine, which still find a role in modern medicine, continue to make important contributions. For example, in the British series, no fewer than four of the six neonatal deaths and another at 3 months of age were due to digoxin. Such cases inevitably raise the spectre of therapeutic mishap [4]; indeed, it is

difficult to conceive how drug deaths at this age could occur otherwise. Mishaps were the cause of eight of the British deaths and of 62% of those below the age of 1 year in a Turkish series [9]. In addition, a very small number of children die after discharge from hospital where they have been treated for poisoning and others occur because the parents fail to react appropriately despite probably being aware that the child has been exposed to a poison [4].

Interpretation of the statistics becomes complicated when older children (up to age 17 or 19 years) are included in mortality series, because an increasing number of the deaths are due to deliberate self-poisoning – intended suicide. For example, 33% of the 24 deaths in a population of poisoned children aged up to 19 years in Maryland, USA, during 1979–82, were due to this cause rather than to accidents [10]. In contrast, all but two of 58 deaths of children aged up to 17 who were admitted to one hospital in Ankara, Turkey, during 1975–84 were considered accidental [9].

17.3 CAUSES AND PATTERNS OF POISONING AT DIFFERENT STAGES OF CHILDHOOD

As has already been indicated, 'childhood' comprises a number of stages of physical, psychological and social development and it is appropriate that poisoning in each of them should be considered separately.

(a) Fetal poisoning

Fetal poisoning cannot occur in the absence of poisoning in the mother and is therefore likely to be the result of deliberate self-poisoning, excessive consumption of alcohol and abuse of substances such as opioid analgesics and volatile substances. Many drugs and poisons absorbed by the mother are able to cross the placenta and enter the fetal circulation to cause subsequent toxicity.

(b) Fetal poisoning secondary to maternal self-poisoning

Little has been written about deliberate self-poisoning in pregnancy other than in relation to intoxication by drugs of abuse (see Chapter 3). The few publications that have appeared have shown most concern for the mother and have paid scant attention to the consequences for the fetus. The only recent review of the subject [11] identified no more than 119 poisonings in pregnancy out of a total of 179 893 (less than 0.1%) telephone inquiries which were made to an American poison control centre over a period of 4 years. Where the information was known, about half of these episodes were found to have occurred during the first trimester with the remainder being fairly equally divided between the second and third. In reality, self-poisoning in the first trimester of pregnancy is almost certainly more common than the statistics would suggest because of the difficulties of diagnosing pregnancy at this stage, particularly on the basis of missed periods. Teenagers featured largely in the American survey (42%); the substances taken in overdosage were most commonly over-the-counter drugs, especially simple analgesics, and others such as tranquillizers, vitamins, iron preparations and antibiotics which one might expect to be prescribed for women of this age. Although figures have not been published, the pattern is probably much the same in the United Kingdom and in other developed countries.

The nature of the drugs taken in overdosage clearly has important implications for the fetus. Two quite separate consequences might be anticipated; first, teratogenic effects – since most self-poisonings in pregnancy occur in the first trimester – and, second, direct damage to maturing organs when it occurs later. Happily, there is no documentary evidence clearly relating tetratogenic effects in humans to acute drug overdosage during pregnancy and it can be deduced that the risk, if any, is very low. Nor have such abnormalities been attributed to antidotes given to protect the mother.

Similarly, reports of direct damage to the fetus are uncommon. Experience with post-natal poisoning strongly suggests that psychotropic drugs would cause transient brain dysfunction in a fetus but would not be expected to produce structural damage any more than in the mother – always assuming that the event is not complicated by factors leading to severe hypoxia or hypotension. On the other hand, drugs such as iron salts and paracetamol (acetaminophen) can cause extensive cell death and there is every possibility that this will occur in the fetus as well as its mother.

Not surprisingly, the data on direct fetal damage is conflicting. There are three reports of significant iron intoxication in pregnancy. Normal children were born following one occurring at about 15 weeks and after another at 34 weeks [12, 13]. The overdose seems to have precipitated spontaneous labour in the latter case and the administration of desferrioxamine in the former did not cause fetal abnormalities. However, concern as to the potential fetal toxicity of desferrioxamine led to it being withheld from a third woman who had clinically severe iron poisoning when about 4 months pregnant. Both mother and fetus died but no information was given about the pathological findings in the latter [14].

The effects of paracetamol overdosage in the fetus might be expected to differ from those of direct cell toxins, such as iron salts, since paracetemol toxicity is due to the action of an intermediary metabolite rather than of the parent drug and the extent of metabolism of this drug by the fetal liver is unknown. However, overdosage sufficient to cause severe but non-fatal hepatocellular necrosis (as evidenced by a peak plasma alanine aminotransferase activity of 4521 iu/l on the fourth day) in a woman who was about 27–28 weeks pregnant led to intrauterine death of the fetus. Labour was induced and histo-logical examination of the fetal liver showed total lysis [15]. Pregnancy in a teenager who was equally severely poisoned with paracetamol (peak alanine aminotransferase 4572 iu/l) at about 20 weeks went to term; the child was jaundiced, but this was not thought to be due to the poisoning [16]. In another case which was similar in respect of the degree of maternal liver damage and stage of pregnancy, the overdose (which included aspirin, caffeine and quinine in addition to paracetamol) precipitated labour. The cord blood showed a paracetamol concentration of 75.5 mg/l; the baby was treated with exchange transfusions and did not sustain liver damage [17]. Two reports of paracetamol overdosage requiring antidotal treatment with *N*-acetylcysteine at 36 and 38 weeks of pregnancy state that there was no damage to the liver of either the mother or the child [18, 19].

Other causes of poisoning in pregnancy have been reported. Overdosage with 20 mg of ergotamine at the 35th week caused intrauterine death some 12 hours later [20], while maternal lead vapour inhalation in the third trimester was held responsible for high blood lead levels in the baby and for the subsequent impaired development of its cognitive skills [21].

(c) The fetal alcohol syndrome

In the past 15 years or so there has been considerable interest in the long-suspected relationship between alcohol consumption during pregnancy and congenital abnor-malities in children. Prenatal exposure to alcohol is now held to be responsible for about 5% of all such abnormalities and the fetal

alcohol syndrome is possibly the leading cause of mental retardation.

The prevalence of the syndrome may be in the range of one to three cases in each 1000 births [22]. The threshold amount of alcohol needed to produce teratogenic effects has not been determined but may be of the order of 90 ml of ethanol per day [23]; the vulnerable period appears to be at about the time of conception. Clinical studies strongly suggest that the severity of the craniofacial abnor-malities is dose-related but correlation between the amounts consumed and the other components of the syndrome is less good [23]. However, excessive alcohol intake during pregnancy is considerably more common than the fetal alcohol syndrome, raising the possibility that other factors determine susceptibility to damage. These have not been identified but black races may be particularly vulnerable [22].

The physical signs of the condition are described in detail in Chapter 3. In general, the severity of growth and intellectual retardation parallels that of the craniofacial abnormalities [24].

(d) Congenital poisoning

The major cause of children showing evidence of intoxication at birth is the therapeutic administration of drugs in the hours prior to delivery. Many drugs cross the placenta and analgesics, sedative drugs and local anaesthetics are among the most important in present-day practice. Their effects are detailed in textbooks of paediatrics [25]. The occurrence of opioid poisoning secondary to administration of these drugs to alleviate the mother's labour pains has been recognized for many years and, provided the possibility is appreciated, it is easily counteracted by adequate doses of the specific narcotic antagonist, naloxone. Similarly, the use of benzodiazepines for neuroleptanalgesia in labour may cause the newborn to be hypotonic and lethargic. Local anaesthetics, particularly lignocaine, which are commonly used for paracervical blocks and other types of regional anaesthesia during labour, can also cause toxicity in the newborn.

Rarely, congenital poisoning is the result of maternal overdosage. The sporadic reports include one of hyperventilation and vomiting in a 20-hour-old baby whose mother had ingested 15–18 g of aspirin 27 hours before the birth. The mother's blood salicylate concentration 20 hours before delivery was 380 mg/l while the admission serum level in the child was 350 mg/l [26]. Another woman ingested 5 g of the non-steroidal anti-inflammatory agent naproxen, 8 hours before completion of a hidden pregnancy. Sixty hours after birth, the baby became floppy, lethargic and disinterested in feeding and was found to have developed severe hypo-natraemia (plasma sodium 118 mmol/l) and fluid retention despite having received no more than the recommended volume of fluid for age and weight. Intoxication was con-firmed by a plasma naproxen concentration of 78 mg/l at age 68 hours [27].

(e) Poisoning in the first year of life

Neonatal poisoning has been reviewed recently by Elhassani [28]. Once born, poisoning can only occur if a toxin is introduced into the body through the gut, skin, lungs or by injection, the latter being a particular risk for neonates who are un-well and who require hospital treatment. Prematurity, in particular, carries additional risks since modern intensive care of the preterm child usually requires indwelling vascular access lines which have to be kept patent; the treatment also takes place in incubators which have relatively confined atmospheres that are liable to contamination. The potential for therapeutic mishaps is clearly high. Appropriate doses of drugs for newborn infants are more difficult to calculate

than they are for older children and errors may be made in drawing up the correct volumes to be injected. More fundamental errors have been recorded. Babies have been given ergonovine instead of vitamin K preparations, occasionally, when it was intended for the newly delivered mother – and reference has already been made to deaths from digoxin due to this cause [4]. Moreover, it is only in recent years that the potential toxicity of some of the inactive constituents of injectable products has been appreciated. These do not often cause problems in adults and older children although they have done so when larger than average amounts are used, e.g. the grey/black urine secondary to the phenol preservative in glucagon given for beta-blocker overdosage. Their presence is, however, considerably more important in neonates in whom they may produce features, the cause of which may go unrecognized unless the possibility is considered. Benzyl alcohol, which is used as a preservative in injectable saline solutions, is an example. When given too often (e.g. as a result of flushing venous lines to keep them open) a 'gasping' syndrome develops which comprises gasping respiration, metabolic acidosis, hypotension and impairment of consciousness.

However, even correct dosage and administration of drugs may cause toxicity. Theophylline and its derivatives, used for the treatment of apnoea in premature babies, have caused increased arousal, vomiting, convulsions and tachycardia while mydriatics instilled into the conjunctival sac have drained into the pharynx and been absorbed leading to anticholinergic features. The grey baby syndrome resulting from the administration of chloramphenicol to premature babies is well known.

Therapeutic misadventure is not confined to the hospital or to the medical and nursing professions. Unintentional exposure of neonates to poisons also happens in the home and no fewer than 29 of 72 enquiries (40%) to the Scottish Poisons Information Bureau about incidents in children aged 3 months or less during 1984–86, concerned the oral administration of surgical spirit in mistake for gripe water. Worry about overexposure to drugs prompted a further 17 enquiries (24%) in this age-group.

The skin of neonates is also a potentially important organ for the absorption of poisons since it is thin and its surface area in relation to weight is comparatively greater than in the case of older children and adults. Indeed, it has been estimated that the systemic availability of substances applied to the skin at this age is increased by a factor of between two and three. The active ingredients of creams and products used to wash nappies may, therefore, be absorbed and cause systemic toxicity. In the past, hexachlorophene absorbed percutaneously from talcum powders has caused extensive neurological damage and deaths, while phenol, dinitro-phenol and pentachlorophenol, used as antiseptics and disinfectants, have caused systemic toxicity after being absorbed from treated nappies. Mercury-containing oint-ments (e.g. merbromin), once popular for application to the umbilical stump, have also caused poisoning particularly when the area of application was abnormally extensive, as occurs with omphaloceles.

Mercury intoxication by inhalation is also recognized as a neonatal risk. Concentrations in excess of industrial threshold limit values have been recorded in the air in incubators and are thought to arise from the use of mercury thermometers.

17.4 POISONING IN THE PRESCHOOL CHILD

(a) Accidental poisoning

The poisons which are most commonly ingested by preschool children are household products and drugs in that order in those under the age of 2 years; the order is reversed over that age [1]. Other substances and plants contribute very much less to morbidity. Unfortunately, the most commonly encoun-tered poisons are all too often stored in homes at floor level and are, therefore, readily accessible to small children who are crawling or who have recently learned to walk. Cupboards beneath kitchen sinks and in bathrooms, and drawers in bedside tables, are common places to find a large number of household products and drugs such as simple analgesics and contraceptive pills. No places could be reached more easily by mobile toddlers who are exploring their environ-ments and using their fingers and mouths as well as their eyes. High storage sites are not invulnerable either, however; the initiative and enterprise of small children attempting to attain attractive objectives is usually underestimated by their elders.

It is extremely difficult to reduce the availability of potential poisons in homes. Few parents would be prepared to deny themselves the advantages and convenience of the numerous modern household products that are available and, although campaigns have highlighted the vast quantities of unwanted medicines in the community, it is unlikely that their retrieval will significantly reduce the prevalence of childhood poisoning. The few studies which have examined this issue have concluded that the drugs involved in poisoning episodes are usually part of current therapy rather than ones from the past and they are, therefore, unlikely to be surrendered. Similarly, the household products involved have usually been found to be in current or recent use.

By contrast, reducing accessibility offers prospects of greater success and much thought and money has gone into this aspect of prevention of childhood poisoning. Not surprisingly, drugs have received special attention. The bottles themselves have been made more opaque to prevent children being attracted by the bright colours of many tablets and capsules and the pleasant flavour of some paediatric medicines has been removed to make them seem less like sweets. In the case of some drugs, the number of tablets which can be sold in one container has been restricted while blister and foil packaging, and a variety of child-resistant bottle tops, have been introduced to reduce the likelihood of a child gaining access to the contents. These packaging techniques vary in the degree of obstruction to opening that they present; child-resistant tops are undoubtedly the most effective [29]. The impact of all these measures is difficult to assess but it has been conclusively shown that the introduction of child-resistant tops has considerably reduced the number of paediatric aspirin poisonings both in Britain and in the United States [29, 30].

Such has been the success of this approach that there have been demands that household products such as detergents and other cleaning liquids should be sold in similar containers. In response, it has been argued that the morbidity and mortality in children from exposure to these products is so low that change is unjustified when the much greater difficulties in designing effective child-resistant closures for this type of product and the enormous expense of altering production lines are considered. There are yet other problems – what could reasonably be regarded as a major public health measure for one section of society can cause difficulties for others. Child-resistant containers defy not only children but, often, adults as well, particularly the elderly and frail and those with arthritic and neuromuscular diseases affecting the hands. As a result, the tops of bottles of extremely toxic drugs – such as cardiovascular and psychotropic agents which many of these patients take on a daily basis and for long periods – may be broken off forcibly or not replaced; the containers are left lying open on mantelpieces and other surfaces

where they can be reached by grandchildren. A recent study from four American poisons centres showed that a mean of 13.5% (range 8–22.7% in the different centres) of children aged less than 6 years who ingested prescribed drugs, took those belonging to grandparents [31]. It is not intended to imply that all of these were due to problems of opening child-resistant closures, but it seems likely that some were.

Accidental poisoning could not occur without toxic products being available and accessible, but its causes are considerably more complex than those factors alone. In particular, it would be wrong to attribute it entirely to irresponsible parents having little concern for the safety and well-being of their offspring. About 20 years ago, two studies carried out in the United States [32, 33] examined the availability and accessibility to children of potential poisons in homes in which a childhood poisoning had occurred and in 'control' homes where there had not been a poisoning but where the families were comparable in terms of size, age distribution and socioeconomic status. A home safety score was devised which allocated the lowest scores to relatively harmless products which were very securely stored and the highest to those which were most toxic and ready to hand. Both studies found that the distribution of home safety scores in the poisoning and control homes was not significantly different. Childhood poisoning, therefore, cannot be entirely blamed on having noxious products available or on failure to store them safely.

Further understanding of the causes of accidental childhood poisoning has come from studies in England. The prevalence of a number of medical and social factors in homes where a child had been poisoned and in comparable control homes was considered. It was found that there were significantly more of the former where there had been a serious family illness in the month preceding the episode, a pregnancy, when one parent was away from home, when there was anxiety and depression in the parents and when there had been a change of home in the preceding 3 months [34]. The concept of the 'sick family' as a cause of childhood poisoning was, therefore, conceived and is important since it identified factors which are potentially correctable and attention to which may prevent further episodes. Presumably, the effect of these factors is to diminish the level of supervision of children in the age-group at risk.

The final component in the causes of accidental poisoning in children is the personality of the victims themselves. In this age-group, boys are more commonly involved than are girls and they have been shown to be more anxious, more active and harder to control. They also tend to cause more worry and to put things other than food in their mouths more often.

(b) Non-accidental poisoning

The description 'non-accidental' is applied to poisoning which results from deliberate, concealed administration of a toxin to a child. It is now recognized as part of the spectrum of child abuse and, like other varieties of this phenomenon, is probably more common than the limited information on its occurrence would lead one to think. The child's mother is most often the offending party. She may gain increased contact and improved relationships with her consort by making the child ill and, thus, a focus of attention and concern. The term 'non-accidental' is not entirely satisfactory as the act is clearly deliberate and has sinister undertones. Care should therefore be taken not to confuse it, as has already happened [35], with intoxication induced unwittingly by over-enthusiastic therapy. However, there may be occasional situations in which the distinction is a fine one.

A variety of substances have been used for non-accidental poisoning including sodium valproate [36], insulin [37] and even naphtha [38]. While the possible toxins are legion in number, drugs which are available to the offender or a close relation are most likely to be involved. This, in turn, places emphasis on the psychotropic drugs and analgesics which are so widely available in society and which are so often prescribed for women with marital, family and social problems. Non-accidental poisoning may be perpetrated on parental visits to hospital as well as in the home and the deviousness is staggering in some cases. The infant who was given naphtha received it by injection into a venous line on at least one occasion when left alone with his mother in hospital and his monitors were first disconnected on another [38].

The clinical manifestations of toxicity in the victim are as protean as is the number of poisons available; this makes diagnosis extremely difficult unless the physician has a high index of suspicion for non-accidental poisoning. Indeed, it is not uncommon for a child to be admitted to hospital on more than on occasion for investigation before the true cause of the illness is suspected. Diagnosis becomes a little easier once suspicion is aroused. Most children can be expected to improve after admission to hospital, at least initially, and it may then be possible to relate relapses, should they occur, to parental visits, particularly if child and parent have been left unobserved for periods. Drowsiness, ataxia and dysarthria may ensue and nystagmus may be present if psychotropic drugs have been used. Positive diagnosis, however, will depend on demonstrating the presence of a potential toxin (which cannot be explained on the basis of therapy) in the child's blood or urine [39]. To minimize technical difficulties for the laboratory and problems in the interpretation of results, it is vitally important to maintain a comprehensive list of all drugs given to the child in the days before samples are taken for analysis – not forgetting those which have been applied to the skin, eyes and mucous membranes. Local anaesthetics in gels used to lubricate bladder catheters and endotracheal tubes prior to insertion seem to be particularly commonly overlooked.

17.5 POISONING IN ADOLESCENTS

In general, poisoning in this age-group only begins to become a problem at about the age of 12 years, although several studies leave no doubt that it occasionally occurs earlier [40, 41]. Poisoning due to accidents is uncommon among adolescents; taking drugs for 'kicks' or in overdosage in response to stress are by far the major causes.

(a) Pleasure-seeking drug use

Adolescence is a time for experimentation, of adaptation to adult customs and, not infrequently, of emotional turmoil. Both the desire to be seen to behave as adults and peer pressure to conform undoubtedly lead some young teenagers to experiment with tobacco and other drugs. Not surprisingly, and despite laws intended to prevent sale to this age-group, alcoholic beverages are often obtained and consumed. Surveys in Glasgow and Nottingham between 1973 and 1984 identified 143 children admitted to hospital for acute alcoholic intoxication; 90 were aged 7–14 and the remainder were even younger. Hypoglycaemia and trauma were important complications while four boys who were made drunk under duress were sexually abused [42].

In recent years, there has been considerable alarm over reports of the use of narcotic analgesics, even intravenously, by young teenagers some of whom finance their habit by stealing. A similar problem in respect of cocaine, previously considered the most expensive of drugs of abuse, has been noted in the United States; increased availability, greater purity of the drug and much reduced cost have been blamed. Car accidents, violent

behaviour, seizures and impaired performance at school are common consequences. The size of the problem of narcotic and cocaine abuse by adolescents is unknown but, while its occurrence will inevitably vary from one country to another, the concern is that it is almost certainly much greater than is realized.

The abuse of volatile substances in the United Kingdom, with death rates highest in Scotland, Northern Ireland and northern England, has also attracted attention. The replacement of the terms 'glue sniffing' and 'solvent abuse' by 'volatile substance abuse' merely acknowledges the fact that products other than glues and solvents are misused for pleasurable purposes. The additional substances include gases, such as butane from cigarette lighter refills and freon propellants (fluorocarbons) in aerosols, and liquids such as petrol. Organic solvents including toluene, trichorethylene and trichloroethane are, however, most commonly abused. Many aspects of the problem were addressed in a recent symposium [43]. The features of intoxication with volatile substances are those of alcohol ingestion but tend to come on more quickly and to resolve faster when inhalation is stopped. The mode of use of these substances, and the consequent disturbed behaviour while under their influence, are the major causes of serious complications and death. Significant hypoxia develops rapidly when a user takes uninterrupted deep breaths from a bag holding the solvent and this may, in turn, lead to cardiac arrhythmias – particularly since some organic solvents sensitize the myocardium to the effects of endogenous catecholamines. Respiratory depression and inhalation of gastric contents are also common causes of death while, in some cases, asphyxia results from the head remaining inside a polythene bag when consciousness is lost.

Abuse of other drugs by teenagers is less well known. Some purchase anti-emetic and sea-sickness remedies which can be obtained from pharmacies without prescription. These drugs include antihistamines (cyclizine in particular) and others, such as hyoscine, which have similarly marked anticholinergic actions when taken in excess. They cause drowsiness, ataxia, dysarthria, dry mouth, dilated pupils and visual and auditory hallucinations. Coma, convulsions and cardiac arrhythmias are rarer, but potentially lethal, complications. Similarly, caffeine, ephedrine, pseudoephedrine and amphetamines are occasionally taken for their effects as central nervous system stimulants.

(b) Self-poisoning in adolescence

Deliberate self-poisoning in teenagers is usually in response to the same impelling emotions and circumstances as in adults. An argument with a key person in the individual's life, often while one or other is under the influence of alcohol, is a common precipitant as, not surprisingly, is breaking up with a boy- or girlfriend. Anxiety about school examinations, possible pregnancy and AIDS is also encountered but psychoses such as depression and schizophrenia are uncommon causes. On the other hand, personality disorder with its frequent background of being brought up in a broken family or, perhaps, in an institution, poor social and financial circumstances, poor educational attainment and emotional lability is common [44]. Not infrequently, teenagers in this group have great difficulty in relating to others and to society in general; they seem to be at war with the world and often with themselves. As a result they are prone to seek solace and oblivion in alcohol and drugs [44, 45] and to take drug overdoses in moments of despair. Unfortunately, many of these underlying factors cannot be corrected; admissions to psychiatric hospitals for cooling-off periods and behavioural therapy may not prevent repetition of self-poisoning, which can occur, occasionally, as frequently as twice or more per week. Family support, if available, and

psychiatric and social work help are given where appropriate but are not always accepted. The risk of dying inevitably increases with the number of overdoses taken but, with patient support, the majority of these adolescents will grow out of this type of behaviour as they reach their middle twenties.

The drugs ingested for this purpose tend to vary from those used by adults because adolescents are less likely to be able to convince doctors that they should be prescribed tranquillizers, sleeping pills and the antidepressants which cause serious morbidity and significant mortality when taken in excess. Drugs of these types are often obtained without consent from others, including members of the family, but simple analgesics such as salicylates and paracetamol are more easily available and are, therefore, more commonly taken in excess. Non-steroidal anti-inflammatory agents, particularly mefenamic acid, are also often taken in overdosage by teenage girls, probably because they are prescribed for menstrual disorders. Indeed, mefenamic acid overdosage is probably now the commonest cause of drug-induced convulsions.

17.6 CONCLUSIONS

In conclusion, the term 'poisoning' must be used and interpreted with care since, in young children at least, most exposures to potential toxins cause neither symptoms nor signs; serious medical consequences and deaths are the exception. Older children and teenagers who deliberately poison themselves in adult manner are undoubtedly at greater risk but, even then, few come to serious harm. The patterns and causes of poisoning in childhood vary according to the age of the child and, although the prevalence and mortality from exposure to toxins seem to be diminishing, accidental 'poisoning' will never completely disappear. Wider use of safety packaging for drugs and, perhaps, for a very small number of household products can be expected to accelerate its decline. By contrast, non-accidental poisonings and those due to therapeutic misadventure, although apparently small in number, will continue to cause anxiety amongst the public and in the medical and legal professions.

REFERENCES

1. Wiseman, H.M., Guest, K., Murray, V.S.G. and Volans, G.N. (1987) Accidental poisoning in childhood: a multicentre survey. 1. General epidemiology. *Hum. Toxicol.*, **6**, 293.
2. Litovitz, T., Normann, S.A. and Veltri, J.C. (1986) 1985 Annual report of the American Association of Poison Control Centers National Data Collection System. *Am. J. Emerg. Med.*, **4**, 427.
3. Cairns, F.J., Koelmeyer, T.D. and Smeeton, W.M.I. (1983) Deaths from drugs and poisons. *N.Z. Med. J.*, **96**, 1045.
4. Craft, A.W. (1983) Circumstances surrounding deaths from accidental poisoning 1974–80. *Arch. Dis. Child.*, **58**, 544.
5. MMWR (1985) Update: childhood poisonings – United States. *JAMA*, **253**, 1857.
6. Pearn, J., Nixon, J., Ansford, A. and Corcoran, A. (1984) Accidental poisoning in childhood: five year urban population study with 15 year analysis of fatality. *Br. Med. J.*, **288**, 44.
7. Proudfoot, A.T., Simpson, D. and Dyson, E.H. (1986) Management of acute iron poisoning. *Med. Toxicol.*, **1**, 83.
8. Vale, J.A., Meredith, T.J. and Buckley, B.M. (1987) Acute pesticide poisoning in England and Wales. *Health Trends*, **19**, 5.
9. Hincal, F., Hincal, A.A., Muftu, Y. *et al.* (1987) Epidemiological aspects of childhood poisonings in Ankara: a 10-year survey. *Hum. Toxicol.*, **6**, 147.
10. Trinkoff, A.M. and Baker, S.P. (1986) Poisoning hospitalizations and deaths from solids and liquids among children and teenagers. *Am. J. Public Health*, **76**, 657.
11. Rayburn, W., Aronow, R., DeLancey, B. and Hogan, M.J. (1984) Drug overdose during pregnancy: an overview from a metropolitan poison control center. *Obstet. Gynecol.*, **64**, 611.
12. Blanc, P., Hryhorczuk, D. and Danel, I. (1984) Deferoxamine treatment of acute iron intoxication in pregnancy. *Obstet. Gynecol.*, **64**, Suppl., 12S.
13. Rayburn, W.F., Donn, S.M. and Wulf, M.E. (1983) Iron overdose during pregnancy: successful therapy with deferoxamine. *Am. J. Obstet. Gynecol.*, **147**, 717.
14. Strom, R.L., Schiller, P., Seeds, A.E. and Bensel, R.T. (1976) Fatal iron poisoning in a pregnant female. *Minn. Med.*, **5**, 483.
15. Haibach, H., Akhter, J.E., Muscato, M.S. *et al.* (1984) Acetaminophen overdose with fetal demise. *Am. J. Clin. Pathol.*, **82**, 240.
16. Stokes, I.M. (1984) Paracetamol overdose in the second trimester of pregnancy. Case report. *Br. J. Obstet. Gynaecol.*, **91**, 286.
17. Lederman, S., Fysh, W.J., Tredger, M. and Gasmu, H.R. (1983) Neonatal paracetamol poisoning: treatment by exchange transfusion. *Arch. Dis. Child.*, **58**, 631.
18. Byer, A.J., Traylor, T.R. and Semmer, J.R. (1982) Acetaminophen overdose in the third trimester of pregnancy. *JAMA*, **247**, 3114.
19. Ruthum, P. and Goel, K.M. (1984) ABC of poisoning: paracetamol. *Br. Med. J.*, **289**, 1538.
20. Au, K.L., Woo, J.S.K. and Wong, V.C.W. (1985) Intrauterine death from ergotamine overdosage. *Eur. J. Obstet. Gynecol. Reprod. Biol.*, **19**, 313.
21. Singh, N., Donovan, C.M. and Hanshaw, J.B. (1978) Neonatal lead intoxication in a prenatally exposed infant. *J. Pediatr.*, **93**, 1019.
22. Sokol, R.J., Ager, J., Martier, S. *et al.* (1986) Significant determinants of susceptibility to alcohol teratogenicity. *Ann. N.Y. Acad. Sci.*, **477**, 87.
23. Enhart, C.B., Sokol, R.J., Martier, S.A. *et al.* (1987) Alcohol teratogenicity: a detailed assessment of specificity, critical period, and threshold. *Am. J. Obstet. Gynecol.*, **156**, 33.
24. Streissguth, A., Clarren, S. and Jones, K. (1985) Natural history of the fetal alcohol syndrome: a 10-year follow-up of eleven cases. *Lancet*, **ii**, 85.
25. Johnstone, F.D. and Forfar, J.O. (1984) Prenatal paediatrics. In *Textbook of Paediatrics*, 3rd edn. (eds J.O. Forfar and G.C. Arneil), Churchill Livingstone, Edinburgh.
26. Earle, R. (1961) Congenital salicylate poisoning – report of a case. *New Engl. J. Med.*, **265**, 1003.

27. Alun-Jones, E. and Williams, J. (1986) Hyponatremia and fluid retention in a neonate associated with maternal naproxen overdosage. *Clin. Toxicol.*, **24**, 257.

28. Elhassani, S.B. (1986) Neonatal poisoning; causes, manifestations, prevention, and management. *South. Med. J.*, **79**, 1535.

29. Wiseman, H.M., Guest, K., Murray, V.S.G. and Volans, G.N. (1987) Accidental poisoning in childhood: a multicentre survey. 2. The role of packaging in accidents involving medications. *Hum. Toxicol.*, **6**, 303.

30. Clarke, A. and Walton, W.W. (1979) Effect of safety packaging on aspirin ingestion by children. *Pediatrics*, **63**, 687.

31. Litovitz, T., Klein-Schwartz, W., Veltri, J. and Manoguerra, A. (1986) Prescription drug ingestions in children: whose drug? *Vet. Hum. Toxicol.*, **28**, 14.

32. Baltimore, C.L. and Meyer, R.J. (1968) A study of storage, child behavioral traits, and mother's knowledge of toxicology in 52 poisoned families and 52 comparison families. *Paediatrics*, **42**, 312; (1969) *Paediatrics*, **44**, 816.

33. Sobel, R. (1969) Traditional safety measures and accidental poisoning in childhood. *Paediatrics*, **44**, 811.

34. Sibert, R. (1975) Stress in families of children who have ingested poisons. *Br. Med. J.*, **3**, 87.

35. Marcus, S.M. (1979) Non-accidental poisoning with salicylate. *J. Med. Soc. N.J.*, **76**, 524.

36. Eeg-Olofsson, O. and Lindskog, U. (1982) Acute intoxication with valproate. *Lancet*, **i**, 1306.

37. Mayefsky, J.H., Sarnaik, A.P. and Postellon, D.C. (1982) Factitious hypoglycemia. *Pediatrics*, **69**, 804.

38. Saulsbury, F.T., Chobanian, M.C. and Wilson, W.G. (1984) Child abuse: parental hydrocarbon administration. *Pediatrics*, **73**, 719.

39. Flanagan, R.J., Huggett, A., Sayner, D.A. *et al.* (1981) Value of toxicological investigation in the diagnosis of acute drug poisoning in children. *Lancet*, **ii**, 682.

40. Hincal, F., Hincal, A.A., Sankayalar, F. *et al.* (1987) Self poisoning in children: a ten year survey. *Clin. Toxicol.*, **25**, 109.

41. Fazen, L.E., Lovejoy, F.H. and Crone, R.K. (1986) Acute poisoning in a children's hospital: a 2-year experience. *Pediatrics*, **77**, 144.

42. Beattie, J.O., Hull, D. and Cockburn, F. (1986) Children intoxicated by alcohol in Nottingham and Glasgow, 1973–84. *Br. Med. J.*, **292**, 519.

43. Symposium (1982) Solvent abuse. *Hum. Toxicol.*, **1**, 201.

44. Crumley, F.E. (1981) Adolescent suicide attempts and borderline personality disorder: clinical features. *South. Med. J.*, **74**, 546.

45. Stephenson, J.N., Moberg, P., Daniels, B.J. and Robertson, J.F. (1984) Treating the intoxicated adolescent. A need for comprehensive services. *JAMA*, **252**, 1884.

CHAPTER 18

The autopsy in the non-accidental injury syndrome

Bernard Knight

The post-mortem examination of a victim of fatal child abuse follows the general pattern of any forensic autopsy [1] but there are some additional aspects which require consideration [2].

THE PRELIMINARIES

18.1 THE SCENE OF THE DEATH

Unlike the requirement in most criminal or suspicious deaths, the pathologist is rarely called to examine the victim of child abuse at the scene of death – although he may well need to inspect the house and its furnishings at a later date.

This lack of opportunity to see the body at the original locus is a direct result of the circumstances of the death which commonly takes place – or is certified – in hospital or at a casualty department. Intracranial or intra-abdominal bleeding frequently takes some hours to reach a fatal outcome; as a result, there is often a delay between the infliction of lethal injuries and death.

When the pathologist *is* called to the scene, his activities there will vary according to the individual circumstances. He should, however, pay particular attention to the relationship of the body to any structures which were alleged to have caused the injuries and, especially, to their physical properties. These include the height and nature of the furniture, the resilience or otherwise of floor coverings and the features of other relevant structures such as stairs, perambulators, push-chairs, toys and the many other objects which are often alleged to have been the cause of accidental injuries – and which may, indeed, have been so.

Although a detailed examination of the body is a matter to be kept for the mortuary, an assessment of the time since death may be an important preliminary in those instances where the pathologist does have the opportunity to see the body at the scene or in a hospital admissions department; this is because of the delay which frequently occurs before battering parents send for assistance. In view of the possibility of sexual abuse, it is not recommended that rectal temperatures should be taken at the scene but a general assessment of skin cooling and of the onset of any rigor should be made. The measurement of hepatic temperature by inserting a Rototherm-type instrument through a stab wound in the upper abdomen is to be deprecated. Apart from the fact that the skin surface – and possibly the clothing and scene – may be contaminated by blood, intra-abdominal injury is an ever-present possibility in child abuse; deep bleeding in the abdominal wall, liver damage and intraperitoneal haemorrhage are to be anticipated, and can be simulated by the insertion of a thermometer. Temperatures can be taken in the axilla or in the nasal or ear passages, although the large errors inherent in such methods must be appreciated. What is being sought is any marked inconsistency between the alleged and the probable time of death.

18.2 IDENTIFICATION

At the mortuary, the first essential preliminary is identification of the body. In every autopsy, whether it be for 'clinical' or for medicolegal purposes, identification of the deceased is essential in order to avoid the infrequent, but regular, distress and embarrassment which is caused by dissection of the wrong body.

In any potentially criminal matter such as fatal child injury, identification is an absolute legal requirement which may have to be substantiated right through to trial in a court of law. There must be an unbroken chain of proof, the so-called 'continuity of evidence', to show beyond any doubt that the body upon which the pathologist carried out his autopsy was, indeed, that of the named victim. This degree of proof applies to all ancillary investigations such as histology, radiology, toxicology and serology.

It is usual for a close relative – other than one likely to be charged with responsibility for the death – to see the child's body in the mortuary chapel before the autopsy and to assure the pathologist categorically that: 'This is the body of John Doe'. A frequently used alternative is for the relative to identify to a police officer, nurse or mortuary technician who then, in turn, identifies the body to the pathologist. Whatever method is employed, the autopsy report must record the place, time and the name of the person identifying the deceased to the pathologist. Those working in Scotland are reminded of the need for corroboration of all evidence in a criminal trial; this applies to evidence of identification – which must, therefore, be corroborated in any case which is likely to come to trial.

Clothing

A record of the clothing worn must be made when the child has come to the mortuary directly from home rather than from a hospital ward. Depending upon the circumstances, forensic scientists, police scenes of crime officers or, in Scotland, members of the identification branch may attend the scene of death or the mortuary in order to collect trace evidence from the clothing and the body surface. Although this is a less common need in cases of child abuse than in those of adult homicide, the clothing must, in any event, be carefully retained; factual or circumstantial evidence collected later may reveal some need for its meticulous examination in the police laboratory. The pathologist should make a general examination of the clothing during removal and should, at the least, note obvious matters such as the position of bloodstaining or physical damage to the fabric.

18.3 PHOTOGRAPHY

Photography often has a prominent role to play in the autopsy. The police will attend and will take their own photographs when criminal charges are in prospect; the direction of the pathologist as to the most appropriate pictures to take will usually be accepted. Photographs are often taken both in monochrome and in colour – many police forces now also take Polaroid or 'instant' photographs and may even use videotape recordings. The pathologist is almost always able to obtain copies for his own use, but many prefer to take their own pictures, especially in the form of colour transparencies for teaching purposes.

Colour photography is far superior to black-and-white reproduction for the recording of skin bruising and other lesions. Care should be taken to obtain correct exposure, as over-exposed or 'highlighted' frames may fail to capture faint surface marks. Colour film, especially when produced as prints as opposed to transparencies, varies considerably in the faithfulness of its rendering of colours, especially of skin and tissues. Even the same film stock will display different hues when either the colour temperature of the illumination varies or when the exposure is outside the optimum. This means that different photographs of the same subject may not be exactly comparable and controversy may arise over the significance of photographs when faint lesions or subtle coloration – such as skin congestion, cyanosis or jaundice – are of importance. Theoretically, a strip of card carrying a set of colour standards should be placed in the field of view of each shot, but the author has never seen this put into practice.

The pathologist should also give tactful advice on the angle of police photographs, as oblique shots may foreshorten lesions and fail to record correctly the size, shape and position of injuries. The camera should be positioned at right angles to the surface, even if the photographer has to use steps or a chair to achieve sufficient elevation; alternatively, a child's body can be placed on the floor if it facilitates better photography. A ruler or scaled tape with clearly visible graduations must be placed near the injuries to indicate their size in the final photographs.

The use of infrared-sensitive film has been advocated to reveal faint bruising invisible on ordinary film. Considerable caution is needed in the interpretation of these photographs as artefacts can produce similar dark areas on the skin. The method seems useful for screening the body surface for faint bruising but confirmation must be obtained by incision into suspect areas.

18.4 RADIOGRAPHY

With the possible exception of gun-shot fatalities, radiography plays a more vital role in the examination of suspected child abuse than in any other type of forensic autopsy [3–7]. The autopsy must be preceded by a full skeletal radiological survey whenever physical injury is suspected of being the cause of or a contribution to a child's death. Some forensic pathologists insist that virtually all infant deaths occurring at home, including presumed 'cot' or 'crib' deaths, should be X-rayed. This counsel of perfection has much to commend it but it must be acknowledged that, in many jurisdictions, logistical or financial restraints make it impossible to implement; the availability of facilities often depends on whether or not the policy of such deaths being investigated by both paediatric and forensic pathologists is applied. It is still possible to halt the procedure and to perform radiography when the autopsy in an originally 'innocent' case reveals some sinister lesion. The results are, naturally, less satisfactory once the thorax or skull has been opened; however, many of the classical stigmata of child abuse are found in the limbs or posterior thorax, areas which are seldom disturbed during a routine autopsy, so retrospective radiography may still be of great value.

Radiography addresses one half of the now famous aphorism of Cameron, Johnson and Camps [8] to the effect that, in child abuse, 'the skin and bones tell a story which the child is too young or too frightened to tell'. As in veterinary pathology, the history in a case of child abuse may be absent, incomplete or deliberately misleading; the investigation must, therefore, be pursued largely through objective findings. Radiology forms a vital element of this objective search and must never be neglected. The topic is discussed fully in Chapter 19 but the major autopsy features are briefly summarized here:

(1) Bony damage in the limbs is seen most often around the metaphyses and epiphyses of growing bones as well as under the periosteal coverings. Cameron and Rae [4] have suggested that metaphyseal fragmentation is virtually pathognomonic of child abuse.

(2) The periosteum is only loosely attached to the long bones of children and is easily elevated by twisting and shear stresses. Blood accumulates under the raised membrane and this calcifies within 7–14 days to give a characteristic radiological picture of a bony shell extending along the shaft [9]. It is often thicker at the extremities, sometimes having a lumpy, irregular profile; this may be seen within 1 week in about half the cases [4]. The calcified rim may extend around the end of the metaphysis and epiphysis or between the two giving a 'bucket handle' appearance on the X-ray films. In young infants, it must be remembered that a breech delivery may sometimes lead to long, smooth periosteal thickening which is caused by subperiosteal bleeding associated with traction on the legs.

(3) The above are the most characteristic radiological lesions seen in child abuse but transverse and spiral fractures of the shafts of the long bones are by no means rare; these fractures were, in fact, found to be more common than metaphyseal damage in a series of 100 cases reported by Kogutt [7]. A spiral fracture of the diaphysis of a long bone in a child must be considered a suspicious injury; such a lesion is likely to have been due to twisting or shearing strains which are uncommon in accidental circumstances.

(4) Fractures of the chest cage are common in abuse, especially of small infants. Apart from a solitary perinatal fracture caused during delivery, accidental damage to the ribs is uncommon in infancy. In abuse, several consecutive ribs may be broken on one or both sides. This damage may be fresh or old and the radiological appearances are quite different. No callus will be seen if such injuries are recent – usually, within 2 weeks – but discontinuity of the bone will be apparent. The usual cause of the injury is the infant being held up by an adult and squeezed around the chest in the axillary region while being shaken – an act which may itself lead to a subdural [10] and intraocular bleeding.

(5) Fractures of the skull may be seen but these will be obvious during the subsequent autopsy. It is not uncommon for fractures found at autopsy to be invisible radiographically, even in retrospect. Skull fractures in child abuse are almost always very recent and, indeed, usually form part of the fatal head injury. Old fractures of the skull rarely show up on X-rays, as they heal in membrane without callus formation.

THE AUTOPSY

The autopsy proper can commence once the preliminaries of identification, examination of clothing, photography and radiography are completed. Hopefully, the pathologist will be in possession of all available history although, by the nature of the syndrome, this is often incomplete and misleading. It is as well for the pathologist to record the time of the start and finish of his examination and to list those police officers and doctors who are observers, as well as to ensure that no unauthorized persons are present.

As with most forensic autopsies, the

external examination is vital and, indeed, may provide more useful information for the investigation than does the internal anatomical dissection. Every part of the infant's body surface should be carefully inspected, not neglecting the scalp beneath the hair, the eyes, the mouth, the axillae and the perineum. When any lesion in or under the scalp is suspected, the hair should be shaved off carefully with a scalpel to expose the underlying skin. It is almost always possible to cover the resultant bald area by judicious arrangement of adjacent hair and to avoid any disfigurement; the cosmetic result after an autopsy on a child is even more important than in adults but it cannot claim priority over the proper investigation of the death.

Although the routine for external examination follows the pattern for an adult autopsy, particular attention should be directed to:

(1) *The lips and mouth*. Bruising, abrasion and laceration resulting from direct and glancing blows or slaps may be seen on the external aspect of the lips. The lips are often forced back against the gums or, if the child is old enough, the teeth. This can bruise or lacerate the inner side of the lips; the external skin may be unmarked and it is essential to evert the lips and to study the whole inner circumference (Fig. 18.1). The gums may be bruised or torn and erupted teeth may be knocked out, chipped, displaced or loosened. Tearing of the frenum, the band of mucosa which joins the upper lip to the gum in the midline, associated, sometimes, with tearing of the adjacent mucosa, is virtually diagnostic of child abuse. It usually results from a 'side-swipe' blow across the mouth which displaces the upper lip violently to one side. The forcible ramming of a feeding-bottle teat into the mouth of a small infant is a less common alternative; the teat misses the gap between the jaws

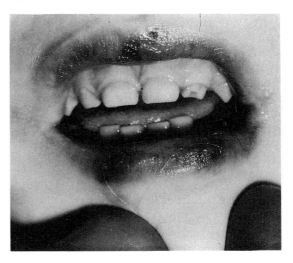

Fig. 18.1 Injuries to the lips following blows to the mouth.

and enters the labiogingival space, impinging on the frenum.

(2) *The eyes*. The examination of the eyes is more difficult but is equally important. It has been found that intra-ocular damage, consisting of vitreous and retinal haemorrhage, lens opacity, optic nerve damage, retinal detachment and displaced lens, is very common in non-fatal child abuse [11–14]. It has been reported that up to 70% of children with subdural haemorrhage also have retinal haemorrhage [11]. Although it is also common as an innocent lesion in newborns after the trauma of birth, retinal bleeding can be caused by shaking, chest compression and by a sudden rise in intracranial pressure. Direct examination is required at autopsy but is often omitted because of the technical difficulty and of the need to preserve the facial appearances. Nevertheless, the eyes should be examined whenever head or facial injuries are present or suspected and some pathologists would recommend this in every case of suspected child

abuse. Two methods are available – enucleation of the eyes with replacement by suitable glass prostheses or partial removal of the globes. The latter is best carried out by removing the floor of the anterior fossa of the skull when examination of the cranial cavity has been completed; the eyes are exposed and the globes may be transected immediately behind the lens, the larger, posterior parts being removed. The orbits must be packed before constituting the head in order to restore the inevitable recession of the front of the eye. However they are removed, the eyes need to be well fixed in formalin before processing for histological sectioning. Apart from seeking intra-ocular damage, the eyelids, conjunctivae and sclerae are examined in the usual way for petechiae which may suggest pressure on the neck.

(3) *Skin bruises* and, more rarely, *abrasions* are the most common indicators of child abuse and must be sought and recorded with meticulous care. The position, size, density and age of each separate lesion needs to be noted. Photography may have been carried out prior to this examination or may be performed as the examination proceeds. The diameter of each bruise is measured to the nearest millimetre and its position is recorded in the text of the autopsy report with reference to nearby anatomical landmarks. For example, a bruise may be described as being: 'an oval, fresh, reddish-blue bruise, 8 by 12 mm, situated on the left side of the front of the chest, 2 cm from the midline and 1 cm below the nipple level'. Note should be made as to whether the lesion is distinct or faint and, if it is not recent, an indication of the colour – such as 'greenish, brown or yellow' – should be recorded.

Particular sites for bruising in child abuse include the ears, as the pinnae form tempting targets for adult blows; small children may also be held up by the ears 'like rabbits'. A common site for centimetre-sized, discoid bruises caused by adult finger-pads is around the large joints of the limbs including the wrist, elbow, upper arm, knee, shin and ankle; these offer convenient 'handles' by which an adult can seize the child and multiple bruises in these sites should arouse grave suspicion. The neck may exhibit bilateral bruises from gripping around the throat; classical strangulation marks are, however, more likely in an acute murder situation than in the more repetitive circumstances of most child abuse. The abdomen, chest, buttocks and thighs are also common sites for bruising. Particular significance must be attached to linear marks on the buttocks, waist, back and thighs which may be due to beating with a strap or stick. A useful and well-referenced survey of bruising sites is given by Macaulay and Mason [15], which notes that a common pattern consists of a thumb bruise on the infant's right temple, with opposing fingermarks on the left side, inflicted in an attempt to cover the face to stop the child from crying. When a very faint lesion is present or when there is doubt as to whether a discoloured area is due to a bruise or hypostasis, an incision should be made into the skin in order to examine the subcutaneous tissues and histology may be useful. This should, however, not be done until all the external appearances have been studied and photography completed.

When many external injuries are present, it is helpful to mark them on a printed body-sketch, numbering them to correspond with the written description in the autopsy report. Sketches intended for clinical neurological use are convenient but often do not portray the lateral aspects of the trunk; in addition, the bodily proportions of an infant are so different from the adult that considerable distortions of distances occur. Specially printed sketches, which include diagrams of infants, are available for medicolegal use*. Injuries marked on such diagrams should have the sizes appended to each lesion and can form a very useful *aide-mémoire* when writing or dictating the full autopsy report after the examination. The sketches should be retained until any criminal proceedings are finished, as the court may require their production. This is an added incentive to make them clear.

18.5 THE PATTERN OF INJURIES

Bruises, especially of the superficial intra-dermal type, and abrasions may well display a pattern which can identify the object which caused them. Although child abuse is usually characterized by manually inflicted injuries, a variety of objects may be used as weapons. These include straps, sometimes with buckles, canes and sticks, all of which may leave a recognizable mark on the skin. One puzzling lesion seen by the author consisted of regular diagonal rows of red dots, which were due to the impact of a hair-brush with stiff nylon bristles.

All patterned lesions should be photographed with a scale alongside and a full, measured description recorded in the autopsy report. This may be vital in confirming or excluding some object later alleged to have been used. Adult fingers and hands can also leave patterned bruises and, occasionally, an unmistakeable imprint of fingers and palm may be seen.

18.6 AGEING OF BRUISES

The age of bruises is a vital observation in child abuse, as the repetitive nature of the

injuries is often the essence of the differentiation from accident [16]. The colour changes of bruising are not a reliable guide as to their absolute age but the well-known sequence is useful in a relative way; bruises of widely differing hues cannot have been caused in the same 'accident' – as is often alleged by the parents. The rate of colour change depends upon the size of bruise, its depth in the tissues and other idiosyncratic factors which differ from child to child. A small fingertip-sized bruise may pass through the spectrum of blue–red–brown–green–yellow to complete fading in 4–5 days, but more extensive collections of blood can last for two or three times that period.

Histology may assist, but many of the claims of exact dating by cellular content cannot be substantiated. Bruises which are obviously of very recent origin may not require histological examination, but older lesions showing colour changes should be sampled; microscopic examination may, at least, show if the cell population is broadly similar or divergent in different bruises if dating becomes a controversial issue.

Faint or doubtful bruises seen on the skin should be incised to confirm or exclude bleeding in the subcutaneous tissues. The pathologist may well be reluctant to do this on areas which will be seen by relatives, especially on the face; an alternative is to reflect the whole skin area and to examine the deeper layers. It can then be replaced entire without any focal incisions which have to be individually sewn up. When racial pigmentation obscures any but the most florid bruises, this flaying technique may have to be carried out over large areas of the body and the inner surface of the skin inspected over the trunk, arms and legs. Long axial incisions down the limbs can be used, these being placed posteriorly or medially so that they are relatively unobtrusive; most of these areas will, however, be covered by the shroud before the body is returned to the family.

* See, for example, *The Police Surgeon Supplement* (1985) **19**, 22, which gives details of supply.

18.7 SEXUAL ABUSE

Sexual abuse of children is not a very common feature in fatalities. This may be because sexual abuse often comes to light early in the case of children who are old enough to protest. It must also be admitted that physical evidence of a minor nature, such as irritative hyperaemia, may not be visible in post-mortem examination.

The autopsy should, however, always include a careful examination of the genitalia and anus. In girls, the standard routine for the investigation of sexual offences should be used if there is the slightest possibility of sexual interference. It is as well always to take a vaginal swab for semen, whatever the history. Examination of the vulva for reddening, abrasions, fingernail-marks and infection should be followed by an inspection by speculum of the vaginal walls and hymen for tears, abnormal dilatation, abrasions, discharge and laceration.

The anus must be examined equally carefully in both girls and boys and, again, a swab taken for semen. Considerable caution must be employed in giving an opinion based solely on the degree of dilatation of the anus, in either sex. A very patulous anus may be a normal condition after death [15]. It habitually relaxes sufficiently for the rectal mucosa to be visible without touching the anal margin and may be of a size which easily admits an adult finger or thumb. It is unwise to speculate that anal penetration has occurred unless hyperaemia, abrasion or bruising of the anal margins are seen – or unless there is a positive semen test in the lower rectum.

18.8 INTERNAL EXAMINATION

As in any forensic autopsy, a full dissection of all organs and examination of all body cavities is essential. Naturally, particular attention will be given to those areas which radiography and/or external appearances have suggested

are most relevant. Direct visual inspection must be made after dissection of old or new fractures which are revealed by X-ray and, where appropriate, samples of tissue should be removed for decalcification and histology. This is particularly important in the case of healing fractures in which a histological estimate of date may be useful.

The configuration of the main incision is partly the personal choice of the pathologist; some will use the usual larynx to pubis incision, while others prefer a 'V-shape' on each side of the neck – or even a wide 'U-shape' across the shoulders in order to avoid stitches being visible on the throat. The importance of the incision is discussed in Chapter 5.

It is often convenient to collect a blood sample – for serological, biochemical and toxicological purposes – from the neck incision before any of the body cavities are opened. By cutting or displacing the sternomastoid muscle, the internal jugular vein can be cut and clean blood collected either directly into a bottle or by syringe from the pool that wells up into the pouch of the neck incision at this site. Blood should never be collected from the body cavities for toxicological estimations after removing the organs, as contamination from the gut is inevitable. It is also prudent to avoid using heart blood wherever possible, as direct diffusion – especially of small mobile molecules such as those of alcohol, electrolytes and barbiturates – can occur from the nearby stomach after death.

(a) Head injuries

The two areas of most concern in fatal child abuse are the head and the abdomen. Head injury constitutes the most common cause of death, followed next in frequency by rupture of an abdominal viscus.

At autopsy, the first major signs of severe

trauma are often seen on reflecting the scalp. Blood may be present over the surface of the skull and fractures may be obvious. These can occur when no external head injury has been apparent and, occasionally, are found quite unexpectedly in an 'innocent' autopsy when no trauma was suspected from the history.

The scalp must be palpated and inspected for swelling, abrasions and lacerations and the hair must be removed as described earlier when any lesions are found. In very young infants, the effects of childbirth upon the scalp must be carefully differentiated from post-natal injuries; a healing cephalhaematoma from parturition may calcify at the rim and present as a suspicious lesion both radio-graphically and at autopsy. Beneath the scalp, haemorrhage, oedema and fractures of the skull must be inspected and described. The state of the fontanelles and sutures should be evaluated in relation to both raised intra-cranial pressure and dehydration.

Fractures of the skull may be found in any position, but the most common in fatal cases are linear cracks across the parietal bone, running either downwards from the sagittal suture or backwards from the frontoparietal suture. These may pass downwards into the temporal bone and, if severe, may extend into the base of the skull. Basal fractures are, generally, rare in child abuse but, if present, usually track across the middle fossa between the sphenoid wing and petrous temporal bone, sometimes entering the pituitary fossa. Parietal fractures are not infrequently bilateral and may be virtually symmetrical. Some-times, a fracture may run up one parietal bone to the sagittal suture and then 'step sideways' for a centimetre or so before continuing down the opposite side. Parietal fractures indicate a blow or fall onto the side or top of the head and, when bilateral, are almost always caused by an impact on or near the vertex (Fig. 18.2). Fractures of the occipital and frontal bones are less common; a focal impact causes a stellate or a depressed fracture and this may,

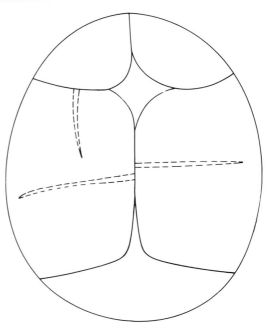

Fig. 18.2 The common patterns of skull fracture in fatal child abuse.

of course, also occur in the temporoparietal area. The fracture line, especially in a young infant, may be visible only on the outer surface of the skull; although there is no true diploe in young infants, the inner table may remain intact. In addition to the bleeding beneath the scalp, blood which has escaped from the osseous vessels may be present beneath the pericranium in the immediate vicinity of the fracture line.

At a criminal trial following the death of a child who has suffered a fractured skull, the pathologist is almost inevitably questioned about the amount of force required and the distance through which a child would, allegedly, have fallen to cause that injury. Such estimates are very subjective and approximate but, in a survey of almost 250 children under five who fell 3 feet (90 cm) or less, and another seven who fell from up to 4.5 feet (150 cm), only three sustained fractured skulls, none of which was bilateral or more than a millimetre wide [17]. Other factors have to be taken into account, including the buffering effect of floor coverings, but, in general, an infant is unlikely to suffer a fractured skull if it falls passively from any height less than adult waist level on to a carpeted floor. Many defences to this type of child injury claim that the infant slipped from the parent's arms or fell from a bed or sofa – such explanations can be accepted only with difficulty if the head injury has been sufficient to cause death.

It should be remembered – and impressed upon lawyers – that unless there is comminution, depression and brain laceration, it is not the fractured skull that kills the baby but the damage to the cranial contents. The importance of a fractured skull is that it provides an index to the severity of the impact which, itself, causes diffuse neuronal damage, cerebral oedema laceration, contusion or intracranial haemorrhage.

The examination of the cranial contents
The calvarium should be removed as gently as possible and the technique used varies according to the age of the child [18]. An ingenious specialized technique is described in Chapter 5 but, for most purposes, pathologists can adopted the 'flower' method in infants up to about 3 months of age. A small incision is made into the anterior fontanelle and, using a strong pair of double-blunt-nosed scissors, the sagittal suture is opened back to the junction with the occipito-parietal suture. The scissor-blades are kept as superficial as possible to avoid digging into the cranial contents. The scissors are then run down each occipito-parietal, inter-frontal and fronto-parietal sutures. At the lower end of each cut, a short cut is made at right angles to allow the flaps of bone to hinge more easily. Each of the bone flaps is then carefully bent outwards to expose the underlying brain. The

dura is more adherent to the inner surface of the skull in infants and one cannot remove the cranium to leave the dura intact. Extradural haemorrhage is, however, uncommon in child abuse and the above technique adequately displays the much more frequent subdural haemorrhage.

When the child is more than 4–6 months old, the skull becomes too robust to remove with scissors and may be removed as in the adult, using a hand or power saw. As the bone is still relatively thin, it may be partly sawn through – either with a delicate touch using a hand saw or setting the minimum depth on the rotary blade-gauge – and the inner layer can then be divided carefully with blunt-nosed scissors.

In very young infants, windows may be made with scissors in each frontotemporo-parietal area, leaving a crest of bone along the sagittal suture. This preserves the sagittal sinus and the falx for examination. However, these then have to be removed to extract the brain, and the method, often used by neonatal pathologists for other purposes, seems to have little advantage over the first method described.

However the skull is opened, the presence of fractures must be recorded photographically and by full description and measurement. Any meningeal bleeding must also be described meticulously, photographed and the volume measured. Subdural haemorrhage is the most common intracranial lesion in child abuse; extradural bleeding is rarely encountered. Subdural haemorrhage formed the basis of Caffey's original paper in 1946 [6], although the same injury was described by Tardieu in child deaths in Paris in the nineteenth century [19, 20]. The bleeding is most often seen in the parietal area, although part of the haemorrhage usually sinks into the base of the skull, especially into the middle fossa (Fig. 18.3). The volume and thickness of the haematoma must be estimated and the effect on the brain, in terms of cortical depression and oedema, noted. Generalized

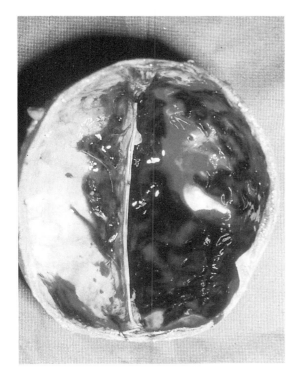

Fig. 18.3 Subdural haemorrhage in an abused child in whom there was no skull fracture.

cerebral oedema is more likely to be due to the diffuse effects of the head injury on the brain, rather than on the space-occupying nature of the haemorrhage. A subdural bleed tends to be more diffuse in infants than is the more focal haematoma of the adult. A widespread thin-film haemorrhage is commonly seen and, although the cause of death is often given as 'subdural haemorrhage', it would probably be more accurate in many instances to ascribe death to cerebral oedema and diffuse neuronal injury. A little subarachnoid bleeding may accompany subdural haemorrhage and is inevitable where there is any cerebral laceration or substantial contusion.

The approximate age of any bleeding must be estimated, both by visual assessment of the colour of the blood or clot and by histology. Blood less than about 4 or 5 days old will remain dark red; a brownish tinge will be apparent after a week, especially on the surface of the dura and on the cortex. Histological dating of subdural haemorrhage is a most inexact and controversial matter and the criteria published by Munro [21, 22] must be followed with reservation. One of the best single markers is the presence of haemosiderin as revealed by Perl's stain; stainable haemosiderin does not appear until a minimum of about 3 days after extravasation of the blood.

The brain itself must be removed with care; the infant brain is always soft and its extraction from the skull and subsequent handling are even more difficult than usual when it is damaged by contusion and has adherent blood clot. It is essential that it be thoroughly fixed in formalin before any attempt is made to slice it to seek internal injuries. The brain should be suspended in a large volume of buffered formalin, using at least ten times its volume of fluid for fixation; it may be suspended by a paperclip hook slipped under a basal artery and hung from a cord stretched across the containing vessel. If this area is too friable or if a sufficiently substantial vessel cannot be identified because of bloodclot, the brain can be supported on a thick pad of cotton wool or cloth on the bottom of the vessel; this will, however, inevitably cause some flattening of the vertex. A further alternative is to make a sling of a large piece of gauze and to use this to support the organ. The time needed for full fixation to the centre of the brain may extend to several weeks but, in spite of pressures from coroners and investigators, the temptation to curtail fixation must be resisted, as an inadequate examination – especially histological – of a crumbling, unfixed central area cannot be justified by haste.

When the brain is examined in detail, attention is directed at finding evidence of:

(1) Cerebral contusion, laceration and infarction.

(2) The presence of oedema which is especially important in infants who survive for even an hour after a head injury. The major features include gyral swelling, sulcal filling, ventricular compression, uncal and hippocampal herniation and cerebellar tonsillar herniation. The brain weight should be measured carefully and compared with age tables for organ weights in order to assess any excess of fluid.

(3) Diffuse neuronal damage is a histological diagnosis which needs expert knowledge and the use of special staining techniques. In all head injuries, death can occur — sometimes vary rapidly — in the absence of any gross brain abnormality and, as in concussion, a generalized disorder of function at neurocellular level must be assumed.

After the brain has been removed, those venous sinuses that could not be examined during the removal of the calvarium are opened, mainly in order to seek ante-mortem thrombus. The dura is peeled from the base of the skull — to which, once again, it is often more adherent than in the adult — to look for fractures of the base or for basal extensions of vault fractures.

The internal ears are examined for blood and sepsis. This can easily be accomplished in infants with a pair of bone forceps: two angled cuts are made into the petrous temporal bone on each side and the wedges of bone removed to reveal the inner ears. An examination of the eyes through the roofs of the orbits may be carried out now. In the posterior fossa, the atlanto-occipital joint is examined for subluxation or dislocation. This is best done by, first, manipulating the joint, taking care not to mistake the mobility which results from the feeble musculature of infants and from the probable absence of rigor mortis for the effects of trauma. The dura should then be incised around the foramen magnum and the joint

and the odontoid process inspected. Radiographs will have been taken before the autopsy and suspicious lesions in these areas may have been noted. In practice, however, films taken primarily to detect fractures of limbs, ribs and cranium may not be the best to reveal occult damage of the cervical spine.

The rest of the neck should be examined and as a counsel of perfection, the spinal cord removed — although this is often omitted unless there is some reason to suspect spinal injury. The least that should be done is a careful examination of the whole spinal column, which should be flexed and extended to reveal any points of abnormal mobility; a vertebral 'slice' is then made with a power saw or sharp chisel through the anterior part of the vertebral bodies and discs. This will display any crushing, fracture or interosseous bleeding in the spine — these are uncommon but, certainly, recorded lesions in child abuse.

(b) Examination of the abdomen

Damage to an abdominal viscus is the second most common cause of death in child abuse, the intestine and liver being by far the most vulnerable organs [23].

The abdomen is opened at autopsy during the main ventral incision but care must be taken not to incise the peritoneum in the initial knife stroke. A very superficial incision is made from the xiphisternum to the pubis as the distance from the skin to the peritoneal cavity may be only a few millimetres. An injudicious knife stroke can easily open loops of bowel, with consequent fouling of the abdominal cavity. This may be extremely disadvantageous if there is also a true rupture of the bowel or if there is a collection of blood in the abdominal cavity. The safest method of opening the infant abdomen after making the initial skin incision is to use a scalpel point to penetrate the peritoneum under direct vision just below the xiphisternum. The small hole can then be cautiously extended with the scalpel or a blunt-pointed scissors until it is large enough to insert the tip of a finger. At this stage, the exposed peritoneal cavity is inspected for any welling up of blood, fibrin, pus or intestinal contents. The finger is then used to lift the anterior parietal peritoneum well clear of the gut, so that the rest of the membrane can be incised down to the pubis with scalpel or scissors. After the abdomen is opened centrally, the skin flaps of both thorax and abdomen are flayed laterally so as to expose the ribs as far back as the posterior axillary line. This carries the abdominal flaps well back, but some dissection posteriorly along the costal margin may be needed to produce the maximum abdominal exposure.

If blood, purulent fluid or intestinal contents are exposed at the initial incision, then cultures are taken for microbiological examination where appropriate, and the volume of blood, clot or other fluid measured before it is lost by wide opening of the abdominal cavity. It is never possible to recover the last drop of blood or fluid for measurement by baling and the purist may wish to complete the task by mopping out with dry sponges and squeezing the residue into the measure; this degree of accuracy rarely contributes much to the eventual interpretation of events.

Many pathologists prefer to make a preliminary exploration of the abdomen to seek any obvious source of free blood or intestinal contents. This is not necessarily due to impatience or insatiable curiosity; a quick confirmation of the basic lesion, before extensive dissection gets under way, may later reassure the pathologist that some damage to the gut or liver was genuine and not merely a post-mortem artefact. However, such a pre-emptive venture should be confined to a gentle displacement of the loops of intestine and omentum; the upper and lower anterior surfaces of the liver, the anterior wall of stomach and the small intestine back to the duodenum can be seen

in this way. If there is a haemoperitoneum with an apparently intact liver, the spleen may be gently lifted forward with a finger to search for obvious rupture, but this must be done very circumspectly, as the infant spleen can be torn at the hilum by only slight traction.

The intestine is removed in the usual way, by cutting through the upper part of the jejunum and dissecting progressively down the mesenteric border of the small intestine to the ileocaecal valve. The upper small intestine is not uncommonly damaged in child abuse; the transection for removing the gut must, therefore, be made only after visual assurance that this area is not involved in trauma. If it is, then the gut is detached from a point lower down the intestine.

The colon is removed in the usual way and either severed at the upper rectum or left in continuity with the loops of bowel displaced on to the autopsy table. Further examination of the remaining abdominal organs is made *in situ* before the chest organs are released and removed in continuity with the abdominal viscera in a modified Rokitansky technique. It is preferable to remove the contents of the chest and abdomen in one mass rather than separate them at the diaphragm, as some abdominal injuries involve the diaphragm or upper surface of the liver and its attachments. It is always bad autopsy technique in either a child or an adult to remove organs *individually* as all anatomical relationships are, thereby, lost.

The major abdominal lesions found in child abuse are:

(1) *Rupture of the liver*. This is the most common fatal injury and can arise as a result of a variety of insults to the abdomen and lower thorax. A direct frontal blow is the most frequent and it cannot be overemphasized that a fatal injury can be sustained with no bruising of the abdominal wall. The liver becomes compressed against the posterior

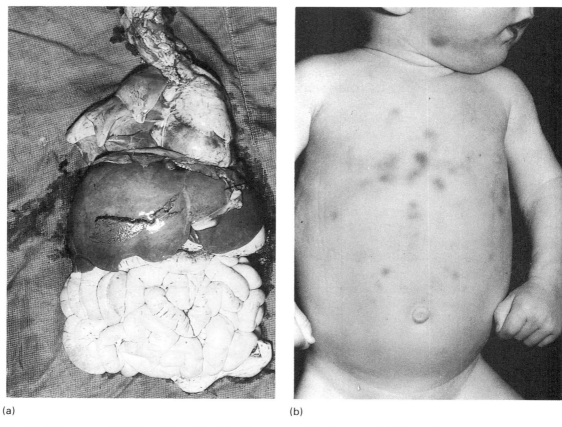

(a)　　　　　　　　　　　　　　　　　　(b)

Fig. 18.4 Rupture of the liver (a), underlying bruises on the chest and abdomen (b).

abdominal wall, usually the vertebral column or rear sections of the lower ribs, and a common injury is a vertical tear on the upper anterior surface, either midline or in the medial part of either lobe. This tear extends deeply in fatal cases and not infrequently extends full thickness through the anterior part of the liver to appear on the undersurface (Fig. 18.4). Bleeding takes place into the general peritoneal cavity or lesser sac and, unless there are other serious injuries, is likely to be the proximate cause of death.

(2) *Injuries of the intestine.* The upper small intestine – and especially the distal duodenum as it crosses the midline – is most vulnerable to severe injury. Here it lies on the vertebral bodies and may be virtually guillotined against the spine when a direct impact is sustained on the anterior abdominal wall. The author has seen two such instances where this part of the intestine was sliced almost as cleanly as if by a scalpel. Shock and early chemical peritonitis due to escape of intestinal contents usually cause death before florid inflammatory and infective changes can develop. Haematomata in the duodenum and jejunum may be found as lesser injuries when death is due to other causes. Bruising and laceration is more common in the rest of the intestine and mesentery

than is transection. Such injury may not be fatal but be discovered as a concomitant finding in death from other severe trauma – on occasions, tearing of the jejunum, ileum and, rarely, the colon may be part of general trauma to the anterior abdominal contents. The mesentery may be torn and fenestrated, with severe bleeding into the peritoneal cavity. There may be thrombosis and infarction of the intestine if death is delayed. The stomach is occasionally ruptured, although this is a rare lesion [24]. It usually happens when the organ is distended with a recent meal and a blow lands over the upper abdomen. A number of cases of 'spontaneous' rupture of the stomach in children have an occult cause and it is very difficult to ascribe these deaths to abuse if neither signs of local damage in the margins of the tear nor signs of other injury are present.

(3) *Other abdominal injuries.* Deep injury to the central abdomen has caused pancreatitis and pancreatic cysts in survivors [9, 25, 26]. Pancreatitis in children under the age of 5 years should raise the presumption of abuse until proved otherwise, although after this age, genuine accidents may often lead to pancreatic pseudocysts. Compared to the frequency of damage to the liver and intestines, rupture of the spleen is surprisingly uncommon in child abuse. Retroperitonal haematoma is seen usually in association with mesenteric and omental bruising and may be a direct extension of bleeding in the root of the mesentery. Perirenal haematomata and more diffuse bleeding around one or both kidneys may also be found in direct continuity with retroperitoneal or deep mesenteric haemorrhage. The kidney may be lacerated in gross trauma but, as with splenic damage, it is not common in child abuse.

(c) Internal chest injuries

Thoracic damage mainly involves the skeletal cage but any of the lesions seen in adults may be present if gross trauma is inflicted.

The most common injuries are bruising and laceration of the lungs. Even though the thoracic cage remains intact, impacts from blows, throwing or falls may cause peripheral bleeding in the lungs, usually of the lateral parts of the lower lobes. Such pulmonary bruising may be severe enough to form haematomata within the lung parenchyma, although this is more likely to accompany direct damage from penetration of the pleura by fractured ribs. Such severe thoracic injuries are uncommon in child abuse, although, when old callused rib fractures are present, lung trauma may have been caused at the time of the original injury. Damage to the heart is very rare in the absence of gross trauma to the trunk.

18.9 BURNS

Thermal injuries are by no means uncommon in abused children and range from extensive areas of burning to small focal injuries [27, 28]. Moist heat causes scalds which may be seen after deliberate immersion of the child into a very hot bath (Fig. 18.5(a)) or where hot water has been tipped or thrown over the infant. The differentiation from accidental scalds is often difficult as this is a common domestic tragedy in which no malice is involved (Fig. 18.5(b)).

At autopsy, the area of the scalds must be assessed in order to determine whether these alone were likely to have been the primary cause of death. Damage to more than about 30% of the total skin surface is unlikely to be compatible with continued life. The configuration of the damaged area should also be evaluated. For instance, the margin of the scalds on the buttocks and feet shown in Fig. 18.5(a) indicates that a horizontal fluid

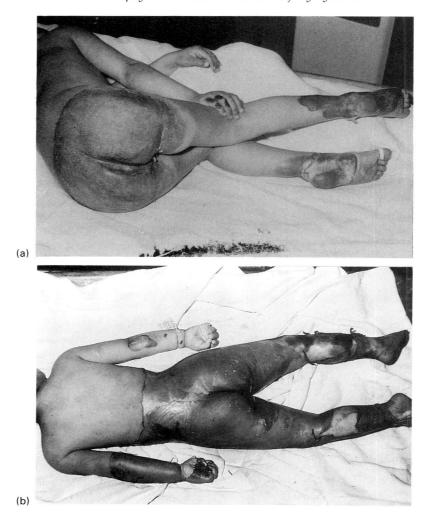

(a)

(b)

Fig. 18.5 (a) Injuries due to dipping in hot water. Compare with (b), accidental scalds in a child left in a hot bath.

level could only be achieved when the child was held under the head and knees, proving that she must have been dipped into hot water, rather than having suffered immersion in any other way. Similarly, trickle marks and shadow areas of undamaged skin may indicate the posture of the child when the injury was sustained.

Death in scalding may be due to shock, fluid and electrolyte disturbances or secondary chest infection, as was the case in the child illustrated. It requires only 30 seconds' exposure to hot water at 54 °C to produce full-thickness scalds; this temperature is usually exceeded in domestic hot-water systems.

Dry burns resulting from child abuse are rarely as extensive as are scalds and are usually due to the application of a hot surface to the skin. Children have been pressed against gas and electric fires, sat on the hotplates of stoves and had hot coal-shovels pressed against their buttocks – the categories of deliberate burns are very wide. In such cases, the burned area is likely to show some shape or pattern which is consistent with the inflicting object. The lesion caused by a lighted cigarette pressed into the skin is particularly associated with child abuse. When fresh, it appears as a red circular mark of 6–8 mm diameter, although, occasionally, a wedge-shaped burn can result when the cigarette is placed obliquely. The burn often has a sharply demarcated rim, outside which is a diffuse flare of erythema which fades rapidly and progressively away from the rim. The surface becomes puckered and rather scaly during healing and a healed burn may present a pink silvery appearance. Cigarette burns may be found on any part of the body, but the backs of the hands, arms, neck, shoulders, back and buttocks are the most common sites.

18.10 BITE-MARKS

Although paediatric forensic odontology is dealt with in Chapter 7, a brief mention must be made of the need for the pathologist to recognize bite-marks at autopsy.

With the possible exception of sexual offences, child abuse provides the majority of examples of human bite-marks [29]. All those seen by the author have been inflicted by the mother, although the literature does not confirm this maternal monopoly. Bites usually appear as bruises – often with an abrasion superimposed. Lacerated human bites are rare and their occurrence may support the frequent claim that the bite was inflicted by an animal, usually the family dog. Human bites usually appear as two partial semicircles, opposing each other in the pattern of the dental arches. They may be very incomplete and one arch may be absent. Individual tooth

impressions may be seen although, again, rarely in a complete pattern. Bruising is a feature of forceful bites and, while the actual bruising is usually continuous, abrasions overlying these may be in the position of individual teeth. Elongated abrasions may be seen where the upper – and sometimes lower – incisors have been scraped down the skin.

A common defence against allegations of biting a child is that another child of the family – or the dog – inflicted the injury. Comparison of the size and shape of the marks and of the individual teeth-marks with the dentition of suspects may clarify the issue. Bites may be inflicted on any part of the body, but the forearms, cheeks, buttocks and thighs seem favourite locations. Wherever possible, the investigation of bite-marks should be carried out by a dentist with forensic experience as described in Chapter 7.

18.11 THE FINAL STAGES

At the completion of the autopsy, full restorative procedures are carried out on the body, preferably by trained mortuary technicians. With care, even the most extensive examination can be completely hidden from view by skilful stitching and the use of prostheses.

The specimens retained at autopsy must be carefully labelled and identified – those going for forensic laboratory examination will usually be handled by the police or by forensic scientists. Histology and microbiology samples are usually dealt with by the pathologist.

A preliminary report may be prepared immediately for the coroner or other law enforcement authority but many pathologists prefer to await all the results of ancillary investigations before issuing a written report. These tests, however, may take days or weeks to be completed and it is essential that the facts of the examination are set down on paper immediately. The court may enquire as to the contemporaneity or otherwise of an autopsy report and demand to see the early notes and sketches, which must always be retained.

It is as well to dictate or write the main report at the end of the autopsy. Some pathologists will tape-record as they go along in the mortuary; many write the report at the end of the examination. Whatever method is used, the report should be completed within 24 hours of the autopsy, even if the final evaluation is left until ancillary investigations are available. The factual part of the report should be followed by a summary which interprets the findings in terms of possible causation, the age of the lesions and the like. An expert witness such as a pathologist has a duty to offer more than a bald, factual account of the lesions discovered – he should interpret them for the benefit of the investigative agency in language that can be understood by lay persons, free of the professional jargon that so often obscures the sense of many medical reports.

REFERENCES

1. Knight, B. (1983) *The Coroner's Autopsy*, Churchill Livingstone, Edinburgh.
2. Norman, M.G., Smialek, J.E., Newman, D.E. and Horembala, E.J. (1984) The postmortem examination on the abused child. *Perspect. Pediatr. Pathol.*, **8**, 313.
3. Ellison, P.H., Tsai, F.Y. and Largent, J.A. (1978) Computed tomography in child abuse and cerebral contusion. *Pediatrics*, **62**, 151.
4. Cameron, J.M. and Rae, L.J. (1975) *Atlas of the Battered Child Syndrome*, Churchill Livingstone, Edinburgh.
5. Smith, F.W., Gilday, D.L. and Ash, J.M. (1980) Unsuspected costo-vertebral fractures demonstrated by bone scanning in child abuse syndrome. *Pediatr. Radiol.*, **10**, 103.
6. Caffey, J. (1946) Multiple fractures in the long bones of infants suffering from chronic subdural hematoma. *Am. J. Roentgenol.*, **56**, 163.
7. Kogutt, M.S., Swischuk, L.E. and Fagan, C.J. (1974) Patterns of injury and significance of uncommon fractures in the battered child syndrome. *Am. J. Roentgenol.*, **121**, 143.
8. Cameron, J.M., Johnson, H.R.M. and Camps, F.E. (1966) The battered child syndrome. *Med. Sci. Law*, **6**, 2.
9. Evans, K.T. and Knight, B. (1982) *Forensic Radiology*, Blackwell, Oxford.
10. Caffey, J. (1972) On the theory and practice of shaking infants. *Am. J. Dis. Child.*, **124**, 161.
11. Tomasi, L.G. and Rosman, P. (1975) Purtscher retinopathy in the battered child syndrome. *Am. J. Dis. Child.*, **129**, 1335.
12. Weidenthal, D.T. and Levin, D.B. (1976) Retinal detachment in a battered infant. *Am. J. Ophthalmol.*, **81**, 725.
13. Eisenbrey, A.B. (1979) Retinal haemorrhage in the battered child. *Child's Brain*, **5**, 40.
14. Friendly, D.S. (1975) Ocular manifestations of child abuse. *Trans. Am. Acad. Ophthalmol. Otol.*, **75**, 317.
15. Macaulay, R.A.A. and Mason, J.K. (1978) Violence in the home, in *The Pathology of Violent Injury* (ed. J.K. Mason), Edward Arnold, London.
16. Wilson, E. (1977) Estimation of the age of cutaneous contusions in child abuse. *Pediatrics*, **60**, 750.
17. Helfer, R.E., Slovis, T.L. and Black, M. (1977) Injuries resulting when small children fall out of bed. *Pediatrics*, **60**, 533.
18. Knight, B. (1983) *The Postmortem Technician's Handbook*, Blackwell, Oxford.
19. Tardieu, A. (1860) Étude médico-légale sur les sévices et mauvais traitments exercés sur les infants. *Ann. Hyg. Publique Méd. Lég.*, **13**, 361.
20. Knight, B. (1986) The history of child abuse. *Forensic Sci. Int.*, **30**, 135.
21. Munro, D. (1934) The diagnosis and treatment of subdural hematoma: report of 62 cases. *New Engl. J. Med.*, **210**, 1145.
22. Munro, D. and Merritt, H. (1936) Surgical pathology of subdural hematoma based on a study of one hundred and five cases. *Arch. Neurol. Psychiatry*, **35**, 64.
23. Touloukian, T.J. (1968) Abdominal visceral injuries in battered children. *Pediatrics*, **42**, 642.
24. Schechner, S. and Erlich, F. (1974) Gastric perforation and child abuse. *J. Trauma*, **14**, 723.

25. Slovis, T., Walter, G., Berdon, E. *et al.* (1975) Pancreatitis and the battered child syndrome. *Am. J. Roentgenol.*, **125**, 456.

26. Pena, S.D.J. and Medovy, H. (1973) Child abuse and traumatic pseudocyst of the pancreas. *J. Pediatrics*, **83**, 1026.

27. Stone, N., Rinaldo, L. and Humphrey, C. (1970) Child abuse by burning. *Surg. Clin. North Am.*, **50**, 1419.

28. Keen, J., Lendrum, J. and Wolman, B. (1975) Inflicted burns and scalds in children. *Br. Med. J.*, **4**, 268.

29. Sims, B., Grant, J. and Cameron, J.M. (1973) Bite marks in the battered baby syndrome. *Med. Sci. Law*, **13**, 207.

CHAPTER 19

Radiological aspects of child abuse

K.T. Evans and G.M. Roberts

There is no doubt as to the importance of radiological examination in the diagnosis of non-accidental injury to infants and children. A syndrome in which fractures of the long bones were associated with subdural haematoma was first described in 1946 [1]; despite the absence of a suggestive history, it was believed that trauma was the cause of the lesions in the long bones and of the intracranial bleeding. The syndrome described was later attributed to ill-treatment by custodians [2, 3]. It was noted that the radiological findings were so bizarre that they would only have been produced by repetitive injuries. Kempe alerted the medical profession and the general public to the problem in a dramatic fashion by coining the term 'the battered child syndrome' [4]. Integral parts of that syndrome are that there is often a delay before the child is taken for medical attention and that, frequently, the history is quite inconsistent with the radiological and clinical findings.

19.1 SKELETAL INJURIES

A skeletal survey is mandatory when screening children who are suspected of having been abused or neglected. Such an examination can provide positive information not only regarding the age of a fracture but also as to the number and sites of bone abnormalities. The radiologist plays a vital role in the diagnosis of child abuse in demonstrating positive radiological evidence of trauma in the growing skeleton. Trauma is often unsuspected by physicians and surgeons and may not be considered unless there is a history of injury. It has been pointed out that the radiologist can safely disregard the clinical findings in such cases as these may be completely misleading [1]. The yield from carrying out skeletal surveys may not be great [5], but new information which is helpful in the detection of abuse is discovered in a number of cases.

Injuries of the peripheral bones are the most common, this being due to the ease with which a child is seized by its arms or legs. Traction or torsion are likely to produce spiral fractures, separation of epiphyses or shearing of the periosteum. Transverse fractures may result from direct blows or from bending of a limb.

It is not always easy to differentiate between accidental and non-accidental injury on radiological grounds. The baby in a cot is, however, much less likely to suffer accidental injury than is the older child. Most children suffering from non-accidental injury are young – almost one-third are aged less than 1 year and about half are under the age of 2.

In a comparison of the patterns of fractures in child abuse and in normal children [6], it was found that no child over the age of 5 had a fracture resulting from abuse, whereas 80% of fractures in abused children occurred when they were less than 18 months of age. Children with non-accidental injuries have an increased prevalence of injury to the face and head and also to the lumbar region [7].

As the periosteum is attached only loosely to the underlying bone in young children, separation due to formation of a subperiosteal haematoma frequently follows trauma. The periosteum may be stripped off the cortex for quite long distances (Fig. 19.1).

Injuries of the metaphysis may result from swinging the baby by its limbs or from forcefully wrenching or twisting the limbs. The metaphyseal lesions in non-accidental injury are highly distinctive. The original descriptions of the pathogenesis of 'corner' and 'bucket-handle' fractures (Fig. 19.2) suggested that these findings are a consequence of avulsion of peripheral metaphyseal fragments at the site of attachment of the periosteum [1] (Fig. 19.1). This hypothesis has now been challenged following a correlative study of radiological and pathological features in autopsy material obtained from abused infants [8]. Histological examination of such cases revealed a series of microfractures in the subepiphyseal area through the most immature portion of metaphyseal bone. A mineralized disc separates and this can be readily demonstrated radiographically; the appearance depends on the severity of the injury and the particular radiographic projection. 'Corner' fractures and 'bucket-handle' appearances derive from the same pathological process. Occasionally, a significant histological abnormality may be present despite apparently normal radiographs [8].

(a) Thickening of the cortex

The outer rim of the periosteum which is stripped from the underlying bone can be identified as a thin bony shell approximately 7–14 days after the injury. This bony shell thickens rapidly and may extend along the whole shaft. Local maturation may be accelerated if the proliferative cartilage in the contiguous epiphyseal plate is injured and this can result in increased growth which is, presumably, due to hyperaemia. The injury to the metaphysis may produce a 'squared'

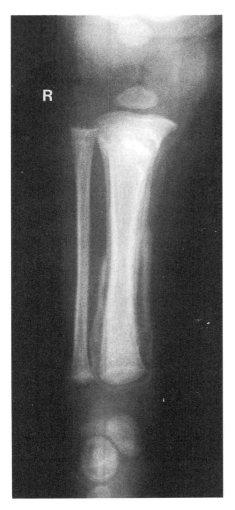

Fig. 19.1 Extensive periosteal elevation and thickening with a metaphyseal lesion.

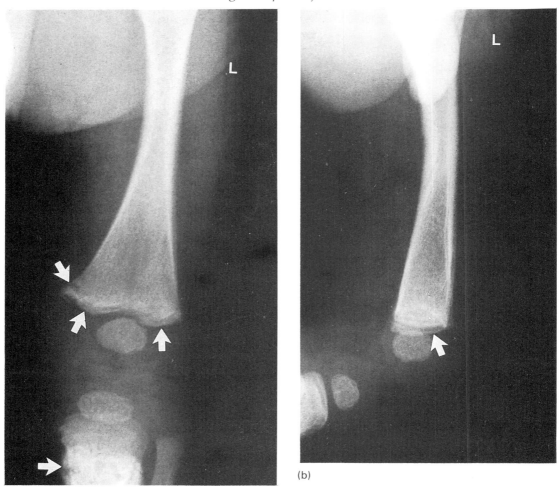

Fig. 19.2 (a),(b) Metaphyseal fracture showing separated fragment. A fracture with extensive callus is also present in the upper tibia.

appearance [1]. Direct injury to the epiphyseal cartilage results in impairment of the blood supply; cupping of the metaphysis follows as the peripheral margin of the cortex continues to grow while there is retardation of longitudinal growth.

(b) Rib fractures

These are sometimes seen in the newborn when they are usually attributed to birth injury. Otherwise, rib fractures are quite uncommon in childhood and the presence of such fractures, without a history of injury, should make the radiologist very suspicious of child abuse.

The rib fractures in child abuse are often multiple and are present most commonly in the posterior and lateral aspects of the ribs. The anterior ends of the ribs may show expansion and sclerosis due to previous separation of the costochondral junctions.

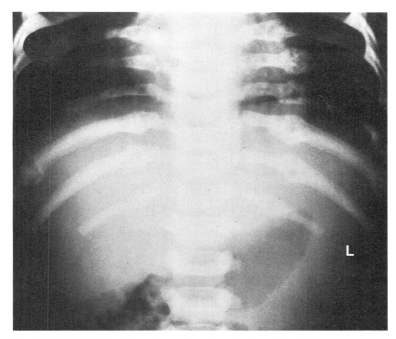

Fig. 19.3 Multiple rib fractures showing 'string of beads' appearance.

The fractures are often bilateral due to adult hands squeezing the chest while shaking. Characteristically, callus formation is abundant and presents as a 'string of beads' in a vertical line (Fig. 19.3).

Although epiphyseal and metaphyseal fractures together with rib fractures are the classic radiographical findings, spiral and transverse fractures of the long bones have been found to be the most common injuries in at least one series [9]. Fractures of the outer end of the clavicle, sternum and scapula were also seen. These are most unlikely to occur in accidental injury in childhood and should arouse suspicion of abuse.

(c) Periosteal thickening

Long, smooth thickening of the periosteum has been described in the legs of newly born infants delivered by breech extraction; this may be the result of normal handling producing small subperiosteal haematomas and consequent periosteal elevation. However, in one series, in which skeletal radiographs taken for a variety of reasons were compared with those of abused children of comparable age, it was found that periosteal thickening was not a normal finding in infancy and should not be regarded as a consequence of normal handling. There was evidence to suggest that the child had experienced abnormal or rough handling in every case in which cortical thickening was present [10]. Care should be taken, therefore, to avoid misinterpretation of the radiological findings.

Serious bone injury may result from passive exercises for presumed muscle tightness which are administered by parents or guardians on medical advice [11]. In such cases, it may be extremely difficult to differentiate the results of overvigorous treatment from non-accidental injury.

19.2 RADIONUCLIDE IMAGING OF THE SKELETON IN CHILD ABUSE

Following intravenous injection, technetium-labelled methylene diphosphonate is selectively localized in areas of active bone growth and repair. This is a sensitive method of detecting osteogenesis but it is not specific to skeletal trauma; areas of increased isotope uptake occur, for instance, in osteomyelitis and tumours. Plain radiographs of the affected parts are then necessary to distinguish between these disorders.

Abnormal isotope uptake can be demonstrated in skeletal trauma earlier than abnormalities can be seen on plain radiography (Fig. 19.4), but abnormal uptake diminishes and ceases long before fractures become completely consolidated; thus, increased isotope uptake is a manifestation of the most active phase of bone repair. A scan may be negative even in the presence of an obvious old fracture.

Normal bone growth and development in infants and children produces areas of high isotope uptake, this being mostly in the ends of the long bones. Pathological uptake in these areas may be masked and, for this reason, plain radiographs of the epiphysis and metaphysis are mandatory. Recent skull fractures

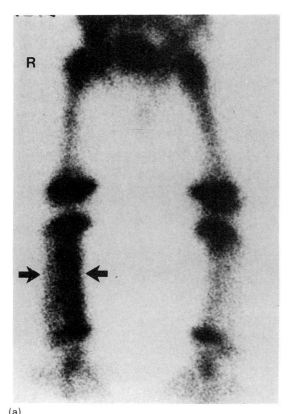

(a)

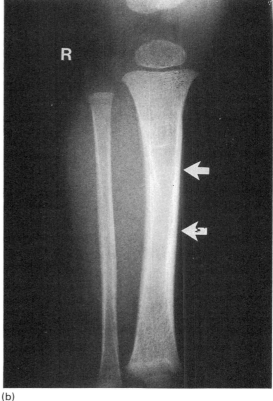

(b)

Fig. 19.4 (a) Marked uptake of radioisotope around the shaft of the tibia. The radiograph at the time was completely normal. (b) Periosteal reaction around the shaft 1 week later.

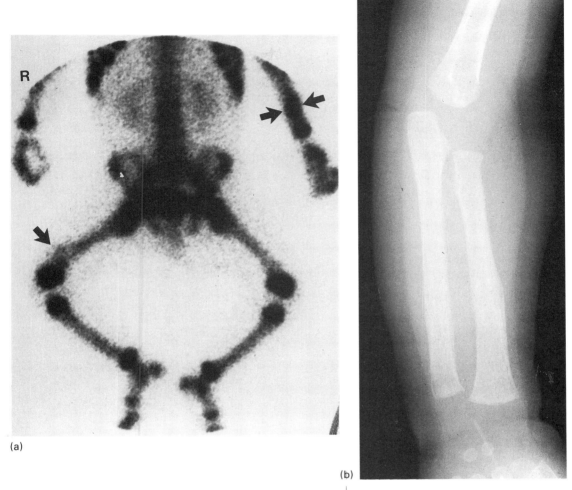

Fig. 19.5 (a) Positive scan of right thigh due to haematoma without a fracture. Increased uptake in left forearm due to injury. (b) Extensive periosteal reaction in forearm corresponding to positive scan in (a).

usually fail to accumulate the isotope. Spurious asymmetry of isotope activity can be caused by restlessness of the infant during scanning; adequate immobilization during the examination is necessary.

Scintigraphy radioisotope bone study has been shown to provide a higher positive and a lower false-negative yield in abused children than does radiography [12]. Scintigraphy was useful in demonstrating lesions not shown radiographically, showing multiple lesions and, also accumulations of isotope in soft-tissue injuries (Fig. 19.5). The dose of radiation to the child was smaller and the technique was generally more sensitive than was radiography.

Skeletal injuries are uncommon in abused children over the age of 2 years [13]. Specific injuries – epiphyseal or metaphyseal fractures and rib fractures – and highly suggestive signs

– occult, multiple or repetitive fractures – are usually confined to infancy. For these reasons, isotope scintigraphy may be used as the primary investigation in such older children who show clinical evidence of musculoskeletal injury and this can be followed by radiography of the areas of abnormal uptake; a full radiographic study can thus be avoided in this group. By contrast, both a full radiographic survey and an isotope study are needed in children under the age of 2 whatever the clinical picture, including neglect; this will safeguard against overlooking bone-end lesions and skull fractures [12].

19.3 CRANIOCEREBRAL TRAUMA

The pattern of skull fracture is very helpful in differentiating those with non-accidental injury from those admitted to hospital with skull fractures sustained in accidents [14]. Fractures in abused children are often complex or multiple (Fig. 19.6), depressed, wide (Fig. 19.7) and, sometimes, increasing in width. The site of the fracture is more often non-parietal in abused children and associated subdural haematoma is more common. Fractures measuring more than 5 mm on presentation are not found after accidental injury.

In the past decade, computed tomography has become the most important diagnostic aid in the evaluation of serious trauma to the head. There is a relatively high incidence of intracranial abnormality in cases of child abuse which is due in part to the increased susceptibility of the infant brain to trauma. Children with fractures or obvious scalp bruises have received direct injuries but

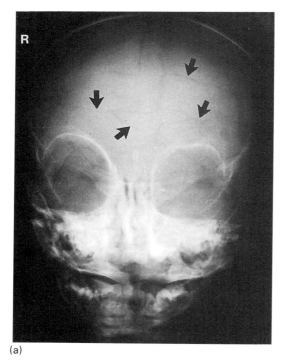
(a)

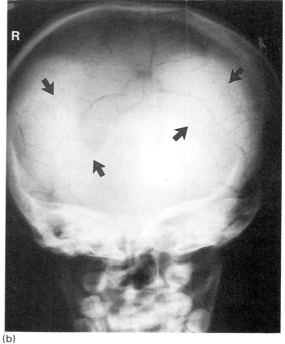
(b)

Fig. 19.6 Trauma and natural disease compared. (a) Complex skull fracture. (b) Wormian bones relating to the sutures (a patient with cleidocranial dysostosis).

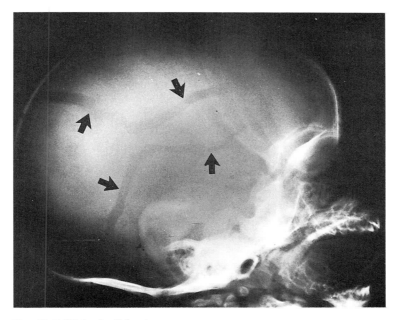

Fig. 19.7 Wide skull fractures.

injuries sometimes result indirectly from severe shaking or 'whiplash'. It has been emphasized that subdural haematomas may arise in the absence of obvious fracture or signs of external injury [15]. 'Whiplashing' of the head on the thorax is clearly more dangerous in infants than in older children as the infantile head is relatively heavier and the neck muscles weaker. Such movements in small children with large fontanelles and open sutures result in excessive shearing forces where vessels are attached to rigid structures such as the falx cerebri. It seems likely that this may well be an important cause of subdural haematomas and of intraocular bleeding (Fig. 19.8).

Computed tomographic findings in one group of 37 children with head injuries resulting from physical abuse revealed that subarachnoid haemorrhage was the most common abnormality and that this was followed by cerebral oedema and cerebral haemorrhage [16]. Nine children had sub-

dural haematoma. Increased vascularity in localized areas of the brain was seen in some initial scans; these areas later showed infarction. The grey matter had lower attenuation than the white matter in some patients who all had irreversible brain damage. Examples are shown in Fig. 19.9.

Interhemispheric subdural haematomas have also been reported in up to 58% of cases of intracranial trauma due to abuse [17]. Up to 95% of serious intracranial injuries are said to be the result of child abuse, and the occurrence of such an injury in the absence of a significant history constitutes grounds for an official investigation [18].

The findings on computed tomography vary considerably with the type of injury. Subdural haematoma occurred in 70% of cases in one series of craniocerebral trauma; the fact that this was associated with a high incidence of skull fractures (45%) suggested a significant role for head injury of impact type [19].

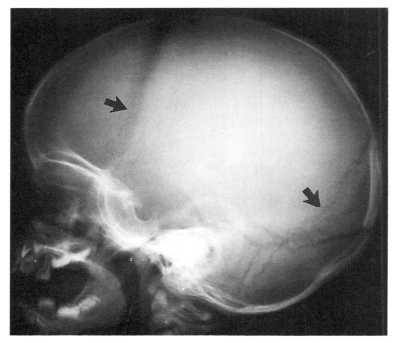

Fig. 19.8 Sutural diastasis. This could predispose to shearing of vessels and intracranial haemorrhage.

19.4 MAGNETIC RESONANCE IMAGING

Although computed tomography has been the accepted method of assessing intracranial injury in child abuse, a recent comparative study has shown magnetic resonance imaging to be superior to computed tomography for the detection of subdural haematomas, intraparenchymal injury and haemorrhage in the posterior fossa [20]. Magnetic resonance imaging is not widely available but it is the method of choice for the detection of intracranial injuries – particularly of those due to shaking.

19.5 ABDOMINAL INJURIES

Deliberate abdominal injury often occurs without any external signs of trauma and, consequently, the diagnosis may be delayed.

A high mortality has been reported in such cases [21].

(a) Aetiology of abdominal injuries

Direct compression tends to produce bursting injuries of the liver or spleen or perforation of a hollow viscus. Such injuries are more common following accidental injury than resulting from child abuse.

. Blunt trauma, such as that arising from kicks or punches, compresses the small intestine and pancreas against the spine. The vulnerability of the small intestine to such injuries is probably due to the retroperitoneal fixation of the descending part of the duodenum and to the fixation of the jejunum at the ligament of Treitz [22]. There may be complete transection of the duodenum or upper jejunum or intramural haematomas may be formed.

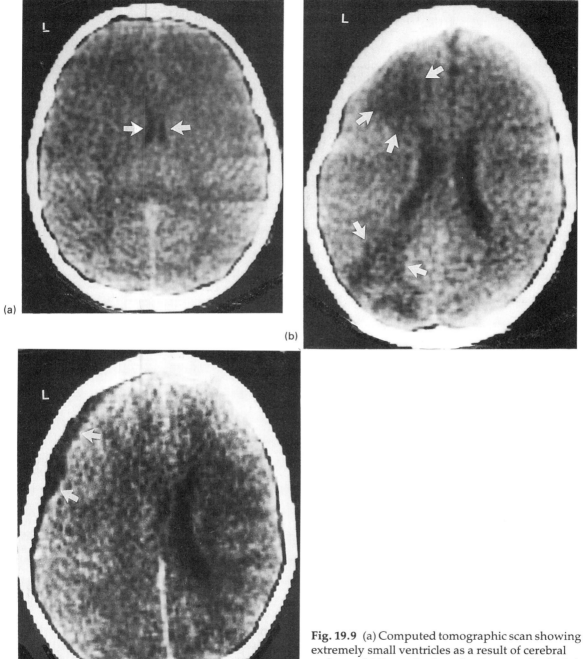

Fig. 19.9 (a) Computed tomographic scan showing extremely small ventricles as a result of cerebral oedema. (b) Extensive low-density areas in the left frontal and occipital regions due to contusion. (c) Chronic subdural haematoma in the left frontal region.

(b) Intramural haematomas of the alimentary tract

Rupture of blood vessels in the mesenteric border may produce a haematoma in the superficial bowel wall. Occasionally, haematomas are found in the muscular and submucosal layers. They are generally encountered in the second, third and fourth parts of the duodenum as well as in the upper jejunum. They may rupture into the peritoneal cavity.

Radiological examination with contrast medium is often valuable in the diagnosis of intramural haematomas. In acute injuries, a smooth obstructing mass may be shown in the second part of the duodenum – most commonly in the lateral wall. The transverse mucosal folds present a 'coiled spring' appearance simulating an intussusception

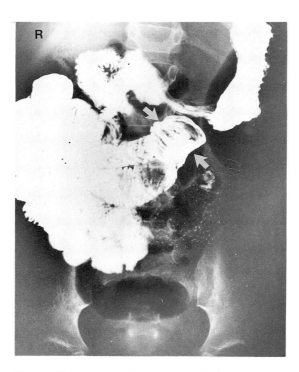

Fig. 19.10 Intramural haematoma in the upper jejunum simulating an intussusception.

[23]; similar appearances are seen in intramural haematomas involving the jejunum (Fig. 19.10). Ultrasonic examination may show an echogenic mass within the duodenum which is elevating the superior mesenteric artery [24]. In the resolving phase, localized masses in the duodenal wall together with prominent mucosal folds indicate previous haemorrhage [25]; child abuse should be suspected in children with these signs and non-specific symptoms.

(c) Injuries to the pancreas

Pancreatitis is much rarer in children than in adults; when it occurs, it is usually acute and is frequently due to trauma. A skeletal survey is advisable in children with pancreatitis and no history of injury as this may show other manifestations of trauma.

Damage to the pancreas arises as a result of compression against the lumbar spine. If the compressive forces are sufficiently severe, pancreatic enzymes are released into the lesser sac resulting in autodigestion of the pancreas and neighbouring tissues. A pseudocyst, which may be filled with clear yellow, haemorrhagic or purulent fluid, results as the sac becomes sealed by fibrous tissue. In one series, nine out of 13 children with proven pancreatic trauma were found to have pancreatic pseudocysts; it was likely that the injury arose from child abuse in three of the children under the age of 3 years [26]. Such cysts have also been reported in association with 'haemorrhagic' ascites, heeling rib fractures and haemorrhagic pleural effusion [27].

A plain radiograph of the abdomen may show an abdominal mass in a patient with a pseudocyst. Ultrasound is probably the method of choice for examining small children; not only will it identify a cystic mass but it can also be used to follow the formation and evolution of a pancreatic pseudocyst. Alternatively, computed tomography can determine the precise situation of the pseudocyst. The use of both modalities is invaluable if the cyst is to be treated by a percutaneous drainage procedure. Foci of fat necrosis have been found in a number of organs at autopsy of patients who have died as a result of pancreatitis. Osseous lesions may develop in both acute and subacute pancreatitis [28]. Multiple punched-out and osteolytic lesions may appear in the long bones and the bones of the hands and feet 3–6 weeks after the acute episode. Periosteal new bone formation occurs and may be followed by the appearance of areas of calcification in the medulla [29]. The bone lesions are generally painful and the radiological appearances are similar to those of leukaemia, sickle-cell infarction or metastatic disease. Occasionally, the lesions are present in both the metaphyses and the epiphyses.

(d) Acute gastric dilatation

Following prolonged starvation due to neglect, the ingestion of a large meal may lead to gross distension of the stomach; this is evident radiologically as is associated displacement of the neighbouring viscera [30].

(e) Traumatic rupture of the liver

Rupture of this organ results from compression injuries to the chest or upper abdomen. Plain radiographs are not very helpful but may show associated rib fractures or changes in the size or shape of the organ. Scintiscanning is a reliable method of detecting hepatic trauma. Localized areas of diminished or absent uptake of sulphur colloid are characteristic. Haematomas or ruptures of the liver are shown as localized areas with low isotope uptake.

(f) Splenic injury

Although the spleen is often injured in major abdominal trauma, it is seldom involved in child abuse. When it is so, plain films of the abdomen are often normal but rib fractures may be present with an associated pneumothorax and elevation of the left dome of the diaphragm. Liver/spleen scintigraphy is a rapid and safe investigation. Computed tomography may also be helpful in demonstrating subcapsular haematoma or intraperitoneal bleeding after contrast medium enhancement. Fractured ribs may also be shown.

(g) Renal injury

A history of haematuria in patients who are known to have been or are suspected of having being injured suggests renal damage. An excretion urogram is an essential first step in the investigation of such cases in order to establish the presence or absence of a normal kidney on the contralateral side.

Ultrasound is valuable in the diagnosis of perirenal collections of blood or urine but the degree of renal damage is best assessed by computed tomography. Renal rupture often appears as an irregular, wedge-shaped, low-density defect which is particularly well shown after enhancement with contrast medium. Avascularity of the kidney can be identified readily in cases with severe damage to the renal pedicle. An isotope renogram will also show the effects of disruption of the renal vasculature at the hilum.

Chylous ascites is a rare manifestation of child abuse [31]. A leak in the abdominal lymphatic system can be identified by lymphangiography. A careful skeletal survey for corroborative evidence of abuse is mandatory in such cases.

19.6 DIFFERENTIAL DIAGNOSIS

(a) Scurvy

Vitamin C deficiency is now a rare condition and one which is uncommon before 6 months of age. The clinical presentation, which includes bruising and painful, swollen extremities, may mimic child abuse. The metaphyses are irregular and subperiosteal haemorrhage is common, the latter also simulating abuse; accidental trauma in such cases adds to the confusion. However, unlike most cases of child abuse, the bones are osteoporotic so that the epiphyses and the patella show a thin dense ring around the transparent bone (Fig. 19.11).

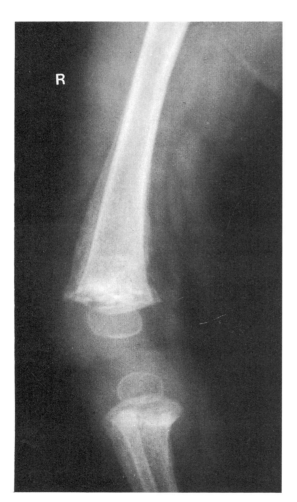

Fig. 19.11 Scurvy showing calcified subperiosteal haematoma, metaphyseal fractures with 'pencilled' outline of the epiphyses due to osteoporosis.

(b) Rickets

Characteristically, the metaphyses in this condition are splayed and irregular and there is an increase in the width of the zone of provisional ossification. The bones are osteoporotic. Fractures are uncommon but, occasionally, there is extensive subperiosteal and metaphyseal calcification which produces an appearance similar to trauma [32]. Widening of the skull sutures, the wrong interpretation of rachitic signs as fractures in the skull and the presence of pseudofractures of the forearm bones led to the incorrect diagnosis of child abuse in one case [33].

(c) Congenital syphilis

Congenital syphilis can mimic the bone lesions of battered children. Periosteal elevation and thickening may be present in both conditions. The laying down of calcium parallel to the shafts of the long bones is widespread throughout the skeleton and involves the long bones symmetrically (Fig. 19.12).

Irregular defects may develop in the shafts and particularly involve the medial aspect of the upper end of the tibia; a pathological fracture may occur through the destroyed bone. The metaphyses of the long bones may also be irregular. Occasionally, a band of increased bone density crosses the metaphysis next to a zone with diminished density producing changes similar to those seen in scurvy.

The differential diagnosis includes rickets, scurvy and leukaemia. In rickets, the metaphyses are cupped and fraying is much less marked than it is in congenital syphilis. Rickets is also uncommon before the age of 6 months while congenital syphilis is usually evident at birth. Subperiosteal haemorrhages are not found in syphilis but are common in scurvy.

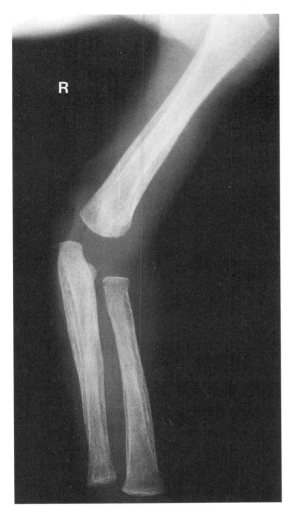

Fig. 19.12 Extensive periosteal thickening of the arm bones in congenital syphilis.

(d) Skeletal lesions produced by drugs

Methotrexate

Children who are on long-term oral maintainance therapy with methotrexate may develop an osteopathy which is characterized by pain in the legs. Radiological examination reveals features similar to scurvy, with periosteal reaction and metaphyseal/epiphyseal fractures [34].

Prostaglandin therapy

Two cases have been reported of cortical hyperostosis simulating child abuse following administration of prostaglandin E_1 for ductus-dependent cyanotic heart disease [35].

Vitamin A intoxication

Extensive cortical thickening occurs in this condition. The history will make differentiation from child abuse easy.

(e) Skeletal lesions following meningococcal septicaemia and disseminated intravascular coagulation

Disseminated intravascular coagulation may develop in meningococcal septicaemia and in association with other severe infections. Occlusion of the blood vessels produces widespread necrotic lesions in many organs.

Skeletal abnormalities have been reported recently [36]. These include destruction of the major epiphyses with disturbance of growth of the adjacent metaphyses. The bone lesions are not specific and may be seen in other conditions such as sickle cell disease, osteomyelitis or trauma. The similarity to the results of child abuse is striking (Fig. 19.13).

(f) Osteogenesis imperfecta

This inherited disorder of collagen is characterized by the presence of brittle bones, blue sclerae and premature deafness. Eighty per cent of affected individuals have relatively mild bone disease and fractures occur mainly in childhood; deformities and scoliosis are minimal and the eventual stature may be nearly normal. This type (Type I) is inherited in an autosomal dominant fashion and abnormalities of extraskeletal, collagen-containing tissues feature prominently – blue sclerae, early deafness, hypermobile joints, rupture of tendons and thin aortic valves which sometimes cause incompetence [37]. The remaining 20% of cases fall into Types II,

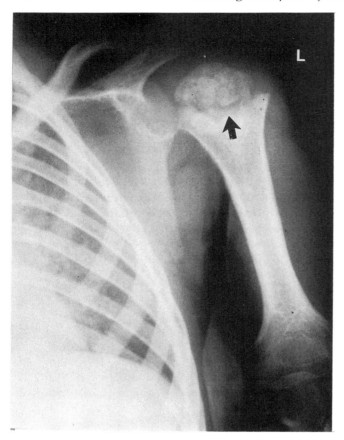

Fig. 19.13 Irregularity in epiphysis and metaphysis of humerus following meningococcal septicaemia.

III and IV. In Type II, the skeleton is grossly abnormal and the condition is lethal at or shortly after birth. Some affected children survive for many months and then behave as if they belong to Type III with progressive skeletal deformities necessitating residential care. The broad, short, featureless bones of Type II should not be confused with the lesions seen in child abuse; the progressive deformities of Type III (Fig. 19.14) are unlikely to be mistaken because growth is severely limited, there is associated kyphoscoliosis and a protruding sternum, and the head tends to be large and asymmetrical. The heterogenicity of osteogenesis imperfecta is emphasized [38] and the recently defined Type IV is the form that is most likely to be confused with non-accidental injury. This is a rare form; inheritance is of autosomal dominant type and the sclerae are white. However, bone disease is more severe than in Type I, the stature is considerably reduced and dentinogenesis imperfecta is more common.

Osteoporosis is a prominent feature of Type IV osteogenesis imperfecta and there is variable deformity of the long bones [38]. The incidence of fracture declines in adolescence and the first fracture occurs at birth more commonly than in Type I [39]. Joint laxity and dislocations are relatively common but bruising and nose-bleeds are less common than in Type I. Although the radiographic

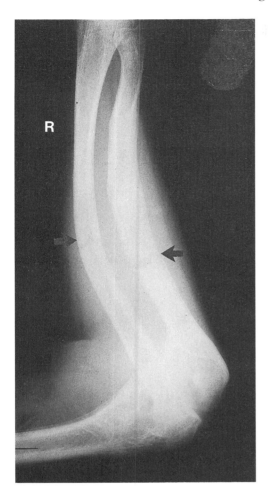

Fig. 19.14 Osteogenesis imperfecta (Type III) showing deformity of the forearm bones with transverse fractures.

appearance of the bones may be normal, the condition may be mistaken for idiopathic juvenile osteoporosis [39].

(g) The kinky hair syndrome

This condition resembles child abuse because periosteal thickening of the shafts of the long bones is present together with symmetrical spurs of the metaphyses [40, 41]. The skull often shows Wormian bones and the anterior ribs are flared. Malformations of the arterial system of the brain and subdural effusions also occur. The abnormality appears to be due basically to a deficiency of copper-dependent enzymes, including ascorbic acid oxidase.

(h) Child abuse and copper deficiency

Distinguishing between the skeletal manifestations of non-accidental injury and those of copper deficiency has provoked considerable controversy [42, 43]. The skeletal abnormalities in copper deficiency occur late and are associated with retarded bone age, osteoporosis, metaphyseal cupping, increased density of the zone of provisional calcification and metaphyseal sickle-shaped spurs [42]. The signs are symmetrical throughout the skeleton; skull fractures are not a feature and rib fractures have been recorded only in premature infants. When the disorder occurs in full-term infants, it is associated with an abnormal diet or with faulty parenteral nutrition. Radiographically normal bones, and a normal bone age, exclude copper deficiency which is of sufficient severity to cause fractures [42]. A diagnosis of non-accidental injury can be made with even more confidence if other signs of copper deficiency – low serum copper, low caeruloplasmin concentrations, neutropenia and hypochromic microcytic anaemia – are absent and when predisposing factors – prematurity, dietary deficiency and total parenteral nutrition – are also absent [42]. The differential diagnosis was discussed in a recent criminal prosecution which was taken to Appeal [44]. The bone density may appear abnormal in some cases of copper deficiency, which suggests the presence of a collagen deficiency [43].

19.7 DATING OF FRACTURES

Dating of fractures on the basis of radiological features is an inexact science. In the normal skeleton, the healing rate depends on several factors. The site of the fracture is particularly relevant in cases of child abuse as fractures of the ribs and upper limb heal more quickly than do those affecting the lower limbs. If the fractures are inadequately immobilized, poor contact may result in non-union or mal-alignment and deformity – this does not, of course, apply to the skull and ribs.

Systemic illness or some metabolic bone disorders may result in unusual healing patterns. Abundant callus is often found in patients with Cushing's syndrome, in those receiving treatment with steroids and in osteogenesis imperfecta. Poor callus formation is a feature of patients with osteo-porosis or osteomalacia.

The healing process can be divided into several stages – resolution of soft-tissue injuries, development of periosteal new bone, loss of the fracture line's definition and the appearance of soft callus.

The assessment of the age of a skull fracture is impossible as the fracture line takes up to 6–8 months to disappear. An absence of periosteal bone in fractures of the long bones usually indicates that the fracture is less than 7–10 days old; a fracture with definite but slight periosteal new bone may be as recent as 4–7 days old. A 20-day-old fracture will almost always have a well-defined periosteal new bone response and also some soft callus formation. A fracture with a large amount of periosteal new bone or callus is more than 14 days old. Loss of the marginal sharpness of the fracture line occurs at 14–21 days [45]. Corner metaphyseal fractures and bucket-handle fractures may persist for longer periods without developing periosteal new bone and can be dated only approximately by loss of marginal definition. In abused children, chronic repetitive trauma and lack of immobilization may delay the resolution of soft-tissue injuries and also affect the development of periosteal new bone. If periosteal reaction is seen in an abused child,

the fracture may be somewhat older than would be expected in a normal skeleton [45]. The quantity, thickness, density and longi-tudinal extent of periosteal new bone are all increased when there is inadequate immobil-ization or repeated injury. Neither radio-nuclide studies nor computed tomography have been found helpful in establishing the age of fractures.

19.8 CONCLUSION

The radiologist has an extemely important part to play in the diagnosis of non-accidental injury in children. It is of the utmost importance that the condition should be considered in the differential diagnosis in children who are suffering from vague or unusual illnesses. A full skeletal survey is recommended if an unexpected fracture is discovered. When children who are suspected of having been abused are referred for radiological examination, each radiograph taken should be verified by the radiographer – and doubly verified in Scotland. This ensures that, in any subsequent legal case, there can be no possible doubt that the radiographs were those of the child in question.

Great care should be taken in the interpretation and recording of all radiological findings, for the radiologist's report may form the basis of a legal statement. Scrutiny of films should be methodical and obsessional. Reports should be *cautious* when it comes to assessing the age of fractures and suggesting the mechanism by which the injuries were sustained.

REFERENCES

1. Caffey, J. (1946) Multiple fractures in the long bones in infants suffering from sub-dural haematoma. *Am. J. Roentgenol.*, **56**, 163.
2. Silverman, F.N. (1953) The roentgen mani-festations of unrecognised skeletal trauma in infants. *Am. J. Roentgenol.*, **69**, 413.
3. Woolley, P.V. and Evans, W.A. (1955)

Significance of skeletal lesions in infants resembling those of traumatic origin. *JAMA*, **158**, 539.

4. Kempe, C.H., Silverman, F.N., Steele, B.F. et al. (1963) Battered Child Syndrome. *JAMA*, **181**, 17.

5. Ellerstein, N.S. and Norris, K.J. (1984) Value of radiologic skeletal survey in assessment of abused children. *Pediatrics*, **74**, 1074.

6. Worlock, P., Stower, M. and Barbor, P. (1988) Patterns of fractures in accidental and non-accidental injury in children: a comparative study. *Br. Med. J.*, **293**, 100.

7. Roberton, D.M., Barbor, P. and Hull, D. (1982) Unusual injury? Recent injury in normal children and children with suspected non-accidental injury. *Br. Med. J.*, **285**, 1399.

8. Kleinman, P.K., Marks, S.C. and Blackbourne, B. (1986) The metaphyseal lesion in abused infants: A radiologic-histopathologic study. *Am. J. Roentgenol.*, **146**, 895.

9. Kogutt, S., Swischuk, L.E. and Fagan, C.J. (1974) Patterns of injury and significance of uncommon fractures in the battered child syndrome. *Am. J. Roentgenol.*, **121**, 143.

10. Tufts, E., Blank, E. and Dickerson, D. (1982) Periosteal thickening as a manifestation of trauma in infancy. *Child Abuse Neglect*, **6**, 359.

11. Helfer, R.E., Scheurer, S.L., Alexander, R. et al. (1984) Trauma to the bones of small infants from passive exercise: a factor in the etiology of child abuse. *J. Pediatr.*, **104**, 47.

12. Sty, J.R. and Starshak, R.J. (1983) The role of bone scintigraphy in the evaluation of the suspected abused child. *Radiology*, **146**, 369.

13. Merten, D.F., Radkowski, M.A. and Leonidas J.C. (1983) The abused child: a radiological reappraisal. *Radiology*, **146**, 377.

14. Hobbs, C.J. (1984) Skull fractures and the diagnosis of abuse. *Arch. Dis. Child.*, **59**, 246.

15. Caffey, J. (1974) The whiplash shaken infant syndrome. Manual shaking by the extremities with whiplash-induced intra-cranial and intra-ocular bleedings, linked with residual permanent brain damage and mental retardation. *Pediatrics*, **54**, 396.

16. Cohen, R.A., Kaufman, R.A., Myers, P.A. and Towbin, R.B. (1986) Cranial computed tomography in the abused child with head injury. *Am. J. Roentgenol.*, **146**, 97.

17. Zimmerman, R.A., Bilaniuk, L.T., Bruce, D. et al. (1979) Computed tomography of cranio-cerebral injury in the abused child. *Radiology*, **130**, 687.

18. Billmire, M.E. and Myers, P.A. (1985) Serious head injury in infants: accident or abuse? *Pediatrics*, **75**, 340.

19. Merten, D.F., Osbourne, D.R.S., Radkowski, M.A. and Leonidas, J.C. (1984) Craniocerebral trauma in the child abuse syndrome: radiological observations. *Pediatr. Radiol.*, **14**, 272.

20. Alexander, R.C., Schor, D.P. and Smith, W.L. (1986) Magnetic resonance imaging of intra-cranial injuries from child abuse. *J. Pediatr.*, **109**, 975.

21. McCort, J. and Vaudagna, J. (1964) Visceral injuries in battered children. *Radiology*, **82**, 424.

22. Haller, J.A. (1966) Injuries of the gastro-intestinal tract in children. Notes on recognition and management. *Clin. Pediatr.*, (*Phila.*), **5**, 476.

23. Stewart, D.R., Byrd, C.L. and Schuster, S.R. (1970) Intramural haematomas of the alimentary tract in children. *Surgery*, **68**, 550.

24. Kirks, D.R. (1983) Radiological evaluation of visceral injuries in the battered child syndrome. *Pediatr. Ann.*, **12**, 888.

25. Kleinman, P.K., Brill, P.W. and Winchester, P. (1986) Resolving duodenal-jejunal haematoma in abused children. *Radiology*, **160**, 747.

26. Peña, S.D.J. and Medovy, H. (1973) Child abuse and traumatic pseudocyst of the pancreas. *J. Pediatr.*, 1026.

27. Hartley, R.C. (1967) Pancreatitis under age of 5 years: report of three cases. *J. Pediatr. Surg.*, **2**, 419.

28. Scarpelli, D.G. (1956) Fat necrosis of bone marrow in acute pancreatitis. *Am. J. Pathol.*, **32**, 1077.

29. Cohen, H., Haller, J.O. and Friedman, A.P. (1981) Pancreatitis, child abuse and skeletal lesions. *Pediatr. Radiol.*, **10**, 175.

30. Franken, E.A., Fox, M., Smith, J.A. and Smith, W.L. (1978) Acute gastric dilatation in neglected children. *Am. J. Roentgenol.*, **130**, 297.

31. Boysen, B.E. (1975) Chylous ascites. Manifestation of the battered child syndrome. *Am. J. Dis. Child.*, **129**, 1338.

32. Radkowski, M.A. (1983) The battered child

syndrome: pitfalls in radiological diagnosis. *Pediatr. Ann.*, **12**, 894.

33. Paterson, C.R. (1981) Vitamin D deficiency rickets simulating child abuse. *J. Pediat. Orthoped.*, **1**, 423.

34. Schwartz, A.M. and Leonidas, J.C. (1984) Methotrexate osteopathy. *Skeletal Radiol.*, **11**, 13.

35. Ueda, K., Saito, A., Nakano, H. *et al.* (1980) Cortical hyperostosis following long-term administration of prostaglandin E_1 in infants with cyanotic congenital heart disease. *J. Pediatr.*, **97**, 834.

36. Robinow, M., Johnson, F., Nanagas, M.T. and Mesghali, H. (1983) Skeletal lesions following meningococcemia and disseminated intravascular coagulation. *Am. J. Dis. Child.*, **137**, 279.

37. Smith, R. (1984) Osteogenesis imperfecta. *Br. Med. J.*, **289**, 394.

38. Sillence, D.O., Senn, A. and Danks, D.M. (1979) Genetic heterogeneity in osteogenesis imperfecta. *J. Med. Genet.*, **16**, 101.

39. Paterson, C.R., McAllion, S. and Miller, R. (1983) Osteogenesis imperfecta with dominant inheritance and normal sclerae. *J. Bone Joint Surg.*, **65B**, 35.

40. Wesenberg, R.L., Gwinn, J.L. and Barnes, G.R. Jr. (1969) Radiological findings in the kinky hair syndrome. *Radiology*, **92**, 500.

41. Adams, P.C., Strand, R.D., Bresnan, M.J. and Lucky, A.W. (1974) Kinky hair syndrome: serial study of radiological findings with emphasis on the similarity to the battered child syndrome. *Radiology*, **112**, 401.

42. Chapman, S. (1987) Child abuse or copper deficiency? A radiological review. *Br. Med. J.*, **294**, 1370.

43. Paterson, C.R. (1987) Child abuse or copper deficiency? (letter) *Br. Med. J.*, **295**, 213.

44. *R* v. *Lees and Lees* [1987] CCA, 24 February.

45. O'Connor, J.F. and Cohen, J. (1987) *Diagnostic Imaging of Child Abuse*, Williams and Wilkins, Baltimore.

CHAPTER 20

Accidental injury and death in children

Alan W. Craft

20.1 INTRODUCTION

Accidents are by far and away the commonest cause of death in childhood and are an equally important reason for the admission of children to hospital. Although accident rates have fallen slowly throughout this century, the decline has not been as dramatic as has been that for the other common diseases of children. Indeed the whole picture of mortality and morbidity in children has changed during this century (Table 20.1) [1]. The previously devastating illnesses in children, which were largely infective in origin, have been conquered so that accidents have become the leading cause of death in children beyond the first year of life. Accidents accounted for one-third of all deaths in this age-group in 1985 (Table 20.2). However, deaths are only the tip of the iceberg. Almost one-fifth of all admissions for children for any reason from birth to the end of childhood are due to accidents and many of these will result in substantial long-term physical and psychological morbidity additional to the distress and anguish caused by the accident itself. Doctors of all specialities are becoming increasingly aware of the problems caused by accidents and path-

ologists are no exception to this. Accidental deaths, by their very nature, occur suddenly and unexpectedly and almost always result in a post-mortem examination being carried out to establish the cause of death. All such accidental deaths in England and Wales must be reported to the coroner who has the power to order an inquest at which the pathologist will often be required to give evidence. Although accidents may be due to a chain of circumstances which are purely accidental, this is not always the case. Their indepth investigation will often reveal causes which may well become the subject of litigation and, in a litigation-conscious society, pathologists can expect to become increasingly involved in cases which may involve either personal or product liability.

Deaths from accidental injury can be due to a variety of causes; the main subgroups are summarized in Table 20.3. Half the 890 accidental deaths which occurred in children in 1984 resulted from road accidents. A majority of the others can be classified as 'home accidents' and these are made up of a variety of other subcategories e.g. burns as a result of fires, falls and poisoning. It can be seen from Table 20.3 that different problems

Table 20.1 Deaths of children aged 1–14 years from various causes

Cause	1911–15		1931–35		1956–60		1970–74		1976–80	
	No.	Rate/10^6	No.	Rate/10^6	No.	Rate/10^6	No.	Rate/10^6	No.	Rate/10^6
Diphtheria	23 380	447	13 820	311	15	0	1	0	0	0
Measles	48 986	936	10 874	254	210	4	111	2	83	1.6
Whooping cough	20 182	385	6071	137	72	1	7	0	10	0.2
Gastroenteritis	25 560	488	3485	78	447	9	487	9	137	2.7
Tuberculosis	46 459	887	14 544	327	306	6	71	1	35	0.7
Scarlet fever	9901	189	2589	58	7	0	0	0	—	—
Rheumatic fever*	3495	67	2465	55	139	3	6	0	35	0.7
Cancer	2388	46	2853	64	3971	83	3743	69	2931	57.3
Pneumonia and bronchitis	76 643	1464	28 226	635	3347	70	2330	43	1454	28.4
Accidents	18 500	353	12 126	273	6736	140	7214	133	5273	103.0

* The figures are not strictly comparable because of revision of the ICD (International Classification of Disease) Code.

Table 20.2 Major causes of death in childhood: England and Wales 1985

	Age-group (yr)									
	0–1		*1–4*		*5–9*		*10–14*		*0–14*	
	No.	*%*	*No.*	*%*	*No.*	*%*	*No.*	*%*	*No.*	*%*
Accidents	119	(1.9)	256	(22.6)	212	(36.1)	357	(44.0)	944	(10.7)
Cancer	37	(0.6)	105	(9.3)	137	(23.3)	141	(17.4)	420	(4.8)
Respiratory disease	429	(7.0)	106	(9.3)	25	(4.3)	28	(3.5)	588	(6.8)
Congenital anomalies	1600	(26.1)	250	(22.0)	79	(13.4)	61	(7.5)	1990	(22.9)
SIDS	1165	(19.0)	30	(2.6)	—	—	—	—	1195	(13.8)
All causes	6141		1135		588		811		8675	

Source: OPCS (1987) Mortality Statistics – Childhood, 1985, E and W, Series DH3 No. 19, HMSO, London.

affect different age-groups. Children under the age of 4 years are much more likely to be injured in the home, while older children are at greater risk from road traffic accidents.

Indeed, overall, the most common childhood accidents occur in the home; national estimates from the Home Accident Surveillance System suggest that some 775 000

Table 20.3 Accidental deaths by cause, age and sex, England and Wales, 1984

	Age-group (yr)								
	0–4		*5–9*		*10–14*		*All ages*		
	M	*F*	*M*	*F*	*M*	*F*	*M*	*F*	*Both*
Road accidents	57	32	105	57	129	68	291	157	448
Fires	34	19	13	9	8	6	55	34	89
Drownings	27	9	13	0	10	5	50	14	64
Inhalation and ingestion	23	21	3	1	4	0	30	22	52
Falls	20	6	12	1	17	2	49	9	58
Mechanical suffocation	16	12	1	1	19	0	36	13	49
Electrocution	0	1	4	0	3	2	7	3	10
Poisoning – medicine	4	4	0	0	0	1	4	5	9
Poisoning – other	1	2	1	2	12	2	14	6	20
Scalds	5	3	1	0	0	0	6	3	9
Other accidents	25	15	15	2	16	9	56	26	82
All accidents	212	124	168	73	218	95	598	292	890
Fatalities per 10 000 population	1.32	0.81	1.12	0.52	1.20	0.55	1.22	0.63	0.93

Source: OPCS (1985) Mortality Statistics: Cause 1984, HMSO London.

children per year in England and Wales sustain injuries in such accidents that are severe enough to bring them into hospital. Burns are the most important single injury in this younger age-group. In addition to road accidents, a significant proportion of injuries in the older age-group occur either at school or when the children are at play.

Road traffic accidents can involve pedestrians, pedal cyclists or occupants of vehicles. Again, the proportions of children affected differ according to age-groups (Table 20.4). Children are far more likely to die as pedestrians than as either car occupants or pedal cyclists. While the death rate for children up to the age of 9 years has fallen steadily over the past 15 years, that for older children, although showing a fall in the mid 1970s, has been increasing steadily since that time (Fig. 20.1). Boys have accidents much more commonly than do girls. This is well demonstrated in the road traffic figures and

Table 20.4 Road accidents to children in Great Britain, 1986

| | Age-group (yr) | | | | | | | | |
| | 0–4 | | 5–9 | | 10–14 | | Totals | | |
	M	F	M	F	M	F	M	F	Both
Pedestrians									
Slight	1 439	806	4 028	2 200	4 148	3 033	9 615	6 039	15 654
Serious	523	264	1 632	718	1 560	1 035	3 715	2 017	5 732
Fatal	40	18	63	36	68	35	171	89	260
Total	2 002	1 088	5 723	2 954	5 776	1 073	13 501	8 145	21 646
Pedal cyclists									
Slight	89	31	1 119	209	3 427	759	4 635	999	5 634
Serious	17	5	295	34	851	143	1 163	182	1 345
Fatal	2	0	3	6	32	8	37	14	51
Total	108	36	1 417	249	4 310	910	5 835	1 195	7 030
Car occupants									
Slight	1 412	1 361	1 565	1 711	1 542	1 874	4 519	4 946	9 465
Serious	181	178	213	183	261	273	655	598	1 253
Fatal	16	15	13	13	11	15	40	43	83
Total	1 446	1 509	1 791	1 907	1 814	2 126	5 214	5 587	10 801
Other road users									
Slight	235	213	194	192	395	476	824	880	1 704
Serious	20	10	32	11	118	43	170	64	234
Fatal	0	0	1	1	6	3	7	4	11
Total	255	223	227	204	519	522	1 001	948	1 949
All road users									
Slight	3 175	2 411	6 906	4 312	9 512	6 142	19 593	12 864	32 457
Serious	1 578	457	2 172	946	2 790	1 494	5 703	2 861	8 564
Fatal	58	33	80	56	117	61	255	150	405
Total	4 811	2 901	9 158	5 314	12 419	7 697	25 551	15 875	41 426

From data provided by 'Road Accidents Great Britain, 1986: The casualty report', Department of Transport: London.

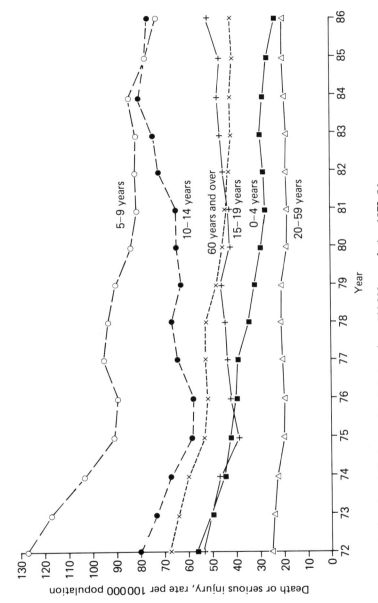

Fig. 20.1 Pedestrians killed or seriously injured per 100 000 population 1972–86.

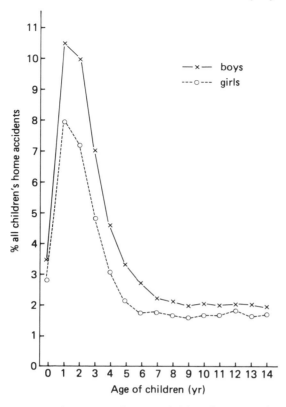

Fig. 20.2 Home accidents to children by age and sex. Sample size 39 099 children. Source: Department of Trade and Industry (1984) The Home Accident Surveillance System, Report of the 1983 data. HMSO, London.

in Fig. 20.2 which shows that, for home accidents, boys are more likely to be involved than girls at all ages and that this is most striking in the first 2–3 years of life.

20.2 CHILDREN IN TRAFFIC [2, 3]

(a) Pedestrians [4]

Pedestrian traffic accidents are the commonest single cause of fatalities in children; approximately 300 such deaths occur each year in Great Britain. Children injured as pedestrians tend to have much more serious

injuries than are seen in other types of accident, simply because of the kinetic forces involved. There is a steadily increasing incidence of death and serious injury from the age of 1 year which reaches a peak at 7 years and slowly declines after that. Boys predominate over girls in a ratio of 2 to 1 but, again, this is greater in the younger age-groups. There are clear socioeconomic factors related to pedestrian accidents. Social class V boys are eight times more likely to sustain a fatal injury than are those in social class I; the ratio for girls is 5 to 1. These differences mainly relate to the degree of exposure – children from more deprived backgrounds are far more likely to be allowed out alone and their only place for play is often a hazardous urban street environment. Socially deprived children are also much more likely to have to cross dangerous roads on the way to school, to the shops and to play facilities. This type of accident occurs less often in the winter than during spring and autumn.

Older children who are struck by a relatively slow-moving car are likely to receive limb fractures – particularly involving the legs. However, life-threatening injuries to the head and, to a lesser extent, the chest and abdomen are likely to be produced in the younger children and in those who are hit by more rapidly moving vehicles. Head injury is the commonest cause of death and serious injury in this age-group, although trauma to the chest and, more especially, the abdomen can also lead to serious morbidity. It has been estimated that up to 10% of children admitted to hospital following pedestrian accidents experience some form of permanent disability, the most common being brain damage, spinal injury with paraplegia, limb deformity or epilepsy.

The causative factors of such accidents can be subdivided into:

(1) *The environment.* Various features of the environment predispose to pedestrian

accidents, particularly in relation to children. These include difficult places for crossing main roads, the obstruction of a small child's view by parked cars and other obstacles, fast open roads traversing residential areas, the density of housing estates and their lack of appropriate play space.

(2) *Parents*. Parents can be partially responsible for such injuries in that their failure to understand child development leads to an overestimation of their child's ability in traffic. They fail to supervise their children or to teach them road drill – and parents tend to set a bad example.

(3) *Drivers*. The main problem relating to drivers is a lack of anticipation and/or understanding of children's behaviour in traffic. One way of overcoming this would be to make some knowledge of children's behaviour a prerequisite before a driving licence was given.

(4) *The child*. Children fulfilling their natural inclinations will run uninhibitedly into the road – for example, after a ball – due to poor understanding of the hazards associated with playing near roads. There are also considerable limitations from the developmental point of view in terms of perception, hearing and judgement.

(b) Accidents to children in cars

In 1986, there were 83 fatalities from this cause in Great Britain; it has been estimated that there may be up to 1000 admissions and, perhaps, 10 000 attendances at accident and emergency departments each year. These accidents are usually caused by someone other than the child himself and it is not surprising, therefore, that there is an equal age and sex distribution throughout childhood except for the early years of life when there is a slightly lower incidence overall. Such accidents are commoner in the summer, this being probably due to increased exposure. There has been a steady fall in the death rate over the past few years and this has been continued following the passage of seat-belt legislation and the introduction of regulations concerning the carriage of children in cars in January 1983 [5]. The main life-threatening conditions which are produced are head injuries, with consequent intra-cranial bleeding, and internal chest and abdominal injuries. Fractures of the long bones, pelvis and spine result in further serious injuries and whiplash injuries to the neck are common. Superficial injuries to the face, from glass, are also common. Children who are unrestrained within cars and who are ejected at impact are at particularly high risk of serious injury or death. Injuries sustained by children in cars rank in terms of severity with those found in pedestrians. The long-term consequences of such injuries are also similar in that there is risk of brain damage, limb deformity and permanent scarring.

(c) Pedal cycle accidents

The number of children injured on pedal cycles has fallen over the past few years and, in 1986, there were only 51 children killed in this way, most of these being in the 10–14-year age-group. Accurate statistics regarding non-fatal injuries are difficult to come by as official police estimates hide a considerable element of under-reporting; it may be that as few as 10% of such accidents are reported to the police and appear in their statistics. Up to 13 000 children may be seriously injured and almost 100 000 attend accident and emergency departments each year. Boys outnumber girls by almost 9 to 1 in respect of fatalities and 5 to 1 for non-fatal accidents. Not surprisingly, there is a marked increase in the summer months. Pedal cyclists are unprotected road users and the majority of deaths are due to serious head injuries. Facial injuries along with limb fractures are common in the non-fatal accidents. The style of bicycles designed for chldren has changed over the past 20 or 30 years and each new style seems to be associated with an increased risk of injury, at least for a period after its introduction. This was well illustrated with the introduction of 'chopper' bicycles in the early 1970s and, more recently, by the BMX bicycle [6,7].

(d) Motorcycle injuries to children

The past few years have seen a considerable increase in the number of children taking part in motorcycling activities; the majority of these involve 'scrambling' off the road. Children are allowed to take part in these events at a surprisingly young age and it is not uncommon for 6- and 7-year-olds to be involved. Injuries to the legs, in particular, and to the arms are the most common but, because the injuries occur off the road, it is uncommon for serious head injuries to be sustained. These injuries are never reported to the police and so do not appear in official statistics [8].

(e) Horse-riding accidents

Although uncommon as a cause of death – only five occurred in 1983 – accidents to children while riding horses are estimated to account for up to 3000 admissions to hospital per year in England and Wales and for five times as many attendances at accident and emergency departments. The injuries occur predominantly in 10–14-year-old girls who outnumber boys by 6 to 1. This is the only type of accident in which girls exceed boys, and this clearly relates to their greater participation in horse-riding activities. It is not surprising that children of the higher socioeconomic groups are most involved and that the peak frequency is seen during the summer months. Injuries are most commonly due to the child falling from the horse; much less often, they are due to being kicked or to the horse falling on the child. Most of the

injuries occurring to such children are minor but head and spinal injuries can have serious consequences which lead either to death or to late sequelae.

20.3 ACCIDENTS IN THE HOME [9]

(a) Falls

Some 70–80 children die each year in England and Wales as a result of falls in the home. The best estimates are that there may be 16 000 admissions and almost a quarter of a million attendances at accident and emergency departments. Falls are particularly common in the age-group 1–4 years and boys predominate over girls in a ratio of 3 to 2. Fatalities are commoner in the lower social classes and accidents resulting in injury are commoner during the summer months. Falls out of windows and down stairs result in serious injuries – intracranial injury and limb fractures. Younger children are more likely to sustain injuries to the head, while lower limb injuries are commoner in older children. The main causative factors differ at the different periods of the child's life. Those under 1 year old are usually injured because they are left unattended in, for example, bouncing cradles or baby walkers; parents underestimate the ability of children to move in these [10]. Between the ages of 1 and 4 years the child has increasing mobility and develops an inquisitive nature; these lead to falls both within the house and from windows. Over the age of 5, falls become due to more boisterous play and the child will not only fall from windows but also from roofs.

(b) Architectural glass accidents

Although uncommon as a cause of death in childhood (five per annum), injuries due to architectural glass can be serious and disfiguring. An example of the type of injury is shown in Fig. 20.3. There are up to 1000

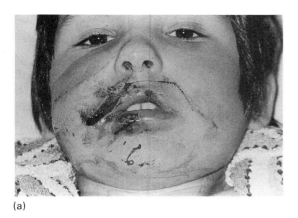
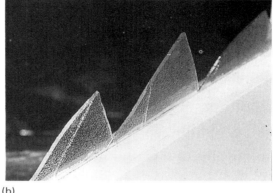

(a)   (b)

Fig. 20.3 (a) Incised wounds likely to be severely disfiguring following a fall through a glass door. (b) It is the remnants of glass within the frame which cause the injuries.

admissions each year in England and Wales and at least 8000 attendances at accident and emergency departments. The greater use of architectural glass within homes has resulted in an increase in the number of such accidents. Severe cuts, particularly to the hands, wrists, arms and face, can result as well as serious internal injuries. Injuries caused in this way are much more likely to involve arteries, nerves and tendons than are other types of cuts and lacerations (Fig. 20.4). The jagged nature of the glass that the child falls through

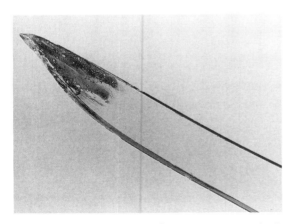

Fig. 20.4 Fragment of glass forming a 'spear' which fatally penetrated the femoral artery.

may cause serious and cosmetically compli-cated injuries; scarring and permanent disability from nerve damage results in some children, and major blood loss and death may occur if a vessel is cut.

All areas of low-level glazing within houses are a hazard; the use of ordinary (annealed) glass in areas of low-level glazing and the proximity of such glass to children's play areas are major causative factors. Prevention of this type of injury is possible if safety glass is used in all domestic areas such as doors and windows, but the use of a polyester plastic film (safety film), which can be fitted over existing glass, may be equally effective [11].

(c) Burns [12]

Almost 100 children die from burns each year in England and Wales; a further 3000 are admitted and 15 000 require attendance at accident and emergency departments. Seventy per cent occur to children under the age of 5 with a peak at 1–2 years. Burns due to flames affect children of all ages, whereas contact burns are only a problem in the very young. Children from the lower socio-economic classes are much more at risk and epidemiological studies have shown a relation with poor housing, overcrowding and family stress. Serious burns occur less commonly in the summer months. There does seem to be a downward trend in the number of deaths from burns and this is almost certainly due to a reduction in the number of instances of clothes catching fire as a result of regulations concerning the protection of fires and the flammability of nightdresses [13]. The move away from open fires to central heating has also helped. Most fatal accidents are due to house fires and the cause of death in these is usually inhalation of smoke and toxic fumes. Injuries to children can be very severe and the long-term consequences include serious physical deformity and disfigurement as well as considerable psychological injury. Repeated admissions for plastic surgery may be necessary following such injuries.

(d) Scalds

Scalds are much less serious in their nature and result in less than 10 deaths per year in England and Wales. However, they are very common as a cause of attendance at accident and emergency departments – there were 31 000 accidents in 1982. Once again, those under 4 years old are particularly at risk and the links with low socioeconomic status, poor housing and family stress are similar to those for burns. Most scalds affect the face, neck, chest and arms and the severity depends on the percentage of the body area affected. It also depends on the ratio of deep to superficial injuries. The major causative factors are either a child pulling a hot liquid on top of himself or being put into a bath which is too hot. Bathwater scalds are particularly dangerous because of the large area of skin which is involved. Serious consequences of such scalds are as for burns with physical deformity, disfigurement and psychological sequelae.

20.4 DROWNINGS AND NEAR DROWNINGS [14, 15]

In 1983, 73 children died from drowning in England and Wales; it is estimated that there are two near drownings which require admission to hospital for every fatal case. Almost half of the children killed are under the age of 5 with, once again, boys predominating 3 to 2; over the age of 5, boys predominate significantly. It is difficult to be clear as to socioeconomic factors. Children from lower socioeconomic groups tend to be drowned in areas available generally to the public – for example, canals and ponds – while those from the higher socioeconomic groups are drowned in private swimming pools. July and August are the commonest periods for such injuries to occur, but this peak is much less pronounced among children under 5 years old. Fortunately, there is a downward trend in the number of drownings, particularly in those children over the age of 5 years. Drowning is, by definition, a fatal event; near drowning usually results in complete recovery although a small proportion of children may be permanently brain damaged and, therefore, handicapped. One-third of such instances occur in rivers, one-fifth in the sea while the remainder arise in swimming pools, lakes, reservoirs and ponds.

20.5 ACCIDENTS AT PLAY

Play is a normal part of child growth and development. As the child gets older he finds himself in increasingly hazardous conditions and it is not surprising that accidents occur (Fig. 20.5). Many are minor but some are serious and even fatal. Boys are more commonly injured than are girls. Injuries sustained during play have been studied in Australia [16] and in playgrounds in the United Kingdom [17].

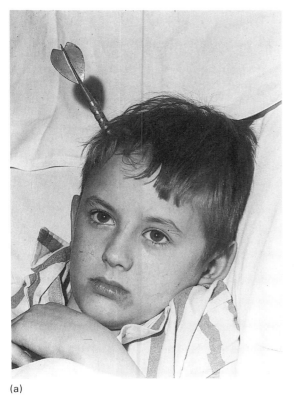

(a)

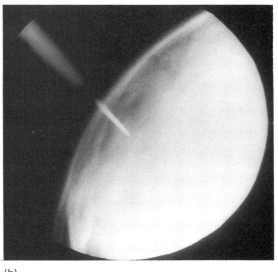

(b)

Fig. 20.5 (a) A dart penetrating a boy's head in the playroom. (b) An X-ray shows the depth of penetration.

20.6 PREVENTION

The prevention of accidents has long been a task delegated to educators and to parents. However, it has become clear over the past two decades that professionals of many types have a real role to play in the prevention of injury and death due to accidents. The designers and maintainers of the environment perform a major role, but they can only act when they are made aware of what constitutes an unsafe environment. Doctors and other health carers are the only people who have a detailed knowledge of the consequences and causes of accidents and it is their responsibility to communicate this to those who can act to prevent the recurrence of similar injuries [18].

Multiprofessional, interdisciplinary teams have come together in many countries to address the problem of the prevention of accidents in childhood. The work and achievements of the Child Accident Prevention Trust in the United Kingdom are a good example of what can be done when professional boundaries are broached [19].

REFERENCES

1. Court, D. and Alberman, E. (1988) Worlds apart, in *Child Health in a Changing Society* (ed. J. Forfar), Oxford University Press, Oxford.
2. Sandels, S. (1975) *Children in Traffic*, Elek Books, London.
3. Jackson, R.H. (1978) Hazards to children in traffic: a paediatrician looks at road accidents. *Arch. Dis. Child.*, **53**, 807.

4. Rivara, F.P. and Barber, M. (1985) Demographic analysis of childhood pedestrian injuries. *Pediatrics*, **76**, 375.

5. Road Traffic Act 1972, s.33B inserted by Transport Act 1981, s.28; Motor Vehicles (Wearing of Seat Belts by Children) Regulations 1982 (SI 1982/1342).

6. Craft, A.W., Shaw, D.A. and Cartlidge, N.E.F. (1973) Bicycle injuries in children. *Br. Med. J.*, **267**, 146.

7. Illingworth, C.M. (1984) Injuries to children riding BMX bikes. *Br. Med. J.*, **289**, 956.

8. Sherman, K. and MacKinnon, J. (1984) Motorcycling injuries to children. *Br. Med. J.*, **289**, 877.

9. Consumer Safety Unit (1987) *Home Accident Surveillance System – Tenth Annual Report*, Department of Trade and Industry, London.

10. Birchall, M.A. and Henderson, H.P. (1988) Babywalkers and infant burns. *Br. Med. J.*, **296**, 1641.

11. Jackson, R.H. (1981) Lacerations from glass in childhood. *Br. Med. J.*, **283**, 1310.

12. Child Accident Prevention Trust (1985) *Burn and Scald Accidents to Children*, Bedford Square Press, London.

13. Heating Appliances (Fireguards) Regulations 1973 (SI 1973/2106; Nightdresses (Safety) Regulations 1967 (SI 1967/839) both made under Consumer Protection Act 1961.

14. Barry, W., Little, T.M. and Sibert, J.R. (1982) Childhood drownings in private swimming pools. *Br. Med. J.*, **285**, 542.

15. Pearn, J.H. (1980) Secondary drowning in children. *Br. Med. J.*, **281**, 1103.

16. Nixon, J., Pearn, J. and Wilkey, I. (1981) Death during play: a study of playground and recreation deaths in children. *Br. Med. J.*, **283**, 410.

17. Illingworth, C.M., Brenan, P., Jay, A. *et al.* (1975) 200 injuries caused by playground equipment. *Br. Med. J.*, **4**, 332.

18. Jackson, R.H. (1988) The doctor's role in the prevention of accidents. *Arch. Dis. Child.*, **63**, 235.

19. Jackson, R.H., Cooper, S. and Hayes, H.R.M. (1988) The work of the Child Accident Prevention Trust. *Arch. Dis. Child.*, **63**, 318.

CHAPTER 21

Death resulting from paediatric surgery and anaesthesia

Kent Mancer

Investigations of death that occur in association with surgery and anaesthesia are the most complex in forensic medicine and pathology. Such deaths may be due primarily to the patient's basic disease or to mishaps that relate to the surgery, the anaesthesia or combinations of these factors.

Therapeutic misadventure includes those deaths that occur unexpectedly during or as a result of medical or surgical procedures. Of cases so categorized in a series from a coroner's office, surgical complications accounted for 36%, anaesthetic accidents for 30%, therapeutic procedures 18%, diagnostic procedures 14% and drug reactions 2% [1].

It has been estimated that one in five anaesthetics is administered to a child. Children have nearly four times the operative mortality rate of adults; 58% of children who die are at low risk, with ASA physical status of 1 or 2 [2]. When death occurs, it is likely to be the result of a surgical or anaesthetic accident. The young infant with life-threatening malformations may not survive operation because of his underlying disease, a risk that he shares with the elderly and the adult with severe coronary artery disease. Generally speaking, the same types of accidents that occur in adults may involve children; the additional

risk for children relates to the special surgical and anaesthetic skills required for their care.

Series of operative deaths that include adults and children have been reported from single institutions [3–9], multiple institutions [10–14], and entire nations [15, 16]. Mortality figures, age incidences and relative incidences of surgical and anaesthetic deaths vary widely depending on the assessors and the means of collection of data. There were very few paediatric deaths in a series which attempted to include all of the experience in Scotland [15]; this was, perhaps, related to the voluntary nature of the reporting. The author pointed out discrepancies related to anaesthesia which were demonstrated between his series and the Confidential Inquiry into Maternal Deaths in England and Wales [17] in which full reports were mandatory. An enquiry into perioperative deaths is currently underway in Britain [18]. Although reporting is voluntary, strict confidentiality has apparently resulted in a high degree of cooperation.

The higher incidence of operative mortality in children has been confirmed repeatedly [4, 8, 10, 11, 16, 19]. It was shown in a report from Finland that it was not until the sixth decade of life that the number of operative deaths surpassed those of the first decade; over half the childhood deaths occurred under the age of 1 year [16].

A particularly high incidence of operative mortality among young children was reported in a series from Thailand. The author considered that inexperience was a major factor and recommended that anaesthesiology trainees, nurse anaesthetists, medical students and student nurses be allowed to manage paediatric cases only under constant supervision. Inexperienced personnel tended to make errors of commission rather than omission in crisis situations [4]. Harrison [5] studied two 10-year periods at a major teaching hospital and credited improved survival in the later period to four factors: improved monitoring during anaesthesia, an increased consultant/trainee ratio approximating 1/1, decrease in caseload per anaesthetist and introduction of recovery rooms within the operating theatre–intensive care area. It was considered that there was an irreducible minimum of about 0.15 deaths per 1000 anaesthetics that related to anaesthetist factors, particularly the need to allow trainees to carry total responsibility in order to achieve competence. As in all medical specialties, excellence cannot be achieved in a state of dependence, but there must be an awareness of limitations.

Operative deaths may occur in the operating theatre, recovery room, intensive care unit or later, when the patient returns to the ward. Although most deaths relate to surgery and anaesthesia, some occur during procedures performed by specialists other than surgeons. Deaths have occurred during anaesthesia covering radiographic techniques, cardiac catheterization and atrial septostomy, procedures that are performed by radiologists and cardiologists. The newly developing field of interventional radiology includes intentional embolization of highly vascular tumors – such as arteriovenous malformations and aneurysms – as an alternative to surgery in high-risk cases. Such emboli may block the wrong vessels, resulting in major infarcts and sometimes death.

Occasionally, operative deaths occur in locations other than the operating theatre, dentist's offices being the most common site outside the hospital. Mishaps in such settings are more likely to result in a fatality even though a qualified specialist in anaesthesiology may be in attendance. Single-handed anaesthetic or intravenous tranquillizer administration in dental surgeries continues to occur and is open to criticism.

A wide variety of delivery of anaesthetic care exists in the world today. In Britain and Sweden, virtually all anaesthetics are administered by physician-specialists trained in anaesthesia or by residents working under their supervision. The practice is similar in the urban areas of Canada but, in smaller communities, anaesthetics may be given by general practitioners, most of whom will have had some specific postgraduate training and who attend periodic refresher courses in anaesthesiology.

There is a wide range of practice in the USA but, in general, nurse-anaesthetists deliver a major portion of anaesthetic care, usually under the supervision of a physician-specialist – or anaesthesiologist. Most or all of the anaesthetics given in large teaching hospitals will be administered by anaesthesiologists or supervised residents. In other large hospitals, there may be nurse-anaesthetists working under supervision. In small communities, no anaesthesiologist may be available and nurse-anaesthetists will function under supervision of the surgeon.

In general, few fully trained physician-specialists in anaesthesiology are available in developing countries. Nurse-anaesthetists may be employed and some anaesthetics may be given by students under supervision. In some countries, major hospitals have no anaesthetists; the surgeon may, then, have to administer local anaesthesia, give sedation and supervise all aspects of the care of the patient as he operates.

21.1 OPERATIVE DEATH DUE TO BASIC DISEASE PROCESSES

Advances in surgical technique have widened the scope of what is considered operable. In the early 1970s, many cases of severe congenital heart disease seen at The Hospital for Sick Children, Toronto, came to autopsy never having had surgery; currently, it is increasingly uncommon to see an untouched cardiac malformation, no matter what its severity. A high operative mortality is considered acceptable for new surgical procedures. Resuscitation by trained paramedics and laymen has resulted in fewer cases of trauma and of natural death being certified dead on arrival at hospital. These factors produce some increase in overall survival but, also, in a greater operative mortality.

21.2 DEATHS DUE TO SURGERY

Although surgical manipulation may be responsible for viscerocardiac reflexes and laryngospasm, most surgical deaths result from demonstrable lesions. Intraoperative deaths due to surgical mishap usually relate to massive haemorrhage from incision of a major vessel. Delayed death may occur when there has been slow haemorrhage in the period following surgery, perforation of a viscus or infarction of a major organ from ligation of its blood supply. The autopsy should provide conclusive evidence of what occurred but, in complex cases, it is helpful to have a member of the operative team available to explain what was done surgically.

Surgery for congenital heart disease often involves placement of patches in sites that are difficult to approach because of the small size of the heart. Sutures may have to be placed close to the coronary arteries and conduction system. Extracorporeal perfusion, with cross-clamping of the aorta to isolate the heart, is needed to achieve a motionless, bloodless surgical field. Currently, the myocardium is being protected from ischaemia by infusion of a 4 °C crystalloid solution or of cooled hyperkalaemic blood to induce cardioplegia. The degree of protection depends upon time and temperature. At a myocardial temperature of 8–10 °C, a cardioplegic time of greater than 85 minutes is associated with a sharp rise in mortality. Overall, 50% of deaths in children undergoing cardiac surgery are associated with inadequate protection of the myocardium from ischaemia [20]. The remainder of deaths relate mainly to difficulties in correcting the defect.

Extracorporeal perfusion (bypass) time is also significant. Bypass ordinarily commences about 15 minutes prior to cross-clamping of the aorta and is maintained for a time after the heart is reperfused – the period of weaning from bypass. Two hours of extracorporeal perfusion is common. More than 3 hours suggests some difficulty, a surgical complication or inability to wean the patient from bypass. Inability to wean implies severe myocardial failure. Some authors consider that death due to surgery should include cases in which the procedure was too lengthy or too extensive to be tolerated by the patient [21].

(a) Haemorrhage

Sudden massive haemorrhage can complicate many surgical procedures. A fatal outcome may be prevented by anticipating situations that are dangerous, having a large-bore intravenous line running and by having adequate supplies of volume replacement available. Blood transfusions are usually given too slowly when there has been unexpected massive haemorrhage during surgery. Infusion pumps should be ready for use in the operating theatre. An apparently small quantity of blood lost may constitute a significant portion of the circulatory volume of an infant. Losses should be monitored intraoperatively and replaced immediately. Blood aspirated from the surgical site is collected and the volume measured; sponges are weighed after use and the total blood loss calculated.

Abnormal bleeding following surgery may result from thrombocytopenia, depletion of other coagulation factors or by disseminated intravascular coagulation, which is often associated with hypovolaemic shock or severe infection. Haemorrhage may occur very slowly in haemophiliacs, an example being a newborn unsuspected haemophiliac who died 1 week following ritual circumcision.

21.3 PATHOPHYSIOLOGICAL FACTORS RELATING TO OPERATIVE DEATH

Hypoxia and cardiac arrest are frequent factors in most anaesthetic and some surgical deaths. The factor common to both is the failure of delivery of adequate oxygen to the brain.

Circulatory arrest for more than 3–4 minutes at normal body temperature results in loss of function and, ultimately, necrosis of cerebral cortical neurones. Restoration of cardiac activity after longer periods is not uncommon as the myocardium can tolerate lack of oxygenated blood for 10–15 minutes. Following successful resuscitation, and despite irreversible brain damage, the heart will continue to beat; ventilator-assisted respiration will be effective until severe pneumonia develops. The maintenance and discharge from artificial ventilation of such patients varies with national medical practice.

Hypoxia with an intact circulation has an effect similar to circulatory arrest, the length of the agonal period depending upon the degree of hypoxia. Ventilation without oxygen results in the steady loss of alveolar oxygen and the oxygen content of the blood decreases dramatically. The time required to cause hypoxic damage will be longer than for cardiac arrest, and ventilation with suboptimal quantities of oxygen will extend the time taken to produce hypoxic damage even further [22].

The brain of the child does not differ significantly from that of the adult in its sensitivity to hypoxia. The brain stem and periventricular regions are most sensitive to hypoxia in children younger than 4–6 weeks of age whereas, later, the cerebral cortex is more likely to be damaged. The unclosed sutures of the young child provide some protection from the effects of cerebral oedema.

(a) Morphological signs of hypoxic injury to the brain

Circulatory arrest and hypoxia generally leave no histological changes in the brain unless there has been a period of survival of 12 hours following the insult. Evidence of cerebral oedema may become apparent earlier but is also dependent upon an interval of survival.

The term 'hypoxic-ischaemic encephalopathy' is used to indicate the central nervous system lesion that has resulted from tissue hypoxia. Changes which are due purely to hypoxia are seldom, if ever, seen. Cerebral oedema inevitably arises during the period of the perfusion of the brain that is necessary for morphological evidence of hypoxic damage to develop. With limitation of space for expansion of the brain, increasing oedema will cause further decrease in its perfusion which, in turn, results in a continuing ischaemic – and, at the tissue level, hypoxic – insult.

The earliest histological signs of hypoxic or ischaemic injury to the central nervous system involve the neurones and consist of cytoplasmic eosinophilia, loss of Nissl substance and nuclear pyknosis (Fig. 21.1). There may be evidence of oedema of the surrounding neuropil.

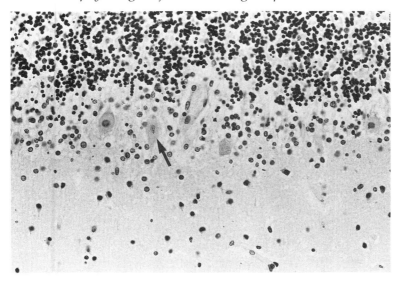

Fig. 21.1 Hypoxic neuronal damage involving Purkinje cells of a 2-year-old boy who died 48 hours following resuscitation. There had been about 10 minutes of asystole prior to restoration of the circulation. The Purkinje cells have lost most of their peripheral basophilia, and the cytoplasm was eosinophilic. Nuclei are shrunken and hyperchromatic. The nucleus of one cell is becoming fragmented (arrow) (haematoxylin and eosin, × 740).

Hypoxic neuronal damage should be differentiated from the shrunken dark neurones that occur as artefacts of handling and which retain cytoplasmic basophilia (Fig. 21.2). Such changes probably occur as a result of injury to the cell membrane, with loss of fluid but not of protein or nucleic acids. The artefact occurs mainly at the surfaces of the intact brain, due to the pressure of handling prior to fixation, and is also commonly seen in brain biopsies – particularly along the edge of the specimen [23].

Subsequent changes in the neurones depend upon longer survival following the hypoxic insult. Nuclear lysis will occur, leaving only the eosinophilic cytoplasm. Later, the neurone disappears entirely and the surrounding neuropil closes the gap. These changes will be accompanied by infiltration of macrophages and proliferation of glial cells, the reparative process that eventuates in the glial scar.

The gross and histological appearances following hypoxic and ischaemic injury to the brain are variable [24]. The mildest insults may involve only a few of the neurones in Somers' sector of the hippocampal uncus. Severe prolonged hypoxia causes generalized cerebral oedema. The increased intracranial pressure may be of such severity that cerebral blood flow ceases. If such a patient survives with ventilator support, autolytic changes will occur *in vivo*, ultimately resulting in the 'respirator brain'. Such a brain is intensely swollen, increased in weight and of a soft, semiliquid consistency. Formalin fixation has little effect in firming the tissue. On histologic examination, the neurones show the autolytic

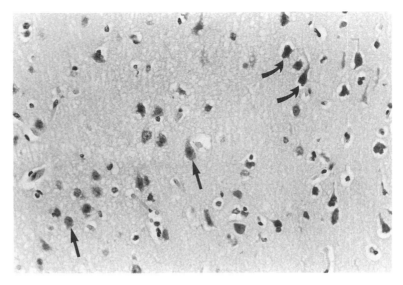

Fig. 21.2 Handling artefact, involving most of the neurones on the right side of the photograph. They are shrunken, have deeply basophilic cytoplasm and hyperchromatic shrunken nuclei (curved arrows). The neurones on the left side are unaffected (straight arrows). Temporal lobectomy specimen from an epileptic 18-year-old male (haemotoxylin and eosin, × 740).

effects of cytoplasmic vacuolation and poor nuclear staining. Despite autolysis, hypoxic-ischaemic changes may still be recognizable if the hypoxic insult was followed by a period of more than 12 hours of effective cerebral perfusion.

Other hypoxia-sensitive tissues include the myocardium, renal cortex and intestinal mucosa. The tips of the papillary muscles of the left ventricle are the most likely regions of the heart to become necrotic. The proximal convoluted tubules of the renal cortex and the mucosal aspect of the intestine are sensitive to hypoxia and ischaemia to a lesser degree.

(b) Cardiac massage

Lesions which arise secondary to cardiac massage should not be implicated as causes of death. External cardiac massage may result in contusions to the endocardium and laceration of the liver, which occurs usually adjacent to the round ligament.

Open cardiac massage is often performed when there has been cardiac arrest during or shortly following cardiac surgery. Acute subdural haematoma is often found in such cases, this being possibly due to pressure being transmitted from the right atrium to the intracranial veins. These haematomas are generally small, less than 1 mm thick, and may be bilateral.

(c) Hypoxia during anaesthesia

Hypoxia may result from inadequate oxygen in the inspired gas, inadequate tidal volume, slow respiratory rate or deficient oxygenation of arterial blood due to abnormalities of lungs, heart or blood. Oxygen deficiency in the inspired gas usually relates to failure of anaesthetic equipment. Decreased tidal volume may be due to leaks or blockage of the airway or, when mask ventilation is used, to excess anaesthetic, laryngospasm, bronchospasm, upper airway obstruction or failure of the respiratory muscles. Inadequate tidal volume is uncommon during manual ventilation of a child. When the patient is being relied upon to ventilate himself, however, the respiratory rate may be slowed or eliminated by narcotics, muscle relaxants and/or anaesthetic gases. Gas diffusion across the alveolar membrane may be defective due to pulmonary oedema, to underlying lung disease that diminishes diffusion capacity or to injury from aspirated vomitus. Anaemia or circulatory shock may result in inadequate transport of oxygen from the lungs to tissues.

Excess of carbon dioxide in combination with hypoxia is more common during anaesthesia than is hypoxia alone and usually results from hypoventilation or from airway obstruction. Carbon dioxide accumulation is insidious and may produce no clinical signs prior to sudden circulatory failure. Increased carbon dioxide in the blood stimulates the cardio-inhibitory centre, causing bradycardia and partial heart block eventuating in cardiac failure and convulsions. Seizures do not occur when there is progressive anoxia alone. A rising level of carbon dioxide in the blood is the most significant factor in causing acidosis in general anaesthesia; there is progressive heart block which is complete when the pH reaches 7.0. Carbon dioxide is a potent cerebral vasodilator and may cause fatal increased intracranial pressure. At autopsy the brain of a patient who has had hypercarbia is likely to be congested and increased in weight.

(d) Autonomic control of the heart and vessels

The parasympathetic nervous system, acting through the vagus nerve, has a slowing effect on the discharge rate of the sinoatrial node of the heart and on the conduction system. Complete block is followed usually by the commencement of a slow ventricular beat – an effect which is known as 'vagus escape', the ventricles being liberated from the depressing action of the vagus. With a strong parasympathetic stimulus, there is a possibility that the vagal escape mechanism may fail and cardiac arrest occur.

The sympathetic nervous system, acting via the hypothalamus, the cervical spinal cord and the cardiac nerves to the sinoatrial and atrioventricular nodes, also acts directly on the ventricle, increasing its rate of contraction. A powerful sympathetic stimulus may cause ventricular fibrillation.

The hypothalamus, which controls the sympathetic and parasympathetic nervous systems, is influenced by the prefrontal cortex and thalamus, this being the pathway by which the emotions influence the autonomic nervous system. To counteract this, the anaesthetist uses premedication to moderate emotional activity.

The peripheral vascular system is controlled by the vasomotor centre of the brain via the sympathetic division of the autonomic nervous system. It is influenced by adrenaline and by anaesthetic agents. The heart does not easily tolerate a sudden increase in peripheral resistance from reflex vasoconstriction. Decreased resistance with drop in blood pressure reduces perfusion of the myocardium and ischaemia, with the possibility of cardiac arrest, may result.

(e) Viscerocardiac reflex

Viscerocardiac reflexes cause slowing of the heart, drop in blood pressure, disturbances in cardiac rhythm and sometimes asystole should the vagal escape mechanism fail. Interpretation of this type of case depends on knowledge of the clinical events surrounding the death. Common causes include intubation

and extubation, tracheal suction, bronchoscopy and manipulation or retraction of
viscera – particularly of the lungs and stomach
[8]. Viscerocardiac reflexes are common at
induction and termination of anaesthesia.
One-third of patients develop some
arrhythmia during induction and some deaths
occur [25].

(f) Cardiac arrest

Cardiac arrest during anaesthesia usually
results from deficient oxygen in the gas
mixture but it may be due to a depressant
effect of the anaesthetic itself. All anaesthetic
agents, with the possible exception of nitrous
oxide, are toxic to the myocardium. They may
affect the heart muscle itself, its conduction
system, the peripheral vascular and autonomic nervous systems and the vascular
supply to the myocardium.

Electrolyte imbalance may produce cardiac
arrest. Excess potassium causes increasing
relaxation of the heart and, eventually, arrest
in diastole. Elevation of ionized calcium
increases the force of contraction and, in
excess, may result in cardiac arrest by
preventing myocardial relaxation. Hypocalcaemia has similar effects to hyperkalaemia. Severe hyponatraemia can also
cause cardiac arrest.

Patients with recent myocardial infarction
have an increased risk of death under general
anaesthesia. Small infarcts are not uncommon
in those with severe congenital heart disease.
Large myocardial infarcts often occur with
truncus arteriosus, because the myocardium
is subjected to greatly increased workload in
the presence of poor coronary perfusion.

Myocardial infarction sometimes develops
during cardiac surgery, due to accidental
interruption or obstruction of major branches
of coronary arteries, particularly from
suturing of large patches high in the
ventricular septum. The obstruction may be
demonstrated post-mortem by probing and
by coronary angiography.

21.4 PHYSIOLOGICAL DIFFERENCES BETWEEN CHILDREN AND ADULTS RELATED TO ANAESTHESIA

A greater technical proficiency is required in
paediatric than in adult anaesthesia because of
the smaller patient and a lesser margin of
safety. Complications occur more rapidly and
with less warning. Infants and children may
not respond to an anaesthetic agent in the
same manner as an adult. Premature infants
differ the most and the child comes to
resemble the adult in his responses with
increasing age [26].

Parasympathetic responses are well
developed in young infants and relatively
large doses of anticholinergic drugs are
tolerated. The sympathetic division is less
developed functionally and vagotonic activity
on the heart predominates; the infant
depends on endogenous catecholamine to
compensate for this.

Young children have a high cardiac output,
which serves to maintain the blood pressure
more significantly than does peripheral
resistance. Consequently, myocardial
depression can produce large drops in blood
pressure and does so more frequently in
children than adults [27]. In addition,
premature infants may lose baroresponse
entirely, and are thus unable to respond to
hypotension by increasing cardiac output
[28].

The blood–brain barrier is not well
developed in infants. Water-soluble agents
are, therefore, taken up better in the infant's
brain than are those with lipid solubility; by
comparison, lipid-soluble agents enter the
adult brain more readily. Possibly as a result of
this, high alveolar concentrations of general
anaesthetic are required to maintain
anaesthesia in the infant. In addition, a
greater proportion of the tissue of the young
patient has a rich vascular supply; this allows
more rapid equilibration of blood and tissue
concentrations and increases the amounts of
agents required to induce and maintain
anaesthesia.

Infants have greater ventilation of alveoli as compared to functional residual capacity and respond to – and emerge from – anaesthesia more rapidly than do adults. They have a relatively large extracellular fluid space for distribution of water-soluble drugs which explains their comparative insensitivity to succinylcholine. The relatively reduced muscle mass of young infants may be responsible for altered responses to the non-depolarizing muscle relaxants.

The fetus is accustomed to a hypoxic state and compensates for it by polycythaemia; this persists for up to 4 weeks, giving the newborn infant the ability to function under hypoxic conditions that would impair an older child. The chronic hypoxia of cyanotic congenital heart disease prolongs this state into childhood.

(a) General anaesthetic agents

All general anaesthetic agents are more or less toxic and can cause cardiac arrest when given in large doses or in hypoxic conditions; all have the property of causing myocardial and respiratory depression as well as the intended effect of depressing the cerebral cortex.

For unknown reasons, halothane-induced hepatitis is extremely rare prior to puberty [29]. Halothane is, thus, still the general inhalation anaesthetic agent which is most widely used in paediatric practice. The related halogenated ethers, enflurane and isoflurane, are now the most popular general anaesthetic agents for adult use. They tend to sensitize the myocardium to catecholamines less than does halothane.

(b) Intravenous barbiturates

Although capable of producing general anaesthesia, barbiturates cause severe respiratory depression in relation to the cerebral cortical depression and muscle relaxation which is achieved. Barbiturate is hazardous in shock states because compensatory vasoconstriction is abolished. Reflex response to painful stimuli is maintained. Adverse effects include laryngospasm, bronchospasm, vomiting, bradycardia, and decrease in cardiac output which relates to peripheral vasodilatation and venous pooling. High concentrations of barbiturate reaching the heart abruptly may cause cardiac arrest by direct depression of the myocardium; this type of death will occur very soon after injection of the drug. Thiopental may be used for induction of anaesthesia in children over 6 months of age, but increased sensitivity to barbiturates is seen in younger children. Barbiturate is contraindicated in obstructive airway disease as apnoea may be induced.

(c) Muscle relaxants

Although Beecher and Todd implicated curare in a high proportion of anaesthetic deaths [11], their interpretation is disputed [21] and the drug continues to be in common use, subject to adequate reversal, for muscle relaxation in lengthy operations.

Succinylcholine is generally used as a muscle relaxant for intubation. Paralysis should pass in 3 minutes provided that plasma cholinesterase activity is normal; deficiency of this enzyme occurs in about 1 in 1500 patients. Respiratory depression occurring from the onset of anaesthesia is more likely to be due to overdosage with barbiturate.

(d) Local anaesthesia

Widely varying death rates have been reported for local anaesthesia. Beecher and Todd reported 1 per 2338 administrations [11], but a figure as low as 1 in 21 000 has been quoted [25]. Simple overdose accounts for most deaths, the primary effect being on the central nervous system.

Toxic effects depend upon the dosage administered, the rate of absorption and the clinical state of the patient. The presence of inflammation will increase the rate of absorption by vessels. Absorption of topically applied local anaesthetics can be very rapid; toxic blood levels can be produced, particularly when the agent is applied to the pharynx, trachea and urethra. Accidental intravenous injection of local anaesthetic, or of the catecholamine that is often combined with it, may constitute a massive overdose as it reaches the heart and cause sudden cardiac failure. Confusion of the names of these drugs, all ending in 'caine' has resulted in many overdoses.

Errors in administration of drugs probably occur much more frequently than is recognized and some result in death. The wrong drug may be given, or the wrong dosage. Quantities meant for adults may be given in error to small children. Accidents of this type are more likely to occur in the operating theatre than the wards because of greater stress in the former situation.

21.5 MALIGNANT HYPERTHERMIA

One per cent of the population are predisposed to malignant hyperthermia and most are unaware of their condition. It is inherited as an autosomal dominant with variable penetrance. Malignant hyperthermia develops in one in 15 000 anaesthetics and involves all age-groups. One-half of cases occur in dental offices and have a higher mortality rate than those in hospitals. The overall mortality is 50% but is decreasing with earlier recognition and treatment.

There is usually no indication of the presence of the disorder until tachycardia, dysrhythmia, blood pressure changes and cyanosis develop during anaesthesia. Hyperthermia is a late sign. The most common precipitants are general anaesthetic agents, such as halothane and halogenated ethers, given in conjunction with succinylcholine.

On exposure to the agent, excessive quantities of calcium ion are liberated in the sarcoplasm, stimulating and maintaining muscle contraction, which causes rigidity, heat production and rising body temperature. Phosphorylase is activated, converting ATP to ADP, and generating heat. Glycolysis occurs in muscle and liver and metabolic acidosis results from the accumulation of lactic acid. Large amounts of carbon dioxide are produced and the soda-lime canister may become too hot to touch. Hypoxia develops because of the increased metabolic state. Other complications include arrhythmias, hypertension, hypotension and hyperkalaemia. The body temperature rises rapidly to very high levels and may reach 44 °C. Arrhythmia or hypoxia are the usual terminal events.

There are no diagnostic signs at autopsy; interpretation depends upon knowledge of the clinical events. Definitive diagnosis requires viable muscle obtained by biopsy of the living patient. The specimen of muscle and a control are placed in a Krebs–Ringer bath and are exposed to caffeine or halothane; contractions occur in cases of malignant hyperthermia [30]. Carriers may have elevated levels of creatine phosphokinase [31].

Malignant hyperthermia can be treated successfully by measures to lower the body temperature, stopping the anaesthetic and ventilating with oxygen. Dantrolene, a skeletal muscle relaxant, given intravenously counteracts the malignant hyperthermia crisis. It should be available in operating theatres and ready for use in any patient having the disease state or known to be closely related to someone diagnosed as having had malignant hyperthermia.

21.6 OBSTRUCTIVE ASPHYXIA

(a) Aspiration of gastric contents

Vomiting is one of the most frequent causes of death during anaesthesia, particularly in children, and accounts for as many as 11% of operative deaths over all age ranges [10]. Vomiting is most likely to occur during induction of anaesthesia if the stomach has not been previously emptied.

Death subsequent to vomiting may be due to airway obstruction by food or, alternatively, the vomitus may have irritated the larynx and caused fatal laryngospasm. Gastric contents which have a pH of 2.5 or less cause chemical damage to small bronchioles, the mucosa of which becomes oedematous, leading to asphyxia; children commonly have highly acid stomach contents [32]. Neutral vomitus does not cause chemical injury but contains viable bacteria; bronchopneumonia may develop later.

The post-mortem diagnosis of aspiration must not depend upon finding food material in the airway. None may be present if there has been laryngospasm due to the irritative effects of vomitus. Conversely, aspiration of vomitus may be no more than an agonal event. The presence of food in the airway may be due to the normal procedures involved in transport of the body to the autopsy table; it has been demonstrated that material from the stomach may pass into the airway and extend as far as alveoli entirely as a post-mortem event [33].

The diagnosis of asphyxia from aspiration of vomitus must take into account known clinical events. An inflammatory reaction to the vomitus is helpful when present but is unlikely if survival was brief following the vomiting episode.

(b) Pharyngeal obstruction

Following tonsillectomy or adenoidectomy, or in cases of basal skull fracture, large pharyngeal clots may be aspirated and cause obstruction of the glottis. The tongue may obstruct the pharynx because of relaxation of muscles of the submental triangle due to anaesthesia, an occurrence which is more common in children than in adults.

A haematoma in continuity with the surgical site may result from surgery to the neck or mouth and obstruct the airway on extubation. At autopsy, it is difficult to quantitate such a haematoma and to estimate its effect on the airway. Radiographic demonstrations should be attempted prior to dissection when obstruction of this type is suspected.

(c) Bronchospasm and laryngospasm

Bronchospasm and laryngospasm frequently occur together and are both common complications of general anaesthesia. They are generally produced by stimuli similar to those that cause viscerocardiac reflexes – most commonly irritation of the bronchial and laryngeal mucosa. The spasm may resolve on removal of the irritant but cyanosis and bradycardia develop if it continues and death may ensue. Ether is notable as an anaesthetic agent that is particularly prone to cause laryngospasm and bronchospasm.

Foreign material on or within the endotracheal tube may cause severe mucosal irritation. Soda lime dust from the carbon dioxide absorption canister is caustic and highly irritative, causing immediate bronchoconstriction and pulmonary oedema. Irritative substances may be produced by the use of irradiation or ethylene oxide for sterilization of polyvinyl chloride endotracheal tubes.

Severe laryngospasm caused by stimulation of the larynx during light anaesthesia is not uncommon in children, particularly in those under the age of 7. It can occur during intubation or after removal of the endotracheal tube. Reflex bronchoconstriction from such afferent stimuli as intubation or traction on viscera may continue in asthmatics long after cessation of the original stimulus.

A period of manual hyperventilation should be given both before attempts at intubation and before extubation to enable the patient to tolerate a period of laryngospasm.

21.7 TRACHEOSTOMY AND BRONCHOSCOPY

A tracheostomy tube which is too short may become dislodged and lie beside the trachea. Most other complications of tracheostomy occur days after placement of the tube. Tracheostomy tubes, being rigid and left in place for prolonged periods, are capable of producing severe erosions through the tracheal wall and into the adjacent innominate artery, causing exsanguination.

Bronchoscopy, also, may be complicated by massive haemorrhage, causing asphyxia or exsanguination. Haemorrhage is most likely to occur on extraction of foreign bodies that have become embedded in the trachea. Penetration of the tracheal wall by the bronchoscope is not uncommon during very difficult procedures. Several deaths in one series were due to syncope, bronchoscopy having been performed with the patient in the sitting position [12].

(a) Endotracheal tubes

Placement of an endotracheal tube in any other site than the tracheal lumen leads to severe hypoxia. The most common abnormal location is within the oesophagus. Death will occur rapidly if a muscle relaxant had been used. Survival has occurred despite oesophageal intubation if the patient has been capable of ventilating himself. The possibility of oesophageal intubation has been recognized by pathologists more frequently in recent years; erosion of the oesophageal mucosa may still provide evidence of misplacement if the tube has been removed prior to autopsy or radiographic study.

Other paratracheal sites include the tube ending in the pharynx, or it may enter a tracheoesophageal fistula resulting in a functional state similar to oesophageal intubation. It may perforate the trachea and enter the mediastinum, a rare occurrence which will result in mediastinal emphysema as well as severe hypoxia.

(b) Obstruction of the endotracheal tube

The endotracheal tube may be obstructed by kinking or twisting, usually just proximal to the connector to the anaesthetic equipment. Kinking may occur at a point of angulation, where the tube passes the incisor teeth or gags for pharyngeal surgery. The tube may be obstructed by doubling back upon itself in the pharynx. Its lumen may be blocked by mucus, pus, blood or foreign material such as a fragment of a broken suction catheter.

A defective cuff of an endotracheal tube, eccentrically inflated, may cause the bevelled end of the tube to lie flat against the inner wall of the treachea. Alternatively the eccentric cuff may, itself, block the orifice of the tube. An old, softened endotracheal tube may be collapsed by overinflation of its cuff.

21.8 MALFUNCTION OF ANAESTHETIC EQUIPMENT

Equipment failure includes malfunction or failure of all anaesthesia-related equipment from the bulk source of gases outside of the building, the pipelines, the gas outlets in the walls, to the anaesthetic machine and the tubing to the patient. Equipment failure is a more frequent cause of death when the patient is under the age of 2 years. It is dangerous to use equipment which is designed for adults in the anaesthesia of small children [10]; too much dead space results in rebreathing, and excessive resistance compromises effective breathing through the device.

Prior to the anaesthetic procedure, the anaesthetist must check the machine by breathing through it himself to make sure that its assembly is correct. Types of malfunction include incorrect flow-meter settings, obstruction to the flow of gases, leaks and failure of oxygen supply. Inadequate oxygen may result from exhaustion of central or machine-mounted oxygen sources, improper placement of gas containers on the anaesthetic machine, mislabelled gas containers and the use of obsolete anaesthetic machines which lack 'fail-safe' devices. Disconnection of the breathing circuit may cause acute hypoxia with irreversible damage to the central nervous system in a few minutes. Disconnections usually occur outside of the body, but Harrison reported one case in which there was unobserved tube disconnection intranasally [5].

Many deaths have occurred as a result of errors in connection of the pipe from central gas supplies. Most commonly, the oxygen and nitrous oxide pipes have been crossed and this is particularly so following repairs to or new construction of operating suites [21].

It is emphasized that the equipment must not be relied upon entirely. The patient must be carefully observed and monitored by the anaesthetist throughout the procedure. Adequate observation and competent management should avert fatal consequences of equipment failure in most situations.

21.9 TRANSFUSION DEATHS

Transfusion reactions are rare causes of operative death. They may result from incorrect blood grouping or, more commonly, from failure to check labels on the transfused blood. Receipt of the wrong blood type results in an immediate haemolytic reaction or agglutination. Death may occur quickly or disseminated intravascular coagulation may develop, and the patient dies in the postoperative period.

Complications of transfusion may also relate to improper storage or administration of blood. Blood that is given to a patient may have already become haemolysed because of overheating, freezing, prolonged storage or the presence of haemolytic bacteria. Blood which is contaminated by bacteria may cause endotoxic shock, disseminated intravascular coagulation or a septic state.

21.10 EMBOLISM

(a) Air embolism

Acute cardiac failure from air embolism may occur during operations involving the larger veins, in open heart surgery, and in neurosurgical procedures done in the sitting position. Air embolism occasionally occurs in small infants, air being accidentally injected when using a syringe for blood transfusion. Significant amounts of air may be trapped in intravenous tubing. Defective infusion apparatus may allow suction of air into the infusion line. When a bolus of air reaches the heart, cardiac action converts the blood and air into a froth which obstructs the pulmonary arterial system, causing acute right heart failure and death within minutes.

A chest radiograph should be taken prior to autopsy and as soon after death as possible when air embolism is suspected. A positive X-ray will provide permanent objective evidence of the condition. The autopsy should be done promptly such that there be no question that bacterial growth may have caused gas to appear in the vascular system. It should be performed with care not to allow artefactual entry of air to the vascular system before the heart and major vessels are examined. A suggested technique is as follows. The large veins of the neck and abdomen should be observed unopened for the presence of air bubbles which will be visible through the vascular wall. The pericardium is opened anteriorly, creating a pocket to be filled with water. The pulmonary artery is opened below the water level and any escaping bubbles noted. The right side of the heart is then opened similarly, followed by the left. Neither opening of the head nor sampling of blood should occur until the foregoing has been completed.

(b) Tissue embolism

Embolism in children may be due to thrombus, tissue, fat, bone marrow, tumour and foreign material.

Although common in adults, massive pulmonary embolism is rare in children. Small thromboemboli are occasionally evident on microscopic examination of the lungs, particularly in patients that have had cardiac surgery or an indwelling catheter, but they are seldom numerous enough to have been an important factor in causing death.

Bone marrow and fat embolism occur less commonly in children than in adults and will seldom be a significant factor in causing death.

21.11 INTRAVENOUS CATHETERS

Central venous and subclavian catheters are being used increasingly for blood pressure monitoring and infusion of fluids. Sometimes they perforate the heart or a large vein, causing haemopericardium and tamponade or massive haemothorax. Haemorrhage in such instances may occur so rapidly that, although it occurs in the setting of the operating theatre, adequate volume replacement may not be possible. Intravenous catheterization is, in practice, commonly done in the emergency room or on the wards where there is less capacity for prompt and effective treatment.

21.12 INVESTIGATION OF OPERATIVE DEATHS

Investigation of a death related to surgery or anaesthesia should be initiated immediately. The investigating officer must instruct those attending the patient to leave everything as it is, and proceed to the scene as soon as possible.

The operative team may use the time interval to write their case notes, which are unlikely to have been maintained from the onset of the crisis. Notes that are made while knowledge is still fresh in the minds of the attending physicians and nurses will prove valuable in the subsequent investigation. Recollections months or years later will be of little value as evidence.

Persons who attended the patient must be instructed to leave all tubes, catheters and intravenous equipment as they were at the time of death. There must be no alterations to the state of the anaesthetic machine or its tubing. An expert in the use of the anaesthetic equipment should be available to explain its functioning and to assist the investigator in a search for possible errors in the arrangement of tubes, connectors, valves and gas sources. An examination of the anaesthetic machine by the manufacturer's service representative may help to determine whether it was functioning properly – impartiality must, however, be ensured.

The entire medical record and particularly the anaesthetic record, nursing notes and record of drugs given preoperatively must be examined and possible overdosage considered. The anaesthetist and each member of the surgical team should be interviewed separately. Questions to be asked include the following: Where was each person at the time of the untoward event? What was each doing? Was there any prodrome to the event? Was there any other unusual episode? What were the vital signs of the patient during the anaesthetic? What procedure was necessary to reverse the untoward event? Was the necessary equipment available? How long did it take to put it to use? What was the result? [34]

Ideally the pathologist who will perform the autopsy will attend the scene or be directly involved in the investigation to this point. Alternatively, a coroner or, in the medical examiner system, a deputy medical examiner will be responsible for this very important aspect of the case; the Scottish system of investigation by the fiscal's medical adviser has much to commend it [35].

Attendance of the surgeon and anaesthetist at the autopsy can be very helpful to the pathologist in terms of showing what was done and explaining the accident that occurred but must be dependent on the permission of the coroner or other legal authority; in England and Wales, however, they or their medically qualified representatives are entitled to be present (Coroners Rules 1984 (SI 1984/552), r.7(3)). Full discussion and careful study of the case by those involved is likely to lead to a diagnosis that is agreed upon by all. The pathologist must remain unbiased and base his diagnosis upon his own observations combined with consideration of all relevant clinical facts.

(a) Reporting of operative deaths

Investigators of such deaths may encounter lack of cooperation on the part of the surgical and anaesthetic team and the institution in which the death took place. Adverse publicity and fear of litigation may be partially responsible for such attitudes. Presently, malpractice suits are becoming more common and damages awarded are increasing. There is an understandable reluctance to be involved in any potentially embarrassing and financially threatening situation.

The rules regarding mandatory reporting of operative deaths should be sufficiently broad as to eliminate doubt that any death occurring secondary to medical mishap will come to the attention of the proper authorities. Knight has provided an excellent discussion of the criteria for reporting of operative deaths in England and Wales [36]; in any event, the Registrar must notify the medical legal authority throughout the United Kingdom if surgical operation or anaesthesia is noted on the certificate of cause of death.

In Ontario, the regulations regarding mandatory reporting are found in the Coroner's Act and include:

> a patient whose death is known or suspected to have resulted from unnatural causes or violence, misadventure, negligence, misconduct, malpractise or by unfair means
> a patient who dies in hospital . . . from any cause other than disease
> a patient whose death occurred suddenly and unexpectedly
> when doubt exists as to the cause of death
> whenever there is any doubt about the necessity of notifying the Coroner's Office.

(b) Transport of the body

The body should be brought to the autopsy room with all of the medical devices in place that had been present at the time of death, apart from the anaesthetic machine, which is disconnected at its junction with the endotracheal tube. It is very important that the endotracheal tube not be removed from the body prior to examination by the pathologist. Autopsy assistants must be trained to leave all medical devices in place until commencement of the autopsy.

(c) Post-mortem radiography

Radiography of the neck and chest should be done prior to autopsy when death is related to surgery or anaesthesia. Appropriate radiographs will allow determination of the position of the endotracheal tube, the location of catheters, the presence of air embolism or foreign bodies and will indicate the extent of any pneumothorax. There should be minimal movement of the body prior to radiography; in particular, flexion or extension of the spinal column and neck, which may alter the location of the endotracheal tube, should be avoided.

(d) The autopsy

The body must be thoroughly examined externally prior to removal of medical devices. A complete internal examination is done and particular attention must be directed to the airway, confirming the site of the endotracheal tube and checking for signs of airway obstruction, interstitial emphysema and pneumothorax. So long as appropriate clinical information has been made available to the pathologist, a thorough autopsy will usually reveal the cause of a death due to a surgical mishap.

Anaesthetic deaths usually relate to a hypoxic episode or cardiac arrest, which leave no diagnostic signs, but the cause may become apparent when an error in administration is discovered or a malfunction found in the anaesthetic equipment. In one study, considerable discrepancy was found between the autopsy diagnosis and post-mortem evaluation by anaesthetist assessors in 251 of 495 operative deaths in which the autopsy routine was not specialized [16]. A thorough investigation of the scene and of the events leading to a death is essential and should minimize such discrepancies.

The autopsy may reveal natural disease of sufficient severity to have caused death – thus minimizing suspicion that surgical or anaesthetic errors had occurred. Deaths which occur as a result of the basic disease usually involve patients in the higher ranges of operative risk.

(e) Post-mortem toxicology in anaesthetic deaths

Toxicology studies are done when there is a question of overdose of any of the drugs used in anaesthesia. The pathologist should communicate with the toxicology laboratory before the autopsy to ensure that specimens are obtained in an appropriate manner.

If such communication is not possible, the following suggestions may be helpful. The most important – and, generally, the only – samples that need be taken are blood and serum. Syringes of blood should be obtained directly from the vascular system and transferred into 10 ml glass tubes with Teflon-lined screw-caps. The tubes should contain a preservative such as sodium fluoride which inhibits enzymic activity. Each tube should be filled so as to leave minimal space into which evaporation of volatile agents can occur. It is best that several such tubes be obtained, one for each drug to be analysed. A specimen of serum should be frozen for subsequent analysis as may be necessary. It is better to have too many than too few specimens on hand.

If the anterior fontanelle is not closed, it is most convenient to obtain blood from the sagittal sinus rather than the heart; much of the blood volume may be obtained by elevating the child's body above the site of sampling. If the blood is clotted, the sample may be obtained by incising the atria and collecting blood and clot in the pericardial sac, from which it may be scooped and placed in the relevant tubes; the pericardial fluid should be removed with clean sponges before incising the heart.

The examination of lung tissue for anaesthetic agents is best achieved by the submission of an entire lung in a tightly sealed jar.

Toxicology tests should be considered for all agents that the patient received that may have contributed to his death, including the properative medication, the short-acting barbiturate used for induction, the muscle relaxant and the general anaesthetic.

The samples should be delivered promptly to the toxicology laboratory together with an explanation of the diagnostic problem.

Interpretation of toxicology data

The gaseous anaesthetic agents are very rapidly eliminated via the lungs, 50% being eliminated in from 1 to 10 minutes for most agents. The resuscitation effort will involve rapid ventilation with 100% oxygen; this is likely to be attempted for at least 10 minutes, thus removing most of the anaesthetic agent from the blood.

Succinylcholine has a short half-life in the body, being rapidly metabolized, and is likely to be undetectable unless there is deficiency of plasma cholinesterase. Levels of most other drugs that are found will generally be reliable indicators of the pre-mortem state. An exception is to be found in deaths that occur during or shortly after administration of rapidly acting barbiturate. The barbiturate may have arrived at the heart in high concentration, caused death by cardiotoxicity and, during resuscitation, become more widely dispersed in the body, so giving toxicology data that do not accurately reflect the status at the moment of death. A similar situation may exist when local anaesthetic has been accidentally injected intravenously.

The most likely agents to have caused a sudden cardiac arrest by overdose are the barbiturate induction agent and the general anaesthetic. Post-anaesthesia deaths that have occurred in the recovery room are commonly due to an obstructed airway or to inadequate reversal of drugs used during surgery, particularly muscle relaxants and potent narcotics such as fentanyl and morphine.

(f) The negative autopsy

It may be very difficult to determine whether surgery, anaesthesia, both or neither caused an operative death. Failure of the pathologist to find anything abnormal at autopsy does not necessarily incriminate anaesthesia as the cause, but it does demand a thorough investigation of the events surrounding the case.

21.13 CENTRALIZED REVIEW OF OPERATIVE DEATHS

In Ontario, deaths that occur in relation to an operative procedure are reported to the coroner's office and investigated by a trained coroner who is also a qualified physician. The coroner orders an autopsy to be performed by one of the designated pathologists for the region. Subsequently, the chief coroner refers each case to a committee of senior anaesthetists who meet as a group, study the available information, ask for any necessary further details and formulate an opinion as to the cause of death. One of the group may act as an expert witness on anaesthesia should there be an inquest. Continuing medical education and publication of results of case studies by this committee serves to educate the medical profession as to operative accidents and is intended to prevent recurrence.

21.14 MEDICOLEGAL CONSIDERATIONS

It has been stated that, for justice to be seen to be done, a pathologist other than a member of the staff of the institution involved should perform the autopsy. Such is not always possible. In our experience, it has not been a significant problem. It is understood that, in the performance of his forensic duties, the pathologist has a separate role from his membership of the hospital staff; he is acting on behalf of the Ministry of the Solicitor General and, in that capacity, is entirely independent.

The pathologist who performs the autopsy must be an unbiased observer. His report should state the findings clearly, concisely and completely. It is best to be conservative in committing one's opinion to print, stating in the report only when is certain – speculations are best left to the courtroom.

The pathology report should not use such judgemental terminology as 'negligence', 'error' and 'misdiagnosis'. 'Therapeutic mis-adventure', although necessary for statistical purposes and appropriate in the reports of coroners and medical examiners, need not appear in the pathology report. The use of such terms is unnecessary and potentially harmful to justice – it is often difficult to eliminate a bias which has been introduced by rash prejudgement.

REFERENCES

1. Murphy, G.K. (1986) Therapeutic misadventure. An 11-year study from a metropolitan coroner's office. *Am. J. Forensic Med. Pathol.*, **7**, 115.
2. Wilson, R.D., Traber, D.L., Priano, L.L. and Evans, B.L. (1969) Anesthetic management of the poor risk pediatric patient. *South. Med. J.*, **62**, 767.
3. Lim, S.M.L., Chew, R.K.H., Foo, K.T. and Foong, W.C. (1986) Mortality review in the University Department of Surgery, Singapore General Hospital: January–December 1981. *Singapore Med. J.*, **27**, 296.
4. Pausawasdi, S. (1986) Morbidity and mortality of Thai patients. *J. Med. Assoc. Thai.*, **69**, 407.
5. Harrison, G.G. (1978) Death attributable to anaesthesia. A 10-year survey. *Br. J. Anaesthesiol.*, **50**, 1041.
6. Marx, G.F., Mateo, C.V. and Orkin, L.R. (1973) Computer analysis of postanesthetic deaths. *Anesthesiology*, **39**, 54.
7. Clifton, B.S. and Hotten, W.I.T. (1963) Deaths associated with anaesthesia. *Br. J. Anaesthesiol.*, **35**, 250.
8. Stephenson, H.E., Reid, L.C. and Hinton, J.W. (1953) Some common denominators in 1200 cases of cardiac arrest. *Ann. Surg.*, **137**, 731.
9. Waters, R.M. and Gillespie, N.A. (1944) Deaths in the operating room. *Anesthesiology*, **5**, 113.
10. Edwards, G., Morton, H.J.V., Pask, E.A. and Wylie, W.D. (1956) Deaths associated with anaesthesia. A report on 1000 cases. *Anaesthesia*, **11**, 194.
11. Beecher, H.K. and Todd, D.P. (1954) A study of the deaths associated with anesthesia and surgery. Based on a study of 599 548 anesthesias in ten institutions 1948–1952, inclusive. *Ann. Surg.*, **140**, 2.
12. Dinnick, O.P. (1964) Deaths associated with anaesthesia. Observations on 600 cases. *Anaesthesia*, **19**, 536.
13. Lunn, J.N. and Mushin, W.W. (1982) *Mortality Associated with Anaesthesia*, Nuffield Provincial Hospitals Trust, London.
14. Gibbs, J.M. (1986) The anaesthetic mortality assessment committee 1979–1984. *N.Z. Med. J.*, **99**, 55.
15. Scott, D.B. (1986) Mortality related to anaesthesia in Scotland. *Health Bull.*, **44**, 43.
16. Hovi-Viander, M. (1980) Death associated with anaesthesia in Finland. *Br. J. Anaesthesiol.*, **52**, 483.
17. Arthure, H., Tomkinson, J., Organe, G. Bates, M., Adelstein, A.M. and Weatherall, J.A.C. (1972) *Report on Confidential Enquiries into Maternal Death in England and Wales 1967–9*, HMSO, London.
18. Devlin, H.B. and Lunn, J.N. (1986) Confidential inquiry into perioperative deaths. *Br. Med. J.*, **292**, 1622.
19. Goldstein, A. and Keats, A.S. (1970) The risk of anesthesia. *Anesthesiology*, **33**, 130.
20. Bull, C., Cooper, J. and Stark, J. (1984) Cardioplegic protection of the child's heart. *J. Thorac. Cardiovasc. Surg.*, **88**, 287.
21. Schapira, M., Kepes, E.R. and Hurwitt, E.S. (1960) An analysis of deaths in the operating room and within 24 hours of surgery. *Anes. Analg. Curr. Res.*, **39**, 149.
22. Ernsting, J. (1966) The effects of hypoxia upon human performance and the electroencephalogram, in *Oxygen Measurements in Blood and Tissues* (eds J.P. Payne and D.W. Hill), Churchill, London.
23. Duchen, L.W. (1984) General pathology of neurons and neuroglia, in *Greenfield's Neuropathology*, 4th edn, Edward Arnold, London, pp. 6–8.
24. Brierley, J.B. and Graham, D.I. (1984) Hypoxia and vascular disorders of the central nervous system, in *Greenfield's Neuropathology*, 4th edn, Edward Arnold, London, pp. 125–145.
25. Keating, V. (1961) Anesthetic Accidents, 2nd edn, Year Book, Chicago.
26. Steward, D.J. (1984) Anesthesia in childhood, in *Textbook of Pediatric Clinical Pharmacology* (eds S.M. MacLeod and I.C. Radde), PSG, Littleton.
27. Nicodemus, H.F., Nassiri-Rahimi, C. and Bachman, L. (1969) Median effective dose (ED$_{50}$) of halothane in adults and children. *Anesthesiology*, **31**, 344.

28. Gregory, G.A. (1982) The baroresponses of preterm infants during halothane anaesthesia. *Can. Anaesth. Soc. J.*, **29**, 105.

29. Goudsouzian, N.G. and Ryan, J.F. (1976) Recent advances in pediatric anesthesia. *Pediatr. Clin. North Am.*, **23**, 345.

30. Britt, B.A., Kwong, F.H.F. and Endrenyi, L. (1977) The clinical and laboratory features of malignant hyperthermia management – a review. In *Malignant Hyperthermia: Clinical Concepts* (ed. E.O. Henschel), Appleton-Century-Crofts, New York, pp. 9–45.

31. Kalow, W., Britt, B.A. and Chan, F.Y. (1979) Epidemiology and inheritance of malignant hyperthermia, in 'Malignant Hyperthermia' (ed. B.A. Britt). *Int. Anesthesiol. Clin.*, **17**, 119.

32. Cunningham, A.J. (1987) Acid aspiration: Mendelson's syndrome. *Ann. R. Coll. Phys. Surg. Can.* **20**, 335.

33. Gardner, A.M.N. (1958) Aspiration of food and vomit. *Q. J. Med.*, **27**, 227.

34. Adapted from Weston, J.T. Lecture notes, Washington DC: AFIP, 1972.

35. Mason, J.K. (1988) *Forensic Medicine for Lawyers*, 2nd edn revised, Butterworths, London, p. 343.

36. Knight, B. (1983) *The Coroner's Autopsy*, Churchill Livingstone, Edinburgh, pp. 143–6.

CHAPTER 22

Parentage testing

Barbara E. Dodd

The advantage of applying blood groups to the solution of parentage problems became evident at the early stages of the discovery of blood group systems once it was shown that they were subject to the Mendelian laws of inheritance. Their value was recognized at a time when it had been barely appreciated that blood grouping and compatibility tests were prerequisites for transfusion therapy. However, it would seem that it was not until 1924 that blood groups were first introduced into Court in Germany. The early history of the whole subject has been well reviewed by Wiener [1].

In the past 30 years or so, there has been a general burgeoning of polymorphisms and many kinds of red and white cell antigens, red cell enzymes and plasma proteins have been shown to exist in allelic forms subject to Mendelian laws of inheritance. Almost all of these can be applied to problems of parentage. Moreover, it has now been shown that genetic variations at the deoxyribonucleic acid (DNA) level are proving to be of extreme importance in their ability to solve questions of parentage, although it seems likely that traditional systems will still have a role.

In parallel with the introduction of so many polymorphisms, there has been a widening of the expertise required for their detection. Besides agglutination and cytotoxicity tests, this now includes electrophoretic procedures of various kinds, including isoelectric focusing (IEF), and culminates in the techniques familiar to those engaged in genetic engineering.

In the space of a short chapter it is impossible to include descriptions of any of these methods, nor is it feasible to describe individual blood group systems or offer any account of elementary genetics. In the ensuing pages, it is assumed that the reader is familiar with the bare bones of both human genetics and of the relevant polymorphisms; it is hoped that the bibliography at the end of the chapter will prove useful.

Since the majority of cases are those in which the maternal–child relationship is accepted and it is the identity of the child's father which is in doubt, all the following descriptions will relate to doubtful paternity although, as will be apparent later, there are situations in which both paternity and maternity have to be questioned.

22.1 SCIENTIFIC BASIS OF PARENTAGE TESTING

There are two main scientific aspects of the subject for discussion. In the first place the ability of blood groups to establish non-paternity and the reliability of such findings must be addressed and, secondly, the question of how far blood group evidence can go towards proof of paternity in the absence of finding an exclusion must be considered.

(a) Exclusion of paternity

A man can be excluded from paternity in any of the following three ways:

Category 1. By finding a gene product in a child which is absent from both mother and putative father. For example, the mother and putative father are both Group O and the child is Group A. Provided the mother–child relationship is not in doubt, the child's A gene is paternal and, therefore, excludes from paternity a man who is Group O.

Category 2. By establishing that genes which the putative father must give to his offspring do not appear in the child. This may be:

a, when he is homozygous for a gene which does not appear in the child. For example, in the Rh system if the putative father has inherited the gene *C* from each of his parents, he is homozygous for *C* (i.e. *CC*) and can give only *C* to his own children. However, if he is alleged to be the father of a child who is homozygous for *c*, the allele of *C*, he is excluded from paternity because he cannot give the child the necessary paternal gene which is *c*.
or
b, when he is heterozygous for two genes, neither of whose products appear in the child. For example, putative father group AB, child group O. The putative father in this case must give either *A* or *B* to his offspring.

The exclusions in Category 2 explicitly exclude the putative father even if the mother is not tested. Exclusions based on 1 and 2b are termed first-order or direct exclusions while those based on 2a are second-order or indirect exclusions. The latter are so named because homozygosity for a particular gene cannot be determined unequivocally by testing but is an assumption (see below under '(c) Reliability of results').

(b) The blood group systems applied to paternity problems

Tests are generally made for red cell antigen systems, serum allotypes, red cell enzyme polymorphisms and the HLA system of the white cells. However, not all laboratories include exactly the same set of systems. A comprehensive list of those which are investigated by most specialists dealing with paternity problems is shown in Table 22.1. The percentage chance which each individual system has to exclude the paternity of a wrongly named man is given, as is the combined chance both with and without the inclusion of HLA – which is the most valuable single system. In the opinion of some workers, the routine inclusion of HLA obviates the need to include more than three or four of the other systems because HLA alone has such a high chance – 90% if tests for A and B loci are included – of excluding a non-father from paternity. However, this practice relies heavily upon the results of one system, albeit one showing extreme polymorphism, and, moreover, reducing the number of systems used lessens the chance of providing evidence for exclusion which is supported by more than one independent system.

Some centres include HLA tests as a routine procedure but omit the enzyme poly-morphisms. In fact, in general, the selection of polymorphisms is influenced not only by the overall capability of the battery of tests chosen to exclude a wrongly named man but also by the available expertise.

Table 22.1 Expected chance of exclusion of white Western European non-fathers

Polymorphism tested	% Chance of exclusion
Red cell antigens	
MNSs	32.1
Rh	28.0
Kidd	18.7
Duffy	18.3
ABO	17.6
Kell	4.5
Lutheran	3.7
Serum proteins	
*Gc (Group-specific component)	30.2
Hp (Haptoglobin)	18.1
PLG (Plasminogen)	16.3
Tf (Transferrin)	15.4
Pi (α_1-antitrypsin)	25.6
Red cell enzymes	
*PGM (phosphoglucomutase)	31.1
EAP (erythrocyte acid phosphatase)	23.4
GLO (glyoxalase)	18.7
*EsD (esterase D)	9.7
ADA (adenosine deaminase)	4.5
AK (adenylate kinase)	3.7
Combined chance	97.3
HLA	90.0
Total all systems	99.6

* Including subtypes differentiated by IEF.

(c) Reliability of results

In considering the reliability of the results obtained it is pertinent to begin with sample taking. Correct identification of the individuals and a technique of sampling which ensures that the right blood sample goes into the right tube are prerequisites of paramount importance because the accuracy of the ensuing investigation depends upon them entirely.

The doctor who samples should be supplied with or, better still, take a photograph of each person from whom he extracts blood, even if the individuals are also identified in other ways, e.g. by an accompanying legal representative.

An error-proof method of labelling each sample correctly must be found. The labelling of tubes with the names of the family members prior to their arrival for blood sampling is unforgivably bad practice as it can result in blood from one person being placed in a container bearing the name of another.

When tests in any blood group system show an exclusion of paternity it is recommended that the critical tests are repeated with fresh aliquots obtained from the original sample tubes. Some workers – for example, those at the University Institute of Forensic Medicine in Copenhagen – recall the family and take new samples in these circumstances.

The interpretation of apparent exclusion results requires expert knowledge of the various polymorphisms investigated because of the existence of rare alleles within each system and, particularly, because of the possible presence of 'silent' genes which may affect the conclusions reached.

Silent genes remain hidden in individuals who are apparently homozygous for a particular normal gene. This is because a silent gene does not have an end-product, so it is masked and remains undetected in the tests if it accompanies a normal gene. The effect that the presence of such a gene might have on the interpretation of the results becomes clear from a study of Fig. 22.1. This shows a polymorphic system containing two common alleles (designated *1* and *2*) so that almost all members of a population are either homozygous for *1* (i.e. *1–1*), homozygous for *2* (i.e. *2–2*) or heterozygous (i.e. *2–1*). Very rarely a silent gene may occur. The universally accepted symbol for a silent gene is *0*; this is not to be confused with group O of the ABO

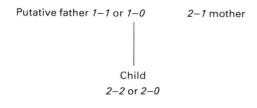

Putative father *1–1* or *1–0*   *2–1* mother

Child
2–2 or *2–0*

0 = silent gene

Fig. 22.1 A family illustrating how a silent gene modifies the interpretation of results.

system which itself is aptly termed 'O' because it also represents a silent gene in the ABO system. A silent gene is not detectable in the routine tests so the putative father in Fig. 22.1, who appears to carry only the product of gene *1* and is, therefore, almost certainly *1–1*, could be *1–0* on rare occasions and, similarly, the child who appears to be *2–2* could be *2–0*. An exclusion is established if the putative father is, in fact, *1–1* and the child *2–2* but, if each possesses a silent gene, far from excluding the putative father from paternity, the results would suggest strongly that they were related. The possibility of the presence of a rare silent gene has to be mentioned in reporting results if a 'back-up' exclusion in another independent system is not obtainable. However, this seldom happens. An indication of the presence of a silent gene may be obtained on occasion by carrying out tests designed to show whether a gene product is present in single or double dose; such tests, however, are not often conclusive.

The question of rare variants also arises. Most of the polymorphisms shown in Table 22.1 have uncommon or rare alternative genes which may occur from time to time at a particular locus on the chromosome. Tests must be designed to detect them as far as is possible – they often yield important results when they occur in paternity problems, either by excluding a putative father from paternity or, because of their low frequency in the

general population, by furnishing very significant evidence in favour of paternity if they appear in both father and child.

The possibility of a mutation occurring and affecting the reliability of results is a question which sometimes arises, although it was more often raised during the earlier years of the application of blood groups to paternity problems. In effect, the question arising is: can a blood group gene mutate (i.e. change) between one generation and the next so that a blood group gene product, which is absent from both parents, appears in a child? No convincing example of a blood group gene mutating between two generations has ever been found.

(d) An example case

An example of an exclusion of a putative father (Mr M) from paternity is given in Table 22.2. This case illustrates all three types of exclusion mentioned earlier. The Rh and EAP systems show first-order exclusions (Category 1 above). The child has the Rh haplotype *CDe* and *EAP-A* which must be paternal contributions since they are absent from the mother. They are also absent in the putative father and, therefore, exclude him from paternity. In the PGM system, Mr M is a heterozygote, *PGM 2 + 1 +*, neither of which genes appear in the child. This is an example of the other type of first-order exclusion (Category 2b). In the Gc system, he appears to be *Gc 1S1S* and the child appears to be *Gc 2–2*. This is a second-order exclusion (Category 2a) because it assumes that the putative father is homozygous for *1S* and that the child is homozygous for *2*, this being on the grounds that no other gene products appear to be present in either the man or the child. Results for a second possible father for the child, who was not excluded from paternity, are also shown in Table 22.2. Methods for calculating the likelihood of his paternity are given below.

Table 22.2 An example case with two possible fathers, one of which is excluded from paternity and the other virtually proven to be the father (see text)

Names	ABO	MNSs	Rh						Duffy		Hp	EAP	GLO	PGM	Gc	EsD	ADA	AK	PLG
			D	C	E	c	C^w	e	Fy^a	Fy^b									
Mr M	B	MNs	−	−	−	+	−	+	+	−	1	B	2.1	2+1+	1S	1	1	1	1
Mrs M	O	NSs	−	−	−	+	−	+	+	+	2	B	2	2−1+	2.1S	1	1	1	2.1
Child M	O	Ns	+	+	+	+	−	+	+	−	2.1	BA	2.1	2−	2	1	1	1	1
Mr G	O	MNs	+	+	−	−	−	+	+	−	1	A	2.1	2−	2.1S	1	1	1	1

For key to systems see Table 22.1.

Table 22.3

	Paternal genes													
	O	Ns	CDe	Fy^a	Hp^1	EAP^A	GlO^1	PGM^{2-}	Gc^2	EsD^1	ADA^1	AK^1	PLG^1	Product
Sperm from Mr G	1	0.5	0.41	1	1	1	0.5	1	0.5	1	1	1	1	0.125 X
Sperm from random man	0.66	0.4	0.41	0.43	0.42	0.36	0.42	0.062	0.27	0.88	0.94	0.95	0.71	2.76×10^{-5} Y
% of men	97	67	65	66	63	59	71	11	44	99	99	99	91	0.3%

To be used in conjunction with Table 22.2 and the text.

22.2 ESTIMATION OF LIKELIHOOD OF PATERNITY

If no exclusion of paternity has been obtained after completing the investigation, a figure is calculated for the likelihood of the putative father's paternity of the child. There are two main ways of doing this: (a) by comparison of sperm and (b) by comparison of men.

(a) Comparison of sperm

In this method, the blood group genes in the child which are seen to be paternal in origin are noted and the chance (X) of the alleged father being able to fertilize an ovum with a sperm carrying them all is calculated. The mere possession by the putative father of the required genes does not mean that all his sperm will carry them all, for this depends on whether he is homozygous or heterozygous for each one. If he is homozygous, all his sperm carry the gene, which therefore scores 100% (or 1); if he is heterozygous, half his sperm will carry the relevant gene, thus scoring 50% (or 0.5). Sometimes, it is not clear whether he is homo- or heterozygous (e.g. if he is group A, the tests do not disclose whether he is *AA* or *AO*); a likelihood calculation then has to be made based on the relative frequencies of homo- and heterozygotes in the general population. The total chance X is the product of the scores for the individual genes in each system. This is compared with the chance (Y) of obtaining a suitable sperm from a random man (RM), a figure which is obtained from the product of the known frequencies of the required genes in the appropriate population (Table 22.3). Then:

X/Y is a balance of probabilities which is internationally known as the paternity index (PI)

A whole range of PI values is possible from those which make no useful contribution

Table 22.4 A range of paternity indices and corresponding RCP values

PI range	Relative chance of paternity (%)
0–10	<91
11–19	91.7–95
20–99	95.2–99
100–399	99.01–99.75
400–999	99.75–99.9
≥1000	>99.9*

* Paternity virtually proven. Some authorities consider that a PI value >400 constitutes proof.

towards proof of paternity to those which offer virtual proof of paternity.

A percentage relative chance of paternity (RCP) can be derived from the paternity index by using the formula PI/PI + 1. Table 22.4 gives a range of PI values and the corresponding values for RCP.

The PI value, in itself, does not constitute a probability of paternity because a realistic estimation of the latter has to include other information besides that which is provided by the blood group investigation. An *a priori* value for chance of paternity may be established from this additional evidence but, since, in practice a realistic *a priori* value is difficult to assess (although some workers attempt it), it is the more general custom to assume an *a priori* value of $P = 0.5$, i.e. there is an equal chance of paternity between the putative father and another man.

An example calculation of a PI value can be made from data obtained from the blood group profile of the second putative father, Mr G, shown in Table 22.2, and from the known paternal genes in the child given in Table 22.3.

The genes for *CDe*, *Hp1*, *EAP A* and *GlO1* are paternal because the mother lacks them. The child is a homozygote for all the others, which fact establishes a paternal contribution for each of them. An X value for Mr G is calculated by noting whether he is homo- or heterozygous for each paternal gene (as described above). The Y value is the product of the individual gene frequencies which, in this case, are those occurring in a Western European population.

$$\text{Thus, PI} = \frac{X}{Y} = \frac{0.125}{2.76 \times 10^{-5}}$$

$$= 4529 \, (\text{approx.})$$

Therefore, the relative chance of paternity (RCP) = 4529/4530 = 99.97%. This constitutes virtual proof of Mr G's paternity of child M provided Mr G's brother is not a contender for paternity of the child.

(b) Comparison of men

This method of establishing the value of the results towards proof of paternity is often preferred by lawyers because they find it more understandable. A calculation is made of the expected percentage of men in the general population who, if subjected to the same set of tests, would not be expected to be excluded from paternity of the child in question; this figure also shows what chance there is of excluding a wrongly named man in any particular case.

Data required for this calculation are also to be found in Table 22.3. For each system, a figure is given for the frequency of all genotypes containing the required gene. The high frequency given for O is because it is not possible to test for O so as to discover which group A and group B people are, in fact, *AO* or *BO*; therefore, all except those who are AB must be considered to be possible possessers of an *O* gene. In the example given, 0.3% of men subjected to the same tests – or approximately one man in 333 – would be expected to have the required genes for fathering child M. Since Mr G has not been excluded, he is among this small proportion of men and is, therefore, highly likely to be the child's true father.

However, calculating the percentage of men in the general population who would not be expected to be excluded does not make the best use of the genetic information available from the results of the tests; comparison of sperm is the preferred method.

The validity of both methods is dependent on any second possible father for the child being unrelated to the named father. If, for example, the putative father's brother is a contender for paternity, comparison with an unrelated man is obviously inappropriate because two brothers inherit their genes from the same small pool of genes present in their parents.

It is also important to take account of the ethnic origin of the family. For example, if a West Indian family is under consideration, blood group gene frequencies for a West Indian population must be consulted in order to obtain the appropriate Y value for the family; similarly, West Indian phenotype frequencies must be used if the method of establishing the percentage of men is requested.

(c) Results from actual cases

An analysis of the findings for 'one man' cases referred to the Serological Unit of the Department of Haematology, The London Hospital Medical College for a 12 month period showed that proof of non-paternity was obtained in 20.3% (1 in 5) cases. Of the cases in which the putative father (PF) was not excluded, 84% showed RCP values over 99% (PI above 100) and 42% of these had RCP values above 99.9% (PI above 1000), which means that paternity was virtually proven in the latter cases.

(d) Presentation of results

The results of a paternity investigation have to be presented at two levels;

REPORT BY TESTER

Ref. No. of Proceedings................   FAMILY LAW REFORM ACT 1969

High Court of Justice, Strand, London W.C.2.

To:—(

(Registrar, ... County Court

(Justices' Clerk, ... Magistrates' Court.

v

Mrs M   Mr M

PART I

I, ..., being a blood tester appointed by the Secretary of State for the purpose of Part III of the Family Law Reform Act 1969, certify that I have carried out a blood group investigation (the details of which are given in Part II of this Report) of the persons named in this direction, viz.,

From the results obtained Mr. ___M___ is excluded/~~XXXXXXXXXX~~ from possible paternity of ___child M___

Reason for conclusion:—

      Mr M is excluded from being the father of child M by the
      results obtained in the Rh, EAP, PGM and Gc systems.
      In these systems the child has inherited the genes CDe,
      EAP A, PGM 2- and Gc 2 from his father. Mr M does not
      possess any of these genes and therefore cannot be the
      father of child M.

Comments on value, if any, of tests in determining whether any person tested is the father of the person whose paternity is in dispute:—

....Signed

....Status

DEPARTMENT OF HAEMATOLOGY
THE LONDON HOSPITAL MEDICAL COLLEGE
TURNER STREET, E1 2AD.

Fig. 22.2 Standard reporting from parentage testing.

(1) They must be intelligible to members of the legal profession who, in respect of these tests, are laymen.

(2) The report must be given in sufficient detail to satisfy a second blood group specialist, as a second opinion is sought occasionally.

In Britain, the report forms introduced at the implementation of Part III of the Family Law Reform Act 1969 are designed to meet both these requirements. Part I of the report summarizes the findings, stating whether or not the putative is excluded from paternity and, if not excluded, a figure indicating the likelihood of paternity is given (Fig. 22.2). Part II allows for a more detailed and technical protocol of the results obtained in each blood group system and this part may be presented in any way chosen by the blood group specialist.

The courts admit the written report as

evidence and the specialist is required to attend court only rarely in difficult or strongly contested cases.

22.3 TYPES OF CASE ENCOUNTERED

(a) Civil cases

Affiliation

In England, these cases are heard in the magistrates' courts. A typical situation is that of an unmarried girl citing a particular man as being the father of her child, which claim he may be unwilling to accept. Unlike the position in some parts of Continental Europe, where the mother is encouraged to name all possible fathers for the child, she is unlikely to win her case in England if she appears to be uncertain about the child's paternity. At present, an affiliation order can be brought against one man only. Thus, only one putative father's blood is available for testing even though in some cases it would have been appropriate to include more than one man in the investigation.

Divorce

These cases are heard in crown courts and usually involve testing two putative fathers – the child's mother's husband and the co-respondent. Experience has proved that it is unwise to assume that, if one of two putative fathers is excluded from paternity, the other is, *ipso facto*, the true father! It is therefore usual to work out a relative chance of paternity for the unexcluded man as in the one-man cases which provide no exclusion (see above).

Private cases

These are cases in which no litigation is contemplated – at least at the time of the request for blood grouping tests. The parties usually wish to resolve a paternity problem for their own peace of mind. Among such cases there will occasionally be father–child

investigations where a sample of the mother's blood is unobtainable – perhaps because she is dead or, for example, because the child's 'father' suspects his wife of infidelity and does not wish her to know this. A father–child investigation precludes the possibility of obtaining a Category 1 first-order exclusion; this reduces the chance of excluding a non-father because, if the husband's suspicions are correct, reliance has to be placed on a Category 2 exclusion alone.

Immigration

In recent years, many requests for a blood group investigation have been received from families in the Indian subcontinent who wish to prove their relationship – usually to the father of the family who has British citizenship and is, therefore, entitled to bring his legitimate wife and offspring into residence in Britain. Maternity as well as paternity may be in doubt in these families since nephews and nieces – of either adult – may sometimes be well integrated in a family unit. In such cases, first-order exclusions such as those described above under Category 1, while proving that one or other is excluded, cannot pin-point which alleged parent is excluded. On the other hand, exclusions under Category 2 show which of the adults is the excluded parent. DNA profiling (see below) is particularly useful in problems of family relationships involving immigrant families [2, 3].

(b) Criminal cases

Incest

Blood groups should be viewed at the level of two generations in these cases. For example, if a father is not excluded from paternity of his daughter's child, it is worthwhile investigating his relationship to his daughter. The author has examined a case in which the accused man, as well as being excluded from paternity of his 'grand-daughter', was excluded also from being the father of his 'daughter'.

Rape resulting in pregnancy

The technical difficulty in this situation is that of obtaining blood from the fetus since, particularly if the victim is a teenage girl, the pregnancy is unlikely to be allowed to proceed; an abortion will be performed early in pregnancy leading to the production of a fetus having very few, if any, red cells. However, there is usually no difficulty in obtaining results for most of the red cell antigens and enzymes if a genuine fetal blood sample can be obtained.

Contamination with maternal blood is always a possibility, so a Kleihauer test is advisable in order to identify the blood as fetal – particularly if the fetal sample does not show any polymorphic characters which distinguish it from one taken from the mother. However, there are more instances in which a clean fetal sample of blood is available in rape cases now that fetoscopy is becoming available.

Legal considerations

Part III of the Family Law Reform Act 1969, which makes provision in England, Wales and Northern Ireland for the use of blood tests in cases of doubtful paternity, became operative in March 1972. For a good many years prior to that, blood group evidence had been accepted by the courts with varying degrees of confidence.

At the present time, although blood tests are not obligatory every time paternity is in doubt (as is the case, for example, in Scandinavia), the court may give a *direction* for a blood group investigation when requested to do so by any party involved in the proceedings. The *direction* is not an *order*, since a blood sample cannot be taken without first obtaining the consent of the individual concerned. However, if there is failure to comply with a direction, the court is at liberty to draw whatever conclusion seems appropriate in the circumstances [4].

When a court direction is made, the clerk of the court is responsible for initiating the proceedings. Special direction forms with attached photographs for identification of each adult – and child, if over 12 months old – are sent to the sampler. Any willing medical practitioner is eligible to take the samples but testing as a result of a court direction is confined to blood group specialists appointed by the Secretary of State. Would-be testers must state their previous experience in the field of haemogenetics and they are requested to submit a list of the polymorphisms they propose to use so that their suitability as testers can be assessed.

Reports are made to the court and the clerk distributes them to each of the parties or their representatives. Not infrequently, a formal court direction is omitted when the mother and putative father both consent to blood tests; arrangements are then made by the solicitors acting on behalf of the parties. This is not considered desirable since the well-designed direction forms are then not used; there is also a loophole whereby individuals, no matter what their lack of credentials and experience, are not debarred from carrying out the scientific work.

The Family Law Reform Act 1969, s.20 has now been amended by the Family Law Reform Act 1987, s.23. One important innovation allows the court, of its own motion, to direct tests to be carried out – that is, the direction no longer has to follow an application by any party to the proceedings but can be made by the court itself. Blood samples from both the husband and the 'other man' may be directed to be taken in divorce cases. Under the 1987 Act, the court now directs the performance of 'scientific tests' rather than of 'blood tests'; the intention here is to allow flexibility so as to take into account any new technology that becomes available.

The Family Law Reform Act 1969 does not run to Scotland where blood testing for paternity has been looked on with some suspicion until recently. The antipathy has rested on the common law principles surrounding consent and evidence and was summed up in a precedental case:

> In these circumstances, the defender is being called upon to provide to the pursuer the basis of evidence from which he has nothing to lose and a great deal to gain while she has nothing to gain and a great deal to lose ... It seems to me that the proposal offends against all conceptions of justice and is contrary to the fundamental principles of our law [5].

The force of this opinion is very much reduced today now that so many polymorphisms are used for testing and high PI values are common, but the possibility of harm being done to a child who cannot consent has also been uppermost in the minds of the courts. Attitudes have, however, changed in recent years and, in 1985, full approval was given to the use of blood tests which were regarded as being completely reliable [6]. Even so, the case was unusual in that two men were actually competing for paternity and the result of the blood tests was thought to promote the welfare of the child; there is, therefore, no certainty that this ruling would be followed in every case.

22.4 DNA POLYMORPHISMS

These are recently discovered polymorphisms at the DNA level which have great potential in the field of parentage problems and the identification of stains, particularly those of seminal origin.

Briefly, isolated DNA is subjected to controlled fragmentation using bacterial enzymes, called restriction enzymes, which cut double-stranded DNA at specific recognized sites along the length of the strand. These restriction fragments (RF) can be separated on the basis of size by electrophoresis on agarose or acrylamide gels. This results in banding; the bands are visualized by the use of a probe which is a radioactively labelled piece of DNA that binds specifically to the target RF by complementary base pairing. The visual appearance is termed an autoradiograph.

Differences in restrictive fragment length can result. There may, for instance, be an alteration in base sequence so that a restriction enzyme recognition site is lost or gained, or blocks of DNA may be inserted or deleted; these variations are expressed in individuals as restriction fragment length polymorphisms (RFLP). Other variation has been found to occur because some regions of DNA have multiple segments of short sequence repeats and the number of repeat segments present can differ.

A special case of multiple band patterns has been described by Jeffreys *et al.* [2,3]. They have used probes against repeat sequences duplicated at many loci along the length of the nuclear genome. The RF patterns contain up to 50 bands of variable intensity and these appear to behave in a Mendelian manner. Because of their variety, these complex patterns appearing on the autoradiograph are believed to constitute individual specific DNA 'fingerprints' – so called because they appear to be as authentically individual as are true fingerprints. In these cases, the autoradiograph resembles the bar codes commonly seen on food packages.

The Jeffrey probes reveal multilocus DNA polymorphisms. In respect of parentage problems, attention is now being focused on single locus DNA polymorphisms, some of which are highly polymorphic. Very significant results are obtained, particularly if several such polymorphisms are used simultaneously. The genetic inheritance of single locus polymorphisms is similar in

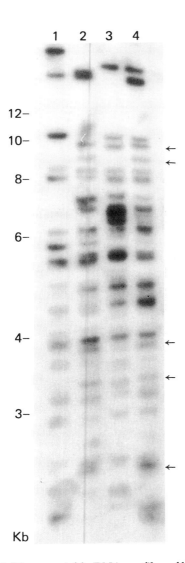

Fig. 22.3 Hypervariable DNA profiles of human DNA. DNA was prepared from whole blood from four individuals named in a case of disputed paternity. The DNA samples were digested with restriction endonuclease *Taq 1*, electrophoresed on a 0.7% agarose gel and Southern blot hybridized with the ^{32}P-labelled DNA probe hMF1 (kindly provided by Dr. D.I. Hoar).

principle to that of the traditional systems described above.

An autoradiograph which establishes non-paternity in a DNA investigation involving two possible fathers and mother and child is shown in Fig. 22.3. Individual 3 is the mother of individual 4 and individuals 1 and 2 are possible fathers. Arrowed bands in the child indicate paternally derived bands present in putative father 2 but absent from putative father 1. This effectively excludes putative father 1 from paternity but not putative father 2.

If the frequency in the general population of any particular band has been established, then the likelihood of paternity of a man who is not excluded by DNA can be calculated – and this often to a very high level, offering virtual proof of paternity.

The place which DNA tests will occupy in the solution of parentage problems in the future is unclear at the time of writing. Some proponents visualize them as entirely replacing the standard grouping tests now operative in the field. Commercial interests, including the granting of patent rights which tend to conflict with the ideals of scientific investigation, are involved and create pressures to establish DNA testing rather more quickly than many scientists consider appropriate. The latter, who include many of those already experienced in the area of forensic blood testing, advise caution – although they agree that DNA profiling has great potential.

Both the American Association of Blood Banks (which is responsible for standards in paternity testing in the USA) and the International Society for Haemogenetics have issued guidelines for the assessment of DNA profiling in parentage problems. Their general conclusion is that DNA polymorphisms need to be further explored. For example, more information is required on gene frequencies, mutation rates and the linkage between genes. It has also been found at the laboratory level that variations in technique can lead to equivocal, or even erroneous, results [7].

Meanwhile, the efficiency of traditional tests must not be overlooked. For example, it can be seen from the analysis of cases on p. 344 that the 20.3% in which non-paternity was proven, together with the 42% of non-exclusion cases in which paternity was virtually established by conventional methods, would not require DNA tests. Moreover, it is doubtful whether many others in which RCP values are >99% could be subjected usefully to DNA testing.

Thus, the whole field of testing for parentage is at a critical stage. By the time this book is published, it may, perhaps, be known whether or not DNA tests are either partially or fully replacing conventional systems.

REFERENCES

1. Wiener, A.S. (1943) *Blood Groups and Transfusion*, 3rd edn, Thomas, Springfield, p. 380.
2. Jeffreys, A., Wilson, V. and Thein, S. (1985) Individual specific 'fingerprints' of human DNA. *Nature*, **316**, 76.
3. Jeffreys, A., Brookfield, J. and Semeonoff, R. (1985) Positive identification of an immigration test case using human DNA fingerprints. *Nature*, **317**, 818.
4. Recently confirmed in *McV* v. *B* [1987] Times, 28 November.
5. *Whitehall* v. *Whitehall* 1958 SC 252.
6. *Docherty* v. *McGlynn* 1985 SLT 237.
7. Rittner, C., Schacker, U., Rittner, G. and Schneider, P.M. (1989) DNA polymorphism in paternity testing: chances, risks and strategies. *Biotest Bull.*, **4**, 27.

FURTHER READING

Boorman, K.E., Dodd, B.E. and Lincoln, P.J. (1988) *Blood Group Serology*, 6th edn, Churchill Livingstone, Edinburgh.
Dodd, B.E. (1980) When blood is their argument. Presidential Address to the British Academy of Forensic Sciences. *Med. Sci. Law*, **20**, 231.
Gaensslen, R.E. (1983) *Sourcebook in Forensic Serology, Immunology and Biochemistry*, US Department of Justice, Washington, DC.
Nijenhuis, L.E. (1984) The use of haemogenetic markers in paternity studies and in the diagnosis of zygosity of twins, in *Immunohaematology* (eds C.P. Engelfriet, J.J. Van Loghem and A.E.G.K. Von dem Borne), Elsevier, Amsterdam.

Acknowledgements

I am indebted to a number of colleagues in the Department of Haematology at the London Hospital Medical College to whom I offer grateful thanks; Dr P.J. Lincoln has read the text and given me helpful criticism. Mr J. Thompson has carried out the DNA profiles shown in Fig. 22.1 using a DNA probe hMF1 generously provided by Dr D.I. Hoar of the Alberta Children's Hospital, Calgary, Canada. Mr C. Phillips has made the analysis of paternity cases submitted to our Unit.

CHAPTER 23

Medicolegal implications of HIV infection in childhood

Layinka M. Swinburne

The acquired immunodeficiency syndrome (AIDS) was first described in adults in 1981. While at first it was recognized in young male homosexuals and in association with intravenous drug abuse and haemophilia, cases were recognized not long afterwards in infants often in association with mothers who were themselves suffering from the disease [1]. These facts, together with the relationship to transfusion of blood and blood products, were evidence of a transmissible agent which was later identified as a retrovirus now known as Human Immunodeficiency Virus (HIV). The earliest perinatally acquired case in the United States has been traced back to 1977 and the earliest case of transfusion-acquired AIDS in a child dates from 1978 [2].

By December 1985 1% of reported cases in the USA were in children under 13 years of age, of whom 80% were under 3 years of age [3]. There were 584 children meeting the criteria for diagnosis of the Centers for Disease in September 1987 [4]; 78% had a parent with AIDS or were exposed to a recognized risk factor for the condition [5]. The number of cases in the UK at this time was relatively small including 13 children of HIV-positive women, six of whom had died. There are reliable figures from very few other countries but the disease is said to be widespread in certain central African states where heterosexual spread is common and the sex ratio in adults is virtually equal. In consequence, many children have been born with human immunodeficiency virus transmitted *in utero*.

From the beginning, ethical and medicolegal problems have added significantly to the difficulties of management and have complicated the lives of these children no less than those of adults. Further problems are created by attempts to control the spread of infection in different countries as the prevalence of AIDS increases worldwide; concomitantly, there is increasing concern over the preservation of human rights.

Although, to date, few of the legal issues have been tested through the courts, a substantial body of experience is being built up and is likely to be supported by new legislation in the future [6–8].

Because of the mode of transmission and the association with intravenous drug abuse, prostitution and the social problems arising out of the disease itself, AIDS will be increasingly a complicating factor in circumstances of violent and criminal behaviour such as child neglect and sexual abuse; it should be added to the repertoire of paediatricians and forensic scientists involved in these areas.

23.1 DEFINITION

Many children remain asymptomatic following infection with HIV. The duration of this period of latency depends on the age at the time of infection and other factors which have not been fully elucidated, such as the presence of other infections and the nutritional status. The virus enters lymphocytes bearing surface markers of type CD-4 and eventually proliferates within the cells so that, in the later stages, more virus is released which can infect further lymphocytes. The cells are destroyed in the process leading to a loss of their normal function (cellular immunodeficiency) and to the possibilities of repeated opportunistic infections due to other organisms and the development of malignant tumours.

The definitions of AIDS and paediatric AIDS which are most widely applied were devised by the Centers for Disease Control, Atlanta [3]. The definition has been widened to take account of newly recognized manifestations [9] so that there has probably been a considerable degree of underreporting of paediatric cases in the past by comparison with later published statistics. There are also children who, although chronically ill in various ways due to the effects of the virus, do not meet the criteria for AIDS or AIDS-related complex (ARC). AIDS is a clinical diagnosis which, in many countries, can be backed up by laboratory findings, including tests of immune status, for the presence of antibody and, more recently, of viral antigen; diagnosis must, however, often be made entirely on clinical grounds in countries where these refinements are not available.

Infants infected *in utero* or in the perinatal period may present with failure to thrive and diarrhoea. Enlargement of the liver and spleen is common. There is a liability to recurrent bacterial infections and severe candidiasis. Others present with thrombocytopenia at an average age of 10 months [3]. Lymphoid interstitial pneumonitis in a child under 13 years of age is included in the definition of AIDS in children. Of interest to forensic pathologists are the cases of cardiac failure and arrhythmias due to myocarditis associated with HIV infection and which are possibly due to the virus itself [10, 11]. Neurological manifestations include progressive encephalitis with learning difficulties accompanied by changes in behaviour and personality which may lead to incontinence and deterioration in the ability to look after personal hygiene [12]. There are many excellent reviews of the clinical and laboratory findings in the children who present as medical problems [13,14].

The recognition of the stigmata of congenital HIV infection in childhood may be useful in pointing to the presence of the condition when it might otherwise not have been suspected in circumstances such as a sudden death in infancy or whenever there is difficulty in ascertaining the background. Reports of dysmorphism in congenitally infected infants [15,16] include growth failure, microcephaly, a prominent box-like forehead, widening of the palpebral fissures, obliquity of the eyes, a flat nasal bridge and scooped out nose, triangular philtrum, short nose and flattened columella. The original descriptions involved a high proportion of black and hispanic children and, although a later report has confirmed the findings on a wider scale [16], there is a need to verify the presence of these features in infants and children of other ethnic backgrounds with differing cephalometric variations. The changes are said to be distinct from dysmorphism due to fetal alcoholism (see Chapter 3). Screening of some of the children showed the presence of heroin and cocaine residues in cord blood, a clear indication of the aetiological significance of intravenous drug abuse in the mother.

23.2 NOTIFICATION

In many countries there is some form of notification both of HIV infection when detected by a positive antibody test and of confirmed cases of AIDS. A review of the situation in the United States [8] describes both administrative regulations and statutes; some form of reporting exists in all 50 states. In Britain, a voluntary system is in operation for the purposes of surveillance; cases may be reported to the British Paediatric Association, to the Haemophilia Centre Directors' Group and to the Communicable Diseases Surveillance Centre (CDSC). The AIDS (Control) Act 1987 places an obligation on Health Authorities to collect data – including the number of those with positive antibody tests and other details related to prevention, health education and treatment. Doctors are invited to submit details of cases in confidence for statistical purposes but AIDS has not been made a notifiable disease. Under the Public Health (Infectious Diseases) Regulations 1985 (SI 1985/43), however, the Secretary of State has assumed powers to order compulsory medical examination, hospitalization and, if in hospital, of detention there in respect of persons suffering from AIDS (r.2(2)); in addition, such a person may be detained in hospital if he or she would not, otherwise, take proper precautions to prevent the spread of the disease (r.3(2)). In Japan, notification was made compulsory in 1987, and in Bavaria this was combined with other strong measures such as a liability to prosecution for knowingly engaging in activity likely to transmit the virus. There is continued debate on the usefulness of notification as an aid to public health measures and planning; it has been claimed that one undesirable effect might be to drive the disease underground.

23.3 TRANSMISSION

In contrast to the predominantly sexual transmission of the virus in adults, the most important modes of transmission in childhood are:

(1) *From mother to infant.* Viral material has been identified in the placenta and in the thymus of a 20-week infant [17]. Perinatal transmission is possible during parturition and cases have been reported of possible transmission by the breast milk of mothers who were transfused at delivery with HIV-positive blood – previous HIV negativity was not, however, proved [18].

(2) *Through blood or blood products* (platelets, clotting factors, etc). The number of haemophiliac children infected varies from country to country according to the use of imported purified clotting factors VIII and IX. About 200 haemophiliac children are known to have been infected in Great Britain, comprising about 30% of children who are severely affected. Blood transfusion accounts for a high proportion of cases reported in the USA. Haemophiliacs formed 4.3% (15 cases) of 345 paediatric patients with the syndrome which had been reported by August 1986 [5]; by contrast, 47 children in the same series were small infants infected through blood transfusion. Further cases of the latter type will come to light due to the prolonged period during which some people remain asymptomatic. This may be 5 years or more and cases are recorded of a lapse of up to 7 years in a child transfused at birth. Since 1985, blood has been screened for antibodies to HIV and blood products derived from large pools of plasma have, in addition, been heat-treated to eliminate traces of virus. The current risk of acquiring the virus from such screened blood has been put at 1 : 1 000 000.

(3) *Children receiving multiple transfusions for the treatment of haemoglobinopathies* have also been at risk. Surveys of the prevalence in thalassaemic children in Europe showed a wide-ranging incidence of positive antibody tests including 2.7% in Greece, 3.7% in one Italian series and 11% in another [19]. The incidence in similar patients at the New York Hospital–Cornell Medical Center was 17.1% [5]. Interesting contrasts have been reported from the Middle East; whilst no cases were reported from Turkey in a collaborative study, it appeared that blood imported from the United States has brought the infection to Qatar where 10 out of 26 samples tested were found to be positive. Blood products which have *not* been implicated include immunoglobulin preparations, albumin, purified protein fraction (PPF) and hepatitis B vaccine. Hepatitis B immune globulin may result in transiently positive tests for HIV antibody [20].

(4) *Through contaminated needles* in areas where re-use of improperly sterilized needles occurs for economic reasons or poor hygiene – such as in a family where a mother gave a vitamin injection to her uninfected child using the same needle as had been used previously on a sibling with transfusion-acquired HIV infection [21].

Other uncommon but possible sources include the various processes of assisted reproduction:

AID (artificial insemination by donor) A number of sexually transmitted diseases due to organisms such as *Neisseria gonorrhoeae, Chlamydia trachomatis* and the virus of hepatitis B have been transmitted by AID. HIV was transmitted to four women out of eight who shared an infected donation [22]. No pregnancy resulted on that occasion but this is clearly a route by which both the prospective mother and infant can be infected; although the British Voluntary Licensing Authority recommends that all donors be tested for HIV, it is not yet a statutory requirement in Britain or the United States [7].

IVF and GIFT (in vitro fertilization and gamate-intrafallopian transfer) Some agencies insist that both partners should be tested for the presence of antibody prior to any of these procedures. The rationale may be both to protect the operators and also to ensure a healthy child. The routes by which the parents might bring a successful action against the obstetrician in the event of the child being infected congenitally and the difficulties in the way of the infant suing for 'wrongful life' are discussed in Chapter 26 [23, 24, 25].

Surrogate motherhood. One case of HIV infection in a surrogate mother is recorded [26]. Testing for HIV antibodies was not deemed necessary prior to the procedure but, after successful insemination using her brother-in-law's semen and 5 months into the pregnancy, the mother admitted that she had previously been an intravenous drug abuser. She was tested and found to be HIV antibody positive. The prospective parents were not told at that stage and the child was found to have antibodies at birth. Neither the donor parents nor the surrogate mother would accept the child. It was too soon at the time the case was reported to assess whether the child was truly infected – passive transfer of maternal antibodies makes it difficult to confirm the fact of transplacental infection until several months after birth.

In all these situations, the mother, semen or ovum donor or the prospective parents should, at least, undergo testing and, depending on the result, should decide whether to go ahead or to abandon the procedure rather in parallel to the choices to be considered in genetic counselling (see Chapter 2). There is a suspicion of an increased rate of fetal abnormality after some of the *in vitro* procedures [27] and it is not clear where the liability would lie after such an occurrence.

The risk that the fetus may be infected by HIV is one which some women deliberately choose to take, even though they have been advised that the chance of producing an infected infant is of the order of 30–50% [28, 29]. The prognosis for the infant is poor – 60% of those with the infection die within the first year. Nor is the effect of pregnancy on the health of the infected woman completely evaluated. Those who have already progressed to a state of immunosuppression may develop opportunistic infections and those who already have AIDS may worsen. More precise studies of antibody levels, antigen and immune status may make it possible to assess the prognosis for these women more accurately in the future, but difficulty will be encountered in assessing the role of other factors such as alcoholism or drug abuse.

These features have been accepted as sufficient grounds for a legal abortion in both the United Kingdom and United States. Such a choice is not universally available and ever-increasing numbers of infected infants are being born. Moreover, in a recent survey [30] of 602 Brooklyn women screened for HIV during pregnancy, only 58% of those who were found to be antibody positive were initially identified as belonging to high-risk groups; the birth of an infected child will increasingly occur unexpectedly and will not be detected until symptoms in the child – or developing later in the mother – or other circumstances provoke investigation.

Bites. Workers caring for children are often concerned about the possible transmission by means of bites. Bites most commonly occur in young children – perhaps as a result of physical abuse, in mentally subnormal people of all ages or in the course of an epileptic fit. So far, transmission has only been reported in one case in which two sisters had a fight – one of them being an intravenous drug abuser and HIV positive. The infected sister had a tooth knocked out and then bit her previously uninfected sister who was found to be sero-converted [31]. Another case in which the infection was possibly transferred by the bite of an infected sibling has been recorded [32]. No seroconversion occurred in another case in which a counter-assistant was bitten by a patient in the course of a fit [33]. One would expect the risk to be very low except when, as in the first case, there is a clear chance of infected blood being introduced into the wound.

Organ and bone marrow transplantation. Cases of transfer of infection by organ transplantation are on record, including infection with HIV. It is clearly the responsibility of the organizers to ensure that the organ donor, whether alive or dead, is free from significant infection. Time factors dictate that, at the present time, reliance must be placed on antibody tests, although, in all situations, including blood transfusion, there is awareness of the so-called 'window' period during which an infected person may be carrying the virus yet may not have developed detectable antibodies. This period varies from a few weeks to many months, which, unfortunately, means that none of the tests currently in general use can guarantee 100% detection of an infected source.

Child sexual abuse. Awareness of sexual abuse (Chapter 15) of children has passed through several cycles of urgency and is currently of worldwide concern. Recognition of a sexually transmitted disease may bring cases to light and the published incidence is disturbing. In series related to the investigation of sexual abuse, the incidence was 11% in the USA and 1% in a similar series in the UK [34]. The infections included gonorrhoea, syphilis, venereal warts and, more recently,

HIV. Both boys and girls are at risk and a few cases have already been reported in the press – one in Australia and three or four in the United States [35, 36] – where children have seroconverted as a result of sexual abuse. According to Hobbs and Wynne, children who are being investigated now ask: 'Will I get AIDS from this?' [37].

Although the exact mechanism of transmission of the virus is not known, there is general agreement that any form of sexual activity which involves trauma – including breach of the mucosal surfaces of the rectum and vagina, of the skin of the perineum or perianal tears or local inflammation from other sexually transmitted infections – is especially likely to favour transmission and such conditions are certainly likely to be found in severe cases of child sexual abuse (see Chapter 15).

Adolescent sexual activity and involvement with intravenous drug abuse and needle-sharing are obvious sources of infection paralleling similar high-risk activities of adults. Special concern arises in cases of mental subnormality when the problem of educating the children and controlling their sexual activities is even greater than in normal adolescents. Teenage prostitution constitutes a serious source of risk in some inner-city areas of the United States.

A proportion of infected children remains for whom no source can be found. Many of these can be reclassified when more persistent investigation brings to light factors previously unknown or not admitted by the parents. There is no foundation for the popular belief that HIV infection can be transmitted by bed-bugs, mosquitoes or other insects.

23.4 FOSTERING AND ADOPTION

In New York, there are numbers of HIV-infected children occupying acute hospital beds for as long as 2 years, unwanted by their families where these exist [38] (cf. Chapter 3).

In other cases, the mother may be ill or have died of AIDS or be incapable of looking after the child because of her own problems of drug abuse. Placing of such children is obviously not easy, but the size and the philanthropic nature of the United States allows the great majority to be absorbed into the community.

A pilot scheme for the care of HIV-infected children has been successful in Scotland [39]. In the series reported, seven out of 33 children who were born HIV positive were in foster care and these included children of drug abusers who were either in prison or who were otherwise incapable of looking after their children. All prospective foster parents were instructed about AIDS, emphasis being placed on the lack of risk of casual transmission of the infection in a household setting other than to sexual partners. Suitable foster-parents emerged who were able to cope with the effects of having an HIV-positive child in their own families; support was provided in preparation for the high probability of illness and eventual death of the child. In the United States, the Centers for Disease Control have made specific recommendations for the education and foster care of children infected with the virus along similar lines [40].

With regard to fostering and adoption in general, it is not recommended that there should be indiscriminate testing of the children in question in areas of low prevalence of HIV infection and where no specific risk factors have been identified [41]. However, it is justifiable to test a child for the virus if the natural mother or father are known to be in a high-risk group. In Scotland, there is a legal obligation to pass on any relevant background information to the prospective foster-parents; there is no such obligation in England where it is a matter for discretion. Where it is necessary, or thought desirable, to pass on the child's status, the prospective parents should be counselled in the light of the result and given a choice – particularly in view of the possible social repercussions in the neighbourhood and the prospects for deterioration of the child's health and possibility of its eventual death.

As to adoption in particular, the requirements of the Adoption Agencies Regulations 1983 (S.I. 1983/1964) include the provision of a medical record of particulars of the parents and the child; the adopters have a right of access to the child's health history, including information on the mother's antibody status provided she agrees to its being passed on for the benefit of the child. In general, prospective adopters should be warned that the babies of some parents are at high risk for a number of diseases but they should not expect specific testing for HIV [41].

23.5 CONFIDENTIALITY

Because of prevailing attitudes it is often decided to keep the HIV status of a child as a confidential matter. The aim is to inform as few people as possible, confining these, say, to the child's doctors and the parents or persons immediately responsible for care. The policy is regularly challenged by various agencies such as school authorities, teachers, or other parents who feel that they have a right to know and to make their own decisions in the light of their knowledge of the disease as to whether the affected child should be allowed to associate with others. Unfortunately, this 'knowledge' is often based on sensational reports in the media and on perpetuated myths and beliefs as to the mode of transmission. The inability of the expert to say with certainty and scientific truth that there is absolutely no risk in certain hypothetical situations means that statements concerning, say, the presence of virus in saliva are often re-interpreted as meaning that there may be some risk; the public then makes the reasonable deduction that the only way to deal with the infection involves some form of isolation.

At one stage, infected persons were advised to tell their ordinary medical practitioners, dentists and other health workers of their antibody status but this sometimes led to a refusal to treat. To obviate this – and the need to set up special precautions in schools and other institutions – the alternative now preferred by the Centers for Disease Control is one of 'universal blood and body fluid precautions' – defined as the routine use of appropriate barrier precautions to prevent skin and mucous membrane exposure when contact with blood or other body fluids of any patient is anticipated [42]. This avoids the need to identify a particular individual and dependence on tests, voluntary declarations or identity cards, except when these are directly necessary for the management of a clinical problem.

As far as possible, confidentiality should be preserved in the case of children to the same degree as it is in adults, although there may be special situations – as in suspected child abuse – where a conflict may arise between the duty to the child and to the parents.

23.6 CONSENT TO TESTING

Testing for the presence of antibodies to human immunodeficiency virus has aroused strong feelings and the recommendation is that, as far as possible, it should only be done with the informed consent of the person being tested. In the case of young children, this implies that consent must be given by the parents or, if they are not available or suitable, by the child's legal guardian or the authority responsible for his or her care. Some legislatures, however, regard the public interest as overriding parental consent. In Rhode Island, for example, state legislation empowers the Director of the State Department of Health to authorize testing of a newborn baby without written permission if there is a high index of suspicion that the child may have contracted the infection [7].

Parents will usually be asked to give consent if the child is under the age of 16 but there seems no reason why the *Gillick* principles [43] should not apply – a child may also be able to consent given a suitable explanation and adequate understanding. In any event, children who are old enough and of sufficient maturity to understand what is happening should be given an explanation of the significance of the test and should be told of the result. Explanations must, however, always be tailored to the degree of knowledge of the child. One 18-year-old boy, who had learned no biology at school, went to give his first donation of blood. As a sample of blood was being taken, he asked if it was to be tested for AIDS and he was told that it would be. He later read the words 'Group O Rh(D) POSITIVE' on his new donor record and spent several weeks in secret misery thinking that it signified that he had AIDS!

Special difficulties arise in cases where the parents have given consent for testing but are unwilling for the child to be given the results; yet the doctor may well feel that it is highly desirable for a boy to be aware of his status in order to protect potential sexual partners [44]. The lay press spotted discussion on this dilemma in a medical journal and followed it with banner headlines 'Our kids have AIDS and don't know it'. As a result one father bluntly told his son that he was HIV antibody positive and then, unable to bear the strain within the family, left the home.

(a) Clinical trials and vaccines

More than 80 drugs and 25 vaccines against AIDS are being tested by the pharmaceutical industry in the United States alone. Many have been approved for clinical trials by the Food and Drugs Administration [45]. Special trials will be needed for those that eventually receive a product licence in order to establish toxicity, effectiveness and suitable dose regimens for children. It is considered ethical for children to participate in trials with the informed consent of parents or guardians when to do so is in the best interests of the child and the potential benefits outweigh the risks (see Chapter 30). Vaccines are being devised with the aim not only of protecting people at risk from acquiring the HIV infection but also of boosting immunity against HIV and prolonging the survival of those already infected.

Some studies in adults have been hampered by the open or surreptitious use of other drugs. There has also been difficulty in recruiting volunteers in sufficient numbers for 'Phase 1' trials on vaccines because they inevitably render the subjects seropositive. The National Institutes of Health have tried to avert the risk of stigmatization and future discrimination by the provision of certificates explaining the circumstances. Such concerns may encourage manufacturers to turn to Third World countries and other risk groups; the World Health Organization has set up a vaccine committee to monitor these activities and prevent exploitation.

23.7 COMPENSATION

A number of legal actions have been instituted in the United States following transmission of HIV infection through blood or blood products. Actions have been brought against doctors, blood banks and commercial plasma fractionating companies [7]. At one time there were estimated to be 90 actions pending against blood banks and blood-product manufacturers.

None of these actions are likely to succeed in countries where commercially prepared clotting factors have been the source of the infection because the viral nature of the disease had not been discovered at the time when most people were infected. The defence has been based on the 'state of the art', i.e. the level of scientific knowledge which prevailed at the time, a defence which is specifically established in the British Consumer Protection Act 1987, s.4(e). It has also been established that the provision of blood and blood products is a service; the products are not drugs and, therefore, the manufacturers cannot be proven to be liable under product liability theory [24]. To be successful, actions in tort would have to prove negligence on the part of the plasma processors or the doctors. Such actions have also been based on a failure to warn the infected person of the risks of transmission or a third party exposed to risk [7]. Another possibility would be to prove the negligent use of unsterilized equipment. Attempts to find the name of individual donors who gave donations of blood later shown to be infective have been rejected, as it has been held that the confidentiality of donors should be protected.

In September 1987, after prolonged representations followed by a brief but determined campaign by the Haemophilia Society, the British government agreed to hand over a sum of £10 000 000 to set up a fund for the relief of hardship and provision of support to the 1200 British haemophiliacs with HIV infection. While this cannot be considered to be compensation in legal terms, and was described as an ex gratia payment, it is a recognition of the fact that some patients were infected entirely inadvertently as a result of essential treatment. Patients who were infected by transfusion of other blood products were not included but it may, nevertheless, have established a precedent. Some 250 of these haemophiliacs were children of school age and below at the time of initial testing in 1984–85.

Children infected by blood and blood products other than purified clotting factors form a much larger proportion of the population of the United States than is the case in the United Kingdom. The prognosis for these children is better than is that for those congenitally infected *in utero*, and in at least one instance there was an interval of 8 years from the time of transfusion in the neonatal period to the onset of symptoms. This means that a number of such cases will remain undetected. Testing of donated blood was introduced in the United Kingdom in October 1985 and in most of the United States and in many other countries at varying times in 1985–86.

23.8 SCHOOLING

In Britain, the Department of Education and Science has issued guidance on 'Children at School and Problems Related to AIDS', stating that:

> since there is no apparent risk on all present evidence of transmitting HTLV/LAV in the school setting and since the benefits for an infected child attending school and enjoying normal social relationships far outweigh the risk of a child with AIDS acquiring harmful infections, infected children should be allowed to attend school freely and be treated in the same way as other pupils.

The Centers for Disease Control stated in their guidance that children with the human immunodeficiency virus, whether asymptomatic or with AIDS or lesser manifestations of the infection, should generally be allowed to attend school in an unrestricted setting [42]. They considered several legal issues, including:

> civil rights aspects of school attendance, the protection for handicapped children under 20 USC 1401 et seq and 29 USC 794, the confidentiality of a student's school record and employee right-to-know statutes for public employees in some states.

Automatic exclusion from school would contravene civil rights but there are some reservations in the case of habitual biters and children who are too young to have complete control of bodily functions. They suggest that such children should not be placed in an unrestricted setting; each case should, however, be assessed on its own merits.

In spite of this, there have been many attempts to exclude children from school, although studies show that the risk of catching AIDS from casual or household contact is negligible [46–48].

Legal actions have been brought by parents to enjoin children diagnosed as having AIDS from attending school in Indiana, New York and New Jersey [7, 48]. The courts have generally held that the child should be permitted to attend school unless such attendance was contrary to medical advice.

In both Britain and the United States, parents of children attending a school where it was known that there was an infected child have reacted by withdrawing their own children until their anxieties might be allayed. Such situations have so far been resolved in Britain by discussions between parents and staff and explanation by experts without recourse to legal action. There have been cases where heavy pressure from the media has stirred up local fear and prejudice even to the point of forcing a family to move house.

23.9 AIDS AND THE FORENSIC LABORATORY

There should be no great risk of acquiring this infection through autopsies or laboratory work provided that normal hygienic precautions are observed. There are no recorded instances of workers in the post-mortem room or forensic laboratory having picked up the infection through their work. There are a few instances on record in which health-care workers have acquired the infection through gross contamination of damaged skin or through accidental injection of a measurable amount of blood. In spite of this reassuring state of affairs, care should always be taken to avoid contamination of skin, especially where it is broken. Precautions should include the use of masks and eye protection if there is a risk of splashing and all specimens of body fluids,

including blood, should be handled with the same care whether they are thought to be infected or not. The recommendations are that the necropsies should be carried out by experienced pathologists and staff wearing masks and eye protection as well as the usual waterproof protective apron and gloves [49].

Exhibits stained with blood or other body fluids needed for production in courts as evidence are now generally sealed in plastic covers so that they cannot be handled directly.

The question is frequently posed: 'How long does the virus take to die?', but there is no clear answer. The virus needs living T lymphocytes to survive and replicate but it can be preserved in some materials for days or weeks and in the freeze-dried state (e.g. in blood products) for years. It is safer to assume that tissue and body fluids remain infective unless they are deliberately heated or otherwise inactivated, even though it is difficult to imagine circumstances in which infection could be transmitted from or by material such as blood stains. To some extent, these precautions may be overzealous, as was the magistrate who cleared the court before hearing a case involving a defendant with HIV infection.

23.10 TESTS FOR HUMAN IMMUNODEFICIENCY VIRUS

A large number of commercial test-kits are available for the diagnosis of infection which are based on detection of antibodies to the various protein components of the virus. Although the tests are increasing in refinement, confirmation should be left to specialized virological laboratories. Full confirmation requires typical ELISA tests of known sensitivity and backed up by Western Blot to identify antibodies – especially those to envelope protein gp120 and core protein p24.

Difficulties in interpretation arise particularly in the case of small infants. Antibodies may be found in cord blood but these may result from passive transfer of maternal IgG antibody through the placenta. Such antibodies may persist for many months – even for as long as 15 months – so that this type of test cannot be relied upon for diagnosis in young children. The virus may sometimes be cultured from lymphocytes and it may be possible to distinguish those infants with latent infection from those with passively transferred antibodies when the more recently developed tests for viral antigens become available generally. The polymerase chain reaction has still to be evaluated in this situation. There is also a quantitative difference in the amounts of antibody of the four IgG subgroups produced. Maternal antibody and adult antibody is predominantly of subclass IgG1 and IgG2, whereas infants show rising amounts of class IgG3 [50].

Sufficient time must be allowed for antibodies to develop before a negative result can be accepted as conclusive when a test is done after possible exposure to the virus – for example, in a case of child sexual abuse. At the beginning, it may be more appropriate to test the perpetrator. When initial tests on the child are negative but there is a serious risk of infection, further tests should be carried out after a few months and repeated at similar intervals for up to a year. The chances of a child being infected in this way are small and there is, as yet, no indication for automatic testing unless the perpetrator is known or suspected to have been particularly at risk.

Studies of cohorts of adults exposed to infection indicate that viral antigens may be demonstrated during the early phases of the infection at a time when the antibody levels are still below the level of detection. These tests have not yet been applied generally for transfusion work or diagnosis and there is debate as to the ideal and most practicable application of current techniques. Antigen tests become negative as the antibody level rises but antigen may again become detectable

in the later stages of the disease when production of antibody to the core protein p24 fails along with the general attrition of immune function. Tests may be carried out on blood or plasma. Tests on other body fluids and immunohistochemical methods which may be used on tissues remain research procedure at present. The amount of virus in infected plasma can be reduced by heating at 60 °C or higher or by the addition of beta-propiolactone before the material is subjected to biochemical or haematological procedures.

23.11 DISPOSAL OF THE DEAD

The bodies of infected children should be disposed of in accordance with the guidance on cases of other transmissible infections such as hepatitis B [49]. In general, embalming is to be avoided because of the necessity to maintain body fluid precautions and the procedure in Britain is to seal the body in a plastic bag before burial or cremation. The undertakers need no more information than that the case is one of suspected or known transmissible infection. It is a requirement in some of the United States that written notification accompany the body to inform funeral directors of the illness for the purpose of observing precautions [88]. A number of legal actions have been brought in California where funeral homes have refused to offer full services such as embalming for fear of AIDS [7].

23.12 REFERRAL TO THE MEDICOLEGAL AUTHORITY

Theoretically, all deaths due to infection transmitted through blood or blood products come under the jurisdiction of the coroner in England and Wales or of the procurator fiscal in Scotland. However, as most cases have been investigated before death as to the source of the infection, there is little to be gained by further enquiries. Several cases have been the subject of a coroner's inquest with jury or of a public inquiry under the Fatal Accidents and Sudden Deaths Inquiry (Scotland) Act 1976.

23.13 CONCLUSION

Many of the special problems that arise in relation to human immunodeficiency virus and AIDS are a result of fear which has been only slightly allayed by public education. Indeed, there was a sharp increase in public anxiety after some of the campaigns and children with the infection have suffered the backlash of general ignorance and prejudice. These attitudes should not be allowed to cloud scientific judgement. A balanced and informed approach must be based on appreciation of the main facts of the disease and its mode of transmission – not on its political implications.

REFERENCES

1. Rubinstein, M.D. (1983) Acquired immuno-deficiency syndrome in infants. *Am. J. Dis. Child.*, **137**, 825.
2. Centers for Disease Control (1987) Human immunodeficiency virus infection in transfusion recipients and their family members. *Morbid. Mortal. Week. Rep.*, **36**, (10).
3. Rogers, M.A., Thomas, P.A., Starcher, E.T. *et al.* (1987) Acquired immunodeficiency syndrome in children: report of the Centers for Disease Control National Surveillance, 1982 to 1985. *Pediatrics*, **79**, 1008.
4. Osterholm, M.T. and MacDonald, K.L. (1987) Facing the complex issues of pediatric AIDS: a public health perspective. *JAMA*, **258**, 2736.
5. Hilgartner, M. (1987) AIDS in the transfused patient. *Am. J. Dis. Child.*, **141**, 194.
6. Kirby, M.D. (1986) AIDS legislation – turning up the heat? *J. Med. Ethics*, **12**, 187.
7. Matthews, G.W. and Neslund, V.S. (1987) The initial impact of AIDS on public health law in the United States – 1986. *JAMA*, **257**, 344.
8. Gostin, O.L. (1989) Public health strategies for confronting AIDS – Legislative and regulatory policy in the United States. *JAMA*, **261**, 1621.
9. Centers for Disease Control (1987) Classification system for human immunodeficiency virus (HIV) infection in children under 13 years of age. *Morbid. Mortal. Week. Rep.*, **36**, 225.
10. Stenherz, L.J., Brochstein, J.A. and Robins, J. (1986) Cardiac involvement in congenital acquired immunodeficiency syndrome. *Am. J. Dis. Child.*, **140**, 1241.
11. Issenberg, H., Charyatan, M. and Rubinstein, A. (1985) Cardiac involvement in children with acquired immunodeficiency syndrome. *Am. Heart J.*, **110**, 710.
12. Belman, A.L., Ultmann, M.H., Horoupian, D., Novick, B., Spiro, A.J., Rubinstein, A., Kurtzberg, D. and Cone-Wesson, B. (1985) Neurological complications in infants and children with acquired immune deficiency syndrome. *Ann. Neurol.*, **13**, 560.
13. Jones, P. and Watson, J.G. (1986) AIDS, in *Recent Advances in Paediatrics* (ed. R. Meadow), Churchill Livingstone, Edinburgh.
14. Falloon, J., Eddy, J., Wiener, L. and Pizzo, P.A. (1989) Human immunodeficiency virus infection in children. *J. Pediatr.*, **106**, 332.
15. Marion, R.W., Wiznia, A.A., Hutcheon, G. and Rubinstein, A. (1987) Fetal AIDS syndrome score. *Am. J. Dis. Child.*, **141**, 429.
16. Iosub, S., Bamji, M., Stone, R.K. *et al.* (1987) More on human immunodeficiency syndrome embryopathy. *Pediatrics*, **80**, 512.
17. Lapointe, N., Michaud, J. *et al.* (1985) Transplacental transmission of HTLV-III virus. *New Engl. J. Med.*, **312**, 1325.
18. Lepage, P., van de Perre, P., Caraël, M. *et al.* (1987) Postnatal transmission of HIV from mother to child. *Lancet*, **ii**, 400.
19. Lefrere, J.J. and Girot, R. (1987) HIV infection in polytransfused thalassaemic patients. *Lancet*, **ii**, 686.
20. Schlech, W.F., Lee, S.H.S., Cook, J. *et al.* (1989) Passive transfer of HIV antibody by hepatitis B immune globulin. *JAMA*, **261**, 411.
21. Koenig, R.E., Gautier, T. and Levy, J.A. (1986) Unusual intrafamilial transmission of human immunodeficiency virus. *Lancet*, **ii**, 627.
22. Stewart, G.J., Tyler, J.P.P., Cunningham, A.L. *et al.* (1985) Transmission of human T-cell

lymphotropic virus type III by artificial insemination by donor. *Lancet*, **ii**, 581.

23. Brahams, D. (1987) Human immunodeficiency virus and the law. *Lancet*, **ii**, 227.

24. Brahams, D. (1987) AIDS and the law. *New Law J.*, **137**, 749.

25. Mason, J.K. and McCall Smith, R.A. (1987) *Law and Medical Ethics*, 2nd edn, Butterworths, London, p. 96 *et seq.*

26. Frederick, W.R., Delapenha, R., Gray, G., Greaves, W.I. and Saxinger, C. (1987) HIV testing of surrogate mothers. *New Engl. J. Med.*, **317**, 1351.

27. Lancaster, P.A. (1987) Congenital malformations after *in-vitro* fertilisation. *Lancet*, **ii**, 1392.

28. Minkoff, H.L. (1987) Care of pregnant women infected with human immunodeficiency virus. *JAMA*, **258**, 2714.

29. Plotkin, S.A. and Evans, H.E. (1988) Perinatal human immunodeficiency virus infection. *Pediatrics*, **82**, 1941.

30. Landesman, S. Minkoff, H.L., Holman, S. *et al.* (1987) Serosurvey of human immunodeficiency virus infection in parturients. *JAMA*, **258**, 2701.

31. Anonymous (1987) Transmission of HIV by human bite. *Lancet*, **ii**, 522.

32. Wahn, V., Kramer, H.K., Voit, T. *et al.* (1986) Horizontal transmission of HIV infection between siblings. *Lancet*, **ii**, 694.

33. Drummond, J.A. (1986) Seronegative 18 months after being bitten by a patient with AIDS. *JAMA*, **256**, 2342.

34. Cain, A.R.R., Osborne, J.P. and Rudd, P.T. (1987) Investigation of sexual abuse. *Lancet*, **ii**, 1218.

35. Leiderman, I.Z. (1986) A child with HIV infection. *JAMA*, **256**, 3094.

36. Berkowitz, C.D. (1986) Sexual abuse of children and adolescents. *Adv. Pediatr.*, **34**, 294.

37. Hobbs, C.J. and Wynne, J.M. (1987) Management of sexual abuse. *Arch. Dis. Child.*, **62**, 1182.

38. Toynbee, P. (1987) The AIDS babies. *The Guardian*, 3 December.

39. Covell, R.G. (1987) HIV infection and adoption in Scotland. *Scott. Med. J.*, **32**, 117. For an interesting journalistic review, see Picardie, J. and Wade, D. (1988) The youngest victims. *The Sunday Times*, 31 January, p. C5.

40. Centers for Disease Control (1985) Education and fostercare of children infected with human lymphocytropic virus type III/lymphadeno-pathy associated virus. *Morbid. Mortal. Week. Rep.*, **34**, 517.

41. White, R. (1987) AIDS: some legal implications for children, in *The Implication of AIDS for Adoption and Fostering*, British Agencies for Adoption and Fostering, London.

42. Centers for Disease Control (1987) Recommendations for prevention of HIV transmission in health-care settings. *Morbid. Mortal. Week. Rep.*, Suppl. 2S.

43. *Gillick* v. *West Norfolk and Wisbech Area Health Authority* [1986] AC 112.

44. Evans, D.I.K. (1987) Human immunodeficiency virus and the law. *Lancet*, **ii**, 574.

45. Cooper, R.M. (1987) AIDS vaccines: liability concerns. *Am. Soc. Microbiol. News*, **53**, 484.

46. Church, J.A. Allen, J.R. and Stiehm, E.R. (1986) New scarlet letter(s), pediatric AIDS. *Pediatrics*, **77**, 423.

47. Rubinstein, A. (1986) Schooling for children with acquired immunodeficiency syndrome. *J. Pediatr.*, **109**, 242.

48. Hilgartner, M.W. (1987) AIDS and hemophilia. *New Engl. J. Med.*, **317**, 1153.

49. Advisory Committee on Dangerous Pathogens (1986) LAV/HTLVIII – The Causative Agent of AIDS and Related Conditions – Revised Guidelines. DHSS, London.

50. Pyun, H.K., Ochs, H.D., Dufford, M.T.W. and Wedgwood, R.J. (1987) Perinatal infection with human immunodeficiency virus. *New Engl. J. Med.*, **317**, 611.

Legal aspects

CHAPTER 24

Legal implications of modern reproductive techniques

J.K. Mason

It is generally stated, albeit with little factual backing, that some 10% of married couples who desire children are unable to have a family by reason of infertility – the underlying cause, whether it be physiological or pathological, being present approximately twice as commonly in the wife as it is in the husband [1]. The longing for children is often intense, and very considerable medical expertise is devoted to the investigation and treatment of the condition. Despite this, no abnormality is discovered in either wife or husband in some 20% of infertile couples.

By and large, the medical or surgical treatment of infertility is a matter between doctor and patient alone. In view of the fact that treatment is directed not only to the well-being of the individual but also to that of the family as a whole, it *may* be good medical practice to involve the normally fertile spouse but there is no law to support an assumption that it is essential to do so. Any adult patient is entitled to confidentiality (the position of minors is discussed in Chapter 28) and, while the courts offer little enough protection against breach of medical confidence [2], the General Medical Council certainly does so; whether or not to treat infertility in strict confidence is a matter for the doctor's own

conscience – he may accept the conditions or refer the patient to another practitioner as he thinks best. Treatment with human gonadotrophins, synthetic antioestrogens and antiprolactins and the like may, however, represent a different situation insofar as an excess of multiple pregnancies may result from successful treatments. It would seem to be only right to involve the husband, whose lifestyle and economic status is likely to be altered greatly, in such circumstances.

There is, moreover, a possible legal problem as to the management of a multiple pregnancy in that the question of selective abortion – or selective reduction of pregnancy – may be raised [3]. In fact, it seems very unlikely that the practice would be regarded as being unlawful. The Abortion Act 1967, s.1(i)(a) enables an abortion to be carried out if the continuance of the pregnancy would involve risk of injury to the physical or mental health of the pregnant woman or any existing children of her family greater than if the pregnancy were terminated. Thus, there could be every reason to invoke the statute in the unlikely event of there being an existing child in the family and, in the absence of such a child, it would not be stretching definition too far to regard an existing fetus as an existing child of the family; moreover, account may be taken of the woman's reasonably foreseeable environment – which would certainly be affected by the arrival of quadruplets. A difficulty can be envisaged in the wording 'continuance or termination of a pregnancy' – it could be argued that the terms relate to the state of pregnancy and not to the presence of a particular fetus; it is, however, difficult to see the law being applied with that degree of pedantry, provided, always, that the operation was performed in good faith. It is also hard to see any ethical objection beyond the quite tenable moral rejection of abortion as a whole; there can be no possible advantage in bringing quintuplets or more to premature term in the near certainty that they will all die amid increasing anguish and wastage of resources when fewer, healthy babies would have resulted from selective reduction of their numbers.

We are, here, concerned, however, not so much with the treatment of infertility as with the treatment of childlessness. It can be argued that there is no right to parenthood [4] and, if that is so, the 'treatment' of childlessness is something of a contradiction in terms; the alternative and, I think, more acceptable view is to compare the process with the 'treatment' of myopia by the provision of spectacles [5]. There can be an ethical objection to reproductive technology only if it is believed that *all* interference with nature is improper – a tenet which would abnegate all operative surgery and which must attract minimal support – or if it considered that sexuality and reproduction constitute a distinct aspect of human physiology with a particular dimension in medical ethics, which would seem to be the position of the Roman Catholic Church [6]. Methods for combatting childlessness are in use everywhere and cannot be intrinsically illegal. The modern techniques do, however, introduce many complications into established family law – and, to a much lesser extent, into the criminal

law – and it is these which this chapter is designed to consider.

24.1 THE REGULATION OF REPRODUCTION TECHNOLOGY

Most advanced countries, and states and provinces within those countries, have set up commissions to look into the legal and ethical issues deriving from the development of human reproductive technology. Unanimity has been a prominent feature of their reports and it is not proposed to deal with each in detail here: Knoppers [7] has presented the details very succinctly. The fundamental and recurring theme has been a recommendation to set up some form of controlling body which will oversee and, if necessary, impose sanctions on medical and scientific activities in the field. Occasionally, notably in Australia, this has now been enacted by statute [8] but, in general, any control of artificial reproduction is, currently, maintained on a relatively unofficial basis.

The United Kingdom response to what has undoubtedly been serious public concern has been expressed through the Warnock Committee [9] which firmly recommended the establishment of a statutory licensing authority to regulate both research and the various types of infertility service which are becoming available. Governments are, however, slow to act and, pending legislation, the Medical Research Council and the Royal College of Obstetricians and Gynaecologists have taken the lead in establishing a Voluntary Licensing Authority (VLA). This body has no executive authority but peer review is a powerful regulator and its recommendations are accepted widely. The VLA has two major functions – to approve a code of practice on research related to human fertilization and embryology and to invite all centres, clinicians and scientists who are engaged in research on *in vitro* fertilization to submit their work for approval and licensing.

At the time of writing, the only United Kingdom legislation attributable to Warnock is the Surrogacy Arrangements Act 1986 (discussed below on p. 377); a wide-ranging consultation paper relating to proposed legislation has, however, been circulated and has been followed by a statement of government intentions (hereafter referred to as the White Paper) [10]. This is an area in which statutory definition of good medical practice is especially difficult. Nevertheless, there is an urgent need for clarification of the way in which the purely legal problems introduced by methods of artificial reproduction are to be solved; perhaps it is even more important that legislation should be coherent and comprehensive – the current piecemeal approach is very unsatisfactory.

24.2 THE INFERTILE HUSBAND

Intrafamilial infertility by reason of male incapacity can be alleviated by artificial insemination. There is nothing new in the technique – it has been practised openly for decades – and it is simple. Indeed, any legislation in the field has to recognize that the process can be carried through in private. There are two main variations – artificial insemination with the semen of the husband (AIH) and artificial insemination with the semen of a donor (AID). The semen of both the husband and a donor are mixed before inoculation in a third variant. This is no more than an attempt at self-deception on the part of the couple – and one which is scarcely justifiable now that non-paternity can be determined so readily (see Chapter 22).

(a) AIH

The circumstances in which AIH might be required are relatively few. Impotence in either partner is probably the least uncommon but it may be a valuable tool when there is antagonism between vagina and sperm; the use of washed and treated sperm may circumvent the condition. A resultant child is indistinguishable from one conceived naturally within the family. Thus, there are no direct legal difficulties involved and ethical problems are minimal; it is unlikely that the process *per se* would ever need to be submitted to public control. AIH has, however, two somewhat unusual side-effects of legal importance.

The first relates to the effect of successful AIH on a petition for a declaration of nullity on the grounds of incapacity to consummate. Consummation of marriage is a matter of adequate vaginal penetration by the male penis; there can, therefore, be no suggestion that artificial impregnation can affect that particular issue. On the other hand, the courts would almost certainly regard submission to AIH as approbation of the marriage; a decree has been refused on these grounds in Scotland [11] and it is very likely that the reasoning would be followed generally.

The more complex situation is that in which a wife wishes to be inseminated after her husband's death with his semen that has been cryopreserved against that eventuality – married couples in the armed forces might well wish to be so self-insured. Certainly, there is no legal bar to a woman having a child be any means or by any man – and this would apply if the man were dead. The legal consequences of a claim by the child to paternity would, however, be very serious in the fields of inheritance and succession; moreover, it is at least doubtful if the deliberate production of a fatherless child is desirable [12]. Posthumous AIH is amenable to control insofar as it involves a technical expertise. There would seem to be an urgent need for a declaration by statute to the effect that insemination by a husband's sperm undertaken when the woman had no cause to believe that her husband was still alive should be treated as if it were an insemination of a single woman by a donor (see below).

(b) AID

Artificial insemination by donor (Fig. 24.1) has been practised for many years and there can be no suggestion that the process is illegal *per se*. The main difficulties, aside from any natural antipathies to masturbation and clinical insemination with the seed of a stranger, have involved the legitimacy of the resultant child and, as a corollary, the parental rights and responsibilities of the donor. These problems were first addressed in the United States and, within the British Commonwealth, in Australia [13]. The general effect of legislation has been to ensure that a child born by consensual AID is to be regarded in law as being the child of that couple and that the person who produced the semen is presumed not to be the father of the child; Australian legislation goes so far as to accept a *bona fide* arrangement as to marriage in the absence of a legal ceremony and has also taken advantage in the various statutes to include ovum donation (see below p. 374) within similar terms.

The English law has recently been similarly brought into line with the undoubted flow of public opinion although, strangely, at the time of writing, there are no comparable provisions in Scotland. The Family Law Reform Act 1987, s.27, now states:

> Where ... a child is born in England and Wales as the result of artificial insemination of a woman who –
> a) was at the time of the insemination party to a marriage ...; and
> b) was artificially inseminated with the semen of some person other than the other party to that marriage, then, unless it is proved ... that the other party to that marriage did not consent to the insemination, the child shall be treated in law as the child of the parties to that marriage and shall not be treated as the child of any person other than the parties to that marriage.

It is to be noted that ovum donation is not included and that the provisions relate only to consensual donations within the bounds of a lawful marriage. Clearly, an AID child born out of wedlock will be illegitimate; while this now carries minimal disadvantages for a child, the donor might, in such circumstances, still be liable for paternal support of the child – which is a powerful argument in favour of anonymity of semen donors and an indication of the difficulties which may be encountered in the artificial insemination of single women (see below p. 371). The new law obviously offends those who seek the purity of truth – the husband of the inseminated woman is *not* the genetic father of the child and to equate social parenthood with genetic parenthood without further qualification is to erect and approve a manifest fiction; nonetheless, regulation of a situation which was open to wide abuse – in particular, in respect of the common false declarations made at the registration of an AID birth – must, on balance, be acceptable on pragmatic grounds.

Consent of the husband is presumed unless proof is adduced to the contrary in any court where the matter is determined. Thus, although the law is now clear so far as it goes, non-consensual AID could still be a legal minefield. The husband would stand in the same position towards the child as any husband who can disprove paternity of this

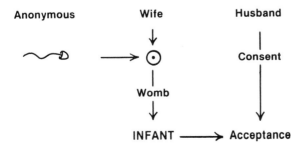

Fig. 24.1 Artificial insemination by donor.

wife's infant. He would not be able to petition for divorce on the grounds of adultery as this requires an act of sexual intercourse [14]; by contrast, a petition grounded in intolerable conduct would certainly be open to him. These considerations alone provide adequate reason for a doctor to refuse AID in the absence of a signed consent by a husband [15].

No case has yet decided the doctor's liability in negligence for the production of, say, a genetically defective or otherwise abnormal infant. Many practitioners attempt a primary screening for this possibility by recruiting donors from those who have been shown in the maternity ward to produce normal offspring. Donors must obviously be vetted for manifest genetic abnormality and should be chosen with a view to ethnic and physical compatibility with the future social father; there is, however, no law on the subject and the normal rules of medical negligence would apply in the event of an unsatisfactory outcome. Under the terms of the Congenital Disabilities (Civil Liability) Act 1976 [16], any right of action would seem to vest only in the mother; it would, it is thought, be impossible to bring an action for 'wrongful life' on the part of the child (see Chapter 26). The uncontrolled and repetitive use of donors also raises the possibility of incestuous matings by half-siblings in later generations; although the chances of that happening, and the likelihood of ill-effects, are slight, there is no doubt that donations should be limited – an arbitrary figure of 10 has been suggested [17].

Thus, despite the recent relaxation in the family law, there remain very good reasons for controlling AID and the Warnock Committee (at para. 4.16) recommended that arrangements for artificial insemination by donor should be subject to the central licensing authority and that its practice outside that control should be an offence; the White Paper indicates that this will be government policy. No limits of availability were laid down in the report but it was considered that, so far as was possible, it was desirable for children to be born into two-parent families (at para. 2.11). It is clear, however, that it is very difficult to criminalize an action which, in theory, requires minimal expertise and which can be accomplished easily in private; while, therefore, it would seem right to incorporate the Warnock Committee's recommendation into statute, it is hard to see that anyone, other than a medical practitioner or other third party, would ever be prosecuted under its terms.

Certain problems of identity still remain. It seems appropriate from every angle that the donor should be anonymous in relation to the social family and this remains true despite the fact that the 1987 Act firmly relieves him of any responsibility. Nevertheless, it is clear from the foregoing that some records must be kept and Warnock has recommended that the child of an AID birth should be entitled to obtain information as to the general nature of his genetic father on reaching the age of 18 years (at para. 4.21). The government intend to follow this recommendation and to leave the door open to an extended form of access. Although this follows the lines of Australian legislation [18] it seems to this author to be unnecessary – an infinitessimal number of children of a united family will doubt their paternity and it is better left that way.

Payment for donation beyond reasonable expenses is already prohibited in the pioneer legislation in New South Wales and, while not going to that extent, Warnock (at para. 4.27) recommended that direct payments should be phased out; the British public is, in general, antipathetic to the sale of human biological materials and it is to be hoped that this will be acknowledged in any future legislation – it is very unlikely that the supply of altruistic donors would be inadequate for therapeutic purposes. The most likely source of pure generosity – fraternal donation – should, however, be strongly discouraged, even if the arm of the criminal law cannot penetrate the privacy of the family; first-cousin marriages are legal in the United Kingdom – insemination by a brother-in-law thus opens the door to involuntary incest in a later generation.

24.3 THE INFERTILE WIFE

Treatment of childlessness by reason of infertility in a woman is, by contrast, generally a matter of great professional expertise and complexity. The necessary procedures are, therefore, amenable to regulation and it is this which, in fact, made up the greater part of the Warnock Committee's report.

The fundamental defect may be treatable by 'infertility drugs' as mentioned on p. 367 above. Such ovulatory therapy is as much a matter between patient and doctor as is any involving the prescription of a medicinal drug. Thus, there are no legal complications other than the largely ethical problems associated with multiple births – which have already been noted and which will be reverted to later.

In other cases, infertility may be due to unresponsive failure to ovulate – including dysgenesis or destruction of the ovaries by disease – or to inability to implant as a result of either tubal inadequacy (15% of all cases of involuntary infertility) or of uterine incapacity. The former group may be alleviated by ovum (female gamete) donation which is, both genetically and legally, the female equivalent of AID; a case complicated by infertility in the husband can be approached via double gamete (or embryo) donation (Fig. 24.2). Tubal insufficiency can, however, be treated without the need for donation as gametes from both parties to the marriage can be made available. Occasionally, multiple abnormalities are present – for example, tubal pathology associated with abdominal disease; the significance of such cases is that ova, although produced, cannot

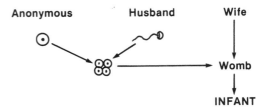

Fig. 24.2 Ovum donation. The husband's semen may be replaced by that of an anonymous donor in embryo donation.

be harvested and the treatment becomes that of anovulatory infertility. Finally, female infertility of certain types – notably those involving uterine defects – can be alleviated by surrogate motherhood; this, alone of the treatments for female infertility, requires no special knowledge or skill and is discussed separately.

(a) *In vitro* fertilization

Strictly speaking, *in vitro* fertilization (IVF) refers only to a technical process – fertilization of an ovum by sperm outside the body – which is common to many of the modern artificial reproductive methods; similarly, embryo transfer (ET) means no more than the movement of an embryo from one place to another. The earliest, simplest and morally least objectionable method introduced was that of harvesting ova from the abdomen of a woman, exposing them to the husband's spermatozoa in the laboratory and implanting the resulting embryo in the wife's womb. Since this is the preferred treatment for childlessness due to tubal obstruction which is not correctable, it is also the commonest technique in use; it has, thus, become accepted practice to refer to this process as a whole as IVF (Fig. 24.3). The method also includes embryo transfer and, here again, the term ET has become synonymous in popular usage with transfer of an embryo from the

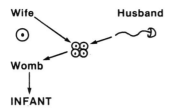

Fig. 24.3 *In vitro* fertilization.

culture medium to the uterus. A more sophisticated variant of the technique is known as gamete intrafallopian transfer in which the fertilization procedure is fabricated within the fallopian tube. Clearly, this method is unavailable in cases of tubal disease and it will be noted that it uses the process of *in vivo* artificial fertilization which is, in some ways, less unnatural than is standard IVF. More specifically, GIFT does not involve embryo transfer. This is of some medicolegal importance as ET dictates manipulation of a developing organism; the possibility of induced developmental abnormality, which could be negligent in origin, is thus raised although, to be fair, there is no convincing evidence that the occurrence of such defects is any higher in babies born as a result of procedures involving ET than that in neonates conceived naturally.

It is clear that there are no problems in family law related to IVF – the process is comparable in every way with successful AIH. Moreover, since the use of frozen ova is, at present, medically unacceptable [19], the possibility of womb-leasing (see below) after death does not arise. The legal complications derive, rather, from that essential element of the technique which involves the production of excess embryos both *in vitro* and *in vivo*.

The latter problem arises by virtue of the fact that the success of IVF is, to an extent, proportional to the number of embryos introduced to the uterus. The legal and ethical difficulties raised by multiple implantations are similar to those discussed above in respect of the use of 'fertility drugs' [20]. The United Kingdom Voluntary Licensing Authority has recommended that no more than three embryos should be introduced [21]; it is the resultant conflict between a general policy and the needs of the individual patient which has provoked the only withdrawal of a licence at the time of writing. The disposal of the excess of embryos produced *in vitro* might, however, have legal implications which would depend entirely on the status conferred on the human embryo by the law. It is not proposed to raise the associated moral problems here, save to note that it is one's attitude to the moral status of the human embryo *in vitro*, which may range from attributing it the status of a full human being to that of a laboratory artefact [22], which dictates acceptance or denial of the morality of the whole IVF programme. Looked at legally, however, it is difficult to see what offence can be committed by the routine disposal of embryos which are surplus to therapeutic requirements. The practice cannot be murder because the embryo *in vitro* could never be regarded as a 'reasonable creature in being'; it cannot be producing a miscarriage because no woman is involved; currently, feticide is not a recognizable criminal offence, and the death of a fetus does not have to be registered. The problem is, therefore, of a purely ethical dimension. It is, however, relatively certain that the introduction of an offence of embryocide – as proposed, for example, in the Unborn Children (Protection) Bill 1985 – would bring *in vitro* treatment of childlessness to a halt; there are suggestions, which are denied by the legislators, that this is already the case in Australia [8, 23]. There is no doubt that some legislation in this area is needed, if only to allay the current wave of public anxiety. All the same, it is difficult to see the logic of this disturbance when the same public is apparently unconcerned that some 170 000 abortions are performed annually in the United Kingdom. As the

Warnock Committee admitted by way of a footnote (at p. 64):

> ... [I]t seems to us totally illogical to propose stringent legislative controls on the use of very early human embryos for research, while there is a less formal mechanism governing the research use of whole live embryos and foetuses of more advanced gestation.

The fact that this referred expressly to research does not stop the same sentiments being applicable to the unwanted and unborn.

[b] Anovular infertility

Infertility deriving from a deficiency of ova can be countered by means of ovum or embryo donation, which differ only in that the husband's spermatozoa are used in the former while those of an unknown donor are required for the latter procedure; both, however, involve the *procedures* of *in vitro* fertilization and embryo transfer. This treatment clearly raises an entirely novel facet of family law – that is, the question of maternity and its legal connotations.

Ovum donation has been distinguished above as the female equivalent of AID but, while this is generally so, the two processes are not necessarily of equal legal importance. We live in a patrilineal society within which, rightly or wrongly, the contribution of the female gamete to parenthood is regarded as being of less importance than is that of the male. The same problems exist as they do in AID but they are less urgent; spousal consent to ovum donation may be desirable but is of a less essential character than applies in AID. The nature of the donor's consent is also slightly different. It is possible that a close friend or relative might wish to donate ova specifically to a named individual, in which case, a very special 'informed consent' may be needed for a procedure which is tedious and invasive and which may have very

considerable psychological repurcussions; the Victoria legislation [8], indeed, requires counselling before all 'fertilization procedures' and it will also be included in United Kingdom policy. The majority of donations will, however, be made anonymously and unemotionally during another treatment; consent is clearly essential – and removal of ova and their use in its absence would certainly be actionable – but it is of a quality different from that required, on the one hand, for a specific operation for donation and, on the other, from the relatively simple *provision* of spermatozoa, consent to the use of which must, in practice, be implied.

There remains only the question of legal motherhood. It is very nearly inconceivable that any adolescent would seek to challenge the identity of his or her mother given a normal family environment; similarly, it is hard to imagine a woman who has carried a child and given birth to it wishing to deny her maternity. For these reasons, it is suggested that there is even less reason in the case of ovum donation to attribute a right to disclosure of artificial conception to the child on reaching maturity than there is in the case of semen donation – openness was recommended by Warnock in both circumstances (paras 4.21 and 6.6). It is, however, desirable that the matter should be decided in law and the adoption of the rule *'mater est quam gestatio demonstrat'* has been suggested [24]; it is, perhaps, worth explaining that this is a personal proposal – the suggested rule does *not*, at least at present, form part of the common law of Scotland as has been implied in some recent writings. It does seem regrettable that the Family Law Reform Act 1987 did not sieze the nettle as has been done in Australia; nonetheless, the White Paper (at para. 89) indicates that it is clearly government policy to apply the same principles as to parentage in the case of ovum or embryo donation as now relates to artificial insemination. It scarcely needs emphasizing that embryo donation, as defined above, provokes questions related not only to maternity but also to paternity as in AID; the position of the genetic father in embryo donation is, thus, now covered in the 1987 Act but that of the mother is not.

(c) Embryo donation

In what must seem to be the unlikely event of a wife being anovular and her husband being infertile – but which, statistically, could exist in some 20% of infertile marriages – the modern reproductive techniques still allow a form of alleviation through the donation of both male and female gametes. These will usually be caused to form an *in vitro* zygote which is, in turn, inserted into the wife's uterus; an alternative method involves fertilization of the ovum within the genital tract of the ovum donor – this process, known as uterine lavage, is so distinct as to be discussed separately below. It will be seen that there is no genetic association between the social parents and the child in either case; the main advantage which embryo donation offers over, say, adoption is the physiological and psychological maternal bonding which accompanies gestation, labour and infant care. Embryo donation is, thus, not easy to justify either in the context of familial ethics or within the framework of the use of scarce resources; nevertheless, it raises no new legal problems *per se* – those that exist have already been covered individually under AID and ovum donation.

Embryos can, however, be preserved in the cold without apparent deterioration. It is convenient to discuss the legal consequences of cryopreservation under the heading of embryo donation, although this is not the only circumstance in which it might be employed. A couple might, for example, wish to preserve their own embryo against the possibility of death or disease in one or other or, more commonly, a woman undergoing *in vitro* fertilization might wish to preserve any excess embryos produced in order to avoid a second episode of enforced superovulation and harvesting; she might even wish them to be preserved as possible donations to other needy couples. In any event, the legal question of ownership is raised together with its associated rights of disposal. In the absence of any definitive law on the point, it is assumed that any such rights should be confined to the couple in whose interest the embryo was formed. Such quasi-property rights must develop despite the fact that the Warnock Committee recommended, rather hopefully, that legislation should be drawn up so as to deny any property rights in the stored embryo (at para. 10.11). Thus far, there is not even a transAtlantic case on which to build a precedent, the only United States case having been decided before the successful use of a stored embryo could be regarded as a practical probability [25]. Currently the government intends to allow storage of gametes and embryos but to vest the right of their disposal entirely in the donors – which seems to be a very questionable policy.

Irrespective of ownership, the embryo itself might claim inheritance rights by reason either of its genetic or social status. Again, this proposition has not been tested but the potential severity of its repercussions has been demonstrated in Australia where the disposal of stored AID-produced embryos following the death of their 'parents' resulted in a legal and moral storm [26]. The White Paper is unclear as to what would be the future position in similar circumstances in the United Kingdom but is biased in favour of donor direction (at para. 60); a firmer view would be that all stored embryos should be destroyed when the marriage of the 'parents' breaks up – for whatever reason. It has been pointed out that the chaos and uncertainty which would result from the absence of some such direction would be intolerable [27].

Uterine lavage, or *in vivo* embryo donation, involves the impregnation of a 'donor' either anonymously or with the spermatozoa of the intending social father, 'flushing out' the resulting zygote and implanting this in the infertile womb. The Warnock Committee (at para. 7.5) recommended that this method of artificial reproduction should not be used on the grounds of the potential dangers to the donor; others would see it as being so close to the farmyard as to be unacceptable in human practice. Most importantly, in the present context, the practice may be illegal. Whether or not this is so depends upon the definition of procuring a miscarriage. If it be accepted that a woman who holds an unimplanted zygote within her womb is pregnant, the uterine lavage contravenes the Abortion Act 1967, first, on the grounds that it is impossible to certify the fact of pregnancy and, secondly, that there are no exisitng statutory grounds for terminating the potential pregnancy. The present author, while disapproving of uterine lavage on the ethical grounds above, is on record as believing that there can be no miscarriage without carriage and that implantation is an essential prerequisite to the latter [28]. If this be so – and the question still remains open, at least at academic level – there is no reason to suppose that uterine lavage is practised contrary to the Offences Against the Person Act 1861, although it will be seen that the possibility of attempted procurement remains open. However, what is apparent is that *in vivo* embryo donation embodies an element of surrogate motherhood and should be considered in that light when legislation is drafted.

24.4 SURROGATE MOTHERHOOD AND WOMB LEASING

We are left with a consideration of the circumstances in which it might be acceptable for a woman who is incapable of producing ova to utilize not only the ova of another

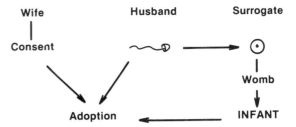

Fig. 24.4 Surrogate motherhood.

woman but also her uterus. The scenario is (Fig. 24.4) that the surrogate is inseminated by a man and carries and gives birth to a baby which is then transferred to the care of its genetic father and his wife. This variant of reproduction and parentage requires no expertise and, certainly, is not to be regarded as a modern technique – there can be few who are unaware of the seemingly 'liberal' behaviour of Abraham, Sarai and Hagar [29]. This does not apply, however, to the extension of surrogate motherhood in which the surrogate carries the fetus resulting from the *in vitro* fertilization of the ovum of the intended or social mother by the semen of her husband. The Warnock Committee made no distinction between the two processes; it is preferred, here, to refer to the latter – and to distinguish it – as womb-leasing (Fig. 24.5) for, clearly, the strict legal status of the infant differs in the two conditions.

There are, in addition, moral distinctions to be made. Both processes may, properly, be accepted as potential treatments for

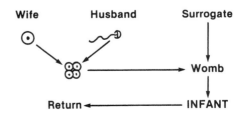

Fig. 24.5 Womb leasing.

childlessness of relatively rare type. Womb-leasing, however, is obviously open to abuse in that it might be employed for purely social reasons – for example, to avert interference with a career; this extension is so parallel to Victorian wet-nursing as to be unacceptable to the majority. A case could, therefore, be made for prohibiting womb-leasing absolutely – and the prohibition could be enforced insofar as the process needs professional involvement. It could, however, be said that womb-leasing has the advantage over surrogate motherhood that the resultant child is wholly the genetic offspring of its intended parents and that this is to its better interest, but it is doubtful if such an end is justified by the means.

This conservative attitude has recently been supported by the announcement that a woman agreed to – and succeeded in – womb-leasing on behalf of her daughter [30]. The difficulty imposed thereby is that, granted the acceptance of the *mater est quam gestatio demonstrat* doctrine, some ludicrous combinations can evolve, e.g. in this particular example, of a woman adopting her legal sister who is, in fact, her genetic child. If this case does nothing else, it should point to the importance of making any form of surrogacy illegal in the direct descendant or ascendant line. The remainder of this section will be confined to surrogacy as it is, not only, commonly understood but, also, as it can be practised without professional help.

The Warnock Committee, despite a dissenting minority [31], recommended that it should be a criminal offence to operate either profit or non-profit making organizations whose purposes include the recruitment of women for surrogate pregnancy or making arrangements for individuals or couples who wish to utilize the services of a carrying mother (at para. 8.18). It is a mark of the emotion which surrounds this particular means of alleviating childlessness that this is the only aspect of the Warnock Report which has led to legislation at the time of writing.

The essence of the Surrogacy Arrangements Act 1985 is that it makes it a criminal offence to interpolate a commercial agency between the infertile couple and the surrogate mother; in accord with the minority view in Warnock, it is positively stated that, in so acting, none of the principals are guilty of an offence (s. 2(2)). It is, of course, a reasonable argument from the feminist viewpoint that a woman should be allowed to dispose of her body as she wishes. To that extent, therefore, the legislation is paternalistic in that it is concerned, first, for the welfare of the resulting infant and, secondly, to protect the vulnerable woman who could be persuaded into surrogacy to her detriment. To which it could be answered that the 'surrogate child' is in a markedly better position than is one who is adopted in the ordinary sense of the word and that there are many other ways in which a woman in need can be exploited without being afforded the protection of statute. More importantly, it would seem that the conditions of the Act, in prohibiting any payment at any time in respect of the arrangement (s.2(3)), excludes assistance from, say, solicitors and doctors [32]. Thus, the only surrogacy arrangements which are currently legal in the United Kingdom are those which are undertaken in a wholly amateurish and uncounselled ambience; this provides the worst of two worlds and, to that extent, the Surrogacy Arrangements (Amendment) Bill 1986, which proposed also criminalizing the actions of the principals, appeared to provide the more consistent view.

There is now good evidence that the British courts are also torn between a conflict of ideals but are, nevertheless, prepared to accept some of the better aspects of surrogacy.

The case of *In re a Baby* [33] was concerned primarily with wardship (see Chapter 29). In that situation, the court was in a position to consider the welfare of the infant as paramount. Accordingly, it was found that, a surrogacy arrangement having been entered into and followed through, no-one else was better equipped to care for the child than the commissioning couple; wardship of the infant was continued but care and control was demitted to its genetic father and his wife on their undertaking to return the baby to the jurisdiction of the court should it so order – and leave was given to take the infant out with the court's jurisdiction.

By contrast, in *Re an adoption application (surrogacy)* [34], the court was able to consider the crucial relationship between surrogacy and adoption, this being because the arrangement has been made on a purely personal basis without benefit of professional advice – it was not until some 2.5 years after the event that the 'parents' realized that adoption was not obviously open to them on the grounds that 'payment or reward' had, arguably, been made to the surrogate mother. The court concluded that, since the payment consisted of no more than recompense for loss of income and amenities, there had been no element of profit or financial reward; moreover, the court had authority to authorize such recompense or reward if it saw fit [35]. As a result, an adoption order was made.

There was harmony between the parties in the above two cases; *P* v. *B* [36], however, illustrates an instance in which the surrogate, having received a donation from her twins' father, refused to hand them over to him and his wife at birth. The twins were placed within the wardship of the court and the disposal of the case then became a matter of custody of the children. In this instance, the judge was concerned with the bonding which had been shown to exist between the children and their natural mother who had 'exercised a satisfactory degree of maternal care'. Custody was, therefore, granted to the surrogate.

The features linking these decisions would seem to be, firstly, that the welfare of the children in being is the overriding factor and

that the courts are prepared to take a liberal view of the existing law in seeking this end; secondly, none of the courts sought to criticize any of the parties to surrogate motherhood. True, the problems of contractual arrangements have not been met head-on; but, granted the absence of any intrinsic impediment to adoption – as evidenced in *Re an adoption* – it seems unlikely that they will wish to do so. The probability is that, in the event of a dispute the rights of a well-intentioned and willing gestational mother will always take precedence over those of a commissioning couple; the sincere motivation of the latter is, however, likely to be appreciated in the absence of conflict as to custody.

This is not to say that legislation is not desirable, because the precise relationship between surrogacy and adoption should be clarified if the former is to be recognized at all. The present writer is on record as believing that surrogate motherhood is an acceptable 'treatment' within the strict confines of certified medical need [37]; there seems no reason why this particular form of artificial reproduction should not be placed under the aegis of any authority that is established to oversee the whole field.

This is not to deny that the minutiae of any surrogate arrangement are bound to be complex – and it is largely for this reason that the White Paper envisages a 'wait and see' policy before any further legislation is contemplated. One particular legal issue is that surrounding the surrogate's right to abortion – a problem which is rather easier to resolve in the context of the medical requirements under the British Abortion Act 1967 than in the United States where the privacy rights of a woman are determinant. Thus, in the remarkable case of *In re Baby M* [38], a clause in the contract which purported to transfer the mother's right to abortion to the genetic father was virtually the only part of the agreement which was declared to be void and unenforceable. The *Baby M* litigation is interesting in that, alone of the comparable decisions which have been taken in the United States, this one was based in the court of first instance on hard, unemotional legal grounds. The case concerned a surrogate who wished to retain her baby after having signed a contract to surrender it to its father – and having received $10 000 for so doing. The court, perhaps a trifle abruptly, dismissed any problems of adoption on the grounds that the State's adoption Acts were drafted before surrogacy was considered as a legal issue and confined itself to contractual considerations and to its powers and duties as *parens patriae*. As to the former, the court concluded that a contract once made was fixed and firm and, as to the second, that it was clearly in the child's interest to be adopted by her father and his wife – a value judgement which was based largely on economics; an order was made that the child be adopted.

The most trenchant words to come from *Baby M* were:

> Melissa needs an end to litigation, she needs to have her parentage fixed, she needs protection from anyone who would threaten her – protection from manipulation and a strong support system to protect her privacy ... Melissa needs stability and peace, so that she can be nurtured in a loving environment free from chaos and sheltered from the public eye.

However much one might agree with such sentiments, the principles of equity must be observed and it is not surprising that the decision in *Baby M* was overturned on appeal to the Supreme Court of New Jersey [39] with the unsatisfactory result that custody rights were given to the genetic father and visiting rights to the natural mother. Perhaps in the end, the major value of legislation would be to remove human reproductive techniques from the adversarial atmosphere of the courts and from the glare of publicity.

REFERENCES

1. Hull, M.G.R., Joyce, D.N. and Turner, G. (1986) *Obstetrics and Gynaecology*, 2nd edn, Wright, Guildford.
2. Mason, J.K. and McCall Smith, R.A. (1987) *Law and Medical Ethics*, 2nd edn., Butterworths, London, p. 136 *et seq*.
3. Craft, I. (1987) When a code catches out the childless. *The Times*, 24 September, p. 16.
4. Mitchell, G.D. (1983) *In vitro* fertilisation: the major issues – a comment. *J. Med. Ethics*, **9**, 196.
5. Singer, P. (1983) Response [to ref. 4 above]. *J. Med. Ethics.*, **9**, 198.
6. Leading Article (1987) Values from the Vatican. *The Times*, 11 March, p. 13.
7. Knoppers, B.M. (1987) Reproductive technology and international mechanisms of protection of the human person. *McGill Law J.*, **32**, 336.
8. Infertility (Medical Procedures) Act 1984, s. 29 (Victoria).
9. Report of the Committee of Inquiry into Human Fertilization and Embryology (M. Warnock, Chairman), Cmnd. 9314 (1984) HMSO, London.
10. Department of Health and Social Security, *Legislation on Human Infertility Services and Embryo Research: A Consultation Paper*, Cm 46 (1986) HMSO, London; Department of Heath and Social Security, *Human Fertilization and Embryology: A Framework for Legislation*, Cm 259 (1987) HMSO, London.
11. *G* v. *G*. 1961 SLT Reps 324.
12. Cusine, D.J. (1977) Artificial insemination with the husband's semen after the husband's death. *J. Med. Ethics.*, **3**, 163.
13. See, for example Status of Children (Amendment) Act 1984 (Victoria); Artificial Conception Act 1984 (NSW): Artificial Conception Act 1985 (WA).
14. *MacLennan* v. *MacLennan (or Shortland)* 1958 SC 105.
15. Royal College of Obstetricians and Gynaecologists (1979) *Artificial Insemination*, March 1979.
16. See also *McKay* v. *The Essex Area Health Authority* [1982] QB 1166.
17. Warnock, ref. 9 at para 4.26.

18. Infertility (Medical Procedures) Act 1984, s. 20 (Victoria).
19. Trounson, A. (1986) Preservation of human eggs and embryos. *Fertil. Steril.*, **46**, 1.
20. Phillips, M. (1984) A testing time. *BMA News Rev.*, **10**,(6), 29.
21. Second Report of the Voluntary Licensing Authority (1987) Annex 1, p. 35.
22. Iglesias, T. (1984) *In vitro* fertilisation: the major issues. *J. Med. Ethics,* **10**, 32; Mason and McCall Smith, ref. 2, p. 49.
23. Trounson, A. (1986) Reported in *Institute of Medical Ethics Bulletin*, no. 19, October, p. 14.
24. Mason and McCall Smith, ref. 2, p. 57.
25. *Del Zio* v. *Manhattan's Columbia Presbyterian Medical Center* 74 Civ 3588 (SD, NY, 1976), discussed by Terry, N.P. (1986) 'Alas! poor Yorick', I knew him *ex utero*: the regulation of embryo and fetal experimentation and disposal in England and the United States. *Vanderbilt Law Rev.,* **39**, 419.
26. Smith, G.P. (1985–86) Australia's frozen 'orphan' embryos: a medical, legal and ethical dilemma. *J. Family Law,* **24**, 27.
27. Brown, H., Dent, M., Dyer, L.M., *et al.* (1986) Legal rights and issues surrounding conception, pregnancy, and birth. *Vanderbilt Law Rev.,* **39**, 597.
28. Mason, J.K. (1989) Abortion and the law, in *Legal Issues in Reproduction* (ed. S.A.M. McLean), Gower, Aldershot.
29. *Genesis* 16:2.
30. Kennedy, R. (1987) Early triplets for first surrogate grandmother. *The Times*, 2 October, p. 9.
31. Expression of Dissent A: Surrogacy, p. 87.
32. Sloman, S. (1985) Surrogacy Arrangements Act 1985. *New Law J.,* **135**, 978.
33. 1985 *The Times*, 15 January. Sub nom *Re C (A minor)* [1985] 2 FLR 846.
34. [1987] 2 All ER 826.
35. Adoption Act 1976, s.7(3).
36. Unreported. See (1987) *The Times*, 13 March, p. 1
37. Mason, J.K. and McCall Smith, R.A. (1987) *Law and Medical Ethics*, 2nd edn, Butterworths, London, pp. 56–57.
38. 525 A 2d 1128 (NJ, 1987).
39. 537 A 2d 1227 (NJ, 1988).

CHAPTER 25

Comparative abortion law; the living abortus

Bartha M. Knoppers

Recent surveys indicate a trend towards the liberalization of abortion legislation in industrialized countries. The motivation behind this movement has been said to include the need to reduce the mortality and morbidity associated with illegal abortion; the provision of access to abortion for those who are economically deprived; and the urge to secure the right of all women to decide on pregnancy and motherhood [1]. Such legislation is, however, usually accompanied by procedural and administrative conditions which effectively limit the actual practice and availability of abortion. At the same time, access to abortion is becoming increasingly restricted during the later stages of pregnancy. According to Leenen [1], this can be 'seen as a balancing of the rights of the woman against the protection of the fetus'. Indeed, postviability protection of the fetus *in utero* only cedes to the overriding right of the woman to treatment where her life is in danger – a right which would be implicit through the general principles of the criminal law even in those countries which permit of no explicit exceptions to the illegality of abortion [2]. Moreover, most countries provide for abortion in the event that there is a serious risk of fetal malformation or abnormality, thus taking into account the interests of the fetus at any stage of development.

While the child once born has the enjoyment of rights vested *in utero*, the sphere of legal protection of the unborn is gradually moving from live birth to the later stages of fetal development *in utero*. This protection derives not only from advances of technology which make possible earlier survival outside the womb, but also from increasingly available scientific knowledge as to the fetal condition [3]. Hence, it is important to understand the legal indications for abortion as they relate to fetal stages of development and, particularly, the legal restrictions on abortion or protections – if there be any – with regard to the living abortus.

COMPARATIVE ABORTION LAW: PROSCRIPTION AND PRACTICE

Even though our examination covers only a few common law (England, Canada, United States) and civil law jurisdictions (France, Belgium), they are indicative of the range of abortion laws. A study of the legislative grounds for abortion, and of the associated procedural criteria, reveals a limited recognition of maternal freedoms and concern for maternal health which, at the same time, serves to protect the fetus indirectly.

25.1 GROUNDS: THE BOUNDS OF RESTRICTION

In the countries under study, the range of legal grounds for abortion vary from restrictive (life), through limitative (life and health), juridical and fetal indications and, finally, to abortion upon request subject to certain conditions.

(a) Life

The 1867 Penal Code of Belgium reflects textually the 1810 French Penal Code in prohibiting abortion. This provision of the 1867 Code is still in force [4]. Numerous bills to reform the law have failed to receive legislative approval. In spite of this prohibition, therapeutic abortions continue to be part of actual medical practice despite the fact that criminal prosecution of illegal abortions was reinstated recently. In 1983, a Belgian court found certain physicians guilty of practising illegal abortions but, nonetheless, acquitted them since the total impunity with which they performed the operations as well as their belief in good faith that reform was imminent, was considered sufficient to ground a defence. In 1985, however, an appeal court condemned a physician for practising illegal abortion and reiterated that necessity – that is, saving the life of a pregnant woman in imminent peril – was the only valid defence [5], and this remains the current state of Belgium law. This increased vigilance over illegal abortions has led to what has been called 'abortion tourism' as Belgian women seek abortions in other more liberal European countries [1]. Such migration is a common result of a restrictive approach to abortion – abortions are totally

prohibited in Eire but Tietze [1] has noted that, when the number of abortions obtained by Irish women travelling to England is considered, the abortion rate among residents of Eire is as high as that of the Netherlands which has, perhaps, the most liberal law in Western Europe.

(b) Limitative

Until 1988, abortion in Canada was penalized under art. 251 of the Criminal Code except where certain conditions were met. The only legal indication was that the continuation of the pregnancy would be likely to endanger the life or health of the women (s.251(4)(c)). This therapeutic indication provided for broad medical discretion and interpretation and resulted in an uneven application of the law [6,7]. No explicit mention was made of the gestational age of the fetus nor of a permissible upper limit.

Most provinces, however, define stillbirths in their vital statistics legislation as the expulsion or extraction of a product of conception showing no signs of life after the 20th week of gestation, while Quebec uses fetal weight (over 500 grams) as the criterion for stillbirth registration. These baselines have spilled over into the abortion domain and, as reflected in a 1976 Canadian study, most abortions for therapeutic indications were performed prior to 20 weeks [6]. Recently, the application of Canada's Criminal Code restriction on abortion was successfully challenged before the Supreme Court of Canada as being a violation of the right to security and liberty of the woman under the Canadian Charter of Rights and Freedoms [8] while, in a contrary case, abortion was challenged under the same article of the Charter as a violation of the unborn child's constitutional right to life [9]. At present, therefore, there is no abortion law in Canada although the federal Minister of Justice has promised new legislation.

(c) Juridical and fetal indications

The jurisdictions under study make no explicit mention of rape or incest as indications for abortion, generally treating them as being included within the permitted therapeutic criteria. Obviously France, which has a 10-week period of abortion upon request based solely on the subjective 'distress' of the pregnant woman [10], would include such indications as would Britain under the broad health indication of the Abortion Act 1967, s.1(1)(a). Access to abortion in the United States is, as is discussed later, largely governed by case law; incest and rape have been designated as causes of pregnancy for which abortion is available through federal funds [11]. Canadian statistics on the actual practice of abortion [6, 7] point to a similar interpretation, even though both juridical and fetal criteria were expressly excluded from the abortion provisions [12].

The risk or presence of congenital or other fetal malformations or abnormalities as indications for abortion are specifically provided for in the British and French abortion legislation. The failure to mention disorders by name would, seemingly, allow for abortion in the case of HIV carriers or AIDS-affected pregnant women (see Chapter 23). Availability is qualified, however, not according to gestational age but according to the risk of occurrence and to the gravity of the handicap itself – the British Act speaks in terms of a *substantial* risk that if the child were born it would suffer from such physical or mental abnormalities as to be *seriously* handicapped while the Code de la Santé Publique has it: '… il existe une *forte probabilité* que l'enfant à naître soit atteint d'une affection d'une *particulière gravité* reconnue comme incurable au moment du diagnostic'. Thus, if these two criteria are met, the French legislation on its face would permit such abortion at any time during a pregnancy. This would not necessarily apply in England,

however, where, although the unsuccessful Infant Life (Preservation) Bill 1987 sought to alter the position, the gestational age limitation imposed by the Infant Life (Preservation) Act 1929, discussed below, is not demitted in the case of fetal abnormality. A difficulty then arises because the use of amniocentesis for the prenatal diagnosis of genetic defects dictates a delay of some 20 weeks before the indications for abortion can be properly assessed (see Chapter 2 for full discussion); this complication lay at the heart of the debate surrounding the similarly unsuccessful Abortion (Amendment) Bill 1987 which was presented to the parliament of the United Kingdom. The fetal indication for abortion is, in most jurisdictions, subsumed within an extended interpretation of the mother's health – the strict interpretation of the British Abortion Act 1967, s.1(1)(b) being that it is the strain on the mother in caring for a handicapped child rather than the child's quality of life which justifies termination [13].

(d) Request (with limited conditions)

The French legislation, in force since 1975 and renewed in 1979, permits an abortion within the first 10 weeks of gestation – under certain medical and administrative conditions – where the woman finds that her pregnancy places her in a situation of distress, the duration of pregnancy being measured as the time since conception which, in turn, is regarded as being 2 weeks less than that of the last menstrual period – a method of counting which differs from that of most countries. Similarly, in Great Britain, termination of the pregnancy is authorized if two medical practitioners agree that its continuation involves a risk to life or injury to the physical or mental health of the woman or to any existing children of her family where such risk is greater than if the pregnancy were terminated. Of greater significance, is the fact that in assessing prospective injury to health, account may also be taken 'of the pregnant woman's actual or reasonably forseeable environment'. While the legislation itself would permit abortions in later gestation, private abortion clinics and the National Health Service have since 1985 voluntarily limited abortions to 24 weeks' gestation. Furthermore, the Infant Life (Preservation) Act 1929 is expressly preserved by the Abortion Act 1967. The 1929 Act makes it a criminal offence intentionally to destroy the life of a child capable of being born alive by any wilful act which causes the child to die before it has an existence independant of its mother. The Act also carries the presumption that a fetus of 28 weeks' gestation is capable of being born alive; thus, 28 weeks becomes the current *legal* limit on abortion in England.

In the United States abortion upon request has been a constitutional right, in at least the first trimester of a pregnancy, since the landmark case of *Roe* v. *Wade* in 1973 [14]. The Supreme Court in that decision held that a right of personal privacy was founded in the Fourteenth Amendment's concept of personal liberty; that right of personal liberty was broad enough to encompass a woman's decision whether or not to terminate her pregnancy. Governmental regulation of a woman's right to choose remains constitutionally permissible in order to further 'compelling' state interests but, according to the court, no compelling state interest exists in the first trimester. Subsequent cases held that the exercise of this freedom did not, however, include mandatory provisions of state funding, nor prevent other state regulation in the second trimester, or state prohibition in the final trimester [15]. Furthermore, the court in *Roe* indicated that state prohibition of abortion in the third trimester – subject, always, to the overriding interests of the preservation of the mother's life and health – could be set to be valid at viability which it estimated could occur at 28 weeks or as early as 24 weeks into a pregnancy. Recently, this reproductive right

to choose abortion was upheld by a bare majority of the court, while the dissent found the trimester approach based on viability 'unworkable' [16]. The 'on request' period under American case law would not, in practice, then extend beyond 24 weeks [40].

This preliminary overview of permissible grounds for abortion and their relation to fetal development reveals, not only a distinction between criminal proscription and actual medical practice, but also a legal recognition of the stages of fetal development in the time limitations imposed. Limiting the grounds for abortion is, however, not the only legal means of recognition of the interests of the developing fetus – procedural requirements which impose their own conditions can also affect the time frame of abortion.

25.2 PROCEDURAL CRITERIA: THE CONSTRAINTS OF FORMALISM

Other legal and administrative conditions serve further to circumscribe, control and limit the availability of, and access to, abortion. These criteria can be divided into, on the one hand, those that are substantive and whose non-fulfilment attract penal sanction and, on the other, those that are only regulatory or administrative in nature, such as those which impose delays for reflection.

With a view to protecting the woman from unsafe practices, one substantive condition common to all jurisdictions is the requirement that the abortion be performed by a medical practitioner. Restrictions also exist as to the place where the abortion is performed and as to the requirement for committee or other medical consultation or approval.

(a) Medical qualifications

Since Belgium totally prohibits abortion except to save the life of the mother, no specific mention is made in the Penal Code of 1867 with respect to a physician, the prohibition applying equally to anyone. France, Canada and Great Britain all limit the practice of legal abortions to qualified medical practitioners as defined by other legislation on professional qualifications [4, 12]. Abortions performed by persons other than 'registered' (Britain) or 'qualified' medical practitioners (Canada) or physicians (United States, France) would be illegal.

(b) Place of abortion

Of the jurisdictions under study, only the United States has no federal criteria as to the place where an abortion must be performed. Nevertheless, state legislation has attempted to control the performance of abortions outside of approved clinics or hospitals; this, however, may not always be successful – in *Akron* [15], for example, an Ohio ordinance which required, *inter alia*, that all terminations of pregnancy after the first trimester be performed in a hospital was held to be unconstitutional.

Legislation on abortion in Britain, Canada and France provides for governmental approval or accreditation of public or private hospitals or clinics offering abortion services. In Canada, however, accredited or approved hospitals were not compelled to provide facilities for abortion; this created problems of inequitable access and availability and accompanying delays which resulted in the legislation being declared unconstitutional as representing a threat to the physical and psychological integrity of the woman. Powell [7], for example, noted that some 2.8 weeks passed between a woman suspecting pregnancy and first seeing a physician; there was, on average, a further delay of 8 weeks before the pregnancy was terminated owing to delays by physicians and hospitals. Tietze [1] estimated that, in both England and in Canada, between 12% and 18% of legal abortions were performed in the second trimester due to delays in the health care

system. In France, public health establishments are listed by the Minister of Health and abortion facilities must be adequate for local needs. Moreover, the number of abortions in any private health establishment in France cannot exceed 25% of the total number of medical interventions in that hospital.

The licensing requirements and systems of control also create bureaucratic problems; moreover, the public hospital services may be physically inadequate to deal with the number of operations sought [17]. Thus, in England and Wales, some 10% of terminations are now publicly funded through private clinics operating on an agency basis and pregnancies of less than 12 weeks' gestation may be terminated in private day-centres. The inherent delays in obtaining termination within the National Health Service may be part of the reason why 50% of the women resident in England and Wales who seek abortion do so at their own expense. Approximately 15% of terminations in England and Wales are carried out in the second trimester.

(c) Approval procedures

Another requirement affecting the range of abortion services, and particularly the time limitations, is the requirement of additional medical or committee approval. The British Abortion Act 1967 dictates the opinion in good faith of two registered medical practitioners, while Canada, at s.251(6) of the Criminal Code, required the approval of a three-member therapeutic abortion committee composed of physicians appointed by the hospital board. Since hospital boards are elected, local sentiments greatly influenced the availability or non-availability of abortions in Canada [6,7]. In this respect, Canadian courts have declined jurisdiction in cases alleging that hospitals' therapeutic abortion committees were too liberal in their interpretation of endangerment of the pregnancy to the life or health of the woman [18]. Yet, this committee approach came under successful constitutional attack before the Supreme Court of Canada [8].

(d) Procedural delays

France is the only country requiring a delay for reflection between the initial medical consultation and the decision to proceed. This is designed to permit the woman to weigh all the factors inherent in the decision to abort following her exchange with the physician who, on his or her part, is required to give the patient information as to the risks of abortion, the availability of social services and assistance, adoption possibilities and a list of establishments performing abortions. A visit with a social worker is also obligatory in France. Written confirmation is required if the woman decides to proceed with her request. Obviously, if this time for reflection would place the woman outside the statutory 10-week legal period (gestational age) for abortion, the physician alone would be the judge of his decision to circumvent this delay. Similar consultation, transmission of information and delays for reflection were legislated into practice by several American States but were subsequently declared unconstitutional in both *Akron* [15] and *Thornburgh* [16].

Summary

Substantive and administrative procedural criteria, although designed primarily to safeguard the medical and psychological environment of abortion, serve to distinguish termination of pregnancy from other medical or surgical procedures and may add to delay in obtaining an abortion. Furthermore, regional and local disparity in the application of procedural criteria creates inequitable conditions for access which cause further delays – especially where the criteria are

substantive in nature. Once the decision to terminate pregnancy has been made, such disparities tend to result in 'abortion tourism' in an effort to find more liberal jurisdictions or a shorter delay – for the woman, herself, realises that the fetus is maturing to the point of viability.

THE LIVING ABORTUS: VIABILITY OR VITALISM?

In order to understand better the dilemmas surrounding the issue of viability and the late abortion debate, it is necessary to consider briefly the various techniques used to induce such abortions, the potential complications associated with each method and the concomitant rate of live births.

The risks of abortion substantially increase with advancing pregnancy; thus, the issue of the woman's safety is intrinsically linked with the type of second trimester technique used. Moreover, the techniques differ markedly in their potential for resulting in live births. Second trimester terminations and those performed late enough for the fetus to be viable usually involve one of the following methods: saline or prostaglandin instillation, dilatation of the cervix and evacuation of the uterus (D & E) or hysterotomy [19].

Saline intra-amniotic instillation is the oldest of these techniques and is highly feticidal. The possibility of a live birth following saline amnioinfusion is extremely remote but, at the same time, it is associated with various maternal risks. The most common complications are haemorrhage and infection, both of which are most likely to occur when an abortion is incomplete. Patients undergoing saline termination also risk cardiovascular effects, coagulation defects, tissue damage and hypernatraemia if saline inadvertently enters the vascular system. In rare cases, uterine injury, including rupture or cervical laceration, and the retention of products of conception may occur. The use of saline is particularly contraindicated in patients with cardiovascular disease, renal disease, sickle cell disease or other severe anaemias. For these reasons, prostaglandin instillation is often used. Theoretically, this is a safer method as there is no risk of hypernatraemia and prostaglandin is eliminated more quickly than is saline; in practice, there are few differences in complication rates between the two methods in the hands of skilled physicians. Prostaglandin is not directly lethal to the fetus; there is, therefore, an increased chance of fetal survival using this method, a possibility which may make physicians reluctant to use the technique after the twentieth week of pregnancy.

Dilation and evacuation (D & E) is now increasingly used and is the most common method of termination of pregnancy in the second trimester. This method necessarily results in fetal death and has a maternal complication rate which is lower than that of the instillation techniques; it may, however, be profoundly disturbing to nurses and other attendants. Finally, hysterotomy involves surgical removal of the fetus without necessarily damaging it but carries serious risks of complications for the woman.

Given the availability of these methods and the different psychological impact of each on the woman seeking termination, on the physician and on the aides performing the operation, it is important to site the debate not only within the framework of fetal viability as legally defined but also within the circumscribed parameters of maternal freedoms and fetal protection, particularly as the matter concerns the living abortus.

25.3 VIABILITY DEFINED: SURVIVAL AND POTENTIALITY

As previously noted, in the countries under study, gestational age limits on abortion are either framed in terms of the risks of pregnancy to maternal life or health or are fixed by statute to a point in time when the risk of maternal complications from abortion is at its lowest. The first subjective criterion used to distinguish the nature of abortion was quickening; special protection for the unborn child once it had 'quickened' was firmly established under the common law from the seventeenth century onwards – destruction of a child of lesser maturity was regarded as being of a different quality. Quickening was, however, abandoned in England as a determinant of culpability or of the severity of punishment for illegal abortion with the passage of the Offences Against the Person Act 1861 which made no distinction as to the gestational age of the fetus. Such a subjective phenomenon as quickening is difficult to prove but it is still often used as the standard for suits under American statutes relating to feticide or wrongful death. In general, however, viability is now adopted as the criterion for regulation of the outer limits of permissible abortion which are based on predictions of fetal maturity.

Various criteria are used in different jurisdictions to define viability; in most instances, the determination is regarded as a medical matter – only in England have the courts attempted a judicial assessment (see below). Kass [20] has described spontaneous circulation, respiration and central nervous system functioning as being essential. A distinction must be made between live birth and viability. An infant is said to be alive if it has one or more of the following attributes: spontaneous muscular movement, response to external stimuli such as touch and pain, elicitable reflexes, spontaneous respiration and spontaneous heart function manifested by cardiac contraction and blood flow. A viable infant, by contrast, must be capable of *living* and it follows that all of these attributes must be present, with or without assistance, for a neonate to be viable. Gestational age, body weight and crown–rump length have also been used but variations in menstrual cycles, racial differences, maternal age, health and nutritional status, ensure that a large grey area surrounds the use of these mathematical assessments. Generally speaking, the extreme immaturity of the lungs and other vital organs make it unlikely that a fetus born before 22 weeks' gestation would be viable [21]; the capacity to breathe may be a decisive and unambiguous criterion for determining viability – it is the inability of the lungs, including a failure to elaborate surfactant, which makes extrauterine survival impossible in the absence of a technology capable of providing an artifical placenta. Notwithstanding that this 22-week cut-off point places the fetus at approximately 500 grams – which corresponds to the preference of the World Health Organization – neonatal survival at this point is, at best, dubious. However, before undertaking an examination of the legal translation and interpretation of the notion of viability by the courts, the relationship of live birth and the crime of child destruction must first be considered.

(a) Live birth and child destruction

Although, under British and Canadian law, the fetus does not come within the ambit of homicide provisions, it is, nevertheless, protected in the later stages of fetal development by the existence of the offence of child destruction. The English Infant Life (Preservation) Act, 1929 s.1, and its counterpart in Northern Ireland, Criminal Justice Act 1945, s.25, stipulate that: 'any person, who with intent to destroy the life of a child capable of being born alive, by any wilful act causes a child to die before it has an existence independent of its mother, shall be guilty of child destruction'; the Canadian parallel is to be found in the Canadian Criminal Code s.221. A separate existence does not depend upon severance of the umbilical connection [22] – a stipulation which is codified in Canada where s.206.1 of the Criminal Code lays it down that: 'a child becomes a human being ... when it has completely proceeded in a living state, from the body of its mother whether or not (a) it has breathed, (b) it has independent circulation, or (c) the naval string is severed' [23]. Thus, before the child has an existence independent of its mother, and provided that the act in question was not necessary to save the life of the mother, the soon-to-be-born fetus is protected from harm.

American case law defines three criteria which are commonly used in making the determination of live birth – the presence outside the womb, an independent circulation and effective respiration [24]. The most exacting live-birth requirements demand that all three criteria be present [25]. In other words, an aborted fetus which exhibits the requisite signs of life would be considered to be born alive provided that it was, at the time, completely outside the mother; this last criterion is of particular interest as to whether the doctor's duty to treat exists only once the fetus is outside the mother or whether such duty prevails even before that moment [26] – the legal criteria for live birth concern only the physical location and the condition of the infant rather than the manner of its exit from the womb.

Turning, then, to the study of the relationship between abortion law and live birth, the British Abortion Act 1967, by specifically preserving the Infant Life (Preservation) Act 1929, makes explicit mention of this protection. Unfortunately, the 1967 Act refers to a viable fetus whereas the 1929 Act speaks of a fetus capable of being born alive; similarly the Births and Deaths Registration Act 1953 makes no mention of viability [27]. The debate as to whether the words 'capable of being born alive' are to be taken as meaning viable – or are to be more restrictively   interpreted   –   is   further complicated by the fact that the 1929 Act itself provides, at s.1(2), that 'evidence that a woman had at any material time been pregnant for a period of 28 weeks or more shall be *prima facie* proof that she was at that time pregnant of a child capable of being born alive'. The converse proposition – that is, that a fetus of less than 28 weeks' gestation is *not* capable of being born alive – is, however, neither stated nor implied. Thus, where the physician intends to cause the death of a fetus *in utero* and it survives to die when fully born, there are two crimes to consider: attempted child destruction and actual homicide – the death of a human being.

The possible conflict between the Abortion Act and the Infant Life (Preservation) Act was the subject of a recent Court of Appeal decision in Britain [28]. The court in that case held that a fetus of 18 to 21 weeks' gestation 'whose cardiac muscle was contracting and which showed signs of primitive movement but which was incapable of breathing was not a child capable of being born alive'. The medical evidence indicated that the termination of such a pregnancy was not an offence under the 1929 Act and the court held that the fetus in question would not, at that stage, 'be capable of breathing, either naturally or with the aid of a ventilator'. In spite of this ruling, there is little doubt that the inconsistencies between the 1929 Act and the Abortion Act 1967 require further clarification; no physician would wish an *ex post facto* legal determination of his medical judgement as to fetal capacity on a case by case basis.

The Canadian Criminal Code not only provides that a 'child becomes a human being ... when it has completely proceeded in a living state from the body of its mother' (s.206(1)), but also that a person commits homicide when 'he causes injury to a child before or during its birth as a result of which the child dies after becoming a human being' (s.206(2)). The fetus at term has been held to be a human being in a charge of criminal

negligence brought against a midwife [29]. Furthermore, in a case in which a 6-month pregnant woman was stabbed, the accused was properly charged and convicted of the manslaughter of the child even though it was born prematurely, lived only for 19 minutes and then died, 'not [being] sufficiently developed' [30].

Given its ordinary meaning, the 'act of birth' begins at the point at which spontaneous or induced labour commences. Actually, such an interpretation permits the use of methods of abortion which would destroy the fetus prior to birth unless live birth were to presuppose the presence of a potentially viable fetus to the extent that any intervention undertaken with the aim of delivering the fetus would be conduct forming part of the 'act of birth' [23]. Such an argument may be impermissible as it confuses the notions of abortion with the act of birth; both concern the expulsion or extraction of the fetus but the proposition makes it impossible for the physician to determine when the abortion has ended and the live birth has begun. Nothing in the British legislation or Canadian Criminal Code indicates that the crime of child destruction during the act of birth is concerned with the delivery of a potentially viable fetus as opposed to a live birth as evidenced by the onset or imminent onset of labour (see below).

Since the French abortion legislation permits abortion beyond the statutory period for serious fetal malformations or grave risk to the life or health of the mother, there could be no crime of child destruction given those conditions. Indeed, the fact of survival did not prevent – and would not now under the 1939 legislation on illegal abortions which is still in force [4] – a charge of attempted abortion when an illegal operation resulted in the premature delivery of a viable child; however, under Belgian law, which follows the exact terminology of the 1810 French Penal Code, there will be no prosecution if the failed abortion results in the premature birth of a viable infant.

Similarly, in the United States, given that, prior to viability, states can only regulate abortion so as to protect the woman's health and given that the fetus *in utero* is not a human being under penal law, until recently, no specific charge of homicide could be brought for the destruction of a child capable of being born alive; the killing of a child in the process of being born could, however, fall within the homicide provision [31]. Thus, a charge of manslaughter following the death of a fetus after an abortion at 21–24 weeks' gestation would be inapplicable and has been found to be so where an infant was dead before being completely extruded from the mother's body [26]; it would follow that homicide liability does not attach in such circumstances. States could, however, extend their homicide statutes by relaxing the requirements for live birth so as to intrude in the actual practice of abortion or they could protect the fetus from intentional killing by creating specific feticide statutes (see below). Late abortions have been further limited in the United States by case law determination of viability.

(b) Viability

The live birth dilemma has arisen both because of changes in abortion techniques and in the development of life-support techniques which are designed to ensure fetal viability. Indeed, attempts to justify maintaining the viability standard serve only to call its utility into question. As a logical justification, viability is a double-edged sword since, if it is to carry great legal and moral weight, it will operate increasingly against late second trimester abortions as the time of viability is pushed back. Physicians may be reluctant to perform such terminations or they will use methods to ensure the destruction of the fetus *in utero* if a duty is imposed to treat viable fetuses which have been aborted when the

prognosis for meaningful survival would be poor.

As mentioned earlier, physicians must depend entirely upon data which indicates the chances of survival at various gestational ages and birth weights, the best parameters being a combination of biparietal diameter of the fetus' head, abdominal circumference and femur length [3]; since neither statistics nor measurements can give a precise answer, there can be no sharp dividing line between viability and non-viability. As related to current technology, some fetuses under 20–22 weeks are clearly not viable, some over 24 weeks are definitely viable while some between 20 and 25 weeks are possibly viable but yet carry a doubtful mental and physical prognosis [32]. Thus, fetal development is a gradual and individualized process and, as the case law will show, is not amenable to the certainty of assessment which is necessary for valid legislation.

Although the debate is relevant for all jurisdictions, viability as a legal issue has been discussed most extensively by the American courts. The 1973 *Roe* v. *Wade* decision of the Supreme Court intrinsically tied the legality of abortion to the medical status of both mother and fetus according to the trimesters of pregnancy. Following that decision, states could not regulate abortion in the first trimester and could do so in the second trimester only in order to protect maternal health; by contrast, all terminations in the third trimester could be proscribed except those which were considered to be necessary to protect a woman's life or health [33]. The Supreme Court justified this trimester system by reference to several medical factors. It was concluded that the state's interest in maternal health becomes compelling at approximately the end of the first trimester because 'of the now established medical fact ... that, until the end of the first trimester, mortality in abortion may be less than mortality in normal childbirth'. Likewise, the state's interest in potential life was thought to become compelling at the end of the second trimester because that is when the fetus becomes viable or, in other words, 'potentially able to live outside the mother's womb, albeit with artificial aid'. The court stated that the point of viability had both 'logical and biological' justifications because a viable fetus presumably has the 'capacity for meaningful life' outside the mother's womb. The court pointed out that viability is 'usually placed at about seven months (28 weeks) but may occur earlier, even at 24 weeks'. It will be appreciated that the trimester schema was premised on the medical facts as they existed in 1973.

The medical nature of the assessment of viability and the necessity of leaving that point flexible as a matter for the judgement of the physician on a case-by-case basis, were emphasized and reaffirmed by the Supreme Court in later cases [34]. It was held that it was not the proper legislative or judicial function to define the term viability in relation to either a specific point in gestation or to an objective standard based on the opinion of a cross-section of the medical community. These affirmations have however played havoc with subsequent definitions. Viability has shifted from potential survival as in *Roe* [33] to the reasonable likelihood of sustained survival as in *Colautti* [34]. The variation in these two definitions is significant in that 'potential survival' implies that any possibility of survival is sufficient while 'reasonable likelihood' implies that the fetus' chances of life must be fairly good. It is arguable that the reasonable likelihood definition should be used as such a standard will generally occur later in gestation [35]. Accordingly, the chances of medical agreement as to whether viability has been achieved will be greater and the physician's fear of the concept of viability will be reduced because, as was said in *Colautti*: 'an erroneous determination of viability could have a profound chilling effect

on the willingness of physicians to perform abortions near the point of viability in the manner indicated by their best medical judgement'.

The difficulties of maintaining a consistent working definition of viability, such as are seen in the decisions of the Supreme Court, are exacerbated by changing medical and scientific developments which affect not only the definition of viability but also the techniques for termination which are to be used; the current framework may be, as was said by O'Connor J in *Akron*[15]:

> ... on a collision course with itself. As the medical risks of various abortion procedures decrease, the point at which the state may regulate for reasons of maternal health is moved forward to actual childbirth. As medical science becomes better able to provide for the separate existence of the fetus, the point of viability is moved further back toward conception.

This is particularly so as regards the latter point. When *Roe* was decided in 1973, viability was generally considered to be around 28 weeks' gestation. Advances in neonatal care have made 24 weeks the generally accepted dividing line, and survival is occasionally possible at 23 weeks' gestation. The World Health Organization have, as previously mentioned, recognized this by establishing 22 weeks as the demarcation point between spontaneous abortion and birth [37]. In short, the interest of the State in maternal health is closing towards its interest in potential life.

In 1986, in *Thornburgh* [16], the Supreme Court took the occasion not only to uphold the *Roe* decision again, albeit by a much narrower margin, but also to recognize the 'undesirability of any trade-off' between the woman's health and additional percentage points of possible fetal survival. It should be noted, however, that this reaffirmation was in the face of particular provisions of state legislation of abortion and not with respect to the trimester format based on the regulation framework of compelling state interest. Moreover, in the strong dissent in the case, the inherent weakness of the viability standard, however interpreted, was again underscored. The dissent maintained that state interest rested in the fetus as an entity – that is, in the potential life of its citizens – and, therefore, did not depend on shifting medical determination. WHITE J argued that state interest in the fetus is equally compelling before and after viability and that medical practice and technology are irrelevant factors. The dissenting opinion, therefore, based its argument on the position that human life begins at conception; the majority opinion rested on the progressive development of the fetus which rendered the establishment of viability as being of particular import. It follows that the dissent would have discarded the viability criterion altogether; note that this, being a 5–4 decision, was greatly dependent on the composition of the court which is always subject to change.

Increasingly, therefore, viability is becoming a statement solely about medical technology and is moving closer to representing the late second trimester, a shift which requires a re-evaluation of its importance. The only remaining justification for viability as a standard is that it symbolizes societal antipathy to late abortion. Arguments for the potentiality of human life are equally compelling before and after viability; once this is accepted, the issue lies between maternal freedoms and fetal protection.

25.4 VIABILITY CIRCUMSCRIBED: MATERNAL HEALTH AND FETAL PROTECTION

Maternal life and health interests have always been the source of abortion regulation. This applies even in countries which prohibit abortion such as Belgium or in those which provide for an early statutory open period of abortion upon request; this is in spite of a corresponding constitutional protection of human life from its commencement [4]. Even where maternal freedoms have prevailed, however, we have seen that they are not absolute in respect of abortion and they may be even less so later in pregnancy where the desire to protect the fetus may affect both the choice of abortion technique and the standard of care of the physician.

(a) Maternal freedoms

Of the countries under examination, none, other than the United States, has considered access to abortion as a constitutional right. There, the court in *Thornburgh* [16] relied on the woman's due process right of privacy and held that the right 'is broad enough to encompass a woman's decision whether or not to terminate her pregnancy' (at p. 153). Recently, the Supreme Court of Canada held the procedural restrictions to abortion under the Criminal Code to be an infringement of the constitutional right to security of the person. Only one judge of the bench of seven, however, held that the liberty interest of the pregnant woman under Article 7 included the right to an abortion [8]. Elsewhere, as, for example, in France and in Canada, while national abortion legislation has been held to be constitutional [36], that is not the equivalent of an unqualified personal right to a termination of pregnancy. Where the therapeutic indications for abortion are based on wide medical and legal definitions of maternal life and health, the general principles governing consent to medical treatment would also imply a right to a choice of abortion technique. The question which thus arises is whether, given the increasing acceptability of a definition of health which is as broad as that of the World Health Organization – 'a state of complete physical, mental and social wellbeing and not merely the absence of disease or infirmity' [37] – may the woman and her physician opt for a method of abortion that is definitely feticidal without state circumscription? In other words, if an abortion is performed because it is needed in order to avoid the burdens that an unwanted pregnancy, childbirth, or motherhood would place on the woman's physical and psychological health, could not her physician assume that it would be best to choose a method which is most likely to ensure fetal destruction?

There is little controversy over the principle that maternal interests should prevail where there would be increased risks to the mother in choosing a procedure that would terminate the pregnancy but not destroy the fetus. Since even postviability abortions are permitted for maternal life or health interests, it would be anomalous if that life or health could be endangered by mandating procedures to save the fetus.

Nevertheless, the woman's health interest does not prevail as clearly where the risks are the same whether the fetus is saved or destroyed. At this extreme, a broad definition of health, including psychological considerations, would still allow the woman's interests to be paramount as interpreted by the medical judgement of the physician. Thus, those very health considerations that justify the abortion decision may also entail the destruction of the fetus.

Furthermore, as we have seen, abortion is generally admissible on the grounds of fetal malformations, and these are not usually detected until late in the second trimester. Whose 'health' considerations are at issue in such abortions? While allowing for fetal destruction for the sake of the woman's psychological and emotional well-being, the state itself has, at the same time, subsumed its compelling interest in potential life in relation to the actual (woman's) or potential (fetus') quality of life. The choice is difficult and it is likely to become more so as prenatal diagnosis becomes more refined; in future it will be possible to detect in the previable fetus not only malformations which are present but also abnormal conditions which will present overtly in later life (see Chapter 2 for full discussion). If abortions for established fetal malformations were to be restricted due to their being detectable only at a late gestational age, abortion of viable fetuses who, if they survived, would live to be handicapped would be prevented while those whose early cells indicated presence of latent disease would be aborted with impunity. A balanced opinion would be struck if there was a possibility of removing a fetus alive without increased danger to the woman. Under such a position, health considerations would only pertain to the decision to abort and would not extend to the separate and distinct issue of the life or quality of life of the fetus. Because a living abortus no longer encroaches on the woman's bodily integrity or privacy, the states' freedom to protect the fetus *in utero* should extend to the abortus *ex utero* in the form of dictating appropriate medical care.

(b) Treatment of the living abortus

Thus far we have examined the extent of the health considerations of the woman. If such a consideration stops at the point of womb-emptying, then the abortus, as an independent biological being, is entitled to treatment akin to that which would be given to a premature or defective newborn. As Rhoden [3] has argued, the physician's duty of care to a child does not change simply because it is unwanted; the same duty is owing to an abortus as to a premature newborn.

Following the earlier American decisions which recognized a compelling state interest in protecting potential life once the fetus becomes viable, subsequent Supreme Court decisions have further supported treatment of the living abortus. Indeed, in *Danforth* [34], the court held that failure to protect a live-born infant is punishable under state law, and in *Ashcroft* [15] it further upheld a state requirement that a second physician be in attendance at postviability termination. Moreover, the court in *Ashcroft* further stated that, while preserving the life of a viable fetus that is aborted is often not possible, the state may legitimately choose to provide safeguards for the comparatively few instances of live birth that occur.

Advances in neonatology have had profound effect on altering the lower limits of viability. Notwithstanding such advances, it is important to be realistic about the relationship of such changes to the prognosis of the child and its 'meaningful survival'. In *Roe's* [14] definition of viability 'meaningful' qualified the state's interest in potential life which constituted the only justification for overriding the woman's right to termination of her pregnancy. A query exists, however, as to whether 'meaningful' in the context of viability is predicated on a 'quality of life' decision; given the high probability of damage to the fetus, it must be asked whether such life-sustaining procedures as are mandated by the state are likely to result in a child capable of a meaningful life.

Finally, when evaluating risk to the mother, the choice of the method of abortion and the standard of care expected of the physician, it may be asked if a statute can mandate the same standard of care towards the living abortus as would be exercised if the fetus were not being aborted? To do so, would limit the choice of technique to one that would provide the best opportunity for the fetus to be born alive so long as a different technique would not be necessary to preserve the life or health of the pregnant woman. However, in *Colautti* [34] such a statute was held to be invalid for having failed to state expressly that the woman's life and health prevailed where they were in conflict with those of the fetus and for failing expressly to permit the physician's exercise in good faith of his medical discretion when faced with such a conflict. A change in the wording of the proposed statute so as to include a specific mention of the physician's

good faith judgement, as well as the preclusion of any abortion technique which would present a significantly greater medical risk to the pregnant woman's life or health, was also struck down in *Thornburgh* [16]. The Court reasoned that these additions, together with the requirement that 'the abortion technique employed shall be that which would provide the best opportunity for the unborn child to be aborted alive' constituted an impermissible 'trade-off' between the woman's health and fetal survival; the statute had, again, failed to require that maternal health be the paramount consideration. Yet, following this reasoning, the future imposition of a duty of care towards the living abortus may not be precluded so long as maternal interests remain paramount; if a future statute were to mandate a certain duty of care of the physician towards the living abortus, it would not be considered unconstitutional so long as it was subject to maternal health. In fact, a number of states have developed statutes relating to feticide and wrongful death of the fetus. Some of these, while expressly excluding legal abortion, apply irrespective of the state of fetal development while others refer only to an unborn 'quick' or viable child. Furthermore, some statutes refer to the twenty-fourth week as that point in a pregnancy at which a woman, herself, may also become liable under these laws [38]. No feticide statute may apply to a termination of a human pregnancy when that is performed in order to preserve the health of the woman or fetus and 'where very reasonable medical effort, not inconsistent with preserving the life of the pregnant person, is made to preserve the life of a viable fetus' [39].

Summary

While this latter discussion has been limited to American constitutional law, it is illustrative of the general debate surrounding the issues of whether the protection of maternal freedoms and health includes a 'right' to choose the destruction of the fetus at a late stage in pregnancy or whether the preservation of potential life requires state intervention to circumscribe that choice. Furthermore, it illustrates the inherent weakness of the viability criterion as a justification for legal or medical intervention, to say nothing of the interpretation of live birth when that is not given its ordinary meaning of the point at which spontaneous or induced labour commences. The impact of such ambiguity on medical care and choice of abortion technique serves to impose unknown duties on the physician, to generate greater maternal health risks and, possibly, to compel the deliberate destruction of the fetus.

25.5 CONCLUSION

This overview of comparative abortion law illustrates the enormous difficulties which are inherent in the issue. The range of approaches illustrated in the proscription of abortion, including limiting the substantive grounds or requiring the adherence to certain procedures, reflects societal interests in maternal well-being as well as in the protection of human life *in utero*. Nevertheless, in practice, both these aims have been undermined by the uncertainty surrounding the interpretation of the law and ensuing medical and administrative delays often result in abortions late in a pregnancy. This poses particular problems now that artificial life-support systems are increasingly able to maintain premature life outside the womb. Such medical intervention raises the same conflicts between vitalism and the quality of human life as does the use of artificial support at the other end of life where it can be used to prolong the process of dying. Hence, there is a need to re-examine and circumscribe the concepts of viability and live birth.

The choice – or lack thereof – of the method of abortion in late gestational stages and the duty of care of the physician towards the living abortus are inextricably linked to the definitions of viability. This brief study has shown that viability is an unworkable legal and medical criterion; both fetal protection from unnecessary destruction and the preservation of maternal health would be better served by an arbitrary, but certain, time limit on late abortions – saving grave danger to the mother's life or health.

Even if, ideally, early abortion decisions could be purely private matters based on individual moral responsibility, late abortions cannot be so regarded. Maternal freedoms, the assurance of medical treatment for the living abortus, the limitation of medical discretion and the *ex post facto* imposition of medical liability, require greater certainty and, hence, legislative intervention.

Acknowledgement
The author is particularly indebted to Ms Lori Luther, LLB, BCL, for her invaluable work and assistance in the preparation of this chapter.

REFERENCES

1. Tietze, C. and Henshaw, S. (1986) *Induced Abortion: A World Review 1986*, 6th edn, Alan Guttmacher Institute, New York. See also Leenen, H.J., Pinet, G. and Prims, A.V. (1986) *Trends in Health Legislation in Europe*, Masson, Paris.
2. For Canadian law and the defence of necessity, see Dickens, B. (1976) The *Morgentaler* case: criminal process and abortion law. *Osgoode Hall Law J.*, **14**, 229.
3. Rhoden, N. 'Some legal considerations', and Stubblefield, P. 'Some medical considerations', both in Note (1985) Late abortion and technological advances in fetal viability. *Fam. Plann. Perspect.*, **17**, 160; Hack, M. and Fanaroff, A. (1986) Changes in the delivery room care of the extremely small infant. *New. Engl. J. Med.*, **314**, 660.
4. Knoppers, B.M. and Brault, I. (1989) *L'Avortement et la loi dans les pays francophones*, Thémis, Montreal.

5. Trib. corr. Bruxelles (8e ch.) 30 Juin 1983 J T 24 Septembre 1983, 105; Cour cass. Neerlandaise (2e ch.) 5 Février 1985 *J des procès*, 3 Mars 1985. But this decision was effectively overturned by the Court of Appeal (Ghent, 14 November, 1988).

6. (1977) *Report of the Committee on the Operation of the Abortion Law* (Badgley Report).

7. Powell, M. (1987) *Report on Therapeutic Abortion Services in Ontario: A Study Commissioned by the Ministry of Health*, Toronto.

8. *Morgentaler, Smoling and Scott* v. *Her Majesty and A-G of Canada* [1988] S.C.R30.

9. *Borowski* v. *Attorney-General of Canada* (1987) 4 WWR 285 (Sask. CA). The question was declared moot by the Supreme Court (March, 1989).

10. Loi no. 75-17 relative à l'interruption volontaire de la grossesse (*Code de la Santé Publique*, arts. 162-163).

11. *Harris* v. *McRae* 100 S Ct 2671 (1980).

12. Knoppers, B.M. (1982) Physician liability and prenatal diagnosis. *CCLT* **18**, 169. See, in general, Dickens, B. and Cook, R. (1979) The development of Commonwealth abortion laws. *Int. Law Q.*, **28**, 424.

13. Rhoden, N. (1984) The new neonatal dilemma: live births from late abortions. *Georgetown Law J.*, **72**, 1451; Dickens, B. (1985) Abortion, amniocentesis and the law. *Am. J. Comparative Law*, **34**, 249; Mason, J.K. (1989) Abortion and the law. In *Legal Issues in Human Reproduction* (ed. S.A.M. McLean), Gower, Aldershot.

14. *Roe* v. *Wade* 410 US 113 (1973).

15. *City of Akron* v. *Akron Center for Reproductive Health Inc.* 103 S Ct 2481 (1983); *Planned Parenthood Ass. of Kansas City, Mo., Inc.* v. *Ashcroft* 103 S Ct 2517 (1983).

16. *Thornburgh* v. *American College of Obstetricians and Gynecologists et al.* 106 S Ct 2169 (1986).

17. Leading Article (1979) No case for an abortion Bill. *Br. Med. J.*, **2**, 230.

18. *Carruthers* v. *Therapeutic Abortion Committees of Lions Gate Hospital et al.* (1983) 6 DLR (4th) 57; *Carruthers* v. *Langley* (1985) 23 DLR (4th) 623.

19. Berger, G.L., Brenner, W.E. and Keith, L.G. (eds) (1981) *Second Trimester Abortion: Perspectives after a Decade of Experience* PSG, Boston; Callahan, D. (1986) How technology is reframing the abortion debate. *Hastings Center*

Report, February, 33; Grimes, D.H. (1984) Second trimester abortions in the United States. *Family Plann. Perspect.*, **16**, 260; Tietze, ref. 1; Wood, M. and Hawkins, L. (1980) State regulation of late abortion and the physician's duty of care to the viable fetus. *Missouri Law Rev.*, **45**, 394.

20. Kass, L.R. (1977) Determining death and viability in fetuses and abortuses. *Bioethics Dig.*, **2**, 1; Rhoden, ref. 13.

21. Dunn, P.M. and Stirrat, G.M. (1984) Capable of being born alive? *Lancet*, **i**, Rhoden ref. 13; Kass, ref. 20.

22. Tunkel, V. (1979) Abortion: how early, how late, and how legal? *Br. Med. J.*, **2**, 253.

23. Somerville, M. (1981) Reflections on Canadian abortion law: evacuation and destruction – two separate issues. *Univ. Toronto Law J.*, **31**, 1.

24. See *People* v. *Hayner* 90 NE 2d 23 (NY, 1949) (complete presence outside the womb); *State* v. *Winthrop* 43 Iowa 519 (1876) (respiration).

25. Sendor, B. (1975) Medical responsibility for fetal survival under *Roe* and *Doe*. *Harvard Civil Rights, Civil Liberties Law Rev.*, **10**, 444.

26. *Commonwealth* v. *Edelin* 359 NE 2d 4 (Mass, 1978).

27. Bowles, T.G.A. and Bell, M.N.M. (1979) Abortion – a clarification. *New Law J.*, **129**, 944.

28. *C* v. *S* [1988] QB 135.

29. *R* v. *Marsh* (1979) 2 CCC (3d) 1 (County Court, Vancouver Island, BC).

30. *R* v. *Prince* (1986) 30 CCC (3d) 35 (SCC).

31. *People* v. *Chavez* 77 Cal App 2d 621 (1947) (fetus in process of being born); *Keeler* v. *Superior Court* 87 Cal Rptr 481 (1970) (destruction of fetus still inside the mother's womb).

32. Yu, V.Y.H. (1987) The extremely low birthweight infant: ethical issues in treatment. *Aust. Paediatr. J.*, **23**, 97.

33. 410 US 113 (1973). For commentaries, see Notes (1976) State protection of the viable unborn child after *Roe* v. *Wade*. How little, how late? *Louisiana Law Rev.*, **37**, 270; Sendor, ref. 25; Wood and Hawkins, ref. 19.

34. *Doe* v. *Bolton* (1973) 410 US 179; *Planned Parenthood* v. *Danforth* (1976) 428 US 52; *Colautti* v. *Franklin* (1979) 439 US 379.

35. Horan, D.V. (1979) Viability revisits the court in *Colautti* v. *Franklin*. *Hosp. Prog.*, February, 20; Nelson, T.A. (1984) Taking *Roe* to the limits:

treating viable feticide as murder. *Ind. Law Rev.*, 1119; Wood and Hawkins, ref. 19.

36. France: Conseil constitutionnel français, 15 Jan 1975, D 1975 II, 529; Canada: see ref. 8; UK: *Paton* v. *United Kingdom* (1981) 3 EHRR 408. Knoppers, B.M. (1985) Modern birth technology and human rights. *Am. J. Comp. Law.*, **33**, 1; Knoppers, B.M. (1987) Reproduction technology and international mechanisms of protection of the human person. *McGill Law J.*, **32**, 336.

37. World Health Organization (1979) *Definitions and Recommendations, International Classification of Diseases*, 9th edn, Vol. 1, WHO, Geneva, pp. 763–768.

38. See, generally (1983 and yearly updates) *Handling Pregnancy and Birth Cases* (Family Law Series), McGraw-Hill, Colorado. Also the recent paper of the Law Reform Commission of Canada. *Crimes Against the Foetus*, 1989.

39. Iowa, s.707.6 (Criminal Law); Arizona, s. 36-2301.01-c.

40. The author points out that, as this book goes to press. *Roe* v. *Wade* is again being challenged: *Reproductive Health Service* v. *Webster* 851 F 2d 1071 (1988). The Supreme Court is likely to rule in mid-1989. See Shapter, D. (1989) *Pediatric News*, March, p. 50 – Ed.

CHAPTER 26

Actions for wrongful life

Barry R. Furrow

26.1 INTRODUCTION [1]

Medicine is at an awkward point in genetic counselling, in transition from a state of ignorance to an intermediate stage at which information as to a spectrum of disorders can be discovered. The ability of physicians to screen the fetus for many genetic disorders such as Down's syndrome has improved, through the use of such testing tools as amniocentesis and through the use of genetic histories, even though no treatment is available [2]. These advances in detection have spawned a new specialization of genetic counselling, the scope of which is discussed in Chapter 2.

Most genetic disorders are, currently, untreatable. The medical profession has, therefore, tended to view such disorders as unfortunate accidents of nature. Recent research developments have raised hopes for the use of the tools of molecular biology to introduce a normal gene into somatic cells, thereby curing a genetic disorder with a single course of treatment [3]. Other techniques are presently effective for disorders such as severe combined immunodeficiency disease and diabetes [4]. Prenatal diagnosis and treatment is thus a sequence of more or less developed therapeutic stages. Stage 1, based on parent or family genetic histories or testing of the parents, allows a genetic disorder to be predicted. Several wrongful birth and life suits have involved failures of doctors to convey correctly to parents the likelihood that their offspring would possess genetically transmitted impairments [5]. Accurate information, when disclosed to the parents, allows them to make a choice whether or not to have a child.

Stage 2, the present state of the art in genetic diagnosis, involves the use of the techniques for prenatal diagnosis in the fetus which have been outlined in Chapter 2 [6]. This stage focuses on the fetus and, therefore, 'treatment' moves from the prevention of conception to the termination of pregnancy through abortion, if the parents find the risks of genetic defects to be unacceptable.

Stage 3, the treatment of genetic disorders *in utero*, is the least developed and is, at present, limited to specific instances such as the treatment of methylmalonic aciduria by administration of vitamin B12 and of rare vitamin-responsive errors of metabolism including galactosaemia, the adrenogenital syndrome and hypothyroidism.

Medical knowledge in this area is in transition, and the legal system is caught on the horns of the dilemma created by current medical limitations. Advances in methods of gene manipulation may portend the use of improved models – including animal models – for understanding human genetic diseases and correcting them [7]. At present, however, prevention of conception and abortion of genetically impaired fetuses remain the two available 'treatments' for genetic defects.

The visible increase in the level of litigation over genetically impaired newborns is not due to American litigation frenzy. Patients have come to expect up-to-date and accurate information about potential genetic defects from their obstetricians and physicians. The availability and legitimacy of abortion as a means of 'treating' genetic defects, even in the absence of medical therapies, has accentuated the value of such information to potential parents. Health-care professionals have conceded their responsibility to meet ordinary standards of care in advising parents about the risks of genetic abnormalities. The increased filing of wrongful life and birth suits has, in practice, been precipitated by a variety of medical errors on the part of obstetricians and testing laboratories in assessing data, testing samples and conveying information.

The courts have grouped genetic impairment suits into two categories: wrongful birth and wrongful life. 'Wrongful birth' suits are brought by the parents seeking to collect the costs incident to the birth, care, and raising of a genetically impaired child. 'Wrongful life' suits are brought by the child itself, through its parents, seeking special damages and recompense for pain and suffering as a result of the injuries sustained. The two actions are distinguished by who brings them – the parents or the child. American jurisdictions treat the two theories of recovery differently. Most American courts have recognized the validity of wrongful birth suits and have imposed no barriers to recovery, although a variety of limitations as to damages have been imposed [8]. 'Wrongful life' suits have proved more troubling and have been allowed by only a handful of courts – and then only with

substantial restrictions on the extent of damages recoverable [9].

Three hypothetical cases involving an impaired newborn may illuminate the roots of the present controversy over the 'wrongful life' suit.

Case 26.1
While in a hospital's newborn nursery, a premature newborn shows symptoms of jaundice from liver malfunctioning. The bilirubin tests results are incorrectly read and the child is released without treatment. The result is bilirubin toxicity and consequent mental retardation of the infant.

Case 26.2
A woman is pregnant with a fetus suffering from methylmalonic aciduria. The condition is not detected by tests that were performed and, therefore, corrective vitamin therapy is not administered. When the child is born, it is retarded.

Case 26.3
A pregnant woman undergoes tests to determine if her fetus is suffering from genetic disorders. Amniocentesis is conducted but the testing laboratory negligently misreads the results, so that Down's syndrome is not detected. Again, the child is born retarded.

In all three cases, the result is a serious impairment of the newborn child. The negligence in all cases involves a similar medical failure to test for defects properly. Why should we allow both the parents and the child to sue in Cases 26.1 and 26.2, but only the parents in Case 26.3? The critical difference lies in the nature of the treatment and its causal relationship to the harm. In Case 26.1, sustained exposure to light will correct the condition and the child will be normal and, in Case 26.2, vitamin therapy may solve the problem. In Case 26.3, however, no treatment, either *in utero* or after birth, can correct the condition. The only means the parents have for dealing with the psychological and monetary costs of an impaired infant will lie in termination of the pregnancy. Abortion is a morally and politically sensitive subject in the United States, and the difference between a medical treatment and a parent's informed choice to abort has caused much distress to the courts. Is the emotional conflict sufficient to justify recovery in Cases 26.1 and 26.2 but not in 26.3? In all three cases, the children are comparably impaired, the parents are subjected to comparable expenses and pain and suffering and the medical personnel are equally culpable. The condition of the third child cannot be described as being qualitatively different, nor is the physician's negligence less objectionable in its case than it is in the first two. The primary difference is that, in Cases 26.1 and 26.2, the physician failed to diagnose and treat, thereby causing the impairment, whereas, in Case 26.3, the physician did not cause the mongolism by failing to treat. By failing to diagnose, however, he denied the parents their option to alleviate the situation by aborting the child. The courts' justifications for distinguishing these situations reveals a deep-seated judicial concern over the devaluation of life which is inferred when seeming to suggest that the life of an impaired child is 'wrongful' – that he or she should not have existed.

26.2 THE JUDICIAL DEBATE

The intensity of the judicial debate over wrongful life suits reflects the highly charged context of the abortion debate and the controversies over treatment and care of handicapped newborns. The American courts discourse on the jurisprudence of wrongful life suits in long and passionate opinions

which are uncharacteristic of most appellate case law. Several major decisions have appeared within the past 4 years. I will summarize briefly some of the recent leading American decisions, the arguments presented against wrongful life suits and possible strategies for avoiding the judicial deadlock that has appeared. My position should be clear from the outset: I see nothing logically or jurisprudentially wrong with the wrongful life suit. If we are going to allow a tort liability system to operate as one of compensation for certain kinds of negligently caused injuries, then it is difficult to distinguish wrongful life suits from others which are brought by parents directly and which serve a valuable function in some situations. I also recognize, however, that the trend in the United States is to disallow such suits both judicially and legislatively – and also to limit the damages which are recoverable in wrongful birth suits.

The legislatures of several American states have expressly prohibited such litigation [10]. American statutes, following the model legislation of the Catholic Hospital Association, generally prohibit actions which are based on the claim that, but for the negligent conduct of another, the child would have been aborted. Minnesota's statute goes so far as to state explicitly that abortion should not be deemed a treatment. It is likely that other states will adopt such limitations on wrongful life – and even wrongful birth suits – over the next few years.

England and Wales have also precluded the possibility of such suits through the Congenital Disabilities (Civil Liability) Act 1976 [11]. The Act defines the conditions under which a child who is born disabled as the result of an occurrence before its birth can sue. Section (2)(b) specifies the occurrence that gives rise to liability as one that 'affected the mother during her pregnancy, or affected her or the child in the course of its birth, so that the child is born with disabilities which would not otherwise have been present'.

Thus, a wrongful life suit cannot be sustained since, in cases giving rise to such action, the child has a congenital disability that would have been present regardless of the negligence of the defendant. The court upheld this clear reading of the Act in *McKay* v. *Essex Area Health Authority* [12], concluding that the possibility of a wrongful life action in England had been extinguished after 1976. The court held specifically, however, that such a novel cause of action is not sustainable. The reasons given by STEPHENSON LJ track the arguments put forward in the American cases – concern about inroads on the sanctity of life, pressure on doctors to counsel abortion and problems in assessing damages.

A close look at the current legal status of wrongful birth and wrongful life suits in America can be taken through some recent cases. *Speck* v. *Finegold* from Pennsylvania [13], the Californian decision in *Turpin* v. *Sortini* [14], *Smith* v. *Cote* [15] and *Azzolino* v. *Dingfelder* [16] present the continuing judicial struggle with such claims in sharp focus. In *Turpin*, the California Court of Appeals for the Fifth District had rejected a claim by the infant plaintiff and had explicitly rejected the holding and reasoning of its sister court which had allowed such an action a year earlier in *Curlender* v. *Bio-Science Laboratories* [17]. Faced with the lower court conflict in *Turpin* and *Curlender*, the California Supreme Court allowed the infant plaintiff to bring a suit on her own behalf, while simultaneously restricting the damages available in the event of a finding of liability. *Turpin* involved a plaintiff, Joy, born with a hereditary hearing abnormality. The complaint alleged that the defendant physicians were negligent in failing to diagnose the defect in the plaintiff's older sister, Hope, and in advising the parents that Hope's hearing was within normal limits when, in fact, a careful examination would have revealed that she was totally deaf. Joy was conceived in reliance on the defendant's diagnosis of Hope. It was alleged that, as a result of the defendant's negligence, Joy was 'deprived of the fundamental right of a child to be born as a whole, functional human being without total deafness, all to her general damages' [14].

The Supreme Court, in a 4–2 opinion, allowed Joy to sue on her own behalf for the costs of special care, training and other exceptional costs that might arise. Potential recovery was denied, however, for general damages (those that cannot be specifically established by medical testimony or tangible proof such as pain and suffering and emotional distress) in an opinion which allowed the cause of action while, at the same time, accepted many of the arguments raised by other courts against the allowance of wrongful life claims [14].

In *Procanik* v. *Cillo* [18], the New Jersey Supreme Court followed California and allowed a wrongful life suit by an impaired child, but only for the 'extraordinary medical expenses attributable to his affliction …' The dependant doctor negligently misinterpreted the results of a rubella titre test which revealed that Mrs Procanik had German measles. He did not order further tests and told her she had nothing to worry about; her son, Peter, was then born with the congenital rubella syndrome. In response to the objection by sister courts that damages are too hard to calculate in the areas of wrongful life and birth, the court stated that extraordinary medical expenses incurred by parents were 'predictable, certain, and recoverable'. The damage to the fabric of the family unit – including the financial impact felt by the injured child, the siblings and the parents – was also recognized. The court did not want to risk the possibility that the parents might not be able to sue on their own behalf, arguing that:

[t]he right to recover the often crushing burden of extraordinary expenses visited by an act of medical malpractice should

not depend on the 'wholly fortuitous circumstances of whether the parents are available to sue'. [18]

Here the parents' claim was barred by the statute of limitations. The court held that:

> a child or his parents may recover special damages for extraordinary medical expenses incurred during infancy, and the infant may recover those expenses during his majority …[18]

As to the claim for special damages, *Procanik* rejected the life/non-life problem:

> … Our decision to allow the recovery of extraordinary medical expenses is not premised on the concept that non-life is preferable to an impaired life, but is predicated on the needs of the living. We seek only to respond to the call of the living for help in bearing the burden of their affliction. [18]

The court, however, rejected the claim for general damages on the grounds that 'there is no rational way to measure non-existence or to compare non-existence with the pain and suffering of his impaired existence'. They were concerned with the capabilities of the jury system and with the policy functions served by tort litigation generally. They held that:

> … it is simply too speculative to permit an infant plaintiff to recover for emotional distress attendant on birth defects when that plaintiff claims he would be better off if he had not been born. Such a claim would stir the passions of jurors about the nature and value of life, the fear of non-existence, and about abortion. That mix is more than the judicial system can digest. [18]

Speck v. *Finegold* [13] involved an infant suffering from neurofibromatosis and a series of medical failures to prevent conception rather than the more common errors of genetic counselling. The father suffered from the disease, their two previous children inherited it and the parents decided not to have more children. The father underwent a vasectomy and was told that he was sterile; nonetheless, his wife subsequently became pregnant. She then sought an abortion, which another defendant physician failed to perform properly; 4 months later, she gave birth to Francine, who had neurofibromatosis. The Pennsylvania Supreme Court held that the parents had a claim against the defendant physicians to recover expenses attributable to the birth and raising of the child, and for mental distress and physical inconvenience related to the birth. The court split evenly on the child's wrongful life claim, however, and the lower court's denial of the cause of action was, therefore, affirmed. In a later case, *Ellis* v. *Sherman* [19], the Pennsylvania Supreme Court explicitly rejected the wrongful life claim, holding that the child could not recover on its own behalf for being born diseased.

Smith v. *Cote* [15] is a 1986 decision of the Supreme Court of New Hampshire. The plaintiff had experienced a rash and fever early in her pregnancy and was treated with antibiotics; she was tested for rubella when she was in the second trimester and was found to be positive. She gave birth to a victim of the congenital rubella syndrome. The mother contended that she would have obtained a termination on eugenic grounds if she had known of the risks. The New Hampshire Supreme Court followed the standard American rule and recognized the wrongful birth claim. It also followed the emerging practice of limiting such damages to 'extraordinary costs', rather than the normal tort rule recovery of the entire cost of raising an impaired child. Such a limitation disallows recovery for the ordinary costs of child raising on the principle that the parents did plan to have the child and that ordinary expenses are the 'price the plaintiffs were willing to pay in order to achieve an expected result' [15].

The wrongful life claim, however, was rejected for the reason that has led most American courts considering it to reject it – the plaintiff's own birth and impairment is not a legal injury:

> The notion that nonexistence may be preferable to life with severe birth defects appears to contravene the policy favouring the 'preciousness and sanctity of human life'. [15]

The court gave three reasons for rejecting such suits. First, courts should not make a decision 'whether a given person's life is or is not worthwhile' [15]. The 'right to die' cases are distinguishable since, in those cases, the courts are simply protecting an individual's right to choose a natural death. The court wrote:

> The necessary inquiry is objective, not subjective; the court cannot avoid assessing the 'worth' of the child's life. Simply put, the judiciary has an important role to play in protecting the privacy rights of the dying. It has no business declaring that among the living are people who never should have been born. [15]

The second reason was that the progress achieved by the handicapped in American society in access to jobs, education and buildings might be set back by a judicial characterization of the life of a disabled person as an injury.

The third reason given by the New Hampshire Supreme Court was that of institutional incompetence. Can the trier of fact – that is, the lay jury in American civil cases – assess damages accurately and fairly? The court was worried that:

> the finding of injury necessarily hinges upon subjective and intensively personal

notions as to the intangible value of life ... The danger of markedly disparate and, hence, unpredictable outcomes is manifest. [15]

The value of the limited damage rule in the cases allowing some recovery in wrongful life cases was recognized. It was further noted that the wrongful life action would make a difference only in those rare cases in which a statute of limitations blocked the parents' right to bring their own wrongful birth suit or when the parents were unavailable to sue. But the court considered that the small benefits of damages being awarded in those rare cases were outweighed by the symbolic effect of judicial recognition of a wrongful life suit.

Two other more recent American decisions have rejected both wrongful life and wrongful birth suits. In *Azzolino* v. *Dingfelder* [16] the North Carolina Supreme Court rejected both theories. The court was worried about encouraging abortions and about exposing obstetricians to excessive liability: 'this will place increased pressure upon physicians to take the "safe" course by recommending abortion' [16]. In *Siemieniec* v. *Lutheran General Hospital* [20], the Supreme Court of Illinois rejected wrongful life as a theory of recovery. The court found that the legislative policy favoured childbirth over abortion, it expressed concern over judicial damage to the principle of the sanctity of life by encouraging such suits and it worried over the line-drawing problems which are inherent in evaluating the life of a genetically impaired infant.

American case law thus appears to be coalescing towards strong opposition to wrongful life suits and to what the courts perceive that those suits represent. Three main areas of dispute emerge: (1) the problem of calculating damages; (2) the logical dilemma of allowing a party to sue when, absent the asserted negligence, the plaintiff would not exist; and (3) the possible devaluation of human life and promotion of abortion as a result of judicial recognition of such actions.

(a) The problem of measuring damages

The first difficulty for the American courts, as the *Turpin* majority put it, is that of 'measuring damages, that is, comparing the value of impaired life against no life' [14]. The first case in which a child's wrongful life claim was rejected, *Gleitman* v. *Cosgrove* [21], is often quoted:

> The normal measure of damages in tort actions is compensatory. Damages are measured by comparing the condition plaintiff would have been in, had the defendants not been negligent, with plaintiff's impaired condition as a result of negligence.

Such a view of damages requires the courts to compare a plaintiff's impaired state to a state of non-existence.

The courts' position is that of logical impossibility, based on a process of deductive reasoning from so-called first principles of damage law. The *Turpin* court, again quoting from *Gleitman*, makes this clear:

> By asserting that he should not have been born, the infant plaintiff makes it logically impossible for a court to measure his alleged damages because of the impossibility of making the comparison required by compensatory remedies. [14]

Justice Krause, writing for the majority in *Turpin*, rejected general damages because of a perception that judges and juries would find it 'simply impossible' to decide if any impaired life is better than no life at all.

A notion of logical impossibility continues to haunt the discussion in the recent cases. The reasoning, however, is problematic. Under our system of jurisprudence, as

Alexander Capron points out: 'subjective calculations about the "value" of lives cut short, of pain and suffering, and of other intangibles, are left to juries and other legal factfinders' even when damages are difficult to assess [22]. The wrongful life cases, like personal injury cases, involve comparisons of states of suffering. Judicial recycling of the sentiments expressed in earlier cases has not advanced the state of the debate. The plurality opinion in *Speck*, advocating recognition of the wrongful life cause of action, described the position of the majority of courts as 'hyperscholastic', ignoring the reality of the existence of the impaired plaintiff:

> Those holding such views are apparently able to overlook what is plain to see: that – in cases such as this – a diseased plaintiff exists and, taking the allegations of the complaint as true, would not exist at all but for the negligence of the defendants. Existence in itself can hardly be characterized as an injury, but when existence is foreseeably and inextricably coupled with a disease, such an existence, depending upon the nature of the disease, may be intolerably burdensome. [13]

Even the California Supreme Court in *Turpin*, by allowing only limited recovery for specifically provable damages, offered no more than a halfway recovery that cannot be rationalized by normal tort principles and functions.

The dilemma of the infant's claim in the wrongful life suits continues to give American courts and state legislatures difficulty. Limiting the rights of the child by toying with damage remedies avoids the central issue of whether or not these suits fit squarely within traditional tort causes of action.

(b) Functions of tort suits: awarding, deterring, validating

A tort suit may serve a variety of functions, including compensating the injured party, deterring future negligence by the defendant and others engaged in the same activity, and articulating and validating social norms [23]. Will a wrongful life suit by the child serve any of these functions or add anything to the wrongful birth suit brought by his or her parents? I suggest that allowance of the child's suit will add a great deal to the possible beneficial efforts of tort litigation in this area.

Compensation is a central function of tort suits. Such suits offer the plaintiff an institutional means of valuing the loss and compelling payment for that loss from the responsible agent. Wrongful birth suits, now allowed by most jurisdictions which have considered the question, entitle the parents of impaired children to sue for their medical expenses, special costs in rearing the child and for the pain and suffering and emotional distress sustained; it is this last aspect which has been the sticking point in many of the cases allowing the wrongful birth action [24]. A wrongful life claim may add an important element of recovery in those cases where the child will incur special expenses, including costs of maintenance, after his age of majority. Since, in many states, the parents' obligation to support will terminate at that age, a child's claim will allow it access to resources from the negligent party. And what if the parents, having recovered their own damages, place a severely impaired child up for adoption? The fund of compensation may not get to the impaired child in such circumstances – this was the situation in *Becker* v. *Schwartz* [25]. Parents may also sit on their rights, tolling a statute of limitations, or lose the right to compensation for their impaired child in other ways. The claim by the child, therefore, serves an important function.

The deterrent function of torts suits results from the coupling of compensation with payment by the party who negligently caused the harm. Awards of damages to plaintiffs arguably 'signal' to defendants such as doctors and inform them as to how much they should invest in order to avoid future accidents [26]. In theory – and, to some extent, in practice – incentives to change can be expected to result [27]. A compensation system for injuries need not necessarily involve such a linkage; indeed, a tax-supported fund from which victims collect, modelled on the New Zealand system, might serve the compensation function more effectively [28]. The state of Virginia has recently enacted a no-fault medical mal-practice scheme which is limited to infant brain damage, creating a state fund into which obstetricians pay and against which parents of brain-injured infants may file a claim. Generally, however, the American approach to medical accidents has been distinguished by the coupling of compensation and deterrence [29]. If the child cannot sue on its own behalf, the true costs of the injury to the family unit are significantly understated and these costs are finally borne in large part by the child and the family rather than by the negligent defendants. At the same time, the defendant, by not bearing the full costs of his negligent conduct, may fail to value properly the costs and benefits of change.

The existence of a full range of causes of action and damages may be more essential in genetic counselling than in other medical areas. First, the field is new; litigation focused on standards of practice will help the field to coalesce around acceptable norms of practice; the pressure of litigation may spur practitioners to reduce the uncertainties by agreeing on norms of practice. Second, the source of the data that the physician or counsellor must interpret and translate for the parents lies in prenatal diagnostic laboratories which are, currently, underregulated and which operate under widely varying standards. Affiliation of laboratories with university medical centres, where peer scrutiny and other constraints are present, has resulted in some control but commercial laboratories are now proliferating and their lack of comparable regulation may pose problems of unacceptable error rates [30].

Concern has also been expressed that quest for profit may dominate quality control [31]. Tort suits involving such laboratories may be a spur to state regulation and are incentive for the commercial laboratories to reduce their error rates.

(c) The problem of the right: a judicial life-negating stance?

The courts in *Azzolino, Siemieniec, Speck* and in most American cases that have considered the issue have extended their objections beyond the logical problems of comparing life to non-life and the practical difficulties in evaluating damages in such cases. The judicial claim is that life is always better than non-life. This operates as a statement of substantive policy, an irrefutable presumption of the intrinsic value of life, no matter how impaired that life may be. The statement in *Berman* v. *Allen* [32] is often quoted:

> No man is perfect. Each of us suffers from some ailments or defects, whether major or minor, which make impossible participation in all the activities the world has to offer. But our lives are not thereby rendered less precious than those of others whose defects are less pervasive or less severe.

The courts are reluctant to take a position which appears to state that a life is 'wrongful', or less valuable than is non-existence. A claim for damages would, indeed, be pointless if any life, no matter how flawed, is always better than non-life. The courts have, however, missed the central issue here for two reasons. First, it is clear that we can imagine situations in which non-life may be preferable: the burn victim with nerves exposed, the elderly patient linked to medical apparatus, even the young person, like Ken Harrison in Brian Clark's play *Whose Life is it Anyway?*, who prefers non-existence to impaired life.

Many courts have, in fact, recognized that life may be intolerable in certain circumstances [33, 34]. Legislatures have taken this one step further by permitting 'living wills' [35]. The newborn nursery has come to present a new paradigm for the tension between impaired life and non-life as parents and medical staff struggle with non-treatment decisions [36]; the vitalist position too rigidly ignores quality issues [37]. Wrongful life cases often trouble the courts because the genetic impairments are not extreme – witness the hereditary deafness of Joy Turpin. Other impairments are, however, horrible and may doom the child to a short and painful existence.

The second error in the courts' arguments is to overstate the right at issue. What is that 'right'? Is the recognition of a cause of action by the impaired child equivalent to acknowledging a legal right not to be born, and is it a short step from there to judicial approval of active euthanasia? The courts fear a slippery slope of incredible angles in which judicial recognition of wrongful life claims equals approval of infanticide. This concern pervades the cases; by authorizing an action by the child, the courts will be adopting a life-negating stance. They will be making, indirectly, a negative 'social worth evaluation' [38]; they will even be encouraging abortion and euthanasia directly. Thus the North Carolina Supreme Court in *Azzolini* v. *Dingfelder* wrote:

> As medical science advances in its capability to detect genetic imperfections in a fetus, physicians in jurisdictions recognizing claims for wrongful birth will be forced to carry an increasingly heavy burden in determining what information is important to parents when attempting to obtain their informed consent for the fetus to be carried to term. Inevitably this will place increased pressure upon physicians to take the 'safe' course by recommending abortion ... Although it is not the controlling con-

sideration in our rejection of claims for wrongful birth, we do not wish to create a claim for relief which will encourage such results. [16]

The courts are struggling to affirm eroding values and to avoid the appearance of making a judgement of individual merit. They do not want to appear to decide against an individual life [39]. As a result, they have engaged in sloppy reasoning.

The 'right' at stake in the wrongful life suit is not a right not to be born; no one seeks the death now of the handicapped plaintiff. If the norm is simply a right not to be born, we find it unpalatable; the suggestion by various commentators that the tort be renamed 'diminished life' recognizes the visceral reaction on the part of courts and legislatures to the phrase 'wrongful life' [40].

The central value in these suits is neither normalcy nor a right to non-existence. Several different norms are involved and deserve judicial annunciation. The first is that of a parental right to information which derives from accepted principles of personal autonomy as reflected, for example, in the doctrine of informed consent. Parents who seek genetic counselling have a right to the communication of accurate information by a physician as to the occurrence of and risk of recurrence of genetic disorders within a family [41]. Wrongful life cases do not fit nicely within this norm, however, since one can hardly say that a fetus has a right to information. This is a weak and derivative rights claim.

The stronger norm at stake for the handicapped infant plaintiff is the right to minimize the damage to one's basic interests at birth – what Joel Feinberg has termed 'birthrights'. The child's birth with severe genetic impairments 'can doom the child's future interests to total defeat' [25]. The child has a right to be 'equipped to meet life on some sort of an equal basis' [42], by means of

compensation for his suffering and necessary medical support. As Feinberg argues:

> Talk of a 'right not to be born' is a compendious way of referring to the plausible moral requirement that no child be brought into the world unless certain very minimal conditions of wellbeing are assured ... When a child is brought into existence even though those requirements have not been observed, he has been wronged thereby; and that is not to say that any metaphysical interpretation, or any sense at all, can be given to the statement that he would have been better off had he never been born [43].

The rights at stake in these cases need to be better articulated, as part of the essential process of setting the boundaries of medical practice in an emerging field.

A second judicial concern is that wrongful life suits could be considered to assert a right to normalcy. This claim could justify state intervention in the form of a bureaucratic system of controls over reproduction so as to ensure an infant's health [44]. This may also encourage parents to adopt a eugenic perspective from which they seek abortion at the slightest sign of abnormality in a fetus. It is unlikely, however, that either circumstances will be fostered by judicial recognition of wrongful life claims of itself. A major shift in political and social attitudes must precede such a change in the regulation of the parent–child relationship. Wrongful life suits do not require or compel such a value shift, since the nature of the claim is not normalcy but, rather, compensation which will enable an impaired plaintiff and his family better to endure a state of incapacity.

REFERENCES

1. For the author's previous thoughts, see Furrow, B.R. (1983) Impaired children and the

emergence of a consensus. *Law Med. Health Care*, **11**, 148; (1982) Diminished lives and malpractice: courts stalled in transition. *Law, Med. Health Care*, **10**, 100.

2. DiMaio, M.S., Baumgarten, A., Greenstein, R.M. *et al.* (1987) Screening for fetal Down's syndrome in pregnancy by measuring maternal serum alpha-fetoprotein levels. *New Engl. J. Med.*, **317**, 342.

3. Hirschhorn, R. (1987) Therapy of genetic disorders. *New Engl. J. Med.*, **316**, 623.

4. Hershfield, M.S., Buckley, R.H., Greenberg, M.L. *et al.* (1987) Treatment of adenosine deaminase deficiency with polyethylene glycol-modified adenosine deaminase. *New Engl. J. Med.*, **316**, 589.

5. *Moore* v. *Lucas* 405 So 2d 1022 (Fla., 1981) (Larsen's syndrome in mother); *Schroeder* v. *Perkel* 432 A 2d 834 (NJ, 1981) (cystic fibrosis in another member of the family).

6. See, generally, Omenn, G.S. (1978) Prenatal diagnosis of genetic disorders, in *Health Care Regulation, Economics, Ethics, Practice* (ed. P. Abelson), American Association for the Advancement of Science, Washington, DC, p. 151.

7. Marx, J.L. (1982) Tracking genes in developing mice. *Science*, **215**, 44.

8. Dobbs, D., Keeton, R. and Owen, D. (1984) *Prosser and Keeton on the Law of Torts*, West Publishing, St Paul, sect. 55, p. 371. See also *American Law Reports* (3d, 1978 and Suppl. 1985) Lawyers Co-operative Publishing Co., New York, **83**, 15.

9. See, generally, Fain, C.F. (1986–87) Wrongful life: legal and medical aspects. *Kentucky Law J.*, **75**, 585. Recent decisions rejecting wrongful life include *Alquijay* v. *St Luke's-Roosevelt Hospital Center* 473 NE 2d 244 (NY, 1984); *Blake* v. *Cruz* 698 P 2d 315 (Idaho, 1984); *James G* v. *Caserta* 332 SE 2d 872 (W Va., 1985).

10. See, for example, Minnesota Statutes, s. 145.424, subd. 2 (1984); Missouri Revised Statutes, ch. 188.130.

11. The Act does not run to Scotland where the common law in this context has not been tested.

12. [1982] 2 WLR 890.

13. 439 A 2d 110 (Penn., 1981).

14. 182 Cal Rptr 377 (1982).

15. 513 A 2d 341 (NH, 1986).

16. 337 SE 2d 528 (NC, 1985).

17. 165 Cal Rptr 477 (1981) (negligently conducted tests on parents for Tay–Sachs disease).

18. 478 A 2d 755 (NJ, 1984).

19. 515 A 2d 1327 (Penn., 1986).

20. 512 NE 2d 691 (Ill., 1987).

21. 277 A 2d 689 (NY, 1967).

22. Capron, A. (1979) Tort liability in genetic counselling. *Columbia Law Rev.*, **79**, 618.

23. See Calabresi, G. (1970) *The Costs of Accidents*, Yale University Press, New Haven.

24. See *Becker* v. *Schwartz* 386 NE 2d 807 (NY, 1978).

25. Discussed in Steinbock, B. (1986) The logical case for 'wrongful life'. *Hastings Center Rep.*, April, **16**, 15.

26. Schwartz, W.B. and Komesar, N.K. (1978) Doctors, damages and deterrence: an economic view of medical malpractice. *New Engl. J. Med.*, **298**, 1281.

27. See Danzon, P. (1983) An economic analysis of the medical malpractice system. *Behav. Sci. Law*, **1**, 39.

28. For example, Kronick, J. (1979) Community responsibility for accident victims. *Hastings Center Rep.*, May, **9**, 11.

29. Institute of Medicine (Division of Legal, Ethical and Educational Aspects of Health) (1978) *Beyond malpractice: compensation for medical injuries; a policy analysis*, Academy of Sciences, Washington.

30. Golbus, M.S., Loughman, W.D., Epstein, C.J. *et al.* (1979) Prenatal genetic diagnosis in 3000 amniocenteses. *New Engl. J. Med.*, **300**, 157.

31. Editorial comment (1979) Prenatal diagnosis of Down's syndrome. *JAMA*, **242**, 2326.

32. 404 A 2d 8 (NJ, 1979).

33. For example, *In re Quinlan* 355 A 2d 647 (NJ, 1976), cert. denied *sub nom. Karger* v. *New Jersey* 429 US 922 (1976).

34. For example, *Satz* v. *Perlmutter* 362 So 2d 160 (Fla., 1978).

35. For example, California Natural Death Act, Cal. Health & Safety Code 7186-95 (West supp. 1977); Ark. Stat. Ann. 82-3801 *et seq.* Generally, Comment (1979) The California Natural Death Act: an empirical study of physicians' practices. *Stanford Law Rev.*, **31**, 913.

36. Shaw, M. (1977) Ethical issues in pediatric

surgery: a national survey of pediatricians and pediatric surgeons. *Pediatrics*, **60**, 588.

37. Rhoden, N. (1985) Treatment dilemmas for imperiled newborns: why quality counts. *South. Calif. Law Rev.*, **58**, 1283.

38. Shapiro, M.H. and Spece, R.G. (1981) *Bioethics and the Law*, West, St Paul, p. 471.

39. See, generally, Calabresi, G. and Bobbitt, P. (1978) *Tragic Choices*, Norton, New York.

40. Others have noted the negative weight conveyed by the attachment of the phrase 'wrongful life' to the child's cause of action. See Capron, ref. 22; Furrow, ref. 1; Mason, J.K. and McCall Smith, R.A. (1987) *Law and Medical Ethics*, 2nd edn, Butterworths, London, p. 100.

41. Healy, J. (1980) The legal obligations of genetic counselors, in Milusky, A. and Annas, G. (eds) (1980) *Genetics and the Law*, 2nd edn, Plenum, New York, p. 131.

42. Per Andreen, J., dissenting, in *Turpin* at p. 135.

43. Feinberg, J. (1984) *Harm to Others*, Oxford University Press, Oxford, p. 101.

44. Annas, G.J. (1981) Righting the wrong of 'wrongful life'. *Hastings Center Rep.*, January, **11**, 8.

CHAPTER 27

The investigation and certification of paediatric deaths

(A) In the United Kingdom

R.M. Whittington

When death occurs, the body must be examined by a medical practitioner and life confirmed to be extinct. As well as searching for signs of trauma or other indications of an unnatural death, the doctor must be satisfied that there is no condition, such as drowning of a child, which may mimic death and which may respond to treatment.

In England and Wales, the certifying doctor, who must be a registered medical practitioner [1], is obliged to issue a Medical Certificate of the Cause of Death to the best of his knowledge and belief. This document has important significance for the relatives and personal delivery with explanation of its contents to the family by the doctor forms an initial stage in bereavement counselling. The certifying doctor must have attended the deceased for the final illness within 14 days of death and he *should* examine the body if the interval is longer. The registrar must inform the coroner if neither condition is fulfilled. Although it is customary and most desirable for the doctor to notify the coroner directly, the legal obligation to do so falls on the registrar if the cause of death is not known or if it may be unnatural, being associated with trauma, neglect, inattention at birth, a therapeutic procedure, drug or poison – including food poisoning. In such circumstances, the registrar cannot register the death without authority from the coroner.

Death certificates may have important legal and epidemiological importance. Thus, trends may be recognized and hypotheses tested – such as a possible relationship between leukaemia in childhood and ambient radioactivity. Accuracy is essential. The immediate cause of death is written first, I(a), followed by any condition leading to I(a), I(b), followed by any condition leading to I(b), I(c). It is important to note that the last entry, whether it is I(a), I(b) or I(c), is recognized statistically as being the cause of death. This is the principle of the 'underlying cause of death', an example of which is shown in Fig. 27.1. Other significant conditions contributing to, but not directly causing, death are listed in Part II. Two causes of death which are considered to be of equal

CAUSE OF DEATH

*The condition thought to be the 'Underlying Cause of Death' should
appear in the lowest completed line of Part I.*

I(a) Disease or condition directly
leading to death† .... Brain abscess ....

  (b) Other disease or condition, if any,
leading to I(a) .... Chronic lung infection ....

  (c) Other disease or condition, if any,
leading to I(b) .... Fibro cystic disease ....

II   Other significant conditions
CONTRIBUTING TO THE DEATH but .... Spina bifida ....
not related to the disease or condition
causing it. ....

Fig. 27.1 Example of certification of death.

importance may be linked, e.g. 'closed head injury and lacerations of the liver'. Legibility and the avoidance of abbreviations or symbols prevent misunderstanding. Many deaths are reported by the registrar to the coroner because the medical certificate is either incomplete or is otherwise inadequate. The value of the certificate is enhanced by precision, e.g. by specifying Fallot's tetralogy rather than congenital heart disease or by indicating the primary site of any malignancy. Terms which merely describe the manner of death, e.g. heart failure or marasmus, should be avoided. Similarly, expressions that may be open to misinterpretation, e.g. asphyxia or septicaemia, need qualification. Completion of these valuable documents should not be delegated to unsupervised junior doctors until they have been thoroughly instructed.

A Certificate of Stillbirth should be completed by the medical practitioner who attended the birth or who examined the body after being informed of its birth or, in the absence of a doctor, by a registered midwife [2]. Alternatively, any qualified informant – that is, a person with immediate knowledge of the stillbirth – may make a declaration, on a distinct form, concerning the stillbirth if neither a doctor nor a midwife was present at the delivery nor was the body examined medically after the event. By definition, a stillborn child is one that issued forth from the mother after the twenty-eighth week of pregnancy and that did not at any time after being completely expelled from the mother breathe or show any other signs of life. A child which shows any signs of life once completely expelled is considered to have lived regardless of the duration of the pregnancy. If the cause of the stillbirth is not known, it may be so stated without any need to refer the matter to the coroner. The certificate of stillbirth is divided into sections which distinguish fetal and maternal causes of death although the completion of both is not mandatory. Conditions which are usually the concern of the paediatrician are considered to be fetal, those of the obstetrician to be maternal. In each section, the most important cause is given first. It is undesirable to give the mode of death, for instance, fetal distress or maceration, as the main cause. Fig. 27.2 shows an example of certification.

Following the death of a neonate, a special certificate called the Medial Certificate of Cause of Death of Live-born Children Dying within the First Twenty-eight Days of Life is used [3]. This combines the features of the medical Certificate of Cause of Death with the Certificate of Stillbirth. The cause of death is ascribed separately to diseases or conditions which affect the fetus and the mother since death under the age of 4 weeks is commonly related to pregnancy (Fig. 27.3).

	CAUSE OF DEATH
a. Main diseases or conditions in infant	Anoxia
b. Other diseases or conditions in infant	Prematurity
c. Main maternal diseases or conditions affecting infant	Pre-eclampsia
d. Other maternal diseases or conditions affecting infant	Spontaneous breech delivery
e. Other relevant causes	No antenatal care

Fig. 27.2 Example of certification of stillbirth.

When cremation is requested, the practitioner who attended the deceased sees and fully examines the body after death; he must give the cause of death on form B [4]. He must question those who were present at the death and those who cared for the patient terminally and he must be satisfied that there is no reason to inform the coroner. Form C, or the confirmatory medical certificate, has to be completed by a practitioner who has been fully registered for at least 5 years and who is neither a relative of the deceased nor of the first doctor – nor, indeed, his partner. He must examine the body either with or without a post-mortem dissection and must agree the cause of death. In the event that the death is the subject of a coroner's inquiry, forms B and C are replaced by the coroner's permission to dispose of the body (form E). Form C may be dispensed with either if the patient died in hospital and a post-mortem dissection was performed by a pathologist of at least 5 years' standing and the result is known to the doctor completing form B or if a post-mortem examination is carried out either by or on behalf of the medical referee. Final

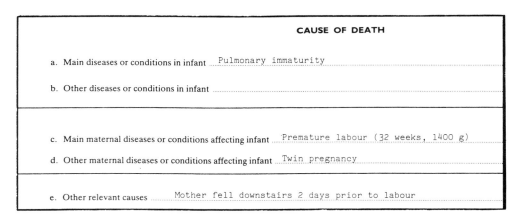

	CAUSE OF DEATH
a. Main diseases or conditions in infant	Pulmonary immaturity
b. Other diseases or conditions in infant	
c. Main maternal diseases or conditions affecting infant	Premature labour (32 weeks, 1400 g)
d. Other maternal diseases or conditions affecting infant	Twin pregnancy
e. Other relevant causes	Mother fell downstairs 2 days prior to labour

Fig. 27.3 Example of certification of the death of an infant dying within the first 28 days of life.

authority to cremate is provided by the medical referee to the crematorium – a senior doctor who is appointed for the purpose by the Secretary of State. If a stillborn child is to be cremated, only one doctor is required to examine the body and to certify the stillbirth; cremation can proceed provided the medical referee is satisfied that no other examination is needed.

In Scotland, the medical Certificate of Cause of Death is similar save that it can be completed by any medical practitioner in the absence of a doctor who attended the deceased; the date on which the patient was last seen when alive is not recorded and, consequently, there is no '14-day rule' comparable to that in England (Fig. 27.4). At the time of writing, there is no certificate

---

MEDICAL CERTIFICATE OF CAUSE OF DEATH   **FORM 11**

This certificate is intended for the use of the Registrar of Births, Deaths and Marriages, and all persons are warned against accepting or using this certificate for any other purpose. See back of this form for notes about registration of a death.

To the Registrar of Births, Deaths and Marriages

I hereby certify that

died at _____ hours _____ on _____ 19 ___
          time   *date*

at _____
                    place of death

and that to the best of my knowledge and belief, the cause of death and duration of disease were as stated below.

Registrar to enter:

Dist No.

Year

Entry No.

CAUSE OF DEATH *(Please print clearly)*		Not to be entered in register		
		Approximate interval between onset and death		
I	I	years	months	days
Disease or condition directly leading to death* a				
due to (or as a consequence of)				
Antecedent causes Morbid conditions, if any, b giving rise to the above cause. the underlying condition to be stated last c	*due to (or as a consequence of)*			
II	II			
Other significant conditions contributing to the death, but not related to the disease or condition causing it				

*This does not mean the mode of dying such as heart failure, asthenia, etc.; it means the disease, injury or complication which caused death.

Please ring appropriate letter and appropriate figure:—
Certified cause takes account of post-mortem information .... A
Information from post-mortem may be available later .... B
Post-mortem not proposed C

Seen after death by me 1
Seen after death by another medical practitioner but not by me 2
Not seen after death by a medical practitioner 3

If deceased was a married woman and death occurred during pregnancy, or within six weeks thereafter, write 'Yes' [ ]

Signature

Date   19

Name in BLOCK CAPITALS

Registered medical qualifications

Address

D2(R)
983

Fig. 27.4 The certificate of cause of death in Scotland.

This Certificate must be delivered to the Registrar of Births, Deaths and Marriages when the still-birth is registered. It is not an authority for burial or cremation. A list of the persons required to give information for the registration of a still-birth is given on the back of this form

CERTIFICATE OF STILL-BIRTH

TO BE GIVEN IN RESPECT OF ANY CHILD WHICH HAS ISSUED FORTH FROM ITS MOTHER AFTER THE TWENTY-EIGHTH WEEK OF PREGNANCY AND WHICH DID NOT AT ANY TIME AFTER BEING COMPLETELY EXPELLED FROM ITS MOTHER BREATHE OR SHOW ANY OTHER SIGNS OF LIFE

Registrar to enter
Dist. No. ....
Entry No......................
Year ....

To the Registrar of Births, Deaths and Marriages...

* *I was present at the still-birth of a* *male/female *child born*

* *I have examined the body of a* *male/female *child which I am informed and believe was still-born*

at............hours, on..............................19............, to..
(*time*)   (*date*)   (*name of mother*)

at...
(*place of birth*)

I hereby certify that the child was NOT BORN ALIVE and that, to the best of my knowledge and belief, the cause or probable cause of death, and the estimated duration of pregnancy of the mother were as stated below

CAUSE OF DEATH (Please print clearly)		Not to be entered in register
I	**I**	**Estimated duration of pregnancy**
Foetal or maternal condition directly causing death	(a).. *due to*	
Antecedent causes *Foetal or maternal conditions, if any, giving rise to the above cause, the underlying condition to be stated last.*	(b).. *due to* (c)..	.... weeks
II **Other significant conditions** *of foetus or mother contributing to the death, but not related to the disease or condition causing it.*	**II**	**Weight of foetus (if known)** .... grammes

Please ring appropriate letter:—

Certified cause takes account of post-mortem information	**A**	*Signature*.. *Date*.......................
Information from post-mortem may be available later	**B**	*Registered Medical Qualifications (or Regd. No. if a certified midwife)*..
Post-mortem not proposed	**C**	*Address*..

* Strike out whichever does not apply.

Fig. 27.5 The certificate of stillbirth in Scotland.

specially designed for neonatal death. The regulations for certifying a stillbirth are the same as those in England; the certificate, however, shows no formal distinction between fetal and maternal causes of death (Fig. 27.5). In Northern Ireland, the medical Certificate of Cause of Death can be issued only by the doctor who treated the deceased for a natural illness within 28 days prior to death. As is the case for a married woman in Scotland, pregnancy or recent pregnancy must be mentioned. A Certificate of Stillbirth is required of a midwife in the absence of a medical practitioner. In the Republic of Ireland, the medical practitioner who attended during the last illness completes the Certificate of Cause of Death. Stillbirths are not registered. Information concerning perinatal deaths is recorded in a section of the Notification of Birth form and is subsequently included in the annual vital statistics.

In England and Wales, coroners are

responsible for the investigation of violent, unnatural and sudden deaths and of deaths of which the cause is unknown [5]. Mediaeval records contain many instances of infanticide and overlaying was common in overcrowded Victorian England. Coroners still enquire into unnatural deaths in many other countries which have English legal traditions, e.g. Australia and New Zealand. Anyone who believes that a coroner should investigate a death has a duty to inform him of the fact. If a child has been brought from one locality to another for treatment, or if the dead body has been moved for some reason, the coroner for the original area, where the significant event occurred, usually holds the inquiry.

Identification is mostly made visually, although special techniques may be required following fire, mutilation or decomposition. The body must be marked with the full name immediately and continuity of identification to the pathologist must be assured (see Chapter 18); the coroner does not now have to view the body personally [6].

Mistakes in identification can happen in a busy mortuary or following a mass disaster. The problems of identifying children following, say, an aircraft accident may be greater than in the case of adults insofar as they are less likely to carry documents, to wear jewellery or to have undergone surgical or dental treatment. It is desirable for one person, probably the coroner, to maintain overall control in a major disaster situation. The bodies should not be removed until the whole area has been mapped and taped according to numbered and lettered squares and they have been photographed *in situ*. All possessions and other items that might be associated with a particular body should be left undisturbed until they have been staked and labelled according to a set routine [7]. The propinquity of a toy or doll may be especially helpful in the case of a child. The bodies should be moved to the body store *together with* the associated possessions. Ideally, one large body store is used rather than dispersal to several smaller areas. Visual identification by relatives is the preferred method although it is not always practical or appropriate. Clothing should always be preserved and may be invaluable. A further photograph should be taken in the body store together with any possessions or artefacts and whilst the body is still dressed. Odontologists may give essential help by comparing previous dental records or orthodontic treatments with their observations in the jaws and, in the case of infants, also by estimating the age from the dentition [8]. The pathologist's findings will be equally important. His report should refer to the height, weight, sex and approximate age of the child. Reference to colour, ethnic group, evidence of previous surgery, congenital anomalies or deformities and the quality of food found in the stomach are other important observations. No details should be omitted – for instance, the colour and quality of hair, whether a boy has been circumcised or whether the finger-nails are bitten. Major conflagrations present the greatest problems. As a result of fire, bodies may be welded together; great care should be taken in their separation and such work should be carried out under the supervision of a pathologist. After a large explosion, a portion of a body, such as a limb, should be treated as if it were a body and be labelled, mapped and photographed so that reconstruction can be achieved.

In general, the bodies of babies and small children should be examined by a paediatric pathologist who is equipped with a knowledge of normal childhood variations. He should assist a forensic pathologist in the investigation of suspicious deaths – an arrangement which is particularly apposite in Scotland where all such autopsies must be performed by two doctors. A full exchange of all available information must be made between pathologists when a second post-mortem examination is performed on behalf of a defendant or other interested party. The mortuary should be equipped with special instruments and scales which are sensitive to small variations in organ weight. Sometimes, only prolonged investigation in the pathological laboratory reveals a cause of death which amends an initial diagnosis of sudden infant death syndrome (see Chapter 10). Parents then need to be informed so that feelings of uncertainty and guilt can be alleviated.

If organ transplantation is contemplated – and this appears to be increasingly the case in paediatric practice – permission from the coroner is not required unless the death is of a type which falls within his jurisdiction. In such an instance, he would need to be satisfied that irreversible brain stem death has been established properly [9]. The coroner may prohibit transplantation of organs but he cannot authorize it; formal sanction must still be obtained from the person in lawful possession of the body, usually the hospital administrator, who must have no reason to believe that there are any objectors within the family [10]. In appropriate cases, it may be helpful to the coroner if his pathologist is present when donor organs are harvested.

One purpose of the perinatal autopsy may be to establish whether one is dealing with a fetal death or a stillbirth. Determination of the age of the subject may be particularly important when the child is killed *in utero*; the offence of child destruction is committed if the fetus is capable of being born alive [11]. The relationship of this to attacks on the mother is referred to in Chapter 27b. An unusual example occurred in England when a dead fetus, believed to be of 24 weeks' gestation, was delivered during emergency hysterectomy after the mother received bullet wounds to the pelvis; the fetus was subsequently shown to be of 27–28 weeks' maturity with a clear potential for a separate existence [12].

The pathologist must be provided with a history of events and should visit the scene in appropriate cases. The presence at the autopsy of any doctor who treated the child and who can explain some of the clinical details is a most valuable adjunct. In this way, suspicious bruises on a baby's face and neck were correctly attributed to hurried attempts at intubation during unsuccessful resuscitation. A whole-body X-ray examination prior to the autopsy may be indicated and is regarded by many pathologists as an essential part of the investigation of apparent cot, or crib, deaths. Organ analysis can be invaluable, especially if the toxicologist's advice is sought at an early stage. The importance of a search for poisons is discussed in Chapter 17 and of the use of biological, as well as toxicological, methods in the investigation of deaths associated with anaesthesia in Chapter 21.

Some babies die from inattention at birth. It is an offence to conceal a birth [13] or for untrained non-professional persons to attend a woman in labour except in an emergency [14]. For inattention at birth to be established as a cause of death, the pathologist must find a condition which might have been prevented by proper obstetric management. The baby must be without significant congenital defects and to be capable of an independent existence. Most cases involve a teenage mother who has either concealed her pregnancy, is unprepared for delivery or fails to recognize the symptoms of labour; prosecutions are very rare.

It is, however, inevitable that the police must investigate the unexplained deaths of babies. Fatal injuries – including those due to suffocation – may not be associated with any external marks. Parental explanations can be notoriously unreliable and child abuse comes in many guises. In one case, in an attempt instituted by a stepfather to stop bed-wetting, a toddler was prevented from drinking and died from dehydration. Infanticide in England and Wales is a specific offence which can only be committed by the mother [15] and is discussed in detail in Chapter 12; otherwise, the killing of a baby is just as much murder or manslaughter as is the killing of an adult and may result from a positive act or from omission. Death caused by lack of care, involving a neglect of duty, is an example of the latter – such as when an epileptic child dies from status epilepticus in a residential institution because of an inexcusable failure to administer prescribed anticonvulsant drugs. Recklessness which results in an unlawful death occurs, for example, when a person follows a course of action knowing that there is a risk of endangering life and heedless of the safety of others. There is often an element of persistence or repetition which is, not infrequently, associated with neglect. The pathologist must look for evidence of such behaviour which is characteristic of many deaths following non-accidental injuries. It is essential that natural disease is excluded in any case in which a charge of murder is contemplated.

An example of the importance of this is to be found in *R* v. *Arthur* [16] which is also referred to in Chapters 8 and 28. In brief, Dr Arthur, who directed that nourishment and medical treatment be withheld from a baby with Down's syndrome while, at the same time, prescribing dihydrocodeine to alleviate the accompanying distress, was charged with murder. The charge was, however, reduced to attempted murder when histological investigations indicated that there was pre-existing natural disease; Dr Arthur was acquitted. This relatively new concept of selective non-treatment, or what might, in some circumstances, be termed iatrogenic neglect, is discussed in depth in Chapter 8.

Fatal injury in a child may be self-inflicted but is not necessarily suicidal. To be so, the child must intend his or her actions, be personally capable of such actions and understand the likely consequences. Children tend to fantasize, to experiment and to be unaware of risks; consequently, suicide is unlikely to be established with any certainty – although older children, say over 14 years, might leave a note of intention. The intention in taking poisons may be naive. In one case, for instance, a child took an overdose of tricyclic drugs in a once-for-all bid to cure his enuresis. In cases of hanging, it must be established that the child was capable of tying the knot and the marks on the body should be carefully matched with the ligature – suicide by children is rare and the practice of sexual asphyxia is unlikely in the prepubertal child. The investigation of accidental deaths in general is discussed in Chapter 20.

The coroner in England and Wales usually only holds an inquest when death is unnatural [17]. Rarely he may need to hear evidence, even if death to be natural, as to whether death was aggravated by lack of care. More often, he may have to adjourn the inquest to allow for completion of tests to confirm the precise cause of death which may, eventually, be shown to have been natural. Normally should a death reported to him be shown as natural, he will notify the registrar so that the death can be registered. It is unusual now for a coroner at an inquest to hear the evidence before a jury. If similar deaths may be preventable, the coroner will notify the appropriate authority so that safeguards may be taken [18]. The investigation of cases of infanticide, murder, manslaughter or causing death by reckless driving is now subject to the authority of the Director of Public Prosecutions (Crown Prosecution Service) to whom the coroner refers the matter even when the possibility of a named person having killed unlawfully only becomes apparent after the inquest has opened [19]. The process of drawing evidence is inquisitorial in nature. Witnesses are questioned by the coroner and are sometimes examined by lawyers or others with an interest. Documents and exhibits, e.g. hospital notes or a faulty child's bicycle, may be produced. Doctors may be summoned to give the cause of death, to give evidence as to how this occurred and, at times, to express an expert opinion. No one is obliged to give evidence that will incriminate him or herself and both witnesses and interested persons may be legally represented. No conclusion should be reached unless it is substantiated by the evidence – for instance, without good cause, no opinion should be expressed that a fourth cot death in a family may not have been natural [20]. The finding of the court is reflected in the verdict which must be expressed without ascribing blame. Following the finding, the coroner issues a Coroner's Certificate of Death after Inquest. The coroner may, as a result of his inquest, announce that he proposes to write to such persons in authority with the power to promote measures to prevent further deaths in similar circumstances [18].

Coroners' decisions may be challenged whether they are taken before or during an inquest. In addition to the verdict of the court, matters such as ordering a post-mortem examination [21] or a refusal to release a body may be affected. An application may be made by an interested party for judicial review by the Queen's Bench Division of the High Court [22]. The potential grounds for review are errors of law, excess or want of jurisdiction, procedural defect, breach of natural justice or unreasonableness. Inquests or other decisions may be quashed or a fresh inquest may be ordered. Alternatively, the Attorney-General may make application to the High Court which, in turn, can order an inquest to be held or a fresh inquest to be convened [23]. The latter may be necessary if fresh evidence has come to light which might have altered the verdict had it been available.

In Scotland, the function of the coroner is filled by the procurator fiscal. Any informed party, usually the doctor but, statutorily, the registrar, can notify him when a death falls into one of those categories agreed between the Crown Office and the Registrar General as falling to be reportable by statute [24] and which, in general, correspond to those reportable to the coroner. The fiscal will then instruct the police and a police surgeon – who may or may not be the fiscal's pathologist – to investigate the death. There will be no suspicious circumstances in the majority of cases and, in such circumstances, the certificate of Cause of Death will be provided either by the police surgeon or by a practitioner nominated by the fiscal. A post-mortem examination will be authorized by the sheriff on the petition of the fiscal if the police surgeon is unable to certify a cause of death or if the fiscal considers that there may be negligence or criminality involved – the autopsy will always be performed by two doctors in the latter case and may be in the former. The cause of death will, then, be certified by the pathologist. There will be no further action in the event of death being due to natural causes; otherwise, the course of action will be determined by the fiscal's precognition of witnesses – a form of inquiry which is taken in private. The whole process is, therefore, free from publicity until there is a definitive hearing, which may be in the criminal court or may take the form of a public hearing under the Fatal Accidents and Sudden Deaths Inquiry (Scotland) Act 1976. The circumstances in which a fatal accident inquiry *must* be held are irrelevant to paediatric practice. An inquiry may be held, however, when it is considered expedient in the public interest on the grounds, *inter alia*, that the circumstances were such as to give rise to serious public concern; a member of the public may also petition the Lord Advocate that an inquiry be held. An inquiry might, therefore, be held if a child was killed in a playground; most commonly, however, one would be precipitated by a death due to medical mishap. The inquiry is before a sheriff who sits without a jury but who may have the help of an expert assessor; unlike the coroner, the sheriff may determine such matters as the factors behind the cause of the accident, the reasonable precautions which might have prevented the accident and whether any persons are to blame. The findings cannot be used in any later civil or criminal proceedings. Something under 2% of cases reported to the procurator fiscal proceed to a fatal accident inquiry but these will include those industrial deaths for which an inquiry is obligatory.

The coroners' system in Northern Ireland is governed by the Coroners Act (Northern Ireland) 1959. Section 7 details the types of death which must be reported. These correspond, in general, to those in England and Scotland but the Act makes it clear that the doctor, and many others involved in the lawful disposal of the body, has a duty to report such a death immediately and directly to the coroner.

(B) In the United States

Boyd G. Stephens

The medicolegal investigation of perinatal deaths in the United States is limited to cases where there is a high probability of death having been directly caused by unnatural, traumatic, chemical or iatrogenic means. Natural deaths are rarely involved in such an investigation.

The laws pertaining to the investigation of death are based on English Common Law and require the coroner to determine the cause, circumstances and manner of certain deaths. Any person having knowledge of an un-natural or sudden and unexpected death is required to report the matter. The certificate of any death which is due either to unnatural cause or manner can only be signed by the coroner or medical examiner, whose jurisdiction starts at the moment of death. On his own authority, he can investigate and, in most states, can perform an autopsy or initiate whatever testing is necessary to determine the facts. The investigation may include an inquest, with or without a jury, but, in either case, the coroner certifies the cause and manner of death in all the cases he investigates. The decision to hold an inquest in a given case rests with the coroner or medical examiner, but some states provide

that other public officials – for example, the district attorney – can instruct him to hold an inquest. In many jurisdictions, the coroner is considered to be a 'law enforcement officer' and, in some regions, the office is under or within that of the sheriff. In most areas, it is a lay position. These relationships reflect the historical background of the office.

There is considerable variation between states both in their laws and in their operation of the coroner's system. Each state establishes its own procedure, and there are no relevant federal regulations. Even within a state, some counties may use a medical examiner while others will prefer the services of a coroner. Moreover, there is some variation within state medical examiner systems which reflect local considerations within the jurisdiction.

Major urban communities excepted, the use of the medical examiner system is still the exception rather than the rule. Most jurisdictions rely on lay coroners and, overall, there is no requirement that autopsies or investigations be performed by a physician with medicolegal training; most state laws simply direct that an autopsy be performed by a licensed physician, without any requirement that the prosector have training in either pathology or forensic pathology. Some lay coroners perform to the same standards as medical examiners but there is wide variation in practice and experience throughout the country. By contrast, it can be firmly said that, despite the absence of any legal requirement, medicolegal autopsies or investigations will always be performed by physicians with medicolegal training within the medical examiner system.

The medical examiner is involved as the sole investigator at the scene of many deaths; however, in cases of suspicious death or possible homicide, he will be present as part of the investigating team of police and crime laboratory personnel. Most medical examiners work closely with the judicial system, and relate medical findings in an unbiased fashion for both prosecution and defence, as appropriate, in criminal cases. A medical examiner is always a physician and is usually board certified in forensic pathology. He derives authority from state laws and, being medically trained, he differs from the coroner in that he is able to perform forensic autopsies and to make medical interpretations and conclusions independently of other support. The district attorney is notified when the coroner or medical examiner makes a finding of death at the hands of another and it is he who takes the final decision on prosecuting the case, based on the evidence at hand.

While the medical examiner system is being adopted increasingly frequently, the majority of the approximately 3000 counties in the United States still use the coroner system under which, in some cases, non-physicians – whose concern is only for the cause of death – perform autopsies. In the worst of these systems, there might be neither an investigation of a perinatal death nor an autopsy because 'nothing would be found'.

Perinatal death investigations require special knowledge and techniques [25]. These cases are among the most difficult to separate as to a natural or unnatural manner, even when they are investigated by an experienced forensic pathologist with both paediatric training and a good understanding of normal and abnormal gestational changes. As has been discussed in Chapter 18, trace evidence plays a less important role in the investigation of infant death than does the gathering and interpretation of medical information yet, unfortunately, paediatric pathology is a young field and forensic paediatric pathologists are rare. It has been said that:

> This field of medicine is different from others in that the cause of death is not best determined by the autopsy, which frequently does no more than demonstrate 'how' the fetus died and not 'why' [26].

A well-defined protocol for a perinatal investigation is an important step for improving both the quality and completeness of the necessary studies [25, 27, 28].

Such a protocol should include a classification of perinatal deaths which is based on the primary cause of death of the fetus or neonate, along with an understanding of the pathophysiology leading up to that death. It should include consideration of intrauterine trauma, both mechanical and chemical, as well as of the complications of labour and delivery. It should also allow for evaluation of the many complications that can become evident in the neonate, thus helping to separate natural from unnatural deaths. The avoidance of such uninformative terms as 'fetal anoxia' by which to describe the mechanism of death leads to a more complete investigation and diagnosis. Besides fulfilling the responsibility for detecting any unnatural death or potential public hazard, accurate information and diagnosis concerning the fetus and placenta are gathered and, thereby, it is possible to identify genetic, toxic or traumatic changes which are of significance to the parents of the dead child or to society as a whole.

Serological tests for paternity and tests for sexually transmitted diseases are important for court presentation when incest or sexual assault is the basis for pregnancy and abortion is, for some reason, not an adopted option. In normal circumstances, the death of such a child from natural conditions would be considered in the same light as that of a child resulting from a normal pregnancy, even through the conception gave rise to a legal problem. The two matters – the conception of the child and its death – would, ordinarily, be handled separately. There is more frequent involvement of the courts when some complication of the pregnancy takes it out of the class of a normal gestation [29].

Once implantation has occurred, a termination of pregnancy is considered to

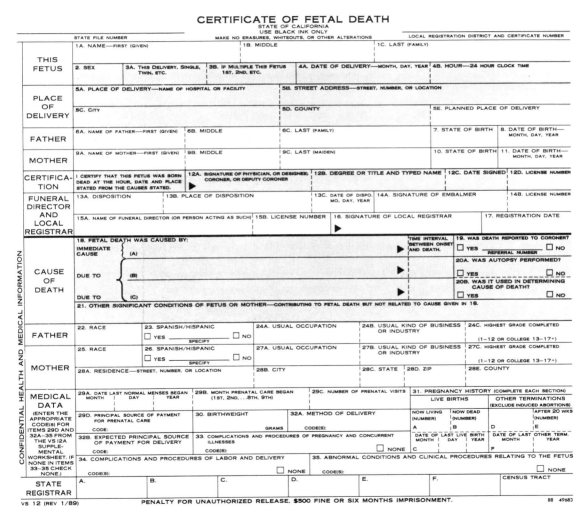

Fig. 27.6 Certificate of fetal death (California).

be abortion [29, 30]. Ending fetal life after the point in time of viability must be justified in the United States by an adequate medical or physical reason if the procedure is to be legal [31]. Medicolegal investigations of abortion are predominantly undertaken when it is illegal; what constitutes legal abortion is regulated by public law or court decisions. The position in the United States is dominated by the decision in *Roe* v. *Wade* (410 US 113 (1973)) [32], as a result of which, the major medicolegal question to be answered is: has the child reached a gestational age which is compatible with life separate from the mother? This age is accepted in the United States as being between 24 and 26 weeks [32] and defines when a death certificate (Fig. 27.6) or non-viable birth certificate must be completed (the definitive time is 20 weeks in California). Prior to this, a simple record of stillbirth is completed and, in some areas, the fetus may be treated as a surgical specimen. The assessment of fetal age is discussed in Chapter 6.

Identifying the parents or the mother of an abandoned fetus is a common problem. Usually, the circumstances of abandonment are such that direct information leading to the mother is lacking. The difficulties have been addressed specifically in Chapter 6. Here, it is only remarked that a search of the community for information on a pregnant girl or woman is sometimes rewarding. Even when such a lead is developed, a court-ordered physical examination or warrant for search of the residence may be needed to show, in the face of denial, that the female has delivered recently. Constitutional rights prohibit self-incrimination in cases of potential homicide; the investigation may be able to proceed only to a certain point and will then become a matter for the courts. In all these situations, the medical examiner plays a part – and, sometimes, a critical part – in collecting evidence and, in particular, providing evidence as to the gestational and develop-mental status of the fetus and as to the presence or absence of a cause of death.

Concealed births resulting in a dead child often occur among juvenile parents who have some reason for not seeking medical care; the issue of distinguishing between stillbirth and infanticide is then raised. Even when the fetus is recovered immediately, the determination of the manner of death is difficult unless the mechanism is obvious – such as blunt or penetrating trauma. Neglect, with attendant hypothermia, is difficult to prove; the demonstration of a single inhalation of breath is seldom easy and the probability of live birth is often supported by no more than normal anatomic findings in the baby, cord and placenta and by the scene investigation. The finding of meconium or squamous cells in the respiratory system may be supportive of intrauterine hypoxia but must be interpreted carefully in the light of all the known facts of the case. If possible, drug analysis should be performed on the infant's tissues in all cases in which an accident or homicide is being considered.

No fetal right to be conceived or carried to completion is recognized in the United States nor is there a clear right to normal development – a matter which has been discussed in some detail in Chapter 26. Nonetheless, reasonable rights against being injured by mechanical or chemical trauma may be guaranteed by the state – as is the right to representation and redress in the courts when those rights are violated. This area of litigation is likely to grow in the civil courts and will occasionally involve the criminal process. Issues of the fetal-alcohol syndrome and of drug dependence raise the potential for a legal obligation on the part of the parents, and, particularly, the mother, to ensure the fetus' well-being (see Chapter 3). Improper care or endangerment of the fetus in this way is sometimes used as a basis for the legal removal of the child from its mother's care after birth [33].

Life within the uterus is a particularly vulnerable time for the child. Totally dependent on the mother, the fetus is subject not only to any toxins assimilated by the mother but also to any trauma delivered to her abdomen [34, 35, 36]. Homicide of the mother, or even major trauma to the abdomen, can result in injury or death of the child; in such circumstances, homicide of the mother can result in allegations of two counts of murder. This issue requires testimony in court supporting three points:

(i) That the fetus has reached the point of viability,
(ii) that the fetus did, in fact, receive trauma or that trauma to the mother was directly proximal to the effects on the child, and
(iii) that trauma was proximal to the death or injury of the child.

Each of these opinions will have to be supported by evidence in court. Killing more than one person carries an increased legal penalty in many jurisdictions, so the issues of viability and of proximal cause are likely to be looked at carefully by the court and by defence counsel. Ageing the fetus in such a case is generally accomplished by measurement of length, head size and weight and by demonstration of centres of ossification as described in Chapter 6; hospital and office medical records are supportive of the date of conception and of normal development until the time under consideration. There must be a reasonable relationship between the trauma and the child's death but it is to be noted that trauma to the uterus which is sufficient to cause intrauterine death of the fetus may not be sufficient to cause recognizable injury to its body. When injury *is* caused, it is usually in the form of intracranial haemorrhage although injuries to solid organs sufficiently severe to cause death from bleeding are also found; the most usual findings, however, are those of abruptio placentae or cord injuries which are sufficient to cause hypoxia.

Penetrating trauma to the fetus is less common but is much easier to relate to cause and effect [34]. Careful attention having been paid to the evidence of injury, intrauterine hypoxia or other traumatic changes, death would then be certified, if appropriate, as to the relative traumatic death and the manner would be listed as an accident or homicide, depending upon the specific circumstances.

Accidental injury of the mother resulting in death of the fetus alone, or the death of both, is investigated in a similar manner. On finding a causal relationship, the fetal death would be certified as accidental. The cause of the trauma, e.g. a car seat-belt, should be noted whenever possible [36, 37]; valuable data are, thereby, gathered for the modification of current design or practice, the ultimate goal being to reduce the potential for future similar injuries. The safety and welfare of the people are directly improved when this information is defined, published and reported to the appropriate regulatory or controlling agencies – and this includes its presentation in court; unfortunately, these opinions are usually advisory only and have little legal force although they may still be used for purposes of bioengineering.

A new dimension to 'fetal rights' is developing along with the increasing capabilities for intrauterine diagnosis and treatment [38]. But, in exercising a right to improved medical care, the fetus also exposes itself to increased risk – and this risk includes the possibility of death. As previously explained, investigations by the medical examiner typically pertain *only* to unnatural death -- and especially to accidental or homicidal death. Whether or not an untoward effect of an intrauterine process which was considered necessary for the survival of the fetus should be classed as an accident may seem to be a minor issue, but it is not. Some of these procedures are extremely experimental and there is little or no precedent by which to judge the correctness of the operator's technique. It will often be the case that a determination as to whether the physician acted properly or not must be based on no more than an assessment of the degree of understanding of the risks by the mother and the gravity of the situation warranting the surgical intervention. Death resulting from the procedure will be an accident but, before it is so classified, the autopsy must demonstrate some reasonable basis on which to associate the invasion directly with the death, such as bleeding from a needle tract; a complication of therapy itself may be registered as an accident without suggesting malpractice.

On the other hand, there is room for comparison of techniques and confidence when a relatively common technique is carried out in a major centre. A finding that the death could have been prevented or that some untoward event caused the death of an otherwise salvageable fetus is potential for finding the death to be accidental.

It is not unheard of for homicide to be a real consideration in perinatal deaths. An uncommon mechanism is the deliberate administration of a drug or toxin to infants. Whatever the reasons, e.g. the so-called 'Munchausen's Syndrome by proxy', these cases are rarely suspected by the initial treating physicians. The motivation for such acts is circuitous and only a high rate of suspicion and the in-depth investigation of unusual clinical presentations or complications can lead to the early detection of such cases which appear to be most common in teaching hospitals. In one instance, a mother repeatedly gave baking powder to one child and then, on that child's death, to another before poisoning was suspected. The resulting hospitalizations and diagnostic procedures employed in order to define the cause of the explosive, life-threating diarrhoea and alkalosis in the first child literally resulted in a 'million dollar' work up. A number of rare secretory tumours and metabolic conditions were considered but the possibility of exo-genous poisoning was not entertained until a second child developed the same symptoms on the anniversary of the first child's death. Careful consideration of the disease process accompanied by a high index of suspicion could have saved the first child [39].

Poisoning of infants from accidental sources – or as an undesirable result of medication – is often not recognized immediately. Usually several children become seriously ill or die before the connection is made between the death and the cause [33, 38, 40–42]. Physicians do not readily include unnatural causes in their differential diagnosis of medical complications even though the literature indicates that the incidence of such events is increasing. Such considerations are warranted in the perinatal period, when no recognized aetiology for the condition is apparent [33, 41, 43].

Delivery by registered midwives is increasing in frequency throughout the United States. There is, however, a contingent of illegal midwives operating whose training, equipment or medical support is inadequate in cases of complicated childbirth. A significant number of perinatal deaths involve the questions: 'Was the child born alive or would the complication leading to the death have been reasonably prevented in the hands of an experienced person?' These cases can be very difficult to investigate as the mother frequently has beliefs which are supportive of the midwife or a fear of the authorities. When the investigation so indicates, these deaths are certified as homicide or accident, depending upon the findings. Depending upon the circumstances, an illegal midwife who is directly responsible for the death of a child may be tried for murder or manslaughter.

Clinical considerations relating to the treatment of defective newborns have been discussed in Chapter 8. Similar problems arising in the United States have led to wide-ranging legal discussion at both court and legislature level. The case of 'Baby Doe'

[44–47] precipitated federal action designed to ensure that handicapped, malformed or otherwise impaired newborns received all possible life-sustaining treatment without any regard to their chances for survival or the quality of that survival. Subsequent court action and Congressional response resulted in the Child Abuse Amendments of 1984 (later, further amended in 1985) which, effectively, stated that withholding medically indicated treatment from a newborn infant would not be child abuse if the infant was in a state of irreversible coma, when treatment would merely prolong dying and when treatment would be futile or inhumane [48]. Since these conditions relate directly to the possibility of a legal charge against a physician or nurse who chooses not to resuscitate or otherwise support a child that he or she deems unlikely to survive, they have considerable impact on the practice of medicine. The legal investigation involves the determining of live birth and a search for evidence of some action taken to either accelerate the death or inaction to prevent it. The physician is now, according to federal law, required to resuscitate and maintain life in cases of significant birth defects not diagnosed *in utero* but which do not meet the criteria of severity outlined above; implementation of the federal Child Abuse Prevention and Treatment Act 1974 is, however, a matter for the individual states.

The administration of narcotics to 'reduce the pain' of the dying infant must be considered carefully. Such procedures should be performed in accordance with an established hospital protocol which delineates the type, amount and frequency of such administrations. The policy also should state the circumstances in which such administration will be allowed and if any other potentiators are authorized. In some cases, large doses of analgesic agents are administered only for their respiratory depressant effects – in order to accelerate death. This may help the family or the emotions of the staff but, even if the practice is acceptable, the use of medication in this way should follow a defined procedure rather than depend upon the decision of an individual. Several such cases have been reported as homicides, usually by a member of staff who is concerned about the ethics of or motivation for such high-dose administration. Currently, euthanasia is not authorized in any jurisdiction in the United States and a homicide charge could be brought against the physician if it was proven that euthanasia was the basis for the drug administration. Each facility should have written policies pertaining to the use of drugs for the dying patient, regardless of his or her age, as well as a policy for high-dose analgesia for patients with malignant disease and others suffering from a temporary or terminal condition in which unusual levels of medication for the relief of pain are considered.

Careful investigation of apparent cases of the sudden infant death syndrome is required because of the effects on the parents, the question about the risk to subsequent children, the potential of a health hazard to other children and, most significantly, the need to delineate an aetiology and, thus, to reduce the loss of life (see Chapter 10). These cases frequently involve suspicion of wrongdoing, of infectious disease or of concern about a recent childhood immunization. Careful investigation, including scene investigation by an experienced person, is essential in order to ensure that no accident or homicide is missed and that the natural death is adequately documented. It is in this type of death investigation that the medical examiner system particularly shows its superiority to that controlled by the US coroner.

Abuse of children in the perinatal period is predominantly associated with lack of care. These cases are often regarded medically as 'failure to thrive' and, indeed, care is required in excluding malabsorption or other natural reason for inadequate growth and development. Direct physical injury is commonly presented as an accidental injury (see Chapter 18) and discretion must be used in accepting statements to that effect without considering the possibility of actions by another party. The proper documentation of bite-marks or other patterned injuries not only allows the medical examiner to consider whether they were caused by another child or animal but also helps to protect the physician in the event of future difficulties. Accidental injuries due to burns, especially those in which there is a pattern, are uncommon in a child who is not yet able to toddle and must always be considered carefully as having been inflicted by another.

The recognition of the consequences of injury to the fetus and abuse of the neonate is rapidly increasing in the United States. The resulting waste of life and the custodial costs to society are great and a new emphasis on improving the quality of developing life and, consequently, ensuring the newborn the best chance of survival in today's world is evolving. The medicolegal system provides a main instrument by which these public demands can be satisfied.

REFERENCES

1. Medical Act 1983, Parts II and III. A doctor in his pre registration year may certify the death of a patient within his care.
2. Nurses, Midwives and Heath Visitors Act 1979, s.10.
3. Registration of Births, Deaths and Marriages (Amendment) (No. 2) Regulations 1985 (SI 1985/1133).
4. Cremation Regulations 1930 (SR & O 1930/1016 as amended); Cremation (Scotland) Regulations 1935 (SR & O 1935/247 as amended).
5. Coroners Act 1988, s.8.
6. Coroners Act 1988, s.11.
7. Mason, J.K. (1978) The aircraft accident as an example of a major disaster, in *The Pathology of Violent Injury* (ed. J.K. Mason), Edward Arnold, London.
8. Ashley, K.F. (1970) Identification of children in a mass disaster by estimation of dental age. *Br. Den. J.*, **129**, 167.
9. Conference of Royal Medical Colleges and their Faculties in the United Kingdom (1976) Diagnosis of brain death. *Lancet*, **ii**, 1069.
10. Human Tissue Act 1961, ss.1(1), (2), (5).
11. Infant Life (Preservation) Act 1929, s.1.
12. *R. v. Pagett* (1983) 76 Cr App R 279.
13. Offences Against the Person Act 1861, s.60.
14. Nurses, Midwives and Health Visitors Act 1979, s.17.
15. Infanticide Act 1938.
16. *R. v. Arthur* [1981] *The Times*, 6 November, pp. 1, 12.
17. Coroners Act 1989 s.19.
18. The Coroners Rules 1984 (SI 1984/552), r. 43.
19. The Coroners Rules 1984 (SI 1984/552), r. 28.
20. *Med. Sci. Law*, 1987, **27**, 68.
21. *R v. Greater Manchester Coroner, ex parte Worch and another* [1987] AC LER 66.
22. Supreme Court Rules, order 53.
23. Coroners Act 1988, s.13.
24. Registration of Births, Deaths and Marriages (Scotland) Act 1965, s. 28.
25. Macpherson, T.A., Valdes-Dapena, M. and Kanbour, A. (1986) Perinatal Mortality and Morbidity: the role of the anatomic pathologist. *Semin. Perinatol.*, **10**, 179.
26. Davies, B.R. and Arroyo, P. (1985) The importance of primary diagnosis in perinatal death. *Am. J. Obstet. Gynecol.*, **152**, 17.
27. Valdes-Dapena, M. and Huff, D. (1983) *Perinatal Autopsy Manual*, Armed Forces Institute of Pathology, Washington, DC.
28. Barson, A.J. (1981) The perinatal postmortem, in *Laboratory Investigation of Fetal Disease* (ed. A.J. Barsen), Wright, Guildford, pp. 476.
29. Kolder, V.E.B., Gallagher, J. and Parsons, M.T. (1987) Court-ordered obstetrical interventions. *New Engl. J. Med.*, **316**, 1192.
30. Munir, A.E. (1984) Perinatal rights. *Med. Sci. Law*, **24**, 31.
31. Samuels, A. (1988) Contraception, pregnancy, childbirth – when things go wrong. *Med. Sci. Law*, **26**, 39.
32. Lenow, J. (1983) The legal ramifications of fetal therapy. In *Perinatal Practice and Malpractice*, Academy Professional Information Services, New York.
33. Hill, L.M. and Kleinberg, F. (1984) Effects of

drugs and chemicals on the fetus and newborn. *Mayo Clin. Proc.*, **59**, 755.

34. Timms, M.R., Boyd, C.R. and Gongaware, R.D. (1985) Blunt and penetrating trauma during pregnancy: four cases. *J. Med. Assoc. Ga.*, **74**, 158.

35. Kiely, J.L., Paneth, N. and Susser, M. (1985) Fetal death during labor: an epidemiologic indicator of level of obstetric care. *Am. J. Obstet. Gynecol.*, **7**, 721.

36. Nichols, M.M. and Weedn, V.W. (1986) Placental laceration and stillbirth following motor vehicle accident: with legal ramifications. *Texas Med.*, **82**, 26.

37. Fakhoury, G.W. and Gibson, R.M. (1986) Seat belt hazards in pregnancy. *Br. J. Obstet. Gynaecol.*, **93**, 395.

38. Robertson, J.A. (1985) Legal issues in fetal therapy. *Semin. Perinatol.*, **9**, 136.

39. Author. Case in preparation for press.

40. Balisteri, W.F., Farrell, M.K. and Bove, K.E. (1986) Lessons from the E-Ferol tragedy. *Pediatrics*, **78**, 503.

41. Hiller, J.L., Benda, G.I., Rahatzad, M. *et al.* (1986) Benzyl alcohol toxicity: impact on mortality and intraventricular hemorrhage among very low birth weight infants. *Pediatrics*, **77**, 500.

42. Sacks, D.A. and Koppes, R.H. (1986) Blood transfusion and Jehovah's Witnesses: medical and legal issues in obstetrics and gynecology. *Am. J. Obstet. Gynecol.*, **154**, 483.

43. Morris, R.A. and Sonderegger, T.B. (1986) Perinatal toxicology and the law. *Neurobehav. Toxicol. Teratol.*, **8**, 363.

44. Angell, M. (1986) The Baby Doe rules. *New Engl. J. Med.*, **314**, 642.

45. Stevenson, D.K., Ariagno, R.L. Kutner, J.S. *et al.* (1986) The 'Baby Doe' rule. *JAMA*, **255**, 1909.

46. Smith, G.P. (1985) Defective newborns and government intermeddling. *Med. Sci. Law.*, **25**, 44.

47. Reynolds, W.B. (1984) Parental rights versus government responsibility for infant medical care. *Conn. Med.*, **48**, 527.

48. Cantor, N.L. (1987) *Legal Frontiers of Death and Dying*, Indiana University Press, Bloomington, pp. 156–170.

FURTHER READING

Bissenden, J.G. (1986) Ethical aspects of neonatal care. *Arch. Dis. Child.*, **61**, 639.

Coulter, D.L. (1987) Neurologic uncertainty in newborn intensive care. *New Engl. J. Med.*, **316**, 840.

Goldsmith, L.S. and Horwitz, B. (1983) Legal aspects of genetic and antenatal counseling, in *Perinatal Practice and Malpractice (Symposium, 1983)*, Academy Professional Information Services, New York, pp. 36–42.

Paul, R.H., Yonekura, M.L., Cantrell, C.J. *et al.* (1986) Fetal injury prior to labor: does it happen? *Am. J. Obstet. Gynecol.*, **154**, 1187.

Perone, N., Carpenter, R.J. and Robertson, J.A. (1984) Legal liability in the use of ultrasound by office-based obstetricians. *Am. J. Obstet. Gynecol.*, **150**, 801.

Sims, M.E., Turkel, S.B., Halaterman, G. and Paul, R.H. (1985) Brain injury and intrauterine death. *Am. J. Obstet. Gynecol.*, **151**, 721.

CHAPTER 28

Parental rights and consent to medical treatment of minors

David W. Meyers

Just as the wishes of parents and of their children may collide, so too may their rights; this is nowhere more evident than in decision-making in the area of medical treatment. It is common practice for parents to consent to medical treatment on behalf of their children because the young child can comprehend neither the nature of nor the consequences of that treatment. However, the child's level of comprehension and understanding expands as he or she grows and matures and, along with this, the ability to choose and consent increases; the need for parental protection and judgement lessens correspondingly. The general purpose of this chapter is to consider whether the right or obligation of the parents to make medical treatment choices for their child diminishes in parallel with the need to do so.

We will see that parents enjoy broad discretion under the law in this respect; but we will also see that certain basic limits are imposed on that discretion on both sides of the Atlantic. We will look at these limits and at the role of parental rights of choice for the medical treatment of their children; in doing so, we will examine the comparative position in the United States and in Great Britain. It will be seen that recent advances in medical

science have had a major impact on this area of the law and that this has resulted in some significant decisions in a field which has, until recently, seen few developments. Some of these decisions have created considerable controversy and, arguably, have raised as many new questions as they have answered.

THE UNITED STATES

28.1 THE BASIS OF PARENTAL RIGHTS TO CONSENT

In the United States, the rights of parents to consent to medical treatment for their minor children derive from the rights of parents to control the upbringing of their children. These rights are constitutional in scope and, as a result, they attract substantial deference. All law, whether statutory or judge made, is subordinate to the Constitution which is the highest law of the land.

Nevertheless, parental rights of control over the rearing of their children are not recognized expressly in the Constitution; rather, they have been recognized judicially as enjoying constitutional protection [1]. This protection flows from the implicit constituional right of privacy which is afforded to all individuals. The right of privacy exists in order to prevent undue governmental intrusion into peoples' private lives. It protects 'fundamental' individual rights from undue scrutiny or regulation by the State. This right of privacy has been extended so as to cover individual choices concerning contraception, marriage, procreation, child rearing, child education and, even, the right to possess pornographic materials in the privacy of one's own home [2]; however, consenting adults have, as yet, no similar right to engage in sodomy in private [3].

In the context of medical treatment, the Supreme Court has decided that this right of privacy grants a woman a right to abort her fetus in certain circumstances [4]. However, it apparently does not give a patient, even one who is terminally ill, the right to obtain drugs which are not yet approved by the government as being safe and effective [5]. Although it has not yet been expressly decided by the Supreme Court, it, nevertheless, seems clear that the right of privacy embraces 'the freedom to care for one's health' within its ambit of fundamental rights [6]; one can think of few more basic rights than those involving health care decision-making, which may well affect one's very survival.

Parents who make medical treatment decisions on behalf of their minor child are, in effect, exercising that child's personal right of privacy. Several limitations apply to this surrogate decision-making. First, parents are given this responsibility only for so long as their child is unable to exercise it personally. Second, the substitute decision must be seen to be in the child's 'best interests'; a right to parental control over medical treatment for children does not permit exposing the child to 'ill-health or death' [7].

The State will step in to protect the child if the parents seek a course of medical treatment or non-treatment which will jeopardize its health or safety. The discretion afforded to parents carries with it the clear responsibility not to make decisions which are contrary to the child's best interests. The State will intervene as *parens patriae*, or substitute parent, if such occurs or is threatened. Child welfare or protective agencies exist in all the United States and the courts have recognized their authority to perform this role for the benefit of the minor – and will continue to do so. The difficulty lies in deciding what precisely is in the child's 'best interests' and, in many cases, this inquiry will boil down to one of medical productivity – do the likely benefits to the child outweigh the pain or risks of undergoing the treatment?

Parents cannot, for example, refuse blood which is needed for a severely traumatized child because of their own religious convictions. The child may or may not share these views when capable of deciding for himself. Accordingly, the courts have consistently overruled such refusals by Jehovah's Witnesses and have ordered treatment for the child. Likewise, parents cannot neglect to provide life-saving medical treatment or nourishment for their child because they believe in faith healing or in divine intervention. A failure to act for the benefit of the child in such circumstances is likely to be regarded as criminal neglect in the form of reckless homicide [8].

The point here is that the right to privacy, like nearly all other personal freedoms guaranteed by the Constitution, is not absolute. A balancing necessarily occurs. Often, the interests of the State will compete with and challenge the exercise of individual liberties. The State's interests will likely take precedence when they are deemed 'compelling' – or fostering a significant government interest. Thus, the State has an interest in preserving and protecting the physical health and well-being of its citizens; this will be particularly so when those citizens are dependent on others because of age or of mental or physical disability. The State's interest in protecting its children becomes compelling when serious disability or death is threatened unless the State intervenes in the medical treatment decision at hand.

Let us now look more specifically at when the child will be allowed to make his or her own treatment decisions. Having done this, we can examine the circumstances in which the State will intervene or override a parental decision on the basis of the child's 'best interests'.

28.2 WHEN CHILDREN MAY DECIDE THEIR OWN MEDICAL TREATMENT

Parents make treatment decisions for any of their children who are unable to give an informed consent. In order to give an informed consent, a minor must be able to comprehend the nature and consequences of the treatment proposed – including the intention behind it, its material risks and the alternatives available. The last include non-treatment, the consequences or risks of which should also be understood.

The question then devolves into whether the child *can* give an informed consent. If so, treatment can proceed in the absence of parental consent. However, because of the deeply ingrained deference which is normally afforded to parental responsibility for their children, efforts will usually be made to locate the parents and to obtain their consent before proceeding. The law considers that consent of the parents is implied by the circumstances when the situation presents as an emergency requiring immediate action to protect the health of the minor; even then, however, the few cases which have considered the issue suggest that, although it may be, perhaps, unnecessary, efforts should still be made to locate an available parent and to obtain his or her consent before proceeding with treatment [9].

Parental consent to the proposed treatment must be obtained when the child is unable to give an informed consent and when parental consent is not implied due to an emergency need to treat:

> A minor of any age who is unable to convince competent medical authorities that she has the requisite understanding and maturity to give an informed consent for any medical treatment, including a therapeutic abortion, will be denied such treatment without the consent of either a parent or legal guardian [10].

The issue of informed consent is one of understanding; it follows that no arbitrary age can be set before which either parental consent is always required or the child's consent is never adequate by itself. Children have different levels of comprehension and understanding at different ages and those of the same age vary widely in their maturity. One child at the age of 12 may be perfectly capable of giving an informed consent to a particular medical treatment whereas the next of the same age may understand neither its nature nor, equally importantly, its consequences, risks and alternatives. Moreover, one form of treatment may be much simpler, more obviously beneficial and less risky than another and, thereby, require a different level of understanding.

The concept of what is sometimes referred to as the 'mature minor' rule has been raised particularly in cases concerned with whether or not abortion is available to a minor in the absence of parental consent. The Supreme Court, concerned to prevent undue interference with or restriction of a woman's right to abort in the exercise of her constitutional right to privacy, has struck down statutes which prohibit abortions for minors without parental consent as being unnecessarily restrictive. However, a statutory requirement that parents be notified before the abortion is carried out is permissible provided that an expeditious court review procedure is readily available to the minor in order to determine whether she is capable of giving an informed consent or whether other good cause supports the abortion despite the parents' opposition [11]. The courts concerned have not specified any particular age which must be attained before the minor's consent alone will be deemed legally sufficient for the abortion to proceed. For example, abortion has been upheld despite the lack of parental consent in several recent cases in which 14- and 15-year-old girls have been adjudged sufficiently mature to make an informed decision. The same result has been obtained in the case of a 12-year-old girl. In this particular instance, however, the pregnancy was rape-induced and its continuance could have endangered the child's life; her best interests thus provided the court with an independent basis on which to authorise the abortion. The reasoning in these cases seems to be equally, if not more, clearly applicable to medical treatment decisions for minors in general since the latter will not involve any possibly conflicting fetal interests.

Some states have recognized that the child's ability to give an informed consent often precedes his or her legal majority at age 18 by a number of years. For example, the California guardianship-conservatorship statute requires the consent of a minor aged 14 years or older to medical treatment unless this is excused by court order or by an emergency necessitating prompt treatment to save life or limb [12]. It would seem that, absent unusual circumstances, the child will be legally presumed to have sufficient understanding of most medical procedures to enable him or her to give (or refuse) consent to them by the age of 14. The presumption, while strong, will, of course, be rebuttable based on the understanding and maturity of the child, his or her physical condition and the nature of the treatment proposed.

Some statutes authorize treatment to proceed on the basis of the minor's consent alone regardless of the child's age. California,

for example, authorizes minors to consent to treatment for pregnancy at any age or to treatment for contagious disease or for any alcohol- or drug-related problem at age 12 [13]. The age of fertility becomes the minimum age of consent in the case of pregnant minors; the courts have, however, imposed the additional requirement that 'the minor must be of sufficient maturity to give an *informed consent* to any treatment procedure' [10]. Thus, where the child cannot give or refuse an informed consent to treatment, it must be given or refused by a parent or a legal guardian. They are substitute decision-makers, their responsibility being to decide what is in the child's 'best interest'. It is here that there may be disagreement between parents, physicians, public agencies and the courts. 'Best interest' is a standard which is easy to recite but one which is, at times, not easy to apply.

28.3 TREATMENT IN THE 'BEST INTERESTS' OF THE CHILD

When the child does not have sufficient comprehension to give an informed consent to medical treatment, the parents are generally considered to have the responsibility to give or refuse consent [10] and their decision will be respected in most cases. However, others may seek to override the parents where they are felt not to be acting in the 'best interests' of the child. The local child welfare agency may be called upon to determine whether the interests of the child require the removal of custodial care and decision-making from the parents and court action for the appointment of a legal guardian may be the result. In other instances, members of the treating team – nurses, doctors or hospital administrators – may petition the local court directly for authority to proceed with such treatment as is considered necessary for the child's welfare.

The strong presumption that the decision of the parents should be respected which exists in American law is rooted in two major principles, one of which is old while the other is quite new. The older principle holds that, so far as is possible, the family as a unit should be able to function as it chooses to do; this is a matter of social policy which is applied in order to foster and promote the family as an independent, self-sufficient entity. The new principle is that embodied in the emerging constitutional right of privacy which has been described on p. 429. The law mirrors the traditional responsibility and privilege of parents to control and shape the nurturing and upbringing of their children. As the Supreme Court has stated:

It is cardinal with us that the custody, care and nurture of the child reside first in the parents, whose primary function and freedom include preparation for obligations the state can neither supply nor hinder [7].

However, strong as the presumption in favour of respect for parental decision making may be, it is circumscribed by the interest of the State – as *parens patriae* of all children among its citizens – to protect and promote the health of those children. In the event of a conflict, the State will intervene when it is clear that respecting the wishes of the parents will expose the child to a serious health risk which is otherwise avoidable. Normally, this will take the form of action by the local child welfare or child protection agency for custodial and guardianship powers. This does not mean that every unwise, unpopular or even unreasonable decision by parents concerning the medical treatment or non-treatment of their child will be subject to challenge. On the contrary, the parents' action or inaction will be supervened only when it is considered to amount to abuse or neglect. In fact, such instances will rarely be reported or opposed and even more rarely will they be determined, following investigation

and/or litigation, to be sufficiently grave to justify the imposition of judicially appointed guardianship. As stated recently by one court:

Inherent in the preference for parental autonomy is a commitment to diverse life-styles, including the right of parents to raise their children as they think best. Legal judgments regarding the value of the child rearing patterns should be kept to a minimum so long as the child is afforded the best available opportunity to fulfill his potential in society.

Parental autonomy, however, is not absolute. The state is the guardian of society's basic values. Under the doctrine of *parens patriae*, the state has a right, indeed, a duty, to protect children. [Citation]. State officials may interfere in family matters to safeguard the child's health, educational development and emotional well-being.

One of the most basic values protected by the state is the sanctity of human life (U.S. Const., 14th Amend., 1.). Where parents fail to provide their children with adequate medical care, the state is justified to intervene. However, since the state should usually defer to the wishes of the parents, it has a serious burden of justification before abridging parental autonomy by substituting its judgment for that of the parents.

Several relevant factors must be taken into consideration before a state insists upon medical treatment rejected by the parents. The state should examine the seriousness of the harm the child is suffering or the substantial likelihood that he will suffer serious harm; the evaluation for the treatment by the medical profession; the risks involved in medically treating the child; and the expressed preferences of the child. Of course, the underlying consideration is the child's welfare and whether his best interest will be served by the medical treatment. [14]

One of the most significant rules which protect a broad range of parental discretion in this area is that which honours the decisions of parents if they are supported by accepted and reasonable medical judgements. It is very unlikely that parents' decisions will be overridden when they have made a choice between accepted schools of reasonable medical practice.

This remains true even when the child's condition is life-threatening. Several recent cases illustrate this. New York's highest court has held that the parents may choose nutritional and metabolic treatment recommended by a licensed physician rather than more conventional and proven but more intrusive chemotheraphy and radiotherapy for their 8-year-old son gravely ill with Hodgkin's disease [15]. The same court has honoured the wishes of the parents of an infant born with multiple defects – which included spina bifida, microcephaly, hydrocephalus, spasticity and brain stem abnormality – to elect against aggressive surgical treatment of the spinal and cerebral malformations [16]. The infant's life expectancy was about 2 years without surgery; with the proposed treatment it was estimated to be about 20 years but would be accompanied by severe retardation, epilepsy, paralysis, frequent infections and confinement to bed. Medical opinion differed as to what level of treatment was appropriate. The parents opted to proceed with conservative, non-invasive treatment – nutritional, antibiotic and hygienic care; the courts refused to overrule their choice because this had been made from among several reasonable medical treatment plans.

Two quite controversial decisions – one from California, the other from Indiana – show that the courts can, at times, be accused of losing sight of the child's best interests when confronted with a parental decision against treatment that is supported by one body of reasonable medical opinion [14, 17]. The US Supreme Court was petitioned in both cases but declined to review either decision, both of which upheld parental decisions against treatment.

In the California case [14], the local child protective agency sought to have the 12-year-old boy in question declared a ward of the juvenile court. California, as do most other states, empowers the local child protective agencies by statute to make custodial guardianship decisions for the child in place of the parents upon a judicial determination that the parents are failing to provide him or her with the 'necessities of life' – which include food, shelter and basic medical care. The subject was a boy with Down's syndrome including a heart defect that was amenable to surgical correction carrying a mortality risk of less than 10%. Without surgery, his life was shortened to about 20 years of slow and painful physical deterioration. His parents, who had institutionalized him many years before, refused consent to surgery. In declining the request for guardianship, the court, presumably, concluded that the productivity – or likely benefit – of the surgery was insufficiently clear to justify removing custody from the parents on the grounds of their failing to provide basic medical care. The decision seems wrong. The reviewing court approached the case too narrowly, only inquiring whether there was some evidence to support the trial judge's decision rather than examining what appeared obviously to be in the child's best interests. Fortunately, although several years later, another court found the latter to be best served by transfer of the boy's custody to foster parents. Although this was partly because of their expressed support for the surgery, it was, by that time, unclear whether his advanced age had rendered the operation no longer feasible [18].

In the Indiana decision [17], the parents of a newborn infant with Down's syndrome refused consent to surgical relief of an intestinal blockage. The operation was not difficult and, without it, the child would die from starvation within a week. Evidently, the child suffered from at least one other serious congenital physical defect, perhaps involving the heart, and differences of medical opinion existed as to whether this was amenable to surgical correction without unacceptable risks. The precise condition and prognosis of the infant are not, however, known as the record in the case was ordered sealed – a practice which is common in those involving minors.

The hospital in which the baby was born sought that surgery be authorized by a court-appointed guardian. The court denied the petition but, at the same time, referred the matter to the child welfare authorities for investigation and such action as was felt necessary; the local agency elected not to intervene. This strongly suggests that substantial and reputable medical opinion supported the decision of the parents. The Indiana appellate courts declined to grant review in the case, as did the Supreme Court – although, by that time, the infant had died.

These cases make it clear that it is highly unlikely that the courts will compel treatment when faced with parental objections which are supported as proper by sound medical judgement, even if the treatment objected to is life-saving in nature. In effect, the courts recognize that they are no more competent to decide such questions than are parents and attending physicians – matters are best left to them except in the case of manifest abuse; except where motive or standard of care are questioned, they are the individuals most directly and intensely concerned with the best interests of the child.

This is not to say, however, that judges will not at times overrule both parents and physicians. The courts are, after all, the final arbiters of what is best for the child, just as they are also the final arbiters of what constitutes acceptable and proper medical practice [19]. Some courts have concluded that medical treatment should be undertaken to improve the physical condition of an infant no matter how hopeless may be the eventual prognosis or how limited is the quality of physiological existence that will result; these cases are, however, noted by their rarity. The reason for the paucity of such decisions is quite apparent. Parents cannot be found unfit, or guilty of neglect or of abuse, when their motives are unquestioned and when their decision is supported by sound and responsible medical opinion. There is little authority for the courts to interfere with the parents' rights of control and decision-making for their own child when no unfitness, neglect or abuse are found. At times, however, the overriding obligation to protect the child's best interests will justify such action [20].

THE UNITED KINGDOM

28.4 INTRODUCTION

While less case precedent has developed in Britain, the legal position as to parental consent rights appears remarkably similar in the United Kingdom and the United States despite the different constitutional frameworks which prevail. In general, the American courts and statutes seem to give minors somewhat greater rights to consent to treatment than is the case in England; historically, however, greater autonomy has been given in Scotland to children who have reached the age of puberty than arises under the common law of either England or the United States.

28.5 THE GILLICK DECISION

The much-discussed *Gillick* case [21] involved the issue of whether the Department of Health and Social Security could rightly advise doctors that they could legally provide birth control or pregnancy advice or treatment to girls under the age of 16 without the consent of their parents. Following conflicting decisions in the court of first instance and in the Court of Appeal, the House of Lords decided that such action was proper in certain circumstances. It also had much to say on the general subject of parental authority over medical treatment decisions for minors.

The Family Law Reform Act 1969, s.8 provides that children over the age of 16 years can give a valid consent to medical treatment in England and Wales. There is no need for parental consent in such circumstances. The Lords rejected the argument that the implication deriving from the statute was that the minor under the age of 16 years was *not* capable of giving consent; in effect, they confirmed the widely held opinion that s.8(3) of the Act reasserts the common law position of the 'mature minor' [22]. An arbitrary age limitation, it was said, should not foreclose the ability to give consent if the minor is 'capable of understanding what is proposed and of expressing his or her own wishes'.

The law lords in *Gillick* considered whether parental 'rights' concerning their children required that the parents' consent be obtained before contraceptive advice or treatment could be given irrespective of the child's level of understanding. Parental rights over their children were seen as existing for the benefit of the children, not of the parents. They exist to the extent necessary to parents to perform their duties of bringing up their children, not so that parents can carry out their own wishes without regard to the best interest of the child. As Blackstone had written (1 Bl. Com., 17th ed., 1830 at p. 452): 'the power of parents over their children is derived from ... their duty'. Custodial rights of parents over their children necessarily carry with them the right to control but, as children mature, so also do their independence and judgement increase –

and the need for and the degree of parental control diminishes correspondingly. The rule has been succinctly stated by LORD DENNING MR as follows:

> ... the legal right of a parent to the custody of a child ends at the eighteenth birthday and, even up till then, it is a dwindling right which the courts will hesitate to enforce against the wishes of a child, the older he is. It starts with a right of control and ends with little more than advice. [23]

Gillick makes it clear that parents do not enjoy absolute rights to decide for their children which are based on the particular age that the child has, or has not, attained. The fact that one child is aged 15 and another 16 does not mean that the consent of the parent is necessary before medical treatment can properly be undertaken in the case of the younger child – and this holds whether it be a matter of giving contraceptive advice or of setting a broken wrist. The determinative factor is whether the child has adequate understanding to consent for himself.

It is further clarified that such parental rights of control over a child as exist are to be exercised for the protection and benefit of the child. The more mature the child, the less is he or she in need of protection and, accordingly, the more limited are the parents' rights and duties to decide on treatment for the child. Lord Scarman summed up the legal position:

> It is that parental right yields to the child's right to make his own decision when he reaches a sufficient understanding and intelligence to be capable of making up his own mind on the matter requiring decision.

Gillick, in effect, concludes that the English legal position, similar to its American counterpart, allows the minor to decide medical treatment decisions below the age of 16 if he is able to give an 'effective consent'. However, this seems to be a rather different concept from both the earlier English and the

American 'informed consent' doctrines and one which arguably turns 'the issue of consent into an issue of wisdom' [24].

The decision reaffirms the basic principle that children can decide for themselves if they are capable of understanding the nature and purpose of the treatment at issue. This is good. It also seems sensible to require that the child understand the risks posed and the benefits anticipated by the treatment, the reasonably available alternative treatments, if any, and their consequences – including the alternative of non-treatment and its consequences. The majority of the Lords in *Gillick*, however, went beyond this definition of 'informed consent'. For example, Lord Scarman suggested that, for a girl's consent to contraceptive advice to be adequate alone, she must understand and appreciate the moral and family questions involved, the emotional impact of pregnancy and its termination and be able to 'appraise these facts'. Williams has commented that '[t]his wraps the notion of consent in considerable murk' [24]. No clear standard of 'effective consent' to medical treatment by minors emerges from the case. As a result, it has been suggested that, in order to avoid liability and to establish certainty, the areas of consent below the age of 16 should be established by statute, similarly to the ability to drive, drink or vote [25].

Lord Scarman's opinion in *Gillick* has potentially broad implications. It suggests an element of a moral awareness in giving consent that could be difficult to find in many cases where the minor may be otherwise perfectly capable of understanding the nature, purpose and risks of the treatment proposed. Lord Scarman stated:

> In light of the foregoing I would hold that as a matter of law the parental right to determine whether or not their minor child below the age of 16 will have medical treatment terminates if and when the child achieves a sufficient understanding of what

is involved to give a consent valid in law. Until the child achieves the capacity to consent, the parental right to make the decision continues save only in exceptional circumstances.

The doctor's responsibility was set out by Lord Fraser in what was, perhaps, the most important speech from the point of view of the profession. He tabled five criteria which had to be met before the doctor would be justified in proceeding without the parents' consent or knowledge:

(1) The girl would, although under 16 years, understand his advice;
(2) he could not persuade her to inform her parents or to allow him to inform the parents that she was seeking contraceptive advice;
(3) she was very likely to have sexual intercourse with or without contraceptive treatment;
(4) unless she received contraceptive advice or treatment her physical or mental health or both were likely to suffer; and
(5) her best interests required him to give her contraceptive advice, treatment or both without parental consent.

Taken as a whole, *Gillick* has done little to ease the lot of either the physician or the patient in the United Kingdom. Thus, the latest authoritative advice to doctors [26] runs:

> When a child below the age of 16 consults a doctor for advice or treatment, and is not accompanied at the consultation by a parent or a person *in loco parentis*, ... the doctor should satisfy himself, after careful assessment, that the child has sufficient maturity and understanding to appreciate what is involved. ...

> If the doctor is satisfied of the child's maturity and ability to understand ... he must nonetheless seek to persuade the child to involve a parent ... If the child

nevertheless refuses ... the doctor must decide, in the patient's best medical interests, whether or not to offer advice or treatment ...

If the doctor is not so satisfied, he may decide to disclose the information learned from the consultation; but if he does so he should inform the patient accordingly, and his judgement concerning disclosure must always reflect both the patient's best medical interests and the trust the patient places in the doctor.

In general, therefore, great discretion is accorded to the physician but the patient can derive little satisfaction from the last possibility which, in effect, puts the onus on the child to prove his or her maturity before being guaranteed confidentiality. *Gillick* does, indeed, seem to have settled very little and there is a real need for clarification. It is noteworthy that, on a simple headcount, more judges favoured Mrs Gillick's position than supported the Department of Health and the diversity of the speeches in the House of Lords undoubtedly complicated the issue. The test of a child's maturity, it seems, should be a simpler more liberal one based on reasonable understanding [24, 27]. It is, however, important to appreciate that *Gillick* was concerned with contraception which is an intensely emotional subject. The judgement can probably be extrapolated to treatments of all types but it seems unlikely that, in doing so, it would be necessary to adopt all the subtleties which the case engendered.

28.6 THE POSITION IN SCOTLAND

It might, indeed, be easier to revert to the common law position which exists in Scotland – where *Gillick* does not state the law. Medical treatment undertaken without consent could constitute unlawful, criminal assault as in England and America. However, the issue of 'informed consent' has not been addressed in the Scottish courts; it is possible that Scots' law would hold that the patient need only understand the nature of the intended medical treatment in general terms for consent to be valid. It is fair to say, however, that some reasonable understanding of the consequences of any treatment would also be needed whether consent was given by an adult or by a child [27].

There is little doubt that a child aged less than 16 may validly consent to medical treatment under Scots' law provided he or she can understand and can know the nature of the act in question. In Scotland, the presumed power of parental control over a child's person has existed historically only so long as the child is a pupil – that is, until reaching minority at the age of puberty, 12 years for girls and 14 for boys [27]. Thereafter, the child, *if capable*, is no longer burdened with the presumption of parental control over personal decisions concerning treatment. Since a girl cannot conceive until puberty, a *Gillick*-type case related to contraception would raise issues only of an intellectual capacity to consent, not of age.

The question is still open as to whether a Scots' pupil could consent to treatment legally. The answer would seem to be that there is no reason why not but this, again, would depend upon the pupil's capacity to understand [28]; clearly, such understanding would be more difficult to show in a prepubertal child and the complexity of the treatment to which valid consent could be given would be correspondingly less – but the principle remains undisturbed.

28.7 THE BEST INTERESTS OF THE CHILD

In the United Kingdom, parental consent to or refusal of treatment will be overruled by the courts even where the child is found incapable of giving consent if such is necessary for his or her physical welfare [29, 30]. The child's best interests are superior to any parental rights of consent. Abortion has been ordered for a 15-year-old girl in deference to her wishes and understanding [29]. Surgery to correct intestinal blockage in a neonate with Down's syndrome has been ordered over parental objection [30]. Sterilization of a seriously disabled 11-year-old girl has been refused despite parental request, yet the operation has been ordered for a severely retarded 17-year-old minor [31].

In the most recent of these cases, the House of Lords concluded that sterilization of a 17-year-old girl was necessary to protect her welfare and best interests. Given a mental age of 5 or 6, she would be unable to comprehend the connection between intercourse, pregnancy and birth; she would be unable to care for a child; and pregnancy posed serious mental and physical risks to her well-being. The Lord Chancellor distinguished an earlier decision in which sterilization was refused as being violative of the woman's right to procreate. It was said that such right existed only when reproduction was the result of informed choice – of which the 17-year-old was not capable. A recent Canadian decision [32], refusing to authorise sterilization of incompetents if this was for 'non-therapeutic' purposes, was rejected as violating the principle of doing what is best for the minor in the particular case.

The Lords concluded that they must authorize the sterilization, to promote the best interests of the unfortunate young woman, as being the only practical means of avoiding 'uncomprehending fear and pain and risk of physical injury' from pregnancy. The case strongly reaffirms the inherent power of the judiciary to require any medical treatment which is shown by the facts to be clearly in the minor's best interests. The difficulty of applying a 'best interests' analysis lies in its subjective element. What constitutes best interest may be unclear when serious quality of life factors enter the picture as, for example,

in the case of defective newborns [14, 18, 30, 33–35]. In such situations, the principle may be interpreted so as to authorize treatment which offers more benefits, more enjoyment of life than the burden it imposes. Yet, at times, this is no easy matter to decide [33].

In a case involving an infant with Down's syndrome, *Re B*, the court made clear that its duty was to determine what was in the best interests of the child, notwithstanding the parents' refusal to consent and the concurring views of the surgeon. Without treatment, the child would die from starvation within a week; the probability was that, given surgery, she would live for 20–30 years. There being no evidence that her disabilities would make her life 'intolerable' (per DUNN LJ) or 'demonstrably ... so awful' (per TEMPLEMAN LJ), the Court of Appeal concluded that it must order treatment. Although 'due weight' was to be given to the decision of the parents, and although medical opinion was divided, the court was required to exercise its own independent judgement as to what was best for the infant's welfare. Her pain, if any, was not so severe and unremitting as to make existence intolerable; surgery was both feasible and productive. Accordingly, the judges had little hesitation in finding that the infant's interests required that it be treated and its life preserved.

Re B is correct. It is also valuable in making it quite clear that mental disability *per se* is an inadequate reason for withholding life-saving medical treatment. Rather, the prospect must be of 'severe' and 'certain' physical pain and suffering before a parental decision to refuse treatment is likely to be upheld. However, this is an area in definite need of more clearly articulated medical treatment standards [35]. The law should strive for consistency and predictability in its application – and these attributes are currently in some doubt given the conflicting results in *Re B* and *Arthur* [30, 34].

CONCLUSION

What strikes one is the similarity of legal analysis and result on both sides of the Atlantic in dealing with parents' rights to consent to or refuse medical treatment for their children. These rights are respected and afforded great deference; they are, however, subject to definite restriction.

First, parents may not abuse or neglect the physical well-being of their children by refusing to consent to necessary medical treatment. The welfare or best interest of the child is given legal priority over the custodial or decision-making rights of parents. What is in the child's best interests may not always be clear. Significant and sincerely held differences of judgement may exist between parents and doctor, or between parents and the state. Nonetheless, as we have seen, broad discretion will be given to both parents and doctors in this sensitive area [14–18, 33].

Second, children may increasingly decide for themselves as they gain the ability to understand the nature and consequences of the treatment proposed. Although the law has set arbitrary age limits for various entitlements, such as marriage, voting, driving and drinking, no particular age can be accepted as proof of entitlement or ability to decide upon medical treatment or be relied upon to deny a minor the right to consent.

The courts will be called upon to decide what is best for the child in cases where doctors and parents do not agree or where alleged child abuse or neglect is reported. If the child is found to understand the nature and consequences of the treatment, then he or she can and should decide. Where such is not the case, the court will decide what is in the child's best interests. In effect, this will mean that such decisions will be based upon what adult judges think most children would want done in the circumstances.

The existing infrastructure of decision-making seems to have worked well and there are few reported cases of abuse. Thus, family- and physician-based decisions should be the norm. Child welfare agencies are available to investigate the concerns of interested parties and to seek guardianship if necessary. Finally, if needed, the courts are available to protect the interests of the child. The courts are equipped to hear and to resolve cases in which parents may have abused their custodial responsibilities and in which informal efforts by other family members, physicians, friends or the welfare authorities to persuade on the proper cause of action have been unsuccessful. In the last analysis, it is they whom society has empowered to strike the balance between the rights of parents and children.

REFERENCES

1. *US* v. *Orito* 413 US 139 (1973); *Meyer* v. *Nebraska* 262 US 390 (1923).
2. *Stanley* v. *Georgia* 394 US 557 (1969).
3. *Doe* v. *Commonwealth Attorney for Richmond* 425 US 901 (1976).
4. *Roe* v. *Wade* 410 US 113 (1973).
5. *US* v. *Rutherford* 442 US 544 (1979).
6. *Doe* v. *Bolton* 410 US 179 (1973) (concurring op. by Mr Justice Douglas).
7. *Prince* v. *Mass* 321 US 158 (1944).
8. *Hall* v. *State* 493 NE 2d 433 (Ind, 1986).
9. *Bonner* v. *Moran* 126 G 2d 121 (DC App, 1941).
10. *Ballard* v. *Anderson* 4 Cal 3d 873 (1971) at 883.
11. The stated rule is that 'the State must provide an alternative procedure whereby a pregnant minor may demonstrate that she is sufficiently mature to make the abortion decision herself or that, despite her immaturity, an abortion would be in her best interests'. *City of Akron* v. *Akron Center for Reproductive Health, Inc.* 462 US 416 (1983) at 439–40. The court cannot deny a minor's petition for abortion for good cause unless it first finds the minor is not mature enough to make her own decision. See *Planned Parenthood Ass'n* v. *Ashcroft* 462 US 476 (1983) at 492.
12. California Probate Code § 2353 (1981).

13. California Civil Code §§ 34.5, 34.7, 34.10.
14. *Re Phillip B* 92 Cal App 3d 796 (1979) at 801, cert. den. 445 US 949 (US S Ct, 1979).
15. *In re Hofbauer* 393 NE 2d 1009 (NY, 1979).
16. *Weber* v. *Stony Brook Hospital* 456 NE 2d 1186 (NY, 1983), cert. den. 104 S Ct 560 (1983).
17. *Infant Doe* v. *Bloomington Hospital* No. 4825140 (Ind. 1982), cert. den. 464 US 961 (US S Ct, 1983).
18. *Guardianship of Philip B* 139 Cal App 3d 407 (1983).
19. *Sidaway* v. *Board of Governors of the Bethlem Royal Hospital and others* [1984] QB 498 (CA), [1985] AC 871 (HL); *Texas and P.R. Co.* v. *Behymer* 189 US 468 (1903).
20. *In re Baby M* 191 Cal App 3d 786 (1987) (emotional harm to child sufficient to deny parental custody without any showing of parental unfitness).
21. *Gillick* v. *West Norfolk and Wisbech Area Health Authority* [1985] 3 All ER 402.
22. For discussion of s.8(3) see Mason, J.K. and McCall Smith, R.A. (1987) *Law and Medical Ethics*, 2nd edn, Butterworths, London, p. 145.
23. *Hewer* v. *Bryant* [1970] 1QB 357.
24. Williams, G. (1985) The Gillick saga – II. *New Law J.*, **135**, 1179.
25. Parkinson, P.N. (1986) The Gillick case – just what has it decided? *Fam. Law*, **16**, 11.
26. General Medical Council (1987) *Professional Conduct and Discipline: Fitness to Practise*, April 1987, paras 83–85.
27. Norrie, K. McK (1985) The Gillick case and parental rights in Scots law. *Scots Law Times*; see also Smith, T.B. (1962) *A Short Commentary on the Law of Scotland*, W. Green, Edinburgh, p. 370.
28. Norrie, K. McK. (1983) Contraceptives, consent and the child. *Scots Law Times*, 285.
29. *Re P (a minor)* (1982) 80 LGR 301.
30. *Re B (a minor)* [1981] 1 WLR 1421.
31. Compare *Re D (a minor)* [1976] Fam 185 (no sterilization) with *Re B (a minor)* [1987] 2 All ER 206 (sterilization ordered).
32. *Re Eve* (1986) 31 DLR (4th) 1.
33. See Meyers, D.W. (1989) Selective non-treatment of handicapped infants. In *Legal Issues in Human Reproduction* (ed. S.A.M. McLean), Gower, Aldershot.
34. *R* v. *Arthur* (1981) *The Times*, 6 November, pp. 1, 12. (Physician who ordered no feeding and drugs for a Down's syndrome infant found not guilty of attempted murder.)
35. Mason, J.K. and Meyers, D.W. (1986) Parental choice and selective non-treatment of deformed newborns: a view from mid-Atlantic. *J. Med. Ethics*, **12**, 67.

CHAPTER 29

The law protecting children

(A) In the United Kingdom

Elaine E. Sutherland

The role of the legal system in attempts to ensure the protection of children has attracted considerable attention of late. It should be borne in mind, at the outset, that the law alone cannot ensure adequate protection. Any approach to the problem must be multi-disciplinary, involving various other professions and the community as a whole. What the legal system can do is to provide a framework – defining standards of protection, mechanisms by which they might be achieved and the roles of the parties involved.

29.1 FROM WHAT ARE CHILDREN BEING PROTECTED?

In attempting to establish a framework for the protection of children, the legal system must first determine what is its objective. Broadly, the child may need to be protected from the actions of others, e.g. physical violence, or from his or her own actions, e.g. consumption of alcohol.

In the former case, the child may be being given protection to which all members of the community, whether adult or child, are

entitled. However, the inherent vulnerability of children and their inability to enforce their own rights may require the legal system to intervene more extensively on this level. In the latter case, the law may be extending its protective function beyond that which is normally applied to adults. Again, it is the child's vulnerability, combined with inexperience, which is used to justify such an interventionist position.

A number of areas of child protection can be identified. First, legislation may deny children access to specific actual or perceived dangers or risks. Thus, a child may not own an air-rifle below the age of 14 [1], buy tobacco below the age of 16 [2] or buy alcohol in a public house below the age of 18 [3]. The lack of any rational structure behind the fixing of particular age limits has been a matter of comment [4]. The criminal law is also invoked so as to deny a child access to dangerous commodities. The supplier of the particular commodity commits an offence [2] by so doing and, frequently, the child also commits an offence [1] by buying or attempting to buy the commodity. Clearly this approach relies on the belief that individuals will desist from conduct simply because it is criminal; a belief which is, at the very least, questionable [5].

Sexual activity requires special mention in the context of protection from specific dangers or risks. No child under 16 can consent to an indecent assault in the United Kingdom [6]. It is an offence to engage in indecent practices with a child below the age of 14 in England [7] or with a child below the age of puberty in Scotland [8]. While, in general, Scots' law regards puberty as occurring at 12 in the case of girls and 14 in the case of boys the issue here is a question of fact to be determined in each case [8]. The question of a woman having sexual intercourse with a boy between the ages of 14 and 16 is unclear. It may be that such conduct could constitute indecent assault.

In both Scotland and England, it is an offence to have sexual intercourse with a girl below the age of 16. Where the girl is under 13, the offence is one of strict liability and carries the potential of imprisonment for life [9]. Where the girl is between the ages of 13 and 16 an offence [10] is again committed unless the man concerned is below the age of 24, and has not been charged with a similar offence before. In this case it is a defence for him to show that he had reasonable grounds to believe that the girl was aged 16 [10]. In addition, it is a defence for the man to show that he had reasonable cause to believe the girl to be his wife [11]. Since marriage is illegal in Britain until each party is aged 16 [12], this defence has little application when the parties have always lived there. However, the defence might be relevant when the parties came to Britain from a country where marriage is permitted at an earlier age.

It is an offence to permit a child under the age of 16 to be in a brothel or on premises for the purpose of having unlawful sexual intercourse with men [13]. In addition, it is a statutory offence to take or to permit the taking of indecent photographs of a person under the age of 16 [14].

A second approach to providing a framework for the protection of children is to ensure that no child is left without a care-taker. Normally, the care-taker will be a parent or guardian and often the child will have two parents fulfilling this role. However, where the child has no effective care-taker, either through the death or disappearance of that person, or where the care-taker is permanently or temporarily incapable of looking after the child, the local authority has a duty to receive the child into its care if it is satisfied that its intervention is necessary in the interest of the child's welfare [15]. This duty applies in respect of all children under the age of 17 and can continue until the child reaches 18.

Initially, this does not give the local authority any power to keep the child in its care if the parent or guardian wishes to resume care. Indeed, the local authority is obliged to ensure that the child's care is taken over by a parent, guardian, relative or friend provided it is consistent with the child's welfare. Once the child has been in the care of the local authority for six months, the parent or guardian must give the local authority 28 days notice of his or her intention to remove the child [16]. The requirement of 28 days notice is designed to afford the local authority the opportunity of invoking other legal provisions to retain control of the child. These provisions are discussed fully below.

The third aspect of the overall approach to protecting children directs itself at the much broader area of what has come to be known as 'abuse and neglect'. This encompasses a whole range of actions and omissions and the phraseology of the law here aims at retaining a flexibility which can meet the variety of situations which present themselves. Extensive discussion of what amounts to abuse and neglect is to be found elsewhere in this book and will not be explored here.

The legal system utilizes both the criminal and civil law in attempting to tackle abuse and neglect of children. In terms of the criminal law, statute [17] provides that it is an offence for any person over 16 who has the custody, care or control of a child to wilfully assault, ill treat, neglect, abandon or expose the child in a way which is likely to cause him or her unnecessary suffering or injury to health. The statutory definition is sufficiently wide to cover all persons having legal control or actual possession of a child.

What amounts to a 'wilful' act or omission is not without its problems. It is questionable that an omission is wilful where a parent's failure to act is due to ignorance of the fact that any action is required. Two cases demonstrate conflicting approaches to the question. In 1968, in the Scottish case of *Clark* v. *HM Adv.* [18], the parents were charged with wilful neglect of their child. The defence sought to introduce medical evidence to the effect that they were 'mentally irresponsible' – an averment which amounted to less than one of insanity or diminished responsibility. It was held that such evidence, although relevant to a plea in mitigation and thus sentence, was irrelevant to the question of guilt or innocence. The court applied an objective standard of the reasonable parent and ignored the state of mind of those actually accused.

This approach was rejected by the House of Lords, by a majority of 3–2 in the more recent English case of *R* v. *Sheppard* [19] in which the parents were convicted initially of wilful neglect of their child. They were of low intelligence and had failed to realize that the child required medical attention. Their conviction was quashed on appeal when the test applied was that, in order for their omission to have been wilful, they must either have been aware of the risk or their ignorance must have been due to their not caring whether or not a risk existed.

The absence of a deliberate intention to harm the child is not alone a defence to a charge of wilful abuse or neglect. This is best exemplified in the case of religious groups who forswear medical treatment in the belief either that it is harmful or that they have a more effective alternative. A number of cases on this point arose at the end of the last century out of the behaviour of a sect known as 'Peculiar People' who believed that prayer was the only acceptable form of 'treatment'. In *R* v. *Senior* [20] a member of the sect was convicted of the manslaughter of his 9-month-old daughter, having failed to seek medical treatment for her pneumonia. The court took the view that the deliberate nature of his behaviour rendered it 'wilful'. Surprisingly, there is no more recent litigation on this point in Britain.

It can be seen that the criminal law plays a significant part in protecting children. This reflects an attempt by society to lay down standards of behaviour. It may also satisfy the apparent public demand for retribution in the most blatant cases of abuse and neglect. The criminal law is, however, something of a blunt instrument when it comes to dealing with the problem. It has already been noted that simply to declare a course of conduct criminal will not necessarily prevent its occurrence. More important is the fact that criminal sanctions will only come to the fore once the offending conduct has taken place. In the most extreme cases, the child will already be dead. While it is true that some of the civil law approaches to child protection require evidence of harm or, at least, a likelihood of harm before they can be invoked, there is a greater emphasis on detection and prevention; the goal of protection is, then, better served by the civil law.

29.2 THE PERSONNEL INVOLVED

Before proceeding to consider the civil legal provisions in respect of child protection, it is useful to identify the agencies and groups involved in the whole field.

(a) The police

Police officers will often be the first people to encounter a situation in which a child requires protection. Quite apart from their ordinary functions in ensuring public order and enforcing the criminal law, they will have to deal with the child's immediate need for protection and ensure that those responsible for the more long-term response are informed. A single constable [21] may remove the child to a place of safety where there appears to be some immediate risk to the child. Thereafter, and in circumstances of lesser immediacy, the local authority or, in Scotland, the Reporter to the Children's Panel, will be informed in order that they can take the appropriate steps.

(b) The NSPCC and the RSSPCC

In England, the National Society for the Prevention of Cruelty to Children, founded in 1884 and, in Scotland, the Royal Scottish Society for the Prevention of Cruelty to Children, founded in 1889, are organizations whose sole aim is the protection of children. To this end they are active in promoting debate and legislation and, at a more grass-roots level, in investigating individual cases of suspected abuse or neglect.

The investigative function is carried out by a large staff of inspectors. Where an inspector is concerned that there is immediate danger to a child, he or she can apply for a care order in the juvenile court [22]. They may also, in common with *any* interested party, apply for a warrant to remove the child to a place of safety [23]. Again, relevant information will be passed on to the local authority, the police and, in Scotland, the Reporter to the Children's Panel.

The Societies' effectiveness is dependent, to a considerable extent, on receiving information from the public. Clearly, members of the public will be more willing to come forward if they are confident that their identity will not be disclosed to those against whom a complaint is laid. The extent to which such confidentiality can be guaranteed was established in *D. v. NSPCC* [24]. In that case, the Society had received a complaint regarding the treatment of D's daughter.

D attempted to recover all the Society's documents on the case and the Society opposed this on the basis that these would reveal the identity of its informant. The House of Lords upheld the Society's right to withhold the relevant documents, thus affording the informant the same protection as that extended to police informants and acknowledging that the public interest was best served by protecting confidentiality in this context. Whether or not RSSPCC informants are guaranteed the same protection has not been decided, but the same 'public interest' argument could apply.

(c) The local authority

Implementation of many of the aspects of child protection is among the functions devolved by central government to the local authorities throughout England and Scotland. The local authority does this through its social work or social services department. The local authority has a general duty to promote the welfare of children in its area [25] and to investigate allegations of abuse or neglect [26]. Again, a warrant may be sought to authorize the removal of a child to a place of safety [22]. Thereafter, the local authority has a wide range of powers and duties in respect of children in need of care. These are discussed fully below.

(d) Other professions

It is in the nature of their work that members of a number of other professions, including physicians, dentists, nursing staff, school teachers and day-care specialists, will encounter cases of suspected abuse and neglect. Social workers apart, no other professionals in Britain are directed by statute to take any particular course of action on the basis of such a suspicion. What the individual professional will do will depend on the ethics of the particular profession and, of course, on the individual's own beliefs. A number of other jurisdictions, including the USA (see p. 461) and Australia [27] have enacted legislation which requires certain professionals to report cases of suspected abuse and neglect on pain of civil and criminal sanctions.

Nevertheless, while a professional who fails to act upon a clear suspicion of abuse or neglect is free from criminal sanction, civil liability may attach. It is a general principle of the law of tort or delict that a professional who is negligent in the exercise of his or her duty will be liable in damages to any person injured thereby, provided that the injury to that person was reasonable foreseeable [28]. Thus, for example, a general practitioner who sees clear indications that a child has suffered repeated physical abuse and does nothing may be liable in damages to the child for subsequent injury caused by a repeat of the abuse. To date, there are no cases reported in the United Kingdom of liability arising in such a situation.

It is essential that all the individuals who encounter suspect abuse or neglect have a clear idea of whom to contact for assistance. To this end, it has been recommended that each local authority should issue guidelines to all the relevant persons in its area [29]. These contain an outline of indicators of abuse or neglect; details of immediate action to be taken; recommended action for specific individual professions; and an outline of emergency legal procedures. It should be borne in mind that guidelines are just that and are not legal requirements. Nonetheless, a professional who is shown to have ignored such guidance might be regarded as being negligent.

As with any other person, a professional may apply to a magistrate for a warrant to remove a child to a place of safety in an emergency [22]. In all other circumstances, the professional may contact the local authority and, in Scotland, the Reporter to the Children's Panel.

Given the range of professionals who may encounter suspected abuse or neglect, it is essential that there should be maximum co-operation between them. The enquiries into cases where the system failed and a child died, from Maria Colwell in 1974 [30] to Jasmine Beckford in 1985 [31], have repeatedly emphasized the lack of co-ordination as a key element in the final tragedy.

(e) The community

Members of the public in Britain are under no obligation to intervene or to report suspected abuse or neglect and, while a number of agencies do receive reports from this source, it is likely that much goes unreported. Failure to report may be attributed to many causes including ignorance, fear of error, fear of the perpetrator and, not least, a desire not to interfere in the life of another family or to 'get involved'. Education can go some way towards removing these causes and there has been a considerable increase in public debate on abuse and neglect through the press and television in recent years.

The introduction of a reporting law compelling everyone to report suspected abuse and neglect might encourage individuals to come forward. In simply obeying the law, the individual might be freed from doubts over 'interfering'. However, such a law would be impossible to enforce and, in effect, would be no more than a cosmetic exercise.

(f) The courts

It will become apparent from the discussion below that the courts play a significant part in the overall process of child care. It is in the courts that disputed facts are decided and specific courses of action ordered. In Scotland, where the Children's Hearing System plays a significant role in the disposal of many of the cases, disputed facts are still resolved in court. It should be borne in mind that, while courts are directed to act in the child's best interest, in practice, the process remains an adversarial one, with evidence being led on behalf of the interested parties involved [32].

It is possible that there will be a conflict between the child's interests and those of the parent or guardian. Throughout Britain there is provision for the appointment of a person, known variously as a guardian *ad litem* or a safeguarder, who protects the child's interest rather than presents the child's instructions [33].

The possibility exists of two separate sets of proceedings before a court in many abuse and neglect situations. There may be a prosecution under the criminal law, where the case against the accused must be established beyond reasonable doubt. In addition, there will often be proceedings aimed at the direct protection of the child; while these proceedings may involve establishing that certain criminal conduct has occurred, they are not, in themselves, criminal in nature. This raises the question of the appropriate standard of proof in such cases. It is outwith the scope of the present discussion to explore the debate amongst lawyers on this point. Suffice to say that the most recent decisions in England [34] and Scotland [35] have taken the view that the proceedings are civil in nature and that proof is on the balance of probabilities. However, in both cases, it was accepted that the weight of evidence required to tip the balance might vary with the gravity of the allegations made. Furthermore, it was accepted that certain alleged conduct, for example, sexual abuse, is unlikely to be corroborated by eyewitnesses. In such cases, the evidence might be enough to satisfy the civil standard for intervention although it might not be sufficient to found a criminal prosecution.

A further problem arises in the choice of expert witnesses in the context of physical and, particularly, of sexual abuse. This has been highlighted more recently in Cleveland, England. Between May and July, 1987, over 200 children were placed in care on the grounds of sexual abuse which was diagnosed by two paediatricians. Many of the children were subsequently returned to their families after court proceedings in which the findings were challenged by others, including police surgeons. A judicial inquiry into the matter has recently issued its report which is discussed in greater detail in Chapter 15. Among the matters ventilated at the hearings was that expert witnesses from the same profession may have different orientations. In short, the police surgeon, being familiar with legal procedures, knows that evidence must be of a particular standard before the courts will act upon it. The clinical paediatrician is primarily concerned with treating the patient and is unfamiliar with the requirements of the law. While there is no simple way to avoid this difference, one point is clear – no child should be subjected to more examinations than are absolutely necessary. This problem could be avoided by having both the clinical paediatrician and the police surgeon present simultaneously.

(g) The Children's Hearing System

The Children's Hearing System came into operation in Scotland in 1971 [36]. The system provides for two broad categories of children: those who offend and those who are offended against. It is based on the premise that all the children concerned, including offenders, may be in need of some kind of non-punitive intervention and, to that extent, all referrals can be seen as being 'protective'. However, the following dicussion will focus on those cases which are aimed at protecting the child from the behaviour of others.

In this context, the system has jurisdiction

where it appears that one of the following situations exists [37]:

(1) The child is falling into bad associations or is exposed to moral danger. This would include, for example, children mixing with others involved in criminality and those in households which exposed them to drugs or prostitution.
(2) A lack of parental care is likely to cause the child unnecessary suffering or serious impairment to his or her health or development. The test of care here is an objective one and no proof of actual harm is required [38]. Thus a newborn infant may be removed on the basis of the parents' previous behaviour [39].
(3) That the child has been the victim of a list of specified offences including physical and sexual abuse [40].
(4) That the child is or is likely to become part of the same household as a person who has committed an offence under (3) above.
(5) That a female child is a member of the same household as a female who has been the victim of incest.

The Reporter is the key figure in the system [41]. He or she receives the initial allegations that one of the grounds of referral exists and there is a requirement to investigate the allegation. Over half of the original referrals proceed no further, either because the allegation is unfounded or because the problem can be resolved by no action or by a voluntary arrangement [42]. However, a children's hearing will be arranged if the reporter is satisfied that there is substance to the allegation. Details of how the Hearing proceeds and the courses of action open to it are discussed later (see p. 453).

The strength of this system lies in the fact that, while disputed matters are subject to all the normal protection afforded by rules of evidence and standards of proof, the final resolution of the case is removed from the adversarial process. Real attempts are made to get to the root of the problem and to find a positive and constructive plan for the future. This is not to suggest that the system is without its flaws. There is the danger that legal procedures will not be observed and that the protection of civil liberties will be eroded in the course of 'helping' [43]. This problem can be resolved in the course of training panel members. In short, one might describe the system as a case conference where *all* the interested parties have an input.

29.3 REGULATION OF VOLUNTARY CARE

Parents are usually best placed and are normally anxious to ensure the best interests of their children [44]. Nonetheless, there are times when they are unable or unwilling to do so. In these circumstances, parents frequently choose to make voluntary arrangements for their children to be cared for by someone else. This section examines the regulation of such forms of care.

(a) Babysitters and day care

Almost all children are placed at some time in the care of a babysitter. The matter is not regulated by statute when this form of care is provided in the parents' home. The parents are bound to take reasonable care in the selection of the babysitter and they may be criminally liable when they fail to do so, e.g. by leaving the child with a 10-year-old or an intoxicated person [45]. In addition, such negligence may amount to neglect and justify investigation and, possibly, intervention.

When the child is cared for outside the parents' home, the situation remains unregulated if the child is cared for in the home of a relative, regardless of the length of time the child lives with that relative [45]. This exemption does not apply where the child is in the care of the local authority or a voluntary organization.

When the child is cared for outside the home of a parent, relative or guardian, registration is required:

(i) of premises, other than private homes, where children are looked after for 2 hours or more in any day or for any longer period of up to 6 days, and

(ii) of persons who receive children under 5 into their homes to be looked after [46].

The local authority may impose conditions regulating the number of children that may be received, the condition of the premises and the number and qualifications of the carers [47]. Failure to comply with the requirements for registration is an offence subject to a penalty of up to 3 months' imprisonment and/or a fine of up to level 3 on the standard scale [48].

Thus, on the face of it, there appears to be protection of children placed in day care. However, unregistered childcare is widespread. While the exact extent of this is unknown, it is not surprising that, in present social conditions, the number of day-care places available is far exceeded by the number of children who require them [49]. Policing the situation is almost impossible. Much as politicians wax lyrical on the subject of adequate care and protection for all children, the necessary resources are not made available.

(b) Foster care

Parents may need to make more long-term alternative provision for the care of a child under 16 than can be arranged through day care. In Scotland, the arrangement is subject to regulation as foster care when the period of care exceeds 6 days [50]. In England, the arrangement is not deemed to be foster care until the period of that care exceeds 27 days [51]; if, however, the carer is already a regular foster parent, care becomes foster care after 6 days [52]. Throughout Britain, there are a number of situations which consitute exceptions to this time-related definition and these include care in the home of an adult relative or guardian, in any home or establishment run by the local authority, in hospital or in a recognized school [53]. Certain persons are prohibited from receiving foster children, unless they disclose the relevant circumstances to the local authority [54]. Broadly, these include persons who have previously had children removed from their care or who have been convicted of specified criminal offences.

In Scotland, the parents must notify the local authority of their intention to place their child in foster care 2 weeks *prior* to the intended placement [55] and the local authority is then under an obligation to assess the suitability of the placement [56]. No parallel regulations have yet been enacted in England although the Secretary of State has the power to do so [57].

The local authority has considerable powers of inspection and visitation so that, as with day care, there appears, on the surface, to be ample regulation to ensure that children placed in foster care are adequately protected. But, while we have come a long way from the 'baby farms' of the eighteenth and nineteenth centuries, the reality is far from ideal. Unregistered fostering occurs and, even where the arrangement is regulated, tragedies can happen. At the time of writing, an incident is reported of a foster parent being accused of killing his foster child – although this was in the context of involuntary fostering [58].

(c) Placement with the local authority

Parents who find themselves temporarily unable to care for their child may place the child in the care of the local authority on a voluntary basis. The local authority is under a duty to receive a child in such circumstances, although the parents may be liable to make a financial contribution towards the child's maintenance.

The parents can usually remove their child from such care on request but the local authority can assume parental rights over the child in certain circumstances when it believes that this would be unsatisfactory; this prevents removal of the child. Parental rights can sometimes be assumed in the face of parental opposition and the matter will be considered below.

29.4 PRELIMINARIES TO COMPULSORY INTERVENTION

(a) Enquiries

The local authority is obliged to investigate a case of suspected abuse or neglect of which it is aware unless it is satisfied that such investigation in unnecessary [59]. Such investigation should include: consulting the child protection register (see below), consulting other agencies which might have knowledge of the child, e.g. school or health visitor, and interviewing the child and the parents. Investigation may also be carried out by NSPCC or RSSPCC inspectors (see p. 444 above). As a result of investigation, it may be decided that further action is required. In an emergency, a warrant can be obtained to remove the child to a place of safety; otherwise, a conference should be called as soon as possible to discuss the case.

(b) The case conference

The aim of the case conference is to bring together the various professionals who may have information about the child and the family and to plan for future action. The Panel of Inquiry into the circumstances which led to the death of Jasmine Beckford expressed the view [31] that the following persons should

be present, where relevant, in addition to the social workers dealing with the case: police officers, health visitors, paediatricians, general practitioners, school teachers and, possibly, home helps, family aides and social work assistants. The Panel acknowledged that the attendance of the parents might be valuable in some situations but, nevertheless, it recommended a flexible approach.

Appropriate action to be taken after the case conference may involve placing the child on the child protection register, starting care proceedings in England or referring the case to the Reporter to the Children's Panel in Scotland.

(c) Child protection register

As a result of advice from central government, local authorities maintain a central register of children in their area who may be at risk of non-accidental injury. These registers are intended as an aid to professionals working in the field of child protection and access is limited to those persons. In deciding whether or not to inform the parents that their child's name has been placed on the register, the key factor is the welfare of the child. There is provision for removal of a child's name from the register where this is initiated by the professionals involved.

The availability of a register is not without drawbacks. In the first place, there is no simple way in which parents who consider themselves aggrieved can have their names removed at their own instigation. Secondly, there is the danger that, being aware of the existence of the register parents will be reluctant to seek medical attention for their children who have been genuinely injured accidentally for fear of a misdiagnosis in favour of non-accidental injury [60]. The only answer to the latter problem is a responsible and sympathetic approach by the professionals involved. (cf. the Cleveland affair, discussed above, p. 446).

29.5 INVOLUNTARY CARE

Various forms of intervention which can take place regardless of parental opposition will be considered in this section. Some of the procedures are substantially the same in England and Scotland and these will be considered in a United Kingdom context. Others are unique to England and Scotland or operate differently in each jurisdiction.

(a) Assumption of parental rights in the United Kingdom

A local authority does not acquire an immediate right to retain a child which it has received into its care. Indeed, it is directed to attempt to find the parents and, where possible, to reunite the child with them or with relatives or friends [61]. However, if the local authority is satisfied that this would not be in the child's interest, and if the child is already in its care, it can pass a resolution vesting parental rights in itself.

The parents can remove their child without notice when the child has been in care for less than 6 months. The question as to whether the local authority can resolve to vest parental rights in itself within that period was discussed in *Lewisham London Borough Council* v. *Lewisham Juvenile Court Justices* [62], but was not resolved. Even if the resolution were held to be incompetent, the local authority could still seek a place of safety order to cover the immediate problem.

One of the following conditions must be satisfied before parental rights can be assumed [63]:

(1) That the child's parents are dead and he or she has no guardian, or
(2) that the child's parents or guardian
    (i) has abandoned him or her, or
    (ii) suffers permanently from a disability rendering him or her incapable of looking after the child, or
    (iii) suffers from a mental disorder rendering him or her unfit to have care of the child, or
    (iv) is of such habits and mode of life as to be unfit to have the care of the child, or
    (v) has consistently failed without reasonable excuse to discharge the obligations of a parent as to be unfit to have the care of the child, or
(3) that a resolution under (2) is in force in relation to one parent who is, or is likely to become a member of the same household as the child and the other parent, or
(4) that the child has been in the care of the local authority throughout the 3 years preceding the passing of the resolution.

The local authority is bound to inform the parents or guardian of the child that it has passed the resolution and must advise them of their right to object by lodging a counter-notice in writing on the local authority within 1 month [64]. If a notice is lodged, the local authority must apply to the juvenile court, in England, or to the sheriff, in Scotland, within 14 days to have the resolution confirmed. The resolution will lapse should the local authority fail to do so. The court will confirm the resolution, provided it is in the child's best interest to do so, if one of the conditions outlined above was satisfied at the time the resolution was passed and one of them remains satisfied. A resolution can continue in force until the young person is aged 18, although it can be rescinded by either the local authority or the court in certain circumstances [65].

The effect of such a resolution is to vest almost all the rights a parent would have in respect of care, control and decision-making in respect of the child in the local authority. At one time, the local authority could even prevent parents from visiting their child [66], but, as a result of legislation passed in 1984 [67], parents who are refused access can now apply to the courts where the local authority's decision may be overturned.

(b) Place of safety order

The aim of a place of safety order is to effect the immediate removal of a child from a situation of risk or to prevent the child's return to such a situation pending further investigation of the case.

In England, involuntary transfer of care is governed by the Children and Young Persons Act 1969. Any person may apply to a magistrate for authority to remove a child to a place of safety and this will be granted if there is reasonable cause to believe that one of the following conditions is satisfied (s.1):

(1) that the child's proper development is being avoidably prevented or neglected or his or her health is being avoidably impaired or neglected or he or she is being ill-treated; or
(2) that the condition set out in (1) has been proven in respect of another child in the same household; or
(3) that a person convicted of one of the offences specified in Schedule 1 to the Children and Young Persons Act 1933 [68] is or may become a member of the same household as the child; or
(4) that the child is exposed to moral danger; or
(5) that the child is beyond the control of his or her parents; or
(6) that the child is of compulsory school age and he or she is not receiving efficient full-time education.

The removal of the child may be for 28 days or such lesser period as is specified.

A police constable may detain a child without specific authorization if he or she believes that one of the conditions (1)–(4) above is satisfied (s. 28(2)). Thereafter, the circumstances surrounding the detention must be investigated by a police officer not below the rank of inspector and the child must either be released or arrangements must be made to detain him or her in a place of safety.

The parent or guardian must be informed and advised of his or her right to apply to a justice for the child's release (s. 28(4)).

The comparable situation in Scotland is governed by the Social Work (Scotland) Act 1968. Authorization to remove a child to a place of safety may be sought from a court or a justice of the peace on grounds similar to those outlined above (s. 37(1)). Again, a police officer may remove a child to a place of safety without specific authorization (s. 37(2)). Thereafter, the Reporter to the Children's Panel must be informed. The detention is initially valid for a maximum period of 7 days and, in any event, the child must be released if the Reporter does not consider it will be necessary to convene a children's hearing (s. 37(3)). If a hearing is deemed necessary, it should be convened on the day following the child's detention and it can authorize the child's detention for up to a further 21 days if it is unable to dispose of the case.

(c) England and Wales

Care proceedings

Care proceedings may be initiated by the local authority, a police officer or an inspector of the NSPCC if one of the conditions outlined above as justifying removal to a place of safety is satisfied (Children and Young Persons Act 1969, s.1).

The court before which the case is brought may make an interim care order when it is not in a position to make a final order – due, for instance, to a lack of information (s. 2(10)). When, however, the court finds that one of the relevant conditions is proven and is satisfied that the child is in need of care or control, it can make one of a number of orders:

(1) It can require that the child's parent or guardian undertakes to take proper care of and to exercise proper control over the child. The order can only be made with the consent of the parent or guardian and

cannot last for longer than 3 years or past the child's eighteenth birthday (s. 2(13)). These orders are rarely used and their abolition has been recommended [69].

(2) It may make a supervision order placing the child under the supervision of the local authority or a probation officer (s. 1(3)(b)). Supervision orders can be varied or recalled and cannot last for more than 3 years or past the child's eighteenth birthday (ss. 15 and 16). They can be replaced by a care order – and this is the only real sanction where the parents or the child do not co-operate with the supervision order.

(3) The court may make a care order placing the child in the care of the local authority (s. 1(3)(c)). This gives the local authority extensive parental rights over the child, including the right to determine the child's residence [70]. The child's parents remain liable to contribute towards his or her support (s. 21A).

In the past, the local authority had considerable discretion to deny or limit parental access to children in care. That system and the procedures for appealing against decisions was criticized by the European Court of Human Rights [71]. Legislative changes by way of the Child Care Act 1980 have strengthened the position of parents who may now apply to a court for an order overriding the local authority's decision to deny them access (s.12(c)). A care order can remain in force until the child is 18 or, if the child was 16 when it was made, until the child is 19 (s.20(3)).

At one time it was thought that parents could use the mechanism of wardship to challenge decisions of the local authority in respect of children in its care. The House of Lords rejected this approach in *A* v. *Liverpool City Council* [72] and *Re W (a Minor)* [73]. As a result of these decisions, challenges to local authority decisions were made by way

of judicial review [74]. However, a recent decision has pointed to the unsatisfactory limitations of this approach and may have reopened the door to wardship [75].

Wardship

The authority to make a child a ward of court has its roots in the sovereign's power as *parens patriae* and is now vested in the Family Division of the High Court. The invocation of wardship has increased in popularity in recent years because of the flexibility it affords [76].

Any person with an interest in the child may initiate wardship proceedings [77]. Consequently, the procedure has been used by a variety of relatives and others with a professional interest in the child [78]. The local authority has used wardship when it doubts that it can satisfy the specific statutory requirements for a care order [79]. Similarly, flexible rules apply to defendants who may include the parents and the local authority. While the child can be separately represented, the current view is that this is necessary only in exceptional circumstances [80].

Wardship will be granted where it is in the child's best interest to do so. The hearing before the High Court is conducted according to the normal rules of evidence, although the judge may assume a more inquisitorial role than is usual [81].

The effect of wardship is to place the child under the control of the Court and no significant decision regarding him or her may be taken without the Court's consent. Thus, the Court can determine the child's place of residence [82], care and control [83] and who may have access to him or her [83]. Since 1969, it has been empowered to place the child in the care of the local authority [84]. Wardship is of considerable use where a specific issue is in dispute – as in the approval of medical treatment for a baby suffering from Down's syndrome [85] or the sterilization of a mentally handicapped teenage girl [86]. Wardship can, however, only continue until the child reaches the age of 18.

(d) Scotland

Children's hearings

The relevant legislation is contained in the Social Work (Scotland) Act 1968. If the reporter decides to take the case to a hearing, the family will be informed and background reports on the child and the family will be gathered (s.39). The hearing consists of a panel of three lay voluntary persons, including one male and one female (s. 34).

Present at the hearing are the child, the parents, the panel members, the reporter, and possibly the social worker involved in the case. Legal aid is not available to pay for a lawyer to represent the parents and most parents are unaccompanied. Where it appears that there may be a conflict between the interests of the parents and those of the child, a separate representative will be appointed for the child (s. 34A).

The panel chairperson opens the hearing by explaining the grounds of referral to the family. If these are accepted as true by them, and provided the child is old enough to understand, the hearing can proceed. Otherwise, the facts must be proven in a court according to the normal rules of evidence (s. 42) and the case is then remitted back to a hearing for disposal. Legal aid is available to provide the parents with legal representation before the court and, if there is a conflict of interest, the child will be separately represented.

In both cases the hearing then moves on to a round-table discussion exploring how the family functions, its problems and possible ways of resolving these. The aim is to involve the family in finding a satisfactory plan for the future.

The panel members then decide, by majority, on the disposal of the case. They may decide that no further action is required and discharge the case. Otherwise they may require that the child should be subject to the supervision of the local authority. This can take place while the child lives at home or in a residential establishment named by panel members. In addition, other conditions of a non-punitive nature may be attached (s. 44).

There is provision for appealing against the decision on the basis that the disposal was inappropriate or on a point of law (ss. 49 and 50). All cases are reviewed annually and the parents and the local authority may request a review at an earlier date (s. 48).

28.6 CONCLUSIONS

A number of issues emerging from the foregoing discussion of the legal framework for child protection deserve emphasis. While standards of protection can include clear and specific rules, there will always be a need for flexible provisions capable of meeting new problems and social change. However, in order that parents should know what is expected of them, this flexibility cannot amount to vagueness.

The system must enable all relevant and interested parties to have an input at both the level of prevention and intervention. An essential element of this is interagency co-operation and co-ordination.

The mechanisms of protection must provide for both emergency situations and future planning for the child. It is essential that action taken in the name of 'protection' should not amount to a denial of the child's rights. In this respect, it might be borne in mind that the overzealous removal of a child from a loving and secure home is, in itself, an abuse of that child.

(B) In the United States
Harold L. Hirsh

To understand better the protection of minors by the law, it is necessary to consider the legal underpinning of the rights of the essential parties: the parents, the child and the state. The earliest legal doctrine affecting this tripartite relationship was the doctrine of *patria potestas* under which the father controlled every aspect of his child's life, including the power over life and death.

29.7 PARENS PATRIAE

Another theory, the doctrine of *parens patriae*, undercut the absolute power of the father and became the cornerstone of contemporary juvenile law. Under this doctrine, state intervention in the parent–child relationship is justified on two grounds: (a) the state will protect all who cannot protect themselves and (b) the state may compel parents and children to act in ways most beneficial to society [87, 88]. Derived from English common law, the doctrine of *parens patriae* has been embraced in the United States for over two centuries and is founded upon the basic concept that the state has a fundamental, legitimate interest in the protection of minor children. Generally, all states have recognized that the primary responsibility for the provision of necessaries plainly rests with the parent but, upon failure of the parent to provide a minimum of care, the state, under its *parens patriae* power, will step in to make such provisions as are necessary to preserve the life, health and welfare of the minor. The justifications for the doctrine are: first, a child's lack of experience and capacity requires that some entity be ultimately responsible for his or her basic needs; second, society as a whole has an interest in the future of its children; third, a delinquent or unstable child can be harmful to others and must be cared for to avoid this harm. There is clearly tension between this theory and the autonomy and liberty interests of the parents but it has been consistently adjudged that the state must intervene on behalf of its citizens who are unable to protect themselves against abuse and neglect.

Parents are the natural care-takers of their children and are held to a strict duty to provide their children with necessary care and nutrition. This duty to act in the best interests of their children is enforced under both criminal and child protection laws. Parents may be prosecuted if their child is injured or dies as a result of inadequate nutrition or of a failure to seek necessary medical care. In exercising ordinary care, parents are expected to be aware of their child's needs and to seek assistance for him or her when warranted.

(a) State intervention: judicial protection

During the nineteenth century, a number of state legislatures enacted statutes authorizing courts to commit to houses of refuge or industrial schools those children whose parents had failed to provide them with food, clothing, shelter or adequate medical care. The traditional notion that a parent is entitled to custody of his child did not, however, disappear. In recent years, a presumption has developed within the law that a child's welfare is best promoted by parental custody and the state may intervene and assert its authority over the child only when it has been shown that the parent is patently unfit. The presumption in favour of parental custody rights soon became well entrenched and a majority of American jurisdictions still apply this presumption [88].

In many jurisdictions, however, statutes permit the state to take custody of a neglected or dependent child, terms that are variously defined [89]. The state through the courts has the right under the doctrine of *parens patriae* to assume guardianship of neglected children and to order such treatment as they may require.

While the various statutes reflect the individual attitudes and concerns of each sovereign state, all contain provisions requiring a parent to provide the minimum of necessaries to the dependent child. In the event of failure, the state, through its variously recognized entities, may step between the parent and child and provide whatever is necessary to preserve the state's interest in the child.

29.8 REFUSAL OF TREATMENT

Parental refusal of medical intervention is most likely to be upheld where the child's condition is not life-threatening, and where the treatment itself would expose the child to great risk. Sometimes, this has been true even when the proposed therapy would offer great benefit to the child; the court may stay its hand if it is persuaded that the child is antagonistic to the proposed therapy and that his co-operation will be necessary to derive any benefit from the treatment. Most of the time, it appears that a court will avoid intervening when the malady sought to be treated is not life-threatening.

(a) Religious beliefs of parents

Where conflict between the parents' wishes and the duties and rights of the state arise, the law must choose between the two [90, 91]. Americans are guaranteed the free exercise of religion under the First Amendment which those who are entirely sincere in their beliefs

may invoke so as to support their desire to withhold treatment from their children. In a variety of circumstances, however, the courts have held that parental rights may be subordinate to the state's interest in the care of children [89, 92]. Parents may be free to become martyrs but it does not follow that they are free to make martyrs of their children before they have reached the age when they can make that choice for themselves. The courts have distinguished two concepts within the First Amendment – the freedom to believe and the freedom to act. The first is absolute but, in the nature of things, the second cannot be. Personal liberty is a relative right which must be considered in the light of the general public welfare. The right to practise religion freely does not include liberty to expose the community or the child to communicable diseases or the latter to ill health or death. Significant neglect may not necessarily be sufficient to sustain a criminal charge but criminal action may be found where a parent's refusal to provide medical care is, in the court's mind, particularly egregious. Religous beliefs are no defence to neglect of this magnitude [7].

The courts do not only weigh the conflicting interests of the state and of parents, but they also are obliged to consider the interests of the children themselves. At least where a child is approaching the age of maturity, and where his life is not in imminent danger, the minor patient himself may have the right to express his own opinion about the morality of any treatment offered and as to his willingness to submit to it. Physicians' opinions are given significant credence.

29.9 THE EMANCIPATED MINOR

The common law has recognized the doctrine of 'emancipation' for many years. This means that the parent has surrendered or forfeited his parental duties and responsibilities and all his rights to control of the minor [94, 95].

In most legal contexts, an emancipated minor is recognized as one who is not subject to parental control or regulation. The precise definition of emancipation varies among states, but an emancipated minor usually does not live at home and is self-supporting. Minors who marry before the legal age of majority are considered emancipated and, hence, are treated as legal adults responsible for their own actions. This is particularly true when the married minor is the head of his own family, and/or who earns his own living and maintains his own home. Minors in military service and, in most situations, college students who are under age 18 but are living away from home, are also considered to be emancipated minors and may consent to medical treatment. The same would apply to youths who have assumed an adult lifestyle in advance of majority.

A runaway child of any age presents a special problem because the child is away from home without parental consent. Thus, the parents have not consented to the child's own decision-making. As a practical matter, runaways who refuse to identify their parents are generally considered emancipated for the purposes of medical care.

Nevertheless, whether a minor is 'emancipated' is a legal question, ultimately to be answered by a court of law. The doctor who, on the basis of a reasoned judgement, gives treatment to a minor believed to be emancipated does so at his own risk, albeit small. Some jurisdictions have passed legislation that specifically entitles a doctor to rely in good faith upon a child's assertion that he is emancipated.

Emancipation may be expressed in partial as well as total terms. Thus, in many states, certain minors – usually stipulated by age – may function as adults in specified limited areas well in advance of majority, e.g. in obtaining a driver's licence, purchasing alcohol, consenting to marriage or to sexual intercourse, and being subject to criminal rather than juvenile court proceedings.

29.10 THE MATURE MINOR

The mature minor rule creates a major exception to the general rule of parental control and consent and tends to overlap the doctrine of emancipation. A 'mature' minor is one who lives at home but is self reliant, and who works and contributes substantially to his own support.

The criteria by which a minor's maturity is judged vary somewhat with the jurisdiction. Although it is difficult to determine eligibility under such an abstract concept, a functional definition which takes into account some or all of the following points can be developed:

— The minor makes most of his own decisions about the conduct of his daily affairs.
— He enjoys substantial independence in his comings and goings from home and moves about easily on his own.
— Even though supported by parents in major matters, he earns his personal expense money and/or manages most of his day-to-day financial matters.

As to medical matters, a mature minor is one who can appreciate and understand the nature of a proposed procedure and its consequences. Nonethless, a physician who offers to treat a minor who appears to satisfy the law's criteria for maturity should do so very cautiously. A doctor's determination of a child's legal capacity to give consent is neither authoritative nor binding. The problems of consent by minors to medical treatment is discussed in detail in Chapter 28.

29.11 THE STATUTORY ADULT

About half the states have legislated that a minor can consent to all treatment so long as he is capable of giving informed consent. In the other states, this right pertains only to limited services: abortion, contraception, drug and alcohol abuse, psychiatric problems and venereal disease. The minor can arrange for treatment by operation of law in a case of immediate threat to health or life.

29.12 SEXUALITY OF MINORS

The sexual affairs of minors are not truly medical although doctors will often be involved in their control. An increasingly liberalized approach is being taken by the courts in these matters and, since 1977, the US Supreme Court has declared that even unemancipated minors have a constitutional right to 'procreative choice'.

(a) Contraception

The right of minors to use contraceptives has also been well established [94]. Distribution of contraceptives to unemancipated minors without notice to parents does not impair parental freedom to exercise the traditional care, custody and control over unemancipated children. Physician reluctance to provide family planning services without parental consent is inappropriate if based upon fear of liability. There can be no imposition of common law tort liability in the situation where services are mandated by federal statute and implementing regulations, and especially where a relationship between a physician and a minor patient is protected by a constitutional privacy right. There has been no judgement against a physician who provided contraceptive services to a minor of any age.

(b) Abortion

Similarly, minors have been held to have a right to an abortion just as adults do and for many of the same reasons [94]. Despite the debate that has raged around the abortion issue, the federal courts have held that the decision to abort is not to be distinguished from other decisions relevant to procreation. The courts have rejected challenges to abortion statutes which have been based on the premise that abortion decisions are different from those relating to other medical treatments [96].

Some states, constitutionally, require parental or judicial consent in the case of unmarried minors. A minor's access to abortion in the absence of parental consent is, thus, governed by the principles detailed in Chapter 28. In summary, the court will grant her application if she can prove that she is mature enough and well enough informed to make her abortion decision, in consultation with her physician, independently of her parents' wishes; or that even if she is not able to make this decision independently, the desired abortion would be in her best interests.

Statutes that require a blanket parental consent in all cases have been struck down and the right of a mature minor to decide to obtain an abortion appears to be secure. As has been stated, a state may constitutionally require a physician to notify, if possible, the parent of an unemancipated, dependent, and non-mature minor before consenting to perform an abortion but a statute imposing civil and criminal sanctions on physicians performing abortions for unmarried minors without parental consent was held to be unconstitutional [97].

Teenage pregnancy has accordingly caught the attention of legislators and legislation has been enacted which may well impact on the laws pertaining to reproductive issues. One such legislative response was adopted by Wisconsin in 1985 when it became the first state to impose financial liability on parents for babies born to their minor children. Grandparents are required under this law to pay the costs of raising the child until the teenparent reaches the age of 18.

(c) Sterilization

Sterilization involves rights which are deemed fundamental by the United States Supreme Court. Although adults are, in general,

permitted to submit voluntarily to sterilization, minors are deemed to be not sufficiently
mature to make such a decision on their own
[87–89, 98]. In the case of minor incompetents,
the disability is two-fold. Most courts hold
that not only do parents lack inherent
authority to consent to the sterilization of
their children but so also do the courts
themselves. In the absence of a statute
explicitly conferring authority, in *some* courts
jurisdictions are generally unwilling to
authorize sterilization of a minor, particularly
one who is mentally incompetent, even with
the consent of the guardian and even where
the procedure is justified both medically and
socially. The judicial authority to exercise
such awesome power, may not be inferred
from the general principles of common
law but, rather, must derive from specific
legislative authorization.

The procedural safeguards attendant to a
sterilization order must be very elaborate.
The standard most commonly demanded by
the courts has been clear and convincing
evidence. Sterilization, even when medically
indicated, will not be permitted on even a
mature minor without the consent of the
parent or one in *in loco parentis*. Finally, there
must be no alternative to sterilization. The
judge must find that all less drastic
contraceptive methods, including supervision, education and training, have been
proved unworkable or inapplicable and that
the proposed method of sterilization entails
the least invasion of the body of the
individual. It must also be shown that the
current state of scientific and medical
knowledge does not suggest either that a
reversible sterilization or other less drastic
contraceptive method will shortly be available, or that science is on the threshold of an
advance in the treatment of the individual's
disability.

Sterilization could be ordered only if it were
determined to be in the best interest of the
incompetent person considering her/his age
and educability, her/his potential as a parent,
the medical indications for the procedure
and the availability of other methods of
contraception. The ground for sterilizing a
mentally retarded, less than 15-year-old,
inhabitant of a state institution, with or
without parental consent, has often been held
to be that of a medical necessity; but this is by
no means uniformly so, especially when it is
the minor's parents who desire the operation.

29.13 PERSONAL FREEDOM

(a) Commitment

Confinement to a state institution for
treatment of mental retardation, mental
illness or for any other reason, does not
deprive a citizen, whether adult or child, of
the right to due process [87–89, 99]. The
Supreme Court, while recognizing that a child
in such circumstances has a substantial liberty
interest in not being confined unnecessarily
for medical treatment, has however, been less
solicitous of the due process of right as to
the institutionalization of children than have
some states. The Court held that state statutes
providing for the commitment of children to
state mental hospitals by their parents
without an adversarial hearing prior or
subsequent to admission are constitutional –
what is best for a child, it was said, is an
individual medical decision that must be left
to the judgement of physicians in each
case. The Court considered that no formal
adversary hearing would be necessary so long
as some kind of inquiry on the questions of
the child's need for hospitalization was made
by a neutral factfinder [100].

Other states still require a full due process
hearing before a minor child can be confined.
The hearing required includes the right to
notice of the allegation, the right to confront
and cross-examine adverse witnesses and,
in addition, a right to counsel and to a
neutral and detached decision-maker. The

discrepancies between the positions of these states and that of the Supreme Court may be confusing to health-care providers who are unaccustomed to interpreting legal decisions. Simply, these states have determined that their constitution requires greater safeguards for committed juveniles than the Supreme Court has determined to be needed by the Federal Constitution. No state in the Union may offer fewer safeguards than the Supreme Court mandates as minimally acceptable; a state in the Union, however, may mandate more – and some, obviously, have done so. Depending on state law, non-institutionalized minors may also be committed to state institutions without parental consent.

(b) Right to refuse treatment

When a minor is committed, he has, in certain circumstances, the right to refuse treatment. This is particularly so in the use of major tranquillizers which can change a patient's behaviour without his co-operation and of electroconvulsive therapy, psychosurgery and the like – at least in non-emergency situations. Possible exceptions to the right to refuse treatment may exist for treatment of communicable diseases or where the patient is a danger to self or others; approval by the courts would be needed.

An institutionalized minor may be able to consent to an additional period of supervision as a juvenile beyond the age of majority, even though such a decision may come at the price of delaying his own liberty, depending upon his age and maturity and on whether he has access to adequate counselling and discussion with his parent or guardian *ad litem*. The patient has a right to petition for release on reaching the age of majority.

29.14 FETAL RIGHTS

Fetal rights were first recognized in property law. At common law a fetus, from the time of conception, could be named an heir to a decedent's estate. The unborn child's property rights, however, only vested upon live birth and if the inheritance inured to its benefit. This eighteenth-century statement of the law has survived essentially intact [101]. Recently a court, in refusing to bestow on an 8-month-old fetus the status of 'a person beneficially interested' in the revocation of a trust, noted that 'a child *en ventre sa mère* is not regarded as a person until it sees the light of day.' The court recognized the existence of fetal property rights, but retained the distinction between recognized and vested rights [102].

Fetal property rights have retained their inchoate character in modern state statutes. Such statutes do not extend full rights of personhood to the fetus; they merely establish a mechanism for protecting the right of the unborn child to inherit property upon birth.

Two major problems complicate any consideration of the legal status of the fetus. First, the undeveloped fetus has been determined by the United States Supreme Court not to be a 'person' as defined by the Federal Constitution. The second problem revolves around the question of when life begins. Certain religions are clear in their belief that life begins at conception. Other philosophies, including that of medicine itself, speak in terms of 'a capacity to be born alive' or 'viability'; the difficulties associated with such concepts are discussed in detail in Chapter 25. The legal status of the fetus as related to its development is equally unclear and past opinions and rulings are rife with contradiction.

An important jurisprudential concept is that 'legal personality' begins only at birth. Legal personality is a grant of the law and is not the same as a potential natural personality. However, as has already occurred in property law, the fetus has been seen to have legal rights vested in it immediately upon conception, provided that it is subsequently born alive. Indeed, actions have been brought against tortfeasors by children who were still *in utero* at the time of their fathers' deaths.

States have long held the power to take custody of children from parents and to appoint guardians when parents refuse to provide them with lifesaving medical care. In effectuating this power, courts override the rights of parents to practise religion and to retain control over their bodies if the best interests of the child are at stake. To that end, recent court decisions have stood for the proposition that fetuses have rights that attach at viability and that mothers have a corresponding duty to ensure live births [103].

Generally, no person has a legal duty to submit to medical treatment for the good of another. The state may insist on medical treatment to parents to prevent the abandonment of minor children but most state juvenile statutes expressly apply to 'children'. Statutory protection of a viable fetus consequently turns on legislative intent. State legislatures may write statutes expressly to include fetuses as well as children, or may otherwise indicate their intent to include fetuses. However, the constitutional limit to the state's ability to grant jurisdiction over a fetus before viability is set by the extent that this would intrude into the woman's rights.

Conflicts among physicians and between the mother and her unborn child that may now arise in the fetal surgery context suggest that viability may be an inadequate benchmark for resolving such conflicts. Current judicial deference to the medical community in determining viability may or may not be adequate for balancing the rights between mother, fetus and health-care provider.

These advances have prompted a spate of difficult questions. If the fetus can be treated, then should it be considered a patient separate from its mother? If, so, does it possess all the rights of postbirth patients? If the treatment of certain conditions *in utero* becomes commonplace, what are the legal implications of a mother's refusal to consent to such treatment? Finally, what decision-making standard should be used in multiple gestation cases, where one fetus may require surgery which would put another at risk? Fundamental to these questions is the issue of whether the mother and the fetus are a single biological entity or two distinct patients. Many obstetricians are disturbed by the notion that maternal and fetal interests can conflict; most prefer to view mother and fetus as a single entity sharing harmonious interests which are furthered by proper maternal care during pregnancy. But physician perceptions may be changing in the light of dynamic advances in fetal diagnosis and care which clearly distinguish the fetus from its mother for treatment purposes.

The live birth limitation on the rights of the unborn in property law is also reflected in criminal statutes. In some jurisdictions, no penalties are imposed for homicide unless the victim has been born. In others, statutes have been construed to punish feticide as murder, manslaughter, or a misdemeanor, depending on whether the child was quick. At the same time, however, such laws expressly exclude abortion procured with the consent of the mother. Efforts to change laws to include abortions under the definition of homicide have, so far, been unsuccessful [101].

'Wrongful death' actions are statutory actions designed to compensate beneficiaries for losses resulting from the death of a family member. Initially, virtually all jurisdictions required live birth as a prerequisite to recovery in a wrongful death action. Several reasons were offered for this requirement. First, an unborn child was regarded as a part of its mother without separate legal personality; courts have relied on scientific and medical support for the proposition that an unborn child, or at least a non-viable one, has no existence apart from the mother. Second, many thought that to permit an action for the loss of the fetus when the mother also receives damages for her injuries is to allow double recovery. Third, pecuniary damages for the lost benefit of an unborn child were considered too speculative. Fourth, wrongful death statutes were created to provide pecuniary assistance to the deceased's survivors, not to punish the tortfeasor. Given that the pecuniary loss for the death of an unborn child is so speculative and that the mother has already recovered for her own injuries, it was believed that recovery in such cases would substitute a punitive purpose for the statute's compensatory goal. Finally, proof of causation was thought to be too difficult when the child was not born alive.

However, the live birth requirement was soon attacked as logically indefensible. To deny a right of action to a stillborn child produces the incongruous result that a tortfeasor would be held liable for injuries to an unborn child later born alive but not for more severe injuries to an unborn child who is later stillborn. This rewards tortfeasors for killing rather than maiming a fetus and also creates an incentive for tortfeasors to withhold efforts to save their victims' lives. Embracing some of these arguments, courts have begun to allow recovery for prenatal death under a wrongful death statute [104]. Where courts allow actions for the wrongful death of a fetus, the actions generally are maintainable for death occurring at any time after the point of viability.

29.15 CHILD ABUSE

Not all parents are reasonable and prudent, let alone loving; a few frankly abuse their children in fits of anger or for other reasons. The legal approach to the battered child syndrome has been to write legislation. By 1967, all 50 states and the District of Columbia had child abuse reporting statutes, codifying a medical diagnosis into a legal framework which in many states defined official

functions for the courts [88]. Not until 1972, did a court decide that parents' right to care, custody and control over their children was no longer absolute [105].

Most child abuse statutes classify failure to report as a misdemeanor usually punishable by up to 1 year in jail, a fine or both. There are two types of liability that a reporter might face unless he is protected by statute: that is, civil or criminal. There might be civil or criminal liability for defamation of character, and civil liability for invasion of privacy by the disclosing of private facts, for malicious prosecution by placing parents in a false light, or for breach of confidence. All Acts, therefore, contain immunity clauses and every state provides immunity in some form for those who report pursuant to child abuse statutes. Immunity from civil liability can be given to mandated reporters so long as reports are made in good faith and without malice. The existence of an immunity clause removes even the remote threat of liability and thereby provides a psychological impetus to report cases of suspected abuse. At present, approximately 40 states have legislation waiving the physician-patient privilege for child abuse. In others, familial and professional-client confidentiality privileges were abrogated. In 32 states, the privilege regarding communication between husband and wife is currently waived by statute for cases involving child abuse.

Several jurisdictions recognize a private cause of action against a physician or hospital for failure to report child abuse. There are two grounds upon which such a suit may be brought: first, common law medical negligence, and secondly, violation of a specific child abuse reporting statute. A common law basis for establishing liability in such a case has been recognized. A defendant's failure to comply with the statute was taken as compelling evidence that he failed to observe the appropriate standard of care.

Most states have created statutory rules of evidence protecting communications between physician and patient. When a communication between a doctor and his patient is protected by law as privileged or confidential, it cannot be presented in evidence in a judicial proceeding. The intent of such statutes is to induce patients to make full disclosure to physicians so that proper treatment may be administered. The privilege is by no means absolute. For example, a physician has a duty to disclose information in the interests of society or the life or well-being of the patient or another person. Clearly, the protection of the life, health, and well-being of an infant may constitute a compelling community interest permitting the disclosure of information.

It is the patient's right to assert the physician-patient privilege. This matter is complicated when the patient is a child, since the right of a minor is often vested in his parents. Nevertheless, numerous courts have held that a parent may not invoke the child's patient privilege, especially when it is being used to shield a person who caused the injury to another. In short, the best interests of the child override the parent's right to assert a self-protective claim on the patient's behalf.

Statutes give juvenile courts jurisdiction over 'neglected' children in every state – and mistreatment, or abuse, is a form of neglect. In some states, the emphasis is on the behaviour of parents, e.g. whether they are cruel to a child. In others, importance is placed on the child's environment and whether it is unsuitable owing to the neglect of one or both parents. The emphasis of a particular state statute is important, since it tells what must be proved to spell out a neglect case. Two questions have to be answered in any neglect or child abuse case: what actually happened? and do the facts presented amount to neglect or abuse? Evidence is a problem, and lack of objective proof means that a situation cannot be remedied through the court. In such

circumstances, the juvenile court may order protective supervision of the child so that his or her situation may be improved through casework techniques and the use of other community resources.

It has been pointed out that a problem arises in ensuring the protection of parents from state power when the allegedly neglected child is offered protective services under laws of the juvenile court. In effecting these, the social worker, who is part of an administrative agency, is authorized to supervise the home as the court may order – and the standards of care expected of the family are set by the agency at its discretion. The presence of a stranger – the agency worker – in the home may deprive the parents of their liberty without the protection of due process of law. In addition, the due process requirement raises the question of the family's right to counsel at a hearing. A defendant in a juvenile court hearing does not have to be provided with the same safeguards as are necessarily provided in a criminal action and it is not mandatory to provide the family with counsel in the form of a lawyer. As a consequence, many feel that the legal maxim – 'every man is entitled to his day in court' – is not carried into effect and that administrative agencies with supposedly benevolent intentions negate legal rights in a number of instances.

There may also be exclusive jurisdiction in the criminal court to try the parents for the assault that may be involved in the abuse, or for the crime of criminal neglect or endangering the welfare of a child. The same conduct and circumstances may be involved in both criminal and juvenile cases. Today 19 states specifically require the appointment of a guardian *ad litem* to represent an abused child's interests in a proceeding for child abuse. Three states permit the court, at its discretion, to appoint a guardian *ad litem* for children in cases of child abuse that result in judicial proceedings.

There are two basic reasons for the

recognition of a child's right to counsel. First, when the state invades the family and conducts a judicial examination of family relations with the implicit power of changing the custody of the child, the due process clause of the Fourteenth Amendment requires representation by counsel as a prerequisite to a fair hearing. Second, the 'best interests of the child', the theoretical guidelines for all child-related judicial proceedings, cannot be adequately ascertained without independent representation of that child's interests.

It is apparent that both society and the professions have now recognized the fact of child abuse and the phenomenon has 'come out of the closet'.

REFERENCES

1. Firearms Act 1968, s.22(2).
2. Children and Young Persons Act 1933, s.7; Children and Young Persons (Scotland) Act 1937 s.18; Protection of Children (Tobacco) Act 1986.
3. Licencing Act 1964, s.169; Licencing (Scotland) Act 1976, s.68.
4. Freeman, M.D.A. (1983) *The Rights and Wrongs of Children*, Pinter, London, p. 7.
5. Walker, N. (1987) *Crime and Criminology: An Introduction*, Oxford University Press, Oxford, Chap. 2.
6. Sexual Offences Act 1956, ss.14(2) and 15(2); Sexual Offences (Scotland) Act 1976, s.5.
7. Indecency With Children Act 1960, s.1.
8. Gordon, G. (1978) *The Criminal Law of Scotland*, 2nd edn, W. Green, Edinburgh, p. 903.
9. 1956 Act, s.5; 1976 Act, s.3.
10. 1956 Act, s.6; 1976 Act, s.4.
11. 1956 Act, s.6(2); 1976 Act, s.4(2)(a).
12. Marriage Act 1949, s.2; Marriage (Scotland) Act 1977, s.1.
13. 1956 Act, s.26; 1976 Act, s.14.
14. Protection of Children Act 1978, s.1: Civic Government (Scotland) Act 1982, s.52.
15. Child Care Act 1980, s.2; Social Work (Scotland) Act 1968, s.15.
16. Child Care Act 1980, s.13; Social Work (Scotland) Act 1968, s.3A.
17. Children and Young Persons Act 1969, s.1; Children and Young Persons (Scotland) Act 1937, s.12.
18. 1968 JC 53.
19. [1981] AC 394.
20. [1899] 1 QB 283.
21. Children and Young Persons Act 1969, s.1(2), Social Work (Scotland) Act 1968, s.37(2).
22. 1969 Act, s.1(1) and S.I. 1970/1500.
23. 1969 Act s.28; 1968 Act s.37.
24. [1978] AC 171.
25. Child Care Act, 1980, s.1; Social Work (Scotland) Act 1968, s.12.
26. 1969 Act, s.2(1); 1968 Act, s.37(1).
27. e.g. Child Protection Act 1974, Tasmania; Child Welfare Act 1977, New South Wales.
28. *Donoghue* v. *Stevenson* 1932 SC (HL) 31.
29. For example, Lothian Regional Review Committee (1983) *Guidelines on Non-Accidental Injury to Children (abuse or at risk to abuse)*, 3rd edn, Lothian Regional Social Work Committee, Edinburgh.
30. (1974) *Report of the Committee of Inquiry into the Care and Supervision of Maria Colwell* (Field-Fisher), HMSO, London.
31. (1985) *A Child In Trust, Report of the Panel of Inquiry into the Circumstances Surrounding the Death of Jasmine Beckford* (Blom-Cooper), Brent Council.
32. (1979) Care Proceedings: the child's interest. *Br. Med. J.*, **1**, 1570. *Humberside CC* v. *DPR* [1977] 3 All ER 964, *per* Widgery CJ.
33. Children and Young Persons Act 1969, ss.32A and 32B; Social Work (Scotland) Act 1968, s.34A.
34. *In re G* [1987] *The Times*, 30 July.
35. *B* v. *Kennedy*, unreported, 5 June 1987.
36. Social Work (Scotland) Act, 1968, Part III.
37. 1968 Act, s.32(2).
38. *M.* v. *McGregor* 1982 SLT 41.
39. *McGregor* v. *L.* 1981 SLT 194.
40. Criminal Procedure (Scotland) Act 1975, Sched. 1.
41. 1968 Act, s.36.
42. 1968 Act, s.39(1) and (2); Social Work Services Group, Statistical Group, Statistical Bulletin, 1987, No. 11, p.12.
43. Martin, F.M., Fox, S.J. and Murray, K. (1981) *Children Out Of Court*, Scottish Academic Press, Edinburgh.

44. Freeman, M.D.A., ref. 4, ch. 7.
45. Nurseries and Childminders Regulation Act 1948, s.4(2); Foster Children Act 1980, s.2(2)(a); Foster Children (Scotland) Act 1984, s.2(1)(a).
46. 1948 Act, s.1(1).
47. 1948 Act, s.2.
48. 1948 Act, s.4.
49. Hoggett, B. (1987) *Parents and Children*, 3rd edn, Sweet and Maxwell, London.
50. Foster Children (Scotland) Act 1984, s.1.
51. Foster Children Act 1980, s.2(3)(a).
52. 1980 Act, s.2(3)(b).
53. 1980 Act, s.2; 1984 Act, s.2.
54. 1980 Act, s.7; 1984 Act, s.7.
55. 1984 Act, s.4; S.I. 1985/1798.
56. S.I. 1985/1798.
57. 1980 Act, s.4.
58. *The Times* (1987) 26 August, p. 3.
59. Children and Young Persons Act 1969, s.2(1); Social Work (Scotland) Act 1968, s.37(1). For recent recommendations on the topic, see Department of Health and Social Security (1988) *Diagnosis of Child Sexual Abuse; Guidance for Doctors*, HMSO, London, and particularly Department of Health and Social Security and the Welsh Office (1988) *Working Together*, HMSO, London.
60. Editorial Comment (1981) Child abuse: the swing of the pendulum. *Br. Med. J.*, **283**, 170.
61. 1980 Act, s.2(3); 1968 Act, s.15(3).
62. [1979] 2 All ER 297.
63. 1980 Act, s.3(1); 1968 Act, s.16(1).
64. 1980 Act, s.3(3); 1968 Act, s.16(6).
65. 1980 Act, s.5; 1968 Act, s.18.
66. *Beagley* v. *Beagley* 1984 SLT 202.
67. Health and Social Services and Social Security Adjudications Act 1984, s.7.
68. The offences specified include; murder, manslaughter and causing bodily injury to a child or young person, incest, neglect or abuse of a child, causing or encouraging the seduction of a girl under 16, permitting a child to be present in a brothel and exposing a child under 7 to the danger of burning.
69. DHSS (1985) *Review of Child Care*, R,176, HMSO, London.
70. Child Care Act 1980, s.10(2).
71. *O, H, W, B, R,* v. *UK* [1987] *The Times*, 9 June.
72. [1982] AC 363.
73. [1985] AC 791.
74. *Re D.M. (a minor)* [1986] 2FLR 122; *R* v. *Bedfordshire County Council, ex p C* (1987) *Fam. Law*, **17**, 55.
75. *R* v. *Newham Borough Council,ex p. McL*, (1987) 137 NLJ 903.
76. 2815 applications for wardship were made in 1985; Judicial Statistics for England and Wales, 1985, Cmnd. 9864.
77. Practice Direction [1976] 1 All ER 828.
78. *Re D (a Minor) (Wardship: Sterilisation)* [1976] 1 All ER 326.
79. *Re JT (a Minor) (Wardship: Committal to Care)* [1986] 2 FLR 107.
80. Practice Direction [1982] 1 All ER 319.
81. Bromley, P.M. and Lowe, N.V. (1987) *Bromley's Family Law*, 7th edn, Butterworths, London, p. 428.
82. *Re H (GJ) (an infant)* [1966] 1 All ER 952.
83. *Re N (care and control: access)* [1983] 4 FLR 150.
84. Family Law Reform Act 1969, s.7(2).
85. *Re D (a Minor) (Wardship: Medical Treatment)* [1981] 1 WLR 1421.
86. *Re B (a Minor) (Wardship: Sterilization)* [1987] 2 All ER 206.
87. Buxbaum, E.R. and Hirsh, H.L. (1983) Minors and health care. *Med. Law*, **2**, 335.
88. Schwartz, A. and Hirsh, H.L. (1982) Child abuse and neglect. *Med. Trial Technique Q.*, **28**, 293.
89. Drews, K-M. (1983) When minors seek medical treatment on their own behalf. *Med. Law*, **2**, 209.
90. Cohn, R. (1985) Minors' right to consent to medical care. *Med. Trial Technique Q.*, **31**, 286.
91. Brackshaw, S.L. (1983) Health care over objections of the parents: clash or right. *Med. Law*, **2**, 221.
92. Hirsh, H.L. and Phifer, H. (1985) The interface of medicine, religion and the law: religious objections to treatment. *Med. Law*, **4**, 121.
93. Gibbs, R.F. (1987) Jehovah's Witnesses and the question of blood. *Legal Aspects Med. Pract.*, **5**, 4.
94. Holder, A.L. (1987) Minors' rights to consent to medical care. *JAMA*, **25**, 3400.
95. Restaino, J.H. (1987) Informed consent: should it be extended to 12-year-olds? *Med. Law*, **6**, 91.

96. *Planned Parenthood of Central Missouri v Danforth* 428 US 52 (1976).

97. *Hallmark Clinic v North Carolina Department of Human Resource* 519 F 2d 1315 (1975).

98. Soskin, R.M. (1983) Sterilization of the mentally retarded: the rules change but the results remain. *Med. Law,* **2**, 267.

99. Hirsh, H.L. (1983) Psychiatric malpractice: liability for suicide and attempted self-destruction. *Urban Health,* **12**, 26.

100. *Parham v J R* 442 US 584 (1979).

101. Goichman, S. and Hirsh, H.L. (1983) The expanding rights of the fetus: an evolution not a revolution. *Med. Trial Technique Q.,* **30**, 212.

102. *State v Willis* 652 P 2d 1222 (NM, 1982).

103. *Taft v Taft* 442 NE 2d 395 (Mass, 1983); *Jefferson v Griffin Spalding County Hospital Authority* 274 SE 2d 457 (Ga, 1981).

104. *Group Health Association v Blumenthal* 453 A 2d 1198 (Md, 1983).

105. *In re Green* 292 A 2d 387 (Pa, 1972); *In re Karwath* 199 NW 2d 147 (Iowa, 1972).

PART 4

Ethical considerations

CHAPTER 30

Research and experimentation involving children

R.A. McCall Smith

The medical need to conduct research on children raises a fundamental and, in many instances, uncomfortable problem – research requires that its subjects should be capable of consenting to participation if it is to be regarded as ethical [1]. This requirement is stated explicitly in all the codes which have been devised to regulate research since the Nuremberg Trials [2]. Thus, captive populations, the mentally ill, the economically desperate and children all fail to meet the criteria necessary for inclusion in medical research programmes to a greater or lesser degree. None of these categories, however, should be excluded automatically; there will be many shades of grey around the black and white cases. Prisoners do participate in medical research – and do so voluntarily; new psychotropic drugs are tested on those suffering from mental illness – and such research is by no means all unethical; there will be some volunteers for whom even a small financial inducement is an important factor in the decision to participate in medical trials; and research in paediatric medicine would come to a halt if doctors were not prepared to use under-age subjects in their projects. In practice, then, those on the margins of eligibility do participate. The problem for those concerned with the ethics

and legality of such participation is one of deciding the point at which the line between the acceptable and the unacceptable is drawn.

30.1 WHY ARE CHILDREN A SPECIAL CASE?

The concept of childhood which is widely accepted in the West in the twentieth century has led to the placing of children in a special category of persons to whom special privileges are accorded. These involve, in particular, protection from certain aspects of adult existence: children are protected from exposure to sexual matters and from certain forms of violence, and, most importantly, they are sheltered from the economic responsibilities of adult life. Child labour is illegal in many Western countries and is regarded with particular distaste by modern social reformers.

It was not always so [3]. It is only in the nineteenth century that we begin to see the emergence of what was initially a middle and upper class notion of a prolonged and privileged childhood. In due course this concept was embraced by the less advantaged sections of the community, who could now afford the luxury of non-working children, and was endorsed by the legal systems and the champions of social and political morality. In 1959, the United Nations Declaration on the Rights of Children stated in Principle 2 that:

> the child shall enjoy special protection, and shall be given opportunities and facilities, by law and by other means, to enable him to develop physically, mentally, morally, spiritually and socially in a healthy and normal manner and in conditions of freedom and dignity. In the enactment of laws for this purpose the best interests of the child shall be the paramount consideration.

The concept of 'sheltered childhood', being a means of protecting children from, economic exploitation, was extended to encompass the protection of children against other forms of abuse by adults. Legislation criminalizing sexual activities with children was passed in the United Kingdom in the late nineteenth century and, during the twentieth century, the courts have steadily eroded parental rights in favour of a form of parental 'trusteeship'. Legally and socially, therefore, children have become a special case. How far should this special status be endorsed and to what extent should it exclude them from participation in medical research? I hope to demonstrate here that, although there are features of the child's position that must give him a special status in some areas, there are some respects in which children may participate in society on the same footing as adults. One implication of this is that researchers are not barred from using children as subjects in research projects purely because they are children.

30.2 THE RESEARCHER'S QUESTION: WHAT CAN I DO?

(a) Ethical restraints

Medical research involving children is subject to the same general restraints as are applied to other forms of medical research. Some of these limitations are specifically legal in origin; others are ethical. Unfortunately, the legal situation sometimes seems as ill-defined as is the ethical position; those engaged in research are, consequently, uncertain as to the extent and nature of the restrictions on what they may do. It would be helpful if one could say that ethical research is always legal and that research which involves illegality will always be unethical. Unfortunately, however, the difficulties of defining what is ethical preclude such a simple solution.

Researchers are assisted by a variety of guidelines set out by a number of national and international bodies. These guidelines do not have the effect of law but must, nonetheless, be observed if a researcher wishes to avoid allegations of unethical practice. Their essential aim is to ensure that the subjects of medical research are not exploited in a way which is harmful to their interests. Existing codes of research ethics recognize that children present special problems. The Declaration of Helsinki (1975) does not exclude the use of children in research projects, but makes specific provision for the consent of the 'responsible relative' to replace that of the subject. More detailed guidance has been provided by the Institute of Medical Ethics, which has recommended rules to be followed by ethics committees in examining proposals for research involving children [4]. The Institute's view is that this is permissible only if it is scientifically valid, cannot be done on adult subjects with the same effect and is potentially of considerable benefit to children. Any benefit obtained from the research should substantially outweigh risks and the only acceptable risks in non-therapeutic research are those which are minimal. The Institute's definition of a minimal risk is one that involves a risk of death lower than one in a million, a risk of a major complication of less than ten in a million or a risk of a minor complication of less than ten in a thousand.

In addition to these requirements, the Institute's guidelines detail certain specifications as to consent. Therapeutic research involving more than a minimal risk should be undertaken only after parents have been given information in writing and have consented after considering this information. Children over the age of 7 should give their own consent to participation; if the child is unwilling, then, provided he is under 14, parental consent may override this unwillingness. A child aged 14 and over should be able to refuse to participate in research irrespective of the parental view, although the consent of parents is recommended until he reaches the age of 16 in the case of therapeutic research or 18 in the case of non-therapeutic research. In effect, then, the Institute's guidelines suggest that no minor should be used in non-therapeutic research unless there is parental consent to such involvement.

The source of these guidelines is an influential body, and they are likely to be applied by many ethics committees vetting research proposals. They are not, however, the last word on the subject.

(b) Legal constraints

The legality of non-therapeutic medical research on children is a subject which has caused considerable concern amongst paediatricians [5]. Some lawyers have commented that all such research on minors is illegal irrespective of parental consent and this view has led to the suspension of a number of research projects involving children [6]. The advice given by bodies concerned with research has been guarded and, sometimes, unhelpful. For example the Medical Research Council's statement issued in 1962 said:

> In the strict view of the law parents and guardians of minors cannot give consent on their behalf to any procedures which are of no particular benefit to them and which may carry some risk of harm. [7]

This statement did not say what was meant by the term 'some harm', but it could be argued that it did not exclude projects where the risk of harm was negligible. Caution was still the keyword a decade later. The Royal College of Physicians stated that children could be used in non-therapeutic research only where there was a negligible risk of harm and 'subject to the provisions of any common or statute law prevailing at the time' [8]. This, however, still left the law undefined and a Department of Health and Social Security circular subsequently further reduced the confidence of researchers by advising that they ought not to assume that the existence of no more than a negligible risk would bring a research project within the law even when it was coupled with parental consent [9].

The grounds upon which these views were expressed – that parents are legally incapable of consenting to anything which is not in the best interests of the child – are now widely discounted. This has been established in a number of decisions in which the courts have indicated that, while the best interests of the child are an important consideration, they are not the only matter to be taken into account and that the general public interest is a factor which enters into the calculations of the responsible parent [10]. The general public interest, however, would be unlikely to prevail if involvement in the research in question were to be found to be clearly damaging to the child's interests. No reasonable parent would consent to the involvement of a child in a programme of research which carried an appreciable risk of damage and it would be unwise for researchers in such circumstances to rely on parental consent.

The question of what would constitute a negligible or acceptable risk is obviously one on which there may be more than one view. There are some procedures in which the risks of anything more serious than minor and temporary discomfort are infinitesimal; most researchers and subjects would undoubtedly regard such risks as negligible. On the other hand, there may be disagreement as to the significance of the risks attached to, say, skin biopsy or procedures involving exposure to even a small dose of investigative radiation. There would probably be near unanimity on the unacceptably high risks entailed in liver biopsy carried out in a non-therapeutic context [11]. The definition of negligible risk suggested by the Institute of Medical Ethics at least has the attraction of mathematical precision.

Even if it is agreed that it is legal to involve minors in non-therapeutic research when parental consent has been given and where the risk is negligible, the question remains as to whether a minor should be able to participate in non-therapeutic research without parental consent or in the face of a parental objection to such involvement. The Institute of Medical Ethics guidelines would preclude this, even if the minor is a week short of his eighteenth birthday and living completely independently of his parents. In such a case one may be tempted to ask why the law should impose such an incapacity, if indeed it does.

The decision of the House of Lords in the controversial case of *Gillick* v. *West Norfolk and Wisbech Area Health Authority and Another* [12] is of some importance in this context, even if it has few implications for the younger child. This case was concerned with the ability of the minor to consent to treatment (the treatment in question being contraception), but it could be argued that the propositions contained in the judgement are applicable to involvement in research as well as to submission to therapeutic procedures. In each case, the matter at issue is the competence of the minor to decide what is done with his or her body within a medical context. Both therapy and non-therapeutic experimentation involve the subjection of the body to procedures which are pro-social in their objective and, if a minor

is competent to make a decision about therapy, he should also be competent to make a decision about involvement in medical experimentation. Both sorts of decision involve assessing risks and acting on the basis of such an assessment.

The essence of the *Gillick* decision is that the minor under the age of 16 may consent to treatment provided he has the ability to understand what is entailed in the treatment. No hard and fast age rule is suggested; competence will be determined according to the characteristics of the child in question. If this approach were to be taken in relation to non-therapeutic research, then whether or not a child under the age of 16 could involve himself in research would depend on the assessment of his ability to comprehend. *A fortiori*, there would be no restriction on the use of children over 16, who are enabled by the provisions of the Family Law Reform Act 1969 to give their consent to medical treatment. The fact that this Act empowers the child over the age of 16 to give a valid consent to medical treatment does not necessarily preclude valid consent to such treatment being given by those under that age, an interpretation of the law which was effectively endorsed by the House of Lords in *Gillick*. The provision in the Act which states that the Act itself should have no bearing on anything which would otherwise have been legal means that the participation of minors in medical research is unaffected by the legislation, provided that it is legal [13].

The difficulty with this analysis is that *Gillick* was solely concerned with decisions as to treatment. It could be argued that the issues involved in participation in medical research are so distinct as to fall outwith the ambit of the principle enunciated by the House of Lords. Acceptance of medical treatment implies a decision that such treatment is in one's best interests, in the sense of protecting one's physical welfare. By contrast, a decision to engage in a potentially hazardous activity does not carry with it the presumption that concern with welfare is the motivating factor.

The majority of the judgements in the House of Lords either implicitly or explicitly rejected the 'extreme' view of parental rights in which the parent is given almost unlimited discretion as to how the child spends his time. The judges were careful, however, not to exclude any parental interest in the matter of medical treatment; it could be argued that involvement in non-therapeutic research is precisely the sort of area where continued parental concern is still appropriate. The presence of risk for no benefit does distinguish such cases from the case of medical treatment; parental involvement might be seen as an important protection for the immature subject. For this reason, it would be safer for researchers not to involve minors in medical research, even if the degree of risk is slight, if the parents have not given their consent to their child's involvement. A broad view of the decision in *Gillick* could suggest otherwise, at least in the case of the more mature minor, but this is not an interpretation of the law on which the researcher could necessarily rely.

Hazardous research on minors is undoubtedly to be avoided, even if the minor is mature and consents and even if the parent has given consent to his child's involvement. The reason for this is that the nature of the consent which the minor can give is subject to an overall public policy limitation. In cases involving negligible risk, the courts may be prepared to accept parental consent or even, on the broad view of *Gillick*, the independent consent of a mature minor; but they would, however, be likely to reject the validity of such consent in a case where the risk of harm was appreciable, on the grounds that consenting to the risk of appreciable harm is something which the law should not allow minors to do. A variety of rationales could be found for such

a refusal – a likely one is the inability of the minor truly to appreciate the implications of such a risk.

The practical consequences of involving children in a medical experiment in circumstances where they or their parents cannot or do not give a valid consent could be serious. A criminal law charge of assault could be competent in such circumstances in that there has been an unlawful touching of the child. A criminal offence, thus, could be committed by a researcher who subjects a child to a hazardous procedure even if both the child and the parents have consented, consent in such a case being irrelevant on public policy grounds. A civil action for damages by the parent would also be legally competent, as would one raised on behalf of the child by his parents or by himself at a later stage.

30.3 THE CURRENT RULES: A CRITIQUE

It is not difficult to identify research projects involving children which will appear controversial according to the ethical criteria identified above. One which enjoys particular notoriety in the literature is the Willowbrook experiment, which was conducted in the United States [14]. In this experiment, which has been widely criticized, mentally retarded children living in an institution – in which various infections were rampant – were deliberately injected with the virus of infective hepatitis in the course of research into the disease. In defence of the project, it was pointed out that the children were actually benefitted by exposure to the virus, as they would subsequently have been in contact with it anyway and it was better for them to develop a subclinical infection under controlled conditions [15]. A more recent European study provides an example of an equally objectionable experiment on children. This project involved the testing by French paediatric cardiologists of a new procedure for the transposition of the great arteries [16]. The existing procedures, which have a mortality of up to 10%, were abandoned in favour of a new procedure which had a mortality of 20% during the first stage of the experiment. Six children died in this stage of the experiment; this did not stop the researchers proceeding, and seven children died in the second stage. Even if justification is seen for the first stage of the experiment, it is difficult to defend the second against such a background of mortality.

It is, perhaps, not surprising to see that the most defenceless of children have also been the most vulnerable. In the recent 'Baby Fae' case in California, a 14-day-old infant with a fatal heart condition received the heart of a baboon [17]. This bizarre operation was performed in the face of overwhelming evidence of the hopelessness of animal-to-human transplantation in current conditions. In spite of the certainty of rejection of the animal organ by the infant's body, it appeared that no effort was made to locate a human heart for transplantation; thus a possible line of treatment was ignored in favour of a procedure which could not possibly prolong the subject's life.

A fourth case demonstrates the touchiness of the issue and the difficulties that may be encountered by researchers who proceed with what they feel is quite ethical research but which is subsequently questioned. An Oxford study was designed to detect whether stress experienced by babies undergoing operations could be alleviated by the addition of a narcotic analgesic to the conventional anaesthetic regimen of nitrous oxide. There were strong parliamentary and press protests over this experiment which were largely concentrated on the fact that some of the babies involved in the study were not given the benefit of the analgesic. The problem with this criticism, however, was that it was directed against an existing practice which had been followed for sound reasons –

namely, because of the belief that the use of deep anaesthesia and narcotic analgesics increases the risk of cardiorespiratory failure in babies undergoing operations. No new discomfort was, therefore, visited on the group of babies operated upon without analgesia.

These cases are out of the ordinary but are worth recalling in order to illustrate how ethical principles surrounding medical research can be tested. It could be argued that, in the first two cases, the health of at least some of the subjects was placed in jeopardy for reasons quite unconnected with the welfare of the children in question. One might go even further in the case of Baby Fae and say that the life of the patient was deliberately shortened in order to obtain whatever data were sought. But would there have been any difference if the subjects in those three cases had been adults?

In the Willowbrook case, had the subjects been mentally defective adults and had the research been viewed as purely non-therapeutic – a difficult question in the circumstances – the project would have been ethically unacceptable on the grounds of the subjects' inability to give a valid consent. The consent of adults to such a procedure would probably have made the Paris cardiological experiment ethically acceptable, but only until the appreciably higher mortality rate was known. Thereafter, the performance of the new procedure on adult patients would have been ethically unacceptable had the motive of the surgeons been that of scientific curiosity rather than therapy. Finally, had Baby Fae been a competent adult, her consent to such a hopeless procedure would not have made it ethical, as the operation was bound to hasten her death and could serve no therapeutic purpose. If, however, such an operation were to give a few extra weeks of life, then a competent consent might render it legitimate.

What is it that is so morally dubious about the first three experiments described above?

The most offensive feature – one which occurs even when we imagine the subjects as adults rather than children – is the fact that the subjects are being 'used'; they are means rather than ends in themselves – and that offends an important moral principle. A person is not used, however, if he freely decides to participate in a project. To decide to participate in a medical experiment involves the exercise of autonomy and it is equally wrong to seek to prevent someone from exercising his autonomy. To what extent, then, do children have an autonomy which they can exercise in this way?

30.4 CHILDREN AND AUTONOMY

The notion of the autonomy of the person is one of the most strongly defended principles in contemporary moral discussion. Full autonomy, however, may be denied to those who are incapable for some reason of exercising it – and children clearly fall into this category.

To say that a person is incapable of exercising full autonomy is not the same as saying that such a person will be incapable of all action. Autonomy cannot be an indivisible concept [18]: for example, the person whose judgement is affected by illness may be incapable of making certain fully informed decisions about treatment but he may be perfectly able to reach a reasonable decision about, say, how to spend his money. In each case, the nature of the action should be considered in the light of what is known about the limitations on the subject's ability to exercise his autonomy.

The child's ability in this context is restricted in certain significant respects. First, his knowledge is likely to be limited. He may also pay more attention to short-term rather than long-term benefit, the immediate good being more attractive than the prospect of later good. There will also be changes of mind:

a body tattoo might seem exciting to the 10-year-old boy but could be an embarrassing disfigurement to the young man of 20.

These factors may be of considerable importance in reaching certain decisions but may be quite irrelevant in others. Consider the case of a child to whom money is given as a present. The child's decision to spend the gift on something which will bring him only short-term benefit – an item which will soon break or be consumed – will seem unwise to the outside observer. To the child, however, it is what he wants, and choosing for himself may be quite important to him. It might be wrong, therefore, to attempt to stop him exercising his autonomy in this way, the decision to 'waste the money' being within the scope of what a person of limited autonomy might properly be allowed to do. A different decision would be reached if the sum involved was considerable. Here we would be inclined to prevent any squandering, justifying our intervention on the seriousness of the damage to the child's interests.

The point of this example is to illustrate the proposition that it is absurd to suggest a blanket denial of autonomy to children. A child should be able to act independently in some matters, while paternalistic intervention is appropriate to stop his acting irresponsibly in others. The factor which distinguishes the two cases in the example cited above is the degree of harm involved. Thus, paternalistic intervention will be appropriate where the course of action undertaken by the child is substantially harmful of his interests – but does this necessarily apply where the action involves a purpose which, while admittedly harmful of the child's interests, is possibly beneficial to others? The answer to this question has a strong bearing on the acceptability of the use of children in medical research because the acceptance of altruism on the part of children must entail allowing children to participate in medical research which carries some degree of risk.

30.5 THE JUSTIFICATION OF PATERNALISM

Let us imagine a case of a child of 12 years of age who has agreed to participate in a clinical trial which involves a risk which, though not great, is nonetheless more than negligible. The issues have been explained to him and he says that he understands. His motive for participation, as far as can be ascertained, is one of a desire to help others.

One approach to such a case is to dismiss his consent to participation as being irrelevant on the grounds of lack of capacity. I have argued above that such a blanket exclusion is wrong in that it offends against the principle of the child's autonomy. A preferable approach is to accept that this sort of activity is within the competence of the child provided that there are no reasons for paternalistic intervention.

The concept which is most central to any philosophical justification of paternalism is that of the existence of a verifiable human good [19]. Human action may help or hinder the attainment of this good and, in the normal case, should be allowed to do either. Ignorance, however, may prevent a person from reaching a judgement as to the effect of his actions in relation to this good and, when this is the case, the paternalist may say that there is a case for intervention. Undoubtedly there will be many children whose ignorance will exclude them from participation in any medical research in which there is more than negligible risk. A child may understand that a procedure carries a risk, for example, of a slight blemish or disfigurement and may discount the seriousness of this. An adult, however, might reach a different view about the seriousness of disfigurement, believing that it is the child's ignorance of the psychological implications of that particular consequence which explains his nonchalant attitude. In such a case, the principle of paternalism justifies vetoing the child's participation in that it may be assumed that

there is a strong possibility that the child will regret consenting to the risk at a later stage. If, however, the risk is one which an adult might be expected to accept, then the case for accepting the child's assumption of that risk becomes stronger.

30.6 THE REALITY OF CONSENT

In the case considered above, it was assumed that the child has been appraised of all the facts and has given a meaningful consent to his participation. Does it make any moral difference if such consent is not present?

The simplest case would be where there is an unambiguous refusal on the part of the child to participate in a non-therapeutic research project. To enforce participation would be totally unacceptable on the grounds that to do so would be to fail to respect the child's autonomy and to treat him as a means rather than an end in himself. On purely pragmatic grounds, too, such a course of action could cause considerable psychological damage irrespective of the physical risks involved.

At the opposite end of the spectrum is the child who appears to understand what is at stake and who gives a ready consent. The significance of this consent will depend to a great extent on the age of the child. There is a widely held view among psychologists that children under the age of 7 are unable to form the necessary judgements to give a meaningful consent to participation in research. It is, furthermore, suggested that, between the age of 7 and 14, the extent of the child's understanding of the issues and his ability to make a considered and informed judgement will be limited [20]. Thus, the issue of the child's consent will be most relevant in the case of children in their mid- to late-teens; prior to that age, the importance of obtaining the child's consent is not so much in order to legitimate his participation but to ensure that no psychological damage results from involvement.

A rather more difficult case is where the child expresses neither consent nor opposition to participation. This may be because the child is too young either to understand what is being done or to express any opinion at all. This case is to be distinguished from that of the consenting child in that, here, there is no exercise of autonomy. Justification of the child's involvement in such a case is likely to be based on the grounds of subsequent consent – namely, that the child may be expected, on reaching a sufficient age, retrospectively to consent to his involvement.

30.7 SOCIAL ARGUMENTS

Consent-based justifications focus firmly on the autonomy of the individual; the social argument, however, rests on the premise that society as a whole has a strong and legitimate interest in the furtherance of medical knowledge. Medical progress is something from which we all benefit and everyone, therefore, has a duty to assist it wherever possible, but it would be difficult to argue that merely by taking the general benefit of modern medicine one has a positive duty to volunteer for medical research. Volunteering to participate is clearly a good thing to do; refusing a specific request for slight grounds is, as has been suggested above, wrong; but merely doing nothing is not something which we would normally be prepared to condemn. We would not impose a duty on people to participate in research in the same way as the state may enforce a duty to pay taxes or serve in the armed forces. Yet, in allowing non-consenting children to participate in medical research, are we not effectively enforcing performance of a social duty? This is undoubtedly a weakness of the social argument: it discriminates against those who are unable to register an opinion. We do not use it to coerce adults and yet, it is used here to coerce children.

One answer to this objection is to argue, as some doctors do, that much research which is prima facie non-therapeutic is, in reality, therapeutic for the participant. This may be upheld by treating all children as a member of a class and by saying that the individual benefits from something which is for the benefit of that class as a whole. Progress in the combatting of a childhood disease may benefit that particular child in the future and is, therefore, therapeutic. Alternatively, research may benefit a sibling, already existing or future, of that child and is, therefore, to the participant's psychological advantage.

These arguments interpret the concept of the child's benefit in an unrealistically broad manner. It would be far more honest to say that the benefit of participation is for the class of children in general and that this is a goal worth achieving even if it involves subjecting individual children to minor risk. This is similar in some respects to the argument which may be used to support large-scale vaccination programmes.

30.8 THE ROLE OF THE PARENTS

In one view, the most important consideration in deciding whether children may be used for medical research is the question of parental consent. The consent of parents is treated by some as a substitute consent, having the same effect as that of the child [21]. The parent may be assumed to act in the best interests of the child and will, therefore, not consent to anything which carries with it any risk of real harm. That parents do not always have the best interest of the child at heart is, however, uncomfortably apparent and, undoubtedly, there will be cases where parents act contrariwise – parents who refuse permission on religious grounds for their children to have blood transfusions provide an example. Alternatively, and perhaps less convincingly, the parent may consent as the person who is most likely to appreciate that to which the child may be expected to give retrospective consent when he reaches an age at which he can understand the implications of his involvement.

Both these justifications are child centred; a quite different tack would be to argue that the giving of parental consent in these circumstances involves the exercise of a power which parents have as parents and that this is justification enough. This is a controversial view which has relatively few supporters, although there are those who stress the importance of parental powers and who seek therefore to minimize state intervention in family matters [22]. The notion of parental power allowing the parent to exercise unrestrained authority over the child belongs to the era of the patriarch and has been replaced by a concept of parental rights in which the parent is regarded as a 'trustee' of the child's interests. As some have put it, the whole point of parental rights is to guide the child to the stage where he can make his own decisions.

This last view of parental rights, focusing on the self-determination of the child, is open to the criticism that it disregards the extent to which the process of bringing up a child involves directional activity. If it were possible to bring up children in such a way that all their important decisions will be deferred until adult life, then that would undoubtedly achieve maximum freedom of the individual. The failure to inculcate values during childhood, however, would surely make them ill-equipped for life as responsible adults. Responsibility to society is clearly such an area, and it could be argued that this is an area in which the exercise of parental power without a requirement of benefit to the child is appropriate because of the very nature of the endeavour.

30.9 CONCLUSIONS

Non-therapeutic medical research involving minors is ethically acceptable provided that the risks involved are minimal. Such research should, in the case of children who are capable of understanding the issues, involve the consent of the child, and should never be undertaken where there is any real opposition on the child's part. The issue of determining what is a minimal risk is one that must be confronted by those who are concerned with ethical restraints on research – preferably by such bodies as research committees which include outside participation. Research involving more than a negligible risk is unethical, even with parental consent, until such time as the child is quite capable of exercising autonomy in relation to a decision of this significance; this will probably not be until the later teen years.

There is now sufficient agreement among lawyers to indicate that the legality of non-therapeutic research on children is something which can be relied upon by the medical profession, provided that the risk is negligible. The consent of the parents is always desirable, although it is possible that a child who is capable of understanding the issues could give an independent consent. This, however, remains legally unresolved and it would, therefore, be safer to obtain parental consent in all cases until the child reaches the age of 18.

REFERENCES

1. For general discussion of the ethical issues surrounding the use of children in research, see van Eys, J. (ed.) (1978) *Research on Children*, University Park Press, Baltimore; Nicholson, R.H. (ed.) (1986) *Medical Research with Children: Ethics, Law and Practice*, Oxford University Press, Oxford.
2. For the texts of the various declarations, see Duncan, A.S., Dunstan, G.R. and Welbourn,

R.B. (eds) (1981) *Dictionary of Medical Ethics* sub 'Declarations', Darton, Longman & Todd, London.

3. Arries, P. (1965) *Centuries of Childhood*, Random, New York; Freeman, M.D.A. (1983) *The Rights and Wrongs of Children*, Pinter, London, pp. 6–26.

4. *Inst. Med. Ethics Bull*, (1986) No. 14, 8; Robinson, R.J. (1987) Ethics Committees and research in children. *Br. Med. J.*, **294**, 1243.

5. For a general survey of the law, see Mason, J.K. and McCall Smith, R.A. (1987) *Law and Medical Ethics*, 2nd edn, Butterworths, London, p. 268 *et seq.*

6. Editorial comment (1978) Research on children. *Br. Med. J.*, **2**, 1043.

7. Report of the Medical Research Council for 1962–3, (1964) Cmnd 2382 (1964) HMSO, London, p. 21.

8. Quoted in Skegg, P. (1984) *Law, Ethics and Medicine*, Oxford University Press, Oxford, p. 64.

9. Department of Health and Social Security (1975) HSC (I.S.) 153.

10. See Dworkin, G. (1978) Legality of consent to nontherapeutic medical research on infants and young children. *Arch. Dis Child.*, **53**, 443. See also Skegg, P., ref. 8, p.66.

11. See Nicholson, ref. 1, p. 76, there is a useful bibliography on risk identification in this work at pp. 121–4.

12. [1985] 3 All ER 402, HL.

13. Family Law Reform Act 1969, s.8 (3).

14. Krugman, S., Ward, B. and Giles, J.P. (1959) Infectious hepatitis: detection of the virus during the incubation period and in clinically inapparent infection. *New Engl. J. Med.*, **261**, 729.

15. Krugman, S. (1971) Experiments at the Willowbrook State School. *Lancet*, **1**, 966.

16. For details see Nicholson, ref. 1, p.28.

17. Schwartz, H.S. (1985) Bioethical and legal considerations in increasing the supply of organs: from UAGA to 'Baby Fae'. *Am. J. Law Med.*, **10**, 397.

18. Haworth, L. (1986) *Autonomy*, Yale University Press, New Haven, p. 55.

19. VanDeVeer, D. (1986) *Paternalistic Intervention*, University Press, Princeton; Culver, C.M. and Gert, B. (1982) *Philosophy in Medicine*, Oxford University Press, Oxford, p. 183 *et seq.*

20. Weithorn, L.A. and Campbell, S.B. (1982) The competency of children and adolescents to make informed treatment decisions. *Child Dev.*, **53**, 285. For discussion, see Nicholson, ref. 1, p. 146.

21. McCormick, R.A. (1982) Proxy consent in the experimental situation. *Perspect. Biol. Med.*, **54**. Contrast, Ramsey, P. (1970) *The Patient as a Person*, Yale University Press, New Haven, pp. 44–7.

22. Goldstein, J., Freud, A. and Solnit, A. (1979) *Beyond the Best Interests of the Child*, The Free Press, London.

CHAPTER 31

Modern paediatric practice: an ethical overview

R.S. Downie

Many of the previous chapters have involved discussions of specific ethical issues in paediatrics such as selective non-treatment of the newborn, consent, parental rights, research and experimentation involving children and so on. The function of an overview is less to add to the discussion of *specific* problems than to provide a survey of the *types* of ethical argument to be found in paediatrics. Accordingly, I will try to fulfil two objectives in this chapter. The first is to draw attention to the all-pervasive nature of value judgements in paediatrics, for it is easy to suppose that values arise only over a small number of identifiable dilemmas and that the rest of paediatrics is technical. The second aim is to discuss, very briefly, the nature of the values which govern medical practice as a whole and then, at greater length, to try to show the special problems which arise when these values are applied in paediatric practice.

31.1 THE TECHNICAL MODEL AND ITS LIMITATIONS

The health-care professions are pre-eminently practical in that they are concerned not simply with adding generally to our knowledge or skills but with carrying out a variety of specific actions and policies which are aimed at effective health care. Moreover, they act in relation to *individual* patients or clients or to *specific* communities. It follows from this that the basic question posed to anyone working in health care is: 'What ought I to do for the best care of this patient or this community?'. In other words, the fundamental question of all caring is individualized and has an 'ought' in it. It is not asking: 'What, in general, *is* the case?'. A question of the latter sort is one for the scientist and is answered by the provision of scientific knowledge, whereas the basic question of care is practical and cannot be answered only by way of information as to what is the case. To answer a practical 'ought' question is to make a *decision* about what ought to be done.

However, there are close links between scientific or technical questions about what is the case and practical questions about what ought to be done – and this applies in many situations besides medical practice. For example, let us imagine that someone who wants to buy a house, or who wants a divorce, goes to a solicitor. The solicitor will decide what ought to be done in the light of his client's wants and of his own knowledge of the law. Thus, we have a professional context in which there are: (i) desires for a given objective and (ii) knowledge of the best available means. A specific decision ought to be taken but it will be taken on a scientific or technical plane; the 'ought' embodies no moral element.

Such a technical model of decision-making is persuasive and is one which is particularly deeply rooted in the health-care professions. It flourishes especially at this time in history when all health-care professions are striving to become more technical and to build up their expertise. Unfortunately, it is not only an oversimplified model but it is also misleading. It conceals from doctors, and from the general public, the pervasive nature of moral and value judgements which are inevitably made in the diagnosis and treatment of patients – and, indeed, in the assessment of the success or failure of such treatments. It is, therefore, important to bring out where the technical model is deficient [1]. This is especially so in paediatrics – an area in which patients and their families are emotionally vulnerable. Let us set out the technical model in a paediatric context:

(1) The paediatrician has relevant scientific knowledge and skills;
(2) the patient needs treatment for a specific problem;
(3) the paediatrician wants to offer treatment.

It seems to follow from these three propositions that the paediatrician ought to take a certain decision in the light of the given situation. But the important complication is that uncertainty, and, therefore, value judgements enter at every step. Take the first step – and let us imagine the following case:

Case report
Jimmy has torn his leg badly on barbed wire. The wound has been cleaned and sutured by the SHO and, 3 days later, the child is brought back to the outpatient clinic. It is noted that both the dressing and the child are in a filthy state giving rise to a risk of infection of the ragged edges of the wound. The limited conversation which the consultant is able to have with an older sister leaves him in much doubt as to whether the usual procedure of leaving the wound uncovered and prescribing an antibiotic spray would work. But he really cannot admit an otherwise healthy boy into an already over-stretched ward. Nor is there any point in asking the health centre to find one of the district nurses to take on the case. They are trying to cover far more urgent cases ...

There is no doubt that the consultant is struggling with a practical dilemma; he is not sure what he ought to do, what might be the best means of doing it or whether he will succeed whatever he decides to do. When he thinks about the problem, he will clearly be assisted by his knowledge of science and economics – but these disciplines cannot, by themselves, determine his decision as to what he ought to do. Let us consider why.

There is a science of bacteriology and a great deal is known about the general circumstances in which a wound becomes infected. But the consultant is not sure if it will do so in this case; his information is incomplete and not entirely certain. This is typical of clinical situations even when they do not have the other complexities of our example. The nature of the available evidence means that a decision, even one based on the purely scientific aspects of a clinical problem, must be tentative – like the propounding of a hypothesis which is to be tested by future observation. Such hypotheses are frequently raised and tested in clinical practice, even in very straightforward situations. For example, the laboratory results suggest that a bacterium cultured from a patient would be sensitive to a particular antibiotic; the hypothesis is tested by prescribing the antibiotic.

This also implies that, in some circumstances, clinical decisions cannot be wholly determined by the scientific evidence, for it is incomplete; a judgement of a wider kind is, therefore, required. To take the example further, suppose the bacterial culture showed that the organism was sensitive to two antibiotics, one of which was cheap but was known to have a 5% risk of side-effects and the other was twice the price but carried a 2% incidence of side-effects. How should the doctor choose? The example also emphasizes that decision-making is associated with probabilities. This is best illustrated by considering the difficult question of prognosis. Take a child with leukaemia in which, say, the recorded prognosis – as judged from observation and a review of the literature – is that he will survive if he is exposed to a course of chemotherapy. This is a probability which must be translated into the particular and communicated to the parents. And to the child? The difficulties with this are apparent but they highlight the problems of translating factual information into clinical decisions.

The discussion so far has concentrated, although not exclusively, on the scientific uncertainties and, therefore, the value judgements which must be made by the *paediatrician*. Let us now look at the situation from the point of view of the *patient's* wants or needs. First, patients of all ages, but especially children, may be confused as to their wants. For example, a child may present with one problem, perhaps, a skin rash, but he may want really to talk about some other matter – maybe that he is unhappy at home; alternatively, the patient may not always realize fully that this is what he wants to talk about. Similarly, a child in hospital may ask a nurse to help with some need or discomfort but is really wanting company for a few minutes. Secondly, the simple model of decision-making presupposes that the patient wants only one thing, whereas he may have several, sometimes incompatible, objectives. For instance, a child may want to go home for his birthday but, at the same time, he wants to please the health-care team by staying in hospital. Thirdly, the needs and wants of other people may be involved. This is particularly important in paediatric practice where parents who are strongly attached to their children may bring pressure to bear to have the child allowed home – or kept in hospital.

Moving, finally, to the third step in the technical model, we can note that, while the paediatrician, by definition, wants to improve the condition of his patients, he will be aware that time spent with one patient may be at the expense of what time or institutional accommodation may be available to others. We have seen this tension in our imaginary case. The paediatrician may also consider that some of his time is needed for research for the benefit of many or, even, for the wants of his own family and friends. Similarly, at the level of health economics, care is a scarce and expensive resource; if there is to be more money for some patients, there may be less available for the needs of others. The original model of decision-making must, therefore, be amended so as to incorporate the complexities of the wants and choices of patients and, also, those of the paediatrician himself.

The doctor's decision in respect of all these uncertainties – whether they be those of diagnosis and prognosis or of choices and objectives – are made in a social context. He will be influenced, first, by his awareness of the professional opinions of his colleagues on cases of the kind with which he is dealing. Secondly, in at least some cases, he will be aware of the state of public or legal opinion. For example, the treatment given to neonates with Down's syndrome reflects not only the practitioner's own views but is bound to take account of those of the parents, his professional peers, the law and the public.

Clearly, then, all three elements of the

technical model of decision-making are considerably more complex than first emerged and, moreover, they arise in an intricate social context. Let us sum up the information which is available to a paediatrician or any health-care worker when faced with a difficult decision. A good and well-informed practitioner can obtain help from the following sources:

(1) Basic sciences – which provide knowledge of the pattern of change and development of injuries, diseases and of all normal and pathological states.
(2) Social sciences – including economics, sociology and psychology – which teach the patterns of human behaviour.
(3) Collective professional opinion on cases of broad types.
(4) Legal opinion.
(5) Public opinion.

A decision must be made in the light of the understanding which comes from all those sources of information. But how? Are the uncertainties to be resolved by quite arbitrary decision? The answer is that a good health-care practitioner will have another sort of understanding of the individual case which is additional to that provided by the natural and social sciences. This second type of understanding involves an awareness of moral values, and it is that which we must now start to analyse.

Scientific understanding is a matter of fitting events into a pattern – of tracing systematic connections. Moreover, scientific understanding is concerned with things in their generality, with the common or universal properties of things or events, or with models. And the same is true of the understanding which the social sciences give of action. They are concerned with what a patient or a disturbed adolescent might do, or with 'children in stress situations' or with the 'one-parent family'. Understanding of this kind, however important, is not the same as

the sort which is involved when we suddenly see, or come slowly to realize, what it means for a specific, named individual, now standing in front of us, to be a patient or to be in a specific situation of stress. Understanding of this latter sort is concerned with actions in their *particularity* – with the uniqueness of situations. We might put the point differently by saying that, whereas science, including the social sciences, gives us *horizontal* understanding, we must supplement this in concrete situations by what we could call *vertical* understanding – the sort of understanding which comes from insight into a personal history.

Moreover, this second type of understanding of human beings, as distinct from the scientific sort, necessarily requires one to have developed within oneself a certain range of moral qualities and, especially, compassion. The claim is that we cannot understand another person properly unless we see him as one who has various wants and values of his own and who calls forth our respect for that reason. The point here is not yet about how we ought to *treat* another person but is, rather, the prior point that an adequate *understanding* of another person requires a moral maturity. This is particularly true in the stressful situations involving children and their parents. The decision reached by a good paediatrician, then, ought to reflect the understanding gained from science and social science. But such understanding will still leave uncertainties in the face of the complexities of actual situations. These uncertainties will be resolved by the good practitioner by the exercise of the second sort of understanding.

The German word *verstehen* is used sometimes in social science to express this concept of understanding. The word, literally, just means 'understanding' but of the kind we aim at when we try to put ourselves on the inside of the actions of others and to capture their meaning for them. Interaction theory sometimes uses the expression *empathy* in attempting to describe the process of understanding an action from the inside. But there is nothing technical or obscure about the idea which is perfectly familiar to us as the kind of understanding which a friend shows to a friend – as we say: 'He is a very understanding person'. This kind of understanding derives from our own moral values and is shown in the quality of our imaginative and sympathetic insights into specific situations. I recall taking part in a seminar entitled 'Helping bereaved parents' in which a participant said that, in her hospital, the ward maid was better at this than was the psychiatrist. Presumably, the maid had this second sort of understanding whereas the psychiatrist had the first and not much of the second. Both are needed – and the second is shaped by our own values.

Note that, in arguing for the fusion of the technical and the value judgement, I am not saying that the paediatrician is agonized in his scientific and moral uncertainties in every case. Often, the diagnosis and prognosis will be clear and the value judgement will go unnoticed because it is uncontroversial; nevertheless, the decisions still result from a fusion of the technical and the moral.

Some doctors may wish to resist this conclusion because they adopt a narrow view of ethics. In the narrow sense, 'ethics' refers to codes or procedures. These are important because they cover the principles which underlie professional activity and they apply across cultural and national boundaries. But it is becoming increasingly recognized that these codes of ethics cannot encompass the range of moral problems which face doctors in modern medical practice.

It is worthwhile stressing the difference between this narrow interpretation of ethics as codified procedures and the broad sense of the term – meaning 'value judgements' – which I have been employing. For example, in the *wide* sense, it is a moral or value judgement

that a given child, all factors considered, ought to be allowed home despite the risk of a recurrence of his problem. But, clearly, this decision does not raise a question of morality or ethics *narrowly* conceived – and it is because some paediatricians take ethics or morality in the narrow sense that they are unaware of the extent to which they are continually making moral or value judgements in the broad sense. There are certainly technical factors – scientific and social – in deciding whether or not a particular patient should be allowed home. But, in the end, the decision about what ought to be done goes beyond the technical and encompasses the paediatrician's overall judgement as to what is for the total good of the patient. Such overall – or all things considered – judgements of the patient's good are what is here meant by moral or value judgements; and one of the central aims of this chapter is to make the paediatrician aware of their all-pervasive nature.

31.2 VALUES IN PAEDIATRICS

This conclusion raises questions concerning the basis of these value judgements which will occupy us for the rest of the chapter. Whose values are the most important in reaching decisions? The paediatrician's own values? Those of his professional peers? The parents'? How far should the child be consulted? Is there one pervasive value, or even one set of values, which dominates health care? If so, does it apply in a straightforward manner to paediatrics? The answers to the last two questions are, respectively, 'yes' and 'no'. Let us examine the typical values in health care and then consider the problems involved in applying them to paediatrics.

The ethical principles which are generally thought to apply to health care, and which can be extracted from traditional codes, are:

Avoid causing harm ('non-maleficence')
Do good if you can ('beneficence')
Act fairly ('justice')

It does not take much reflection to see that these very general principles govern many of the more specific ethical guidelines for medical practice – such as the importance of confidentiality, of obtaining consent for invasive treatments, of spending time with each patient in an equitable manner and so on [2]. Many writers on ethics try to sum up these principles in a single supreme value: that patients ought to be respected as ends. This principle, which derives from the philosophy of Kant, is sometimes called the principle of autonomy. Persons are autonomous – or self determining and self governing – by their very nature and, since health care impinges on this autonomy in an essential way, the relationship of doctor to patient is bound to raise ethical issues.

Before examining the complexity of this widely accepted idea as it relates to paediatrics, let us look at a difficulty which applies generally – that the ethics of health care have developed around the face-to-face or one-to-one model. There is, however, another dimension to modern health care – the socioeconomic. This has become important because doctors now have available a wide range of treatments and technologies, many of which are very expensive. The resource implications of this require justification, and the ethical justification for such large commitments of resources brings in the principle of utility – 'produce the best consequences for the majority'. Whereas in the past the doctor's ethical concern was directed exclusively to the patient in front of him, it must now be directed, also, at society in general. Many doctors will resist this way of putting the matter, for they will see economics as an intrusion in the relationship with the patient – health economics, they hold, will damage our health! I believe that this point of view, while being understandable, is mistaken. Resources directed to one patient are, by that token, being denied to others; that is what economists call 'opportunity cost'.

We must, therefore, add utility to non-maleficence, beneficence and justice as a further principle of medical ethics. I will not address the question of whether utility can be derived, like the others, from the principle of respect for the autonomous individual in this paper; rather, let us turn to the difficulties in applying this brief, and dogmatically stated, account of medical ethics to paediatrics.

One complexity, of course, lies in the wide age range confronting the paediatrician – from neonates to those who are on or over the edge of full maturity. Nevertheless, the basic ethical question which runs through all paediatrics is: 'when is an infant, minor or child a person in the sense of being an autonomous individual?' There are really two points here, the first of which concerns the normal, competent child. The focus is then on such matters as when do children achieve sufficient maturity to give consent to treatment, to request treatment without their parents' knowledge and the like.

Leaving the law out of it, there can be no firm guidelines because children vary so much in their general maturity. It is likely, however, that the ingrained paternalism of the medical profession will be especially encouraged when treating minors. Moreover, there may well be a tacit conspiracy between the parents or relatives and the paediatrician with a view to protecting the child from anxiety. In other words, beneficence is very likely to override respect for autonomy in a health-care situation which involves a child. This is extremely probable when the prognosis is not good. It is still very much the case that the full truth is not always disclosed to adult patients even when they show signs of wanting it. This is all the more liable to be so when the patient is a child. In addition to (often mistaken) beneficence, an additional motivation for concealing the truth from a child lies in the difficulty of communicating it – both in the sense that it is emotionally difficult to do so and also that it may not be easy to find forms of words which a child can assimilate. Studies have, however, shown that a child can have a conception of death and that children can come to terms as well as can adults with bad news which is communicated within a trusting and loving relationship.

The second part of the question is, in some ways, harder to answer philosophically and is just as emotive as is the first – it concerns the status of a brain-damaged neonate or child. If we accept the premise that to be a person is to have the abilities to be self determining and self governing, it follows that the brain-damaged child is not a person and probably, is not even a potential person. Does it then follow that such a child should be allowed to die if he or she catches an infection and the parents refuse consent to treatment? Should such a neonate be denied life-preserving surgery?

Although I shall assume for present purposes that the neonate is not a person in the full sense, it does not follow that there should be no life-preserving treatment [3]. That would only follow if we also accepted that having a right to life is necessarily tied to being a person. But, while being a person may be a sufficient condition of having a right to life, it is not obvious that it is a *necessary* condition. Indeed, it could hardly be a necessary condition for owning rights, otherwise the undisputed actual rights of normal children and babies would depend upon a mere potentiality for becoming a person in the future – but the actual cannot depend upon the possible! What, then, are the conditions needed for being an owner of rights?

It might be suggested that having rights presupposes having desires and that the function of rights is to protect those desires. It would follow from this that a severely brain-damaged neonate would not have the right to life to the extent that it could not have desires – although it might have needs – for one cannot have desires without being aware that one has

them or what their objects are, and a brain-damaged neonate would not have this sort of awareness. But this criterion is unsatisfactory; it is possible to have rights that one does not know about and, therefore, does not mind about – for example, a person may be unaware that he has a right to claim certain tax benefits. It is more plausible to argue that rights protect *interests*, or, at least, important interests. On this criterion, *things* cannot have rights because they cannot have interests, whereas babies have interests to the extent that they have a welfare – they can be happy or miserable – regardless of whether they are, or are ever likely to be, persons in the full moral sense; it follows that they can have some rights. Obviously, they cannot have all the rights of an adult, such as the right to vote or to get married, but they can, at least, have the right to life. Does it follow that this right must, at all times, be given paramount consideration?

Various types of argument could be advanced in support of this thesis and it might be helpful to classify them in an 'overview' [4]. They are based, essentially, on three different moral assumptions. The first of these holds that the *basis* of a decision to withhold life-preserving treatment will always be *uncertain* or *subjective* or *irrelevant*. It will be uncertain if the basis for the decision is sought in scientific or medical 'facts', such as poor prognosis, for how certain can one be of these 'facts'? An extreme version of this position is that, even if the patient appears to be dead, the criteria for death are too controversial to be given credence. It is likely that doctors can make mistakes and there may be an unforeseen turn of events, including what religious-minded people might call a 'miracle'. The basis will be *subjective* if it involves an assessment of the potential quality of life for the neonate who is not to be treated – for any assessment of the quality of life by the health-care team will always be subjective. If the basis for the decision not to treat is that the provision of treatment and continued care for the child are too expensive, then those who insist on a right to life in all instances will hold it to be *irrelevant*.

The force of all three points concerning the *basis* of a decision to withhold treatment can be exaggerated. I have already discussed the uncertainties of applying medical science to particular cases but, very often, the scientific facts can be established beyond reasonable doubt and an assessment of the quality of life is not entirely subjective. There are some human qualities, such as having a functioning brain or being more than a vegetable, that must be assumed in any account of quality of life and the case for not treating is overwhelming when they are absent. I have already insisted that the principle of utility expressed via health economics is not irrelevant to the morality of health care – resources diverted to X are moved at the expense of resources for Y. The case for diverting resources to X must, therefore, be made if the decision to do so is to be morally sound, and it is difficult to make out a case for the continued care of patients with severe brain damage.

The second assumption holds that, although the scientific or economic basis for rejecting a right to life and withholding treatment may be sound, the *decision* to deny the right to life is always wrong in itself. One relevant point of view is that of those who hold a fundamental religious position as to the sanctity of all forms of human life. This line occasionally merges into that of the doctor's inherent or sacred duty to maintain life at all cost; failing to do so, it might be said, is negating the very essence of being a doctor. Complementary to this argument, we can appeal to the rights of the patient. If the doctor *qua* doctor has a duty to maintain life, so also can we say that the patient *qua* patient has a right to treatment – in this case, life-preserving treatment.

In assessing such arguments, we encounter the near impossibility of convincing those who are deeply committed to religious positions. It should, however, be pointed out that, whatever may be true of Buddhism, the Judaeo-Christian tradition is not one stressing the sanctity of life but is, rather, one stressing the creation of man in the image of God. It is the person who is sacred, not the corrupt body; there is no mandate in the Scriptures for maintaining the body on a ventilator or in a vegetative state. The associated arguments, that the doctor *qua* doctor has a duty to maintain life at all costs and that the patient *qua* patient has a right to receive treatment at all costs, are seriously confused. In the first place, the definition of the role of the doctor offered – to maintain life – is one-sided; there is no reason to accept it any more than that the doctor, by definition, relieves suffering. Secondly, nothing of any moral substance follows from a definition, for a definition simply reports or recommends a word-use – and it does not make any moral sense to decide what someone ought to do by looking up a dictionary.

The third type of argument for the view that we ought always to defer to the right to life comes from those who, while conceding that the basis for the decision not to resuscitate may be sound and that the decision itself may not be intrinsically wrong, hold that the *consequences* of such decisions are always bad. There are various ways in which consequences may be invoked. First, it might be said that public awareness of the fact that paediatricians do not always treat may undermine confidence in the profession. Secondly, the 'slippery slope' argument may be used – if particular kinds of patient are 'allowed' to die today, who will it be tomorrow? A third extension of this fear of generalizing consequences is expressed in the suggestion that patients who are identified as receiving 'nursing care only' may, generally, receive less attention and care than they would if they were not so labelled. A fourth consequentialist argument refers to the role of the family. If a doctor tries to share responsibility for the decision not to treat with the patient's family, they may be likely to agree for the wrong reasons – for their own interests rather than those of the child. If, on the other hand, the family accept non-intervention for apparently good reasons, they may still be left with life-long guilt or doubt as to whether they acted in the right way.

None of these arguments in favour of never withholding treatment is entirely convincing. That derived from public confidence cuts both ways. Even if it were true that some members of the public become anxious in believing that brain-damaged children are not always treated, others are relieved to hear that this is so, for there is sometimes a fear that severely handicapped neonates are treated officiously when the relatives might wish that they should be allowed to die. Again, the 'slippery slope' argument, as with all uses of it, is effective only if we have good reason for believing that there is a slope and that it is slippery.

The third and fourth arguments are stronger. There is clearly a psychological danger that nursing staff, knowing that a patient is not to be treated, will not give attentive nursing care; this is a danger which the nursing staff can guard against. Families should certainly be consulted and counselled but there is no need to suppose that the medical staff will concur in a family wish for no treatment unless this course is indicated medically.

The conclusion, then, is that the provision of treatment for brain-damaged neonates does not depend upon their being persons or potential persons but on their having interests which others can protect, interests expressed in the claim that they have a 'right to life'. But this right to life is not absolute and must be observed in a context where other rights may be involved, such as those of the parents or other members of the family – and, ultimately, society itself which may be the paymaster of the treatment. Moreover, and this may be the fundamental ethical point, if a right to life is based on the idea of the infant's best interests, then, sometimes, those best interests may be to be allowed to die; in such circumstances, its right to life would not, thereby, be violated.

It may be appropriate to conclude an 'overview' of ethical arguments in paediatrics by examining three issues which are often addressed in the context of ethical discussions: acts and omissions, the slippery slope and the doctrine of double effect.

Let us assume that a neonate has a right to life which can only be overridden when it is in the infant's best interests not to continue in life. The usual assumption when this is so is that the death of the infant will come about through non-treatment and the provision of nursing care only. Now, many might argue that it is not in the infant's best interests to have its suffering prolonged when a lethal dose could put an end to those sufferings speedily and painlessly. This, of course, is at the centre of the question of 'acts and omissions'. Whereas many doctors are prepared to allow death to occur as a result of non-treatment, they are, at the same time, unwilling to bring about death by doing something actively. Others will argue that there is a kind of hypocrisy here because you are, in effect, bringing about the infant's death by failing to do something which would preserve its life. Why not, then, implement a decision to allow the child to die in as quick and humane a way as is possible? The logic of this argument is strong and its failure to be effective in practice is a sign of the emotional involvement of paediatricians and family with the infant; not wishing the suffering to be prolonged, they are, nevertheless, psychologically unwilling to take the step that would end it. We are, here, noting a deep human inhibition which it might be unwise to tamper with in the name of logic.

It might be argued that a non-emotional reason for shunning active, non-voluntary euthanasia – which is what 'acts', as distinct from 'omissions', would amount to – is that it starts us on a 'slippery slope'. If we kill hopelessly brain-damaged infants, it will be no time before we are killing those who are less severely brain-damaged, and then it will be the senile ... . Utility will have got out of hand and will be dominating the more traditional values of health care and of society as a whole. In assessing this kind of argument, we must, as was noted earlier, be sure that there is a slope and that it is slippery; otherwise, we shall be refusing to do something which is admitted to be morally good on the vague possibility that it might lead to something bad. But it may be that an inhibition against actively killing infants, even those who are brain-damaged, ought to be maintained as a fence against a slippery slope beyond.

There is, however, another way of looking at this situation. The 'acts and omissions' argument, coupled with that of the 'slippery slope', may lead us to regard it as wrong to accept active, non-voluntary euthanasia. But only under that description. There may be another way of describing the situation which will enable us both to reject active, non-voluntary euthanasia and also to bring about the death of an infant for humane reasons. The relevant argument is known as that of 'double effect'. It is used, particularly, in some religious contexts; it stresses the moral importance of intentions and draws a sharp distinction between intended *ends* of actions and foreseen, but unintended, *consequences*. For example, I am morally permitted to use force to defend myself if I am attacked; 'defending myself' is the intended and morally permissible end of my actions. In doing so, I may, correctly, foresee the unintended consequence that my assailant will be injured or killed; but I am not *morally* guilty of his injury or death – provided the force I used was not excessive – because that was not my intention.

The argument can be used in various health-care contexts. Let us assume that euthanasia is morally wrong. The double-effect argument can be used to justify a massive dose of pain-killing drugs for someone who is dying, say, from an agonizing cancer. The morally permitted intention is to relieve pain and it is a foreseen, but unintended, consequence that the patient dies. Again, even if we assume that abortion is always wrong, we may still operate on the uterus of a pregnant woman in order to remove a malignant growth; the death of the fetus will be foreseen but not intended.

In assessing the double-effect argument, note, first, that it assumes that there are certain sorts of policy which are always wrong in themselves, such as abortion, suicide or euthanasia. There is no *need* for double-effect arguments in the absence of this assumption. But not everyone would agree that certain sorts of action are always wrong, or right, *whatever the consequences*. Secondly, the argument assumes that we can always distinguish between what is intended and what is merely foreseen and that such a distinction is always morally relevant. But, if an obstetrician operates on the uterus of a pregnant, but seriously ill, woman, *can* we distinguish between saying, on the one hand, that the intention was to save the life of the woman and that the death of the fetus was a foreseen, but unintended, consequence and, on the other hand, that the intention was to procure an abortion in order to save the life of the woman? And, supposing that we could draw this distinction, is it morally relevant in any case? Captain Oates walked into the snow but it does not seem to matter morally whether we say he intended to walk on his own to prevent himself from being a burden to his companions and, in doing so, foresaw his certain death, or whether we say that he intended to commit suicide in order to save his companions; either way, it can be seen as a gallant action and only those who maintain that suicide is wrong whatever the consequences will prefer the first description. The double-effect argument is useful only to those holding absolutist principles, such as support for an absolute right to life, and the danger of the argument is that it encourages moral dishonesty. But it is employed in paediatrics – as are those relating to acts and omissions and to the slippery slope.

To sum up, I have identified and criticized the technical model of decision-making in health care. What has emerged is the pervasive nature of value judgements – a feature of decision-making which is not always noticed because doctors tend to assume a narrow view of ethics. The dilemmas facing paediatric practitioners are especially difficult, partly because the emotions of parents and of society in general are deeply engaged, but mainly because the typical patients are infants or children below the age of consent and the ethics of decision-making are, therefore, complex. As a consequence, paediatricians are forced to consider such matters as the nature and the extent of the moral rights of brain-damaged neonates and how those rights are to be balanced against those of the parents and of society. Paediatricians, in particular, cannot escape the need to engage in moral arguments; the purpose of this chapter has been to outline the nature and validity of some of these.

REFERENCES

1. The technical model of decision-making is discussed in more detail in Downie, R.S. and Calman, K.C. (1987) *Healthy Respect*, Faber and Faber, London.
2. For a general discussion of the ethical principles of health care, see Beauchamp, T.L. and Childress, J.F. (1983) *Principles of Biomedical Ethics*, (2nd edn), Oxford University Press, Oxford; Harris, J. (1985) *The Value of Life*, Routledge and Kegan Paul, London.
3. See Steinbock, B. (1985) Infanticide, in *Moral Issues in Mental Retardation* (eds R.S. Laura and A. Ashman), Croom Helm, Sydney; Campbell, A.G.M. and Duff, K.C. (1979) Deciding the care of severely malformed or dying infants. *J. Med. Ethics*, **5**, 65; Kuhse, H. and Singer, P. (1985) *Should the Baby Live?*, Oxford University Press, Oxford.
4. For discussion of the logic of medical reasoning, see Downie and Calman, ref. 1; Gillon, R. (1986) *Philosophical Medical Ethics*, John Wiley, Chichester.

APPENDIX A

List of cases

UNITED STATES

Table of statutes

Standard growth charts

Standard growth charts in current use throughout the United Kingdom for infants from 24 weeks' gestation to age 2 years (Revised edition (1988) of Gairdner, D. and Pearson, J. (1971) A growth chart for premature and other infants. *Arch. Dis. Child.* **46**, 783). (Reproduced by permission of Castlemead Publications).

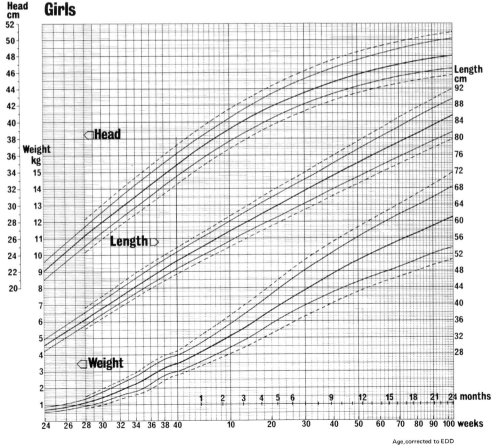

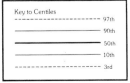

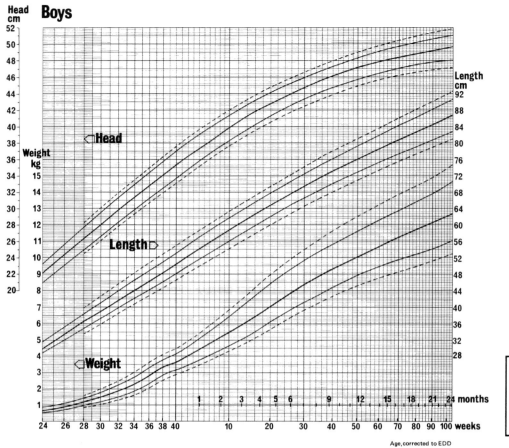

Boys

Head cm / Weight kg / Length cm / Age, corrected to EDD

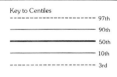

Key to Centiles
- ----------- 97th
- ——————— 90th
- ——————— 50th
- ——————— 10th
- ----------- 3rd

Fetal foot length and sitting height

End of week	Mean sitting height	Mean foot length	Minimum foot length	Maximum foot length	Percentage mean foot length: sitting height
	mm	mm	mm	mm	p. ct.
8½	27	4.2	3.8	4.6	15.6
9	31	4.6	4.2	5.0	15.0
10	40	5.5	5.0	6.0	13.8
11	50	6.9	6.0	7.8	13.8
12	61	9.1	7.5	10.8	15.0
13	74	11.4	9.8	13.0	15.4
14	87	14.0	12.5	15.5	16.0
15	101	16.8	15.2	18.5	16.6
16	116	19.9	18.2	21.6	17.0
17	130	23.0	21.0	25.0	17.7
18	142	26.8	24.8	28.8	18.9
19	153	30.7	28.5	33.0	20.0
20	164	33.3	31.0	35.7	20.0
21	175	35.2	32.5	38.0	20.0
22	186	39.5	36.0	43.0	21.0
23	197	42.2	39.0	45.5	21.4
24	208	45.2	42.0	48.5	21.8
25	218	47.7	44.5	51.0	22.0
26	228	50.2	47.0	53.5	22.0
27	238	52.7	49.0	56.5	22.0
28	247	55.2	51.5	59.0	22.3
29	256	57.0	53.0	61.0	22.3
30	265	59.2	55.5	63.0	22.3
31	274	61.2	57.5	65.0	22.3
32	283	63.0	59.0	67.0	22.3
33	293	65.0	61.0	69.0	22.2
34	302	68.2	64.0	72.5	22.6
35	311	70.5	66.0	75.0	22.6
36	321	73.5	69.0	78.0	23.0
37	331	76.5	72.0	81.0	23.0
38	341	78.5	74.0	83.0	23.0
39	352	81.0	76.0	86.0	23.0
40	362	82.5	77.5	87.5	23.0

Fetal foot length and its proportion to sitting height. From: Streeter, G.L. (1920) Weight, sitting height, head size, foot length, and menstrual age of the human embryo. *Carnegie Inst. Pubs.* **274**, 143.

Index

Page numbers in *italic* refer to Figures and page numbers in **bold** refer to Tables.